Qin Bowei
Guide to Clinical Practice

Qin Bowei

Translated by Gao Xianli

CHICAGO ACADEMIC PRESS

Qin Bowei Guide to Clinical Practice

Author: Qin Bowei

Translator: Gao Xianli

Language: English

Word Count (for space of all pages): 596 thousand words

Publisher: Chicago Academic Press

Number of Pages: 694

ISBN: 978-1-965890-43-1

Publishing Chicago Academic Press

5923 N Artesian Ave

Chicago IL 60659

Email contact@chicagoacademicpress.com

Website http://chicagoacademicpree.com/

Book Size 6X9 inches

First Edition: September, 2025

Translator's Profile

Gao Xianli (b. 1971), Master of Arts, is an Associate Professor in the School of Foreign Languages at Guangdong Pharmaceutical University. His research focuses on foreign language education, medical and pharmaceutical English, teacher development, and innovation and entrepreneurship education.

Professor Gao teaches courses including College English, Medical English, Pharmaceutical English, and Medical Literature in English.

He has led and completed two collaborative education projects supported by the Ministry of Education of the People's Republic of China, one research project funded by the Guangdong Provincial Philosophy and Social Science Planning Office, one project funded by the Guangdong Provincial Education Science Planning Office, and one teaching reform project under the Provincial-Level Teaching Quality and Reform Project for Undergraduate Universities in Guangdong Province. Additionally, he has participated in five provincial-level research projects.

He has published 30 academic papers in domestic and international journals, including Foreign Language and Literature Studies, Chinese Journal of Applied Linguistics, Journal of Zhejiang International Studies University, Medicine, and Psychological Reports. Professor Gao serves as chief editor of two digital textbooks (e-textbooks), contributor to five additional textbooks, and translator for two academic translations.

Notes from Standing in the Snow——A Preface

Mr. Qin Bowei was a renowned traditional Chinese medicine (TCM) scholar and educator. He was erudite, skilled in medical practice, and prolific in writing, earning him the status of a leading figure in the TCM field. He made outstanding contributions to TCM education, clinical practice, scientific research, and the development of TCM undertakings.

Since the 1980s, with the progress of the times, Mr. Qin Bowei's position in the history of TCM development has been highlighted again. Along with this, more and more articles about his life story and TCM academic thoughts have been written. Although we have written some recollections and commemorative articles successively, we always feel that we have not fully expressed our thoughts. This time, we have compiled Mr. Qin's relevant articles and medical manuscripts into a large collection, which we believe will contribute to the research on Qin Bowei and TCM. This piece of notes mostly contains some little-known materials recorded when we were studying under his mentorship. Taking this opportunity, we record them here, hoping to provide some small but true materials for later learners to fully understand Mr. Qin's life.

I. Mr. Qin's Lifelong Love for Lotus

Mr. Qin's given name was Zhiji, styled name Bowei, and art name Qianzhai. He was born on the 16th day of the sixth lunar month in 1901 in Chenjiahang (also known as Chenxing Town), Pudong, Shanghai. Since he was born in the Chenshi period (7-9 a.m.), he would get up very early on his birthday every year to sort out his articles, reading notes and other writings from the past year. On this day, the whole family would accompany Mr. Qin to eat light vegetarian food. In the evening, he would always write a small poem to encourage himself. A line he often chanted,

"June lotus blooms on my birthday", also frequently appeared in his own calligraphy and paintings. Mr. Qin loved lotus all his life. In his poems, he often praised the lotus for "being cleansed in clear ripples without being charming", and placed his own pursuits in it. To commemorate his love for lotus, at our suggestion, the fourth reprint of *Introduction to Traditional Chinese Medicine* by People's Health Publishing House in January 1981 and its Japanese version both used a lotus pattern on the cover.

II. Notes on Mr. Qin's Family Affairs

Mr. Qin was born into a family with a long tradition of TCM. His grandfather, QinDiqiao, whose given name was Naige and art name Youci, was a talented scholar in the Jiangnan region at the end of the Qing Dynasty. He was famous for his literary works and had written books such as *Collected Manuscripts from Yuping Flower Studio* and *Yu Quyuan's Medical Notes*. He was also skilled in medical practice. Mr. Qin once said that his grandfather "was proficient in poetry, ancient prose and ci poetry, and dabbled in medicine as a secondary pursuit, saving many lives". Therefore, in Mr. Qin's compiled book *Essence of Medical Cases of Famous Doctors in the* Qing *Dynasty*, 31 medical cases of Mr. Diqiao were selected (all included in *Lectures on* Qin *Bowei's Medical Cases* in this series as an appendix).

Mr. Qin's father had knowledge of medicine but did not practice it. Unfortunately, his father passed away when Mr. Qin was 16 years old.

Mr. Qin studied in a private school for several years. From an early age, he read extensively through medical books, inheriting his family's academic tradition. In 1920, he became a disciple of Ding Ganren, a master of the Menghe School, and emerged as an outstanding student among Ding's disciples.

Mr. Qin married Qiao Peiheng in 1933. They had five children, among whom the fourth and fifth died in infancy, leaving one son and two daughters. The son was named Xiaoqian, taking the character "Qian" from Mr. Qin's art name "Qianzhai". The daughters were named Xiaopei and Xiaoheng, each taking one character from Qiao's given name "Peiheng". After the victory of the War of Resistance against Japanese Aggression, he separated from Qiao in 1945. He met Wang Lianbi in 1947. At that time, the Qin family disapproved of his relationship with Wang, so it was not until March 26, 1950 that Mr. Qin formally married Wang. They temporarily lived in Cuihua Hutong, Beijing, and hosted a banquet for three tables at Cuihualou Restaurant in Beijing. Famous figures in the Beijing TCM circle, such as Shi Jinmo, Kong Bohua, Xiao Longyou, Zhao Shuping, and Yuan Hechai, attended to offer their congratulations. After living in Beijing for three months, they returned to Shanghai. From then on, Mr. Qin lived with Wang until his death, and they had no children. Mr. Qin kept in touch with Qiao and their children and provided them with living allowances.

III. Mr. Qin's Employment in Beijing

After the liberation, Mr. Qin worked at the 11th Hospital in Shanghai. In 1953, Mr. Guo Zihua, then Vice Minister of the Ministry of Health of the People's Republic of China, visited Mr. Qin's home on behalf of the ministry's leadership to invite him to serve as a TCM consultant at the Ministry of Health. Mr. Qin was reluctant to move north because he had lived in the south for a long time. Vice Minister Guo Zihua went to his home almost every evening to persuade him. Due to the trust of the organization and the persuasion of the leadership, Mr. Qin had to agree. After arriving in Beijing, he lived in the dormitory of the Ministry of Health on Gulou West Street.

In 1956, Beijing University of Chinese Medicine was formally established in Haiyun Cang, Dongzhimen. For the convenience of teaching at the university and working at its affiliated hospital, he moved from the dormitory of the Ministry of Health to the university dormitory in Dongzhimennei, which is about 50 to 60 meters west of the north gate of the China Academy of Chinese Medical Sciences today. After Wang Lianbi came to Beijing, she worked in the neighborhood. In 1959, the leadership of the Ministry of Health had a talk with Wang, saying, "To enable Mr. Qin to work better, taking good care of his life and health is your job." From then on, Wang resigned from her job and took care of Mr. Qin's household chores and daily life, becoming a rare life companion.

On March 4, 1963, the Beijing TCM Association held a banquet to welcome the famous veteran TCM doctors who came to Beijing to work at the research institute. Mr. Qin improvised a poem:

Answering the motherland's call, I gladly come to this ancient capital.

Gathered here for a grand occasion, all around are renowned figures.

Zhao and Dong are pioneers highly regarded,

Yuan and Shi are senior and respected.

Raising the cup, emotions run deep,

Hoping to fulfill a lifetime's aspirations.

Qin's note: Zhao refers to Zhao Shuping, then Chairman of the Beijing TCM Association. Dong refers to Dong Demao, then Editor-in-Chief of the *TCM Magazine*. Yuan is Yuan Hechai, and Shi is Shi Jinmo. The elders Yuan and Shi were famous veteran TCM doctors in Beijing. Despite their advanced age, they still participated in hospital work.

IV. Before and After Mr. Qin's Death

In 1964, arranged by the central government, Mr. Qin stayed in the 301 Hospital of the People's Liberation Army for a comprehensive physical examination, and the result was "healthy" with all indicators normal. After the Cultural Revolution, his home was ransacked, and he was forced to live in the Gongzi Building of the College of Chinese Medicine, which is about 500 meters west of the east gate of Dongzhimen Hospital Affiliated to Beijing University of Chinese Medicine today. The room was about 9 square meters with a west-facing window, so it received no sunlight all day long.

In 1967, Mr. Qin suffered from lobar pneumonia, yet he was still subjected to struggle sessions all day long and could not receive timely treatment. Moreover, because Wang Lianbi came from a landlord family background and was categorized as one of the "five types of elements" (landlords, rich peasants, counter-revolutionaries, bad elements, rightists), she was sent back to her hometown. Mr. Qin was left alone in Beijing with no one to take care of him. At that time, Wang Fengqi's mother, elder sister, etc., lived in Jishikou outside Chaoyangmen, which was not far from Dongzhimen. Despite their own financial constraints, Wang Fengqi's mother and elder sister saved money by living frugally to make nutritious food and supplements for Mr. Qin. Wang Fengqi's nephews and nieces, such as Shi Huiping, Miao Junyuan, and Shi Baogang, were able to often walk to deliver meals to Mr. Qin because their schools were closed. Mr. Qin, when not being struggled against, could also walk to Wang Fengqi's mother's home. Every two or three weeks, he would have his hair cut by an old barber in Jishikou Hutong, chat, and play chess with him.

On March 9, 1968, Wang Lei, the son of Wang Fengqi and Wu Dazhen, was born and grew up at his grandmother's home in Jishikou. Mr. Qin, though ill, came to see the child with pleasure. During a medical examination in 1968, it was found that he had lung cancer. By early December 1969, his condition worsened, and he could barely move. Wang Lianbi was recalled to Beijing to take care of him. By January 1970, Mr.

Qin was bedridden. At 8 p.m. on January 27, Mr. Qin's heart stopped beating in the internal medicine ward of the former Dongzhimen Hospital (i.e., the red building east of the north gate of the present China Academy of Chinese Medical Sciences). Thus, a generation of renowned masters passed away. Later, his ashes were placed in Room 4, Deputy Room 4, No. 27 of Babaoshan Martyrs' Cemetery in Beijing, where he rests in the same room with famous old Chinese medicine practitioners such as Shi Jinmo and Fang Shishan.

At that time, Mr. Zhang Cansen from Shanghai wrote a commemorative article and submitted it to the "Health News" for publication, but it was not published due to various reasons. On July 29, 1979, "Health News" reprinted an article by Mr. Qin entitled "From Jealousy to Affection" which he had published in "Health News" on February 8, 1957, and also published a commemorative article by Comrade Zhang Enrong, "Rereading His Articles Is Like Seeing the Man—In Memory of Mr. Qin Bo".

V. Mr. Qin's Life Hobbies

Mr. Qin liked drinking, but he was not a heavy drinker nor did he indulge in alcohol. He would drink one or two *liang* (a unit of weight, 1 *liang* ≈ 50 grams) every night, and sometimes one or two cups during lunch. His favorite was Wuliangye. During the Cultural Revolution, he often went to Wang Fengqi's home. Since there was no Wuliangye there, he had to drink Beijing Erguotou, but he was still happy. However, he would never drink "sweet potato wine", saying that this kind of wine would cause a headache after drinking. He preferred light dishes and disliked greasy food, but he really liked to have pig's head meat as an accompaniment to wine. It was best to have one or two small cold dishes with each meal. He had a small appetite and liked some vegetables and bean products. Among fruits, he loved pears the most, saying that the power of pears to nourish yin and promote the production of body fluids was stronger than any Chinese herbal medicine. In particular, "Laiyang pears" were soft, sweet, and very delicious. On September 7, 1959, Beijing Evening News published an article written by Mr. Qin in praise of pears, entitled "Pear" (included in Article 32 of "Qin Bowei's Supplementary Qianzhai Medical Lectures" in this series). Mr. Qin was very fond of tea. He did not like the old Beijing jasmine tea very much, but only loved the stronger "Biluochun". He often said, "This is the tea named and loved by Emperor Kangxi."

Mr. Qin was addicted to smoking, about two packs a day. From his small - scale daily records during the Cultural Revolution, it can be seen that there was a record of two packs of cigarettes every day. Of course, he also said, "I am a person living in a cloud of smoke, and the cigarette boxes are the cards on which I record my learning experiences." However, considering that he finally suffered from lung cancer, it is hard to say that it has nothing to do with smoking. It is better to smoke less or not at all.

Mr. Qin was also proficient in poetry, calligraphy, painting and chess. His poetry, calligraphy and paintings were already well - known in the field of TCM, and almost everyone knew about them. But fewer people knew that he was good at chess. He had a high - level chess skill in both Go and Chinese chess. During the Cultural Revolution, when Wang Fengqi returned to Beijing, or when Wang Fengqi's father and Wu Dazhen's father came to Beijing, they often accompanied Mr. Qin to play chess, chat and relieve boredom, and often played a game or two after meals. In a letter to Wang Fengqi and Wu Dazhen on July 2, 1968, Mr. Qin wrote a wonderful passage. He said, "When will you be able to come back? The whole family is looking forward to it. When you come back, we should have a good discussion and then play three games. I think playing chess is an art of struggle. If you send out a large number of 'troops' and only want to checkmate the opponent, without considering the emptiness inside your own 'camp', you will be completely defeated when you can't stand the counter - attack. This is also the same as treating this kind of disease (referring to the medicine prescribed by the doctor after Mr. Qin got sick). It is necessary to suppress the symptoms and consider the patient's physical strength. Otherwise, just a few doses of Puji Xiaodu Yin (a TCM formula) will not only fail to relieve the symptoms, but also cause loss of appetite and loose stools..."

Mr. Qin seemed to be talking about chess skills here, but in fact, he was talking about the principles of TCM.

VI. Mr. Qin's Unforgettable and Hard - to - find Photos

In the 1950s, when Chairman Mao Zedong met with more than 100 experts from all walks of life in Huairen Hall, Beijing, Mr. Qin attended as a representative of the TCM community. He had two photos taken with Chairman Mao Zedong. In one photo, he was shaking hands with Chairman Mao Zedong, and Premier Zhou Enlai was smiling and looking at him beside them. In the other photo, he was sitting at the same table with Chairman Mao Zedong at a banquet. He had always treasured these two photos, but they were confiscated during the Cultural Revolution. He had more interactions with Premier Zhou Enlai. At a national political consultative conference in the 1950s, Premier Zhou Enlai saw Mr. Qin holding a fan with lotus flowers painted by Mr. Qin on it. Premier Zhou Enlai said, "Mr. Qin, your paintings and calligraphy are very good, and can be compared with those of calligraphers and painters." Mr. Qin quickly said, "I dare not, I dare not. Premier, you praise me too much." Premier Zhou Enlai smiled and joked, "Can you paint one for me?" Mr. Qin said excitedly, "If Premier doesn't mind, I will surely show my poor skills." The two smiled at each other. Premier Zhou Enlai said, "Good, good. Thank you in advance." After returning home, Mr. Qin spent a week painting a fan - shaped painting of narcissus and inscribed words on it, and presented it to

Premier Zhou Enlai. After receiving it, Premier Zhou Enlai replied with thanks and inscribed the words “The spring in the medical field is warm” and presented it back to Mr. Qin. Unfortunately, the inscription by Premier Zhou Enlai treasured by Mr. Qin was burned to ashes during the ten - year turmoil. Whenever this matter was mentioned, Mr. Qin would just slightly shake his head and sigh.

In 1963, Premier Zhou Enlai sent a special plane to Shanghai several times to have Mr. Qin diagnose and treat leaders such as Ke Qingshi and Liu Yalou.

During the Cultural Revolution, Beijing carried out several population evacuations. Most veteran TCM doctors from Beijing University of Chinese Medicine were sent down to other places outside Beijing, and Mr. Qin was assigned to Shijiazhuang, Hebei Province. When Premier Zhou Enlai learned about this, he informed the Ministry of Health: Mr. Qin must not be sent down and must stay in Beijing. Mr. Qin talked to us about this matter many times, always saying emotionally: I am grateful to the Premier, who still thought of me in such a complicated situation...

Mr. Qin had extensive interactions with central leading comrades such as Dong Biwu, Lin Boqu, Wang Zhen, and Chen Yi, as well as with figures like Wu Han, Deng Tuo, Liao Mosha, Xia Yan, and Tian Han.

Internationally, Mr. Qin went to the Soviet Union twice to treat Mikoyan’s wife for hemophilia, achieving excellent results. Mikoyan’s wife was Lenin’s granddaughter. He also went to the People’s Republic of Mongolia several times to diagnose and treat Chairman Choibalsan.

All these precious photos of these interactions were burned to ashes during the ten-year turmoil, which is truly regrettable.

The Editors

January 2014

I. Before and After the Publication of Introduction to TCM

In 1959, People's Health Publishing House reprinted Mr. Qin Bowei's famous work *Introduction to Traditional Chinese Medicine*. In just one or two years, it sold 380,000 copies, which was a leader among medical publications at that time.

In 1959, we had just been admitted to Beijing University of Chinese Medicine. At that time, the university had no complete and systematic textbooks, only two kinds: one introductory book called *An Outline of Traditional Chinese Medicine*, and the printed lecture notes of the main teachers of various subjects.

As Mr. Qin later told us, *An Outline of Traditional Chinese Medicine* was organized by Jiangsu Provincial School of TCM, the predecessor of Nanjing University of Chinese Medicine, with Teacher Yin Huihe as the writer, and Mr. Qin participated in its review. Mr. Qin said: "That outline is well written, but it is a bit too complicated for beginners. I suggest you take time to read my *Introduction to Traditional Chinese Medicine*." Over the years, we have increasingly realized that *Introduction to Traditional Chinese Medicine* is indeed a representative work of Mr. Qin's academic thoughts, which shows that Mr. Qin put a lot of effort into this book. Although *Introduction to Traditional Chinese Medicine* has only 86,000 words, it is concise, to the point, and succinctly summarizes the four core elements of TCM: theory, method, prescription, and medicine.

In April 1989, Professor Iwahashi Nobutane, Executive Director of the Oriental Medical Promotion Foundation, a Japanese friend, talked to us about the fact that the Japanese Kampo medicine community liked Mr. Qin Bowei's medical works very much, and especially hoped that we could help them choose a representative work. At that time, there were two books to choose from: Qi*anzhai Medical Lectures* and *Introduction to Traditional Chinese Medicine*. However, we felt that it was more difficult to translate Qi*anzhai Medical Lectures* into Japanese, so we recommended translating *Introduction to Traditional Chinese Medicine*. Mr. Iwahashi Nobutane kept saying: "Good, good, and please write a preface for us." Our classmate and Japanese language expert Wu Ruimin did the Japanese translation, which took half a year to complete. We suggested that the cover of the book should preferably have a "lotus" pattern. Mr. Iwahashi Nobutane asked why? We said that Mr. Qin Bowei was born on the 16th day of the sixth lunar month in China, when lotus flowers were in full bloom in the south of the Yangtze River. Therefore, Mr. Qin loved lotus all his life, took lotus as the theme in many of his calligraphy and paintings, and always encouraged himself with the spirit of lotus "growing out of the mud without being stained". Mr. Iwahashi Nobutane said: "Good, well said, we will definitely do it as you suggest." (See the photo of the Japanese version of *Introduction to Traditional Chinese Medicine*)

The book's launch ceremony was held in Miyazaki Prefecture, Japan, on May 14, 1990. Professor Wu Ruimin and we were invited to attend and received a warm welcome from our Japanese colleagues.

We are very fortunate that through our efforts, we have been able to translate *Introduction to Traditional Chinese Medicine*, a representative work embodying Mr. Qin's academic thoughts, into Japanese, enabling TCM academic insights to be shared with Japanese colleagues. If Mr. Qin were to know this in the afterlife, he would surely smile with contentment.

II. Anecdotes about Essentials for Clinical Practice of TCM

One evening after dinner in 1968, Mr. Qin said to us: *Essentials for Clinical Practice of Traditional Chinese Medicine* is not a representative work of my academic ideas. It merely aims to open up some ideas for ordinary TCM practitioners and provide them with a "follow-the-map-to-find-the-steed" approach to learning and application.

Inspired by Mr. Qin's ideas, we collaborated with Professor Sun Guangrong to compile *TCM Differentiation and Treatment of Inflammation*, which was published by China Medical Science and Technology Press in 1989. In October 1992, it won the Second Prize of National Excellent Science and Technology Books and was also published in traditional Chinese characters by Zhiyin Publishing House in Taiwan.

Mr. Qin stated that *Essentials for Clinical Practice of Traditional Chinese Medicine* was based on the lecture notes he gave to Li Yan, Zhang Tianren, and Wei Zhizhen, Communist Party members among the first batch of students (admitted in 1956) of Beijing University of Chinese Medicine. He lectured for one or two hours every evening for approximately one to two months. These lecture notes were later compiled into a book and published by People's Health Publishing House in September 1963.

III. The Origin of New Principles of Treatment

As early as the 1930s, Mr. Qin was inspired by *Insights into Medical Learning*, which states, "Diseases in the human body are nothing but internal injuries and external contractions. Wind, cold, summer heat, dampness, dryness, and fire are external contractions; joy, anger, worry, thought, sadness, fear, shock, yin deficiency, and improper diet are internal injuries. In total, there are nineteen characters, from which all the ever-changing diseases arise." He was also inspired by Mo Meishi's *Words on Studying Classics*, which notes, "There are eight causes of all diseases: first, pathogenic qi; second, water dampness; third, ghosts and spirits; fourth, insects and beasts; fifth, objects; sixth, food and drink; seventh, medicinal stones; eighth, human affairs." Drawing on these, he wrote and published *New Principles of Treatment* (published by Shanghai TCM Publishing House in 1932), which became a guiding prescription book for TCM clinical practice at that time.

Mr. Qin explained "principles" as follows: "The term 'lü' (principles) here refers to rules and patterns. These rules govern the methods, guide the use of prescriptions, dictate the administration of medicines, and determine modifications. They adapt to the syndrome and change accordingly, embodying flexible and ingenious methods that generate thousands of formulas and approaches to cope with various diseases. There are fifty-six principles, categorized under thirteen main headings. They encompass both classical prescriptions and contemporary formulas, cover cold damage and warm diseases, include external contractions and internal injuries, transcend the boundaries of *zang-fu* organs and meridians, and integrate the treatment principles of various schools into one."

In March 1955, *New Principles of Treatment* was reprinted by People's Health Publishing House. In the preface to the reprint, Mr. Qin wrote: "Undoubtedly, the content of this book consists of outdated theories, and it seems unnecessary to reprint it. However, some colleagues believe that TCM treatment methods are too complex, and since it is temporarily impossible to standardize them, having such a pamphlet as a guide for clinical prescribing, while using the original features of TCM as a new reference, is still necessary."

By 1961, to facilitate people's learning and mastery, Mr. Qin, integrating his clinical practice, revised and adjusted the content into thirteen outlines for syndrome differentiation, including wind, cold, summer heat, dampness, dryness, fire, qi, blood, phlegm, deficiency, food retention, worms, and pestilence. Under each of the thirteen outlines, there are four or five treatment methods, followed by syndrome differentiation, commonly used medicines, prescriptions, explanations of prescriptions, modifications, and summaries, etc. Entitled "Outline of Syndrome Differentiation and Treatment", it was published in the first issue of *Journal of Beijing University of Chinese Medicine*.

Subsequently, under the title "Outline of TCM Syndrome Differentiation and Treatment", it was serialized in issues 1, 2, and 3 of *TCM Magazine* in 1961, which was more comprehensive and systematic than *New Principles of Treatment*.

In 1962, it was published by People's Health Publishing House under the title *Outline of TCM Syndrome Differentiation and Treatment*. When talking about this during his lifetime, Mr. Qin once said that the academic development of TCM should be continuously improved and deepened, and one should not stick to established rules, for standing still means falling behind.

This reprint is not a simple repetition of the 1955 edition of *New Principles of Treatment*, but an enhanced version supplemented with later articles. To more truly reflect Mr. Qin's academic thoughts, we still use the title *New Principles of Treatment*.

Collators

January 2014

Introduction to Traditional Chinese Medicine

Recently, there are many people learning TCM, and everyone has a common request: how to start learning? And they hope to learn better in a relatively short period of time. Therefore, there is a great need for a simple reference book that includes the basic theories and knowledge of TCM, so that one can start from here and gradually improve. This is a very natural thing.

The main way for TCM to treat diseases is based on a set of medical methods that combine theory, method, prescription, and medicine. Personally, I think that understanding the features of TCM and mastering the laws of its disease treatment from these four aspects is a relatively correct way to learn TCM. Therefore, this book is divided into four parts: theory, method, prescription, and medicine, and each part isfurther divided into several items for more detailed introduction.

I also believe that learning TCM theory must be combined with clinical experience of TCM, so that the learning can be more solid. Therefore, when introducing the basic theories of TCM in this book, many cases of common diseases are cited for explanation, so that one can learn while connecting with practice.

Learning any knowledge requires great efforts, and learning TCM is no exception. Whether learning comprehensively or learning a subject or a disease, one cannot do without theory, method, prescription, and medicine. However, it is not necessary to regard it as too difficult, nor to estimate it as too simple. As long as one proceeds step by step, starting from the basics and then improving, it is not difficult to learn.

Under the leadership of the Party, I am willing to contribute my humble opinions to help readers solve some practical problems in learning. It is hoped that through this book, readers can have a preliminary concept of TCM and lay a foundation for further learning. However, due to my limited level, there must be shortcomings and mistakes, and criticisms and corrections are welcome.

Qin Bowei
September 1959

Contens

Chapter One Theoretical Part

Section 1 Features of Traditional Chinese Medicine

I. Concept of holism

In treating diseases, TCM takes a holistic perspective. First, it regards the relationships between the internal organs of the human body and various tissues and organs on the body surface as indivisible. At the same time, it holds that changes in the environment have a significant impact on human physiology and pathology. Therefore, it emphasizes the unity within the human body and also attaches importance to the unity between the human body and the external environment. Thus, in clinical practice, problems are always considered comprehensively, not only from the perspective of the affected part, but also by observing the season, climate, and local conditions, and paying attention to the patient's emotions and living habits, etc. This holistic concept is the basic concept of TCM in treating diseases, which will be explained in several aspects as follows.

1. Organic wholeness of the human body

TCM believes that all parts of the human body are organically connected. First, the twelve internal organs are regarded as twelve kinds of functions, called the "twelve officials"; they are also divided into six *zang*-organs and six *fu*-organs. Functionally, each *zang*-organ is combined with a *fu*-organ, called "interior-exterior relationship". This classification of internal organs is not meant to imply that they act independently; on the contrary, it is to understand physiological activities or pathological changes as having an inseparable relationship with each other. This relationship is not only manifested in the *zang* and *fu*organs, but also in the relationship between the *zang*and*fu* organs and various tissues and organs of the body. For example, the heart governs the blood vessels and the tongue; the liver governs the tendons and the eyes; the spleen governs the muscles and the mouth; the lung governs the skin and hair and the nose; the kidney governs the bones and the ears; furthermore, the spleen governs the limbs, the kidney controls urination and defecation, and so on. All these illustrate the functions of the *zang-fu* organs and their relationships with the body. More importantly, the meridians are distributed systemati cally throughout the body, circulating repeatedly, serving as the connecting channels between the interior and the exterior of the body, thereby maintaining the overall internal and external correlation of the human body in terms of function. Precisely because of this, in treatment, for diseases of the internal organs, treatment is not limited to a single affected organ, and even not focused on the diseased organ itself; instead, cure can be achieved by treating other internal organs. For instance, stomach diseases can be treated concurrently with spleen regulation; lung diseases can be addressed by treating the spleen and stomach to indirectly enhance the lung's resistance. Particularly notably, for local disorders of the body, TCM often adopts methods of treating the internal organs for cure. For example, wind-fire red eyes can be treated with methods that clear the liver; deficient-fire toothache can be treated with methods that warm the kidney; another example is gangrene (which can cause the ten toes to fall off), for which Western medicine often performs amputation, while TCM achieves good results with methods that promote blood circulation and warm the meridians. In addition, for external conditions such as skin diseases, swellings, and ulcers, TCM mostly uses internal medications to reduce swelling, discharge pus, or promote healing.

2.The human body and climate

All things in nature, especially the survival and development of living organisms, are directly affected by the objective environment. TCM attaches great importance to this relationship, believing that human health is inseparable from the climate, and that only by adapting to the natural environment can one stay healthy and live a long life. Therefore, it identifies the characteristics of the four seasons in a year, such as spring warmth, summer heat, autumn coolness, and winter cold, as well as the changing laws of the six different climates in the four seasons: wind, cold, summer heat, dampness, dryness, and fire. It also points out the ways to adapt to the objective environment and the diseases that may be incurred by going against climate changes. Based on these principles, it further deduces diagnostic and therapeutic methods. For example, when a climate occurs at an inappropriate time,i.e., in spring, which should be warm, it is instead cold or hot, which is considered an abnormal qi, called "pathogenic factors and evil winds".These improper qi must be avoided in a timely manner. As for the regular changes in the climate of the four seasons, they are beneficial to the human body and are called "healthy qi". Therefore, people often take advantage of the normal changes in the climate of spring, summer, autumn, and winter to nurture health and treat diseases. To take a simple case, phlegm-fluid cough and asthma, which are common in the elderly, tend to ease in spring and summer and worsen in autumn and winter. The reason is that the spleen and kidney yang are deficient, and damp turbidity condenses into phlegm. In clinical practice, warm medicines are often used for nurturing, and it is advocated to take advantage of the period when yang qi is most vigorous in summer for conditioning and prevention. Another example is that patients with blood deficiency and hyperactive liver yang are prone to symptoms such as dizziness, distending headache, blurred vision, tinnitus, and mental fatigue in spring. The occurrence of such symptoms is closely related to the climate, so tonifying in winter can reduce the chance of onset. From these examples, we can understand that TCM pays close attention to the mutual adaptation of the internal and external environments in health preservation and disease treatment.

3. Geo-adaptive Physiology

Different water and soil, as well as different living habits, can lead to different diseases. China has a vast territory. The northwest region has a cold climate, with high terrain and dry conditions; the southeast has a mild climate, with low terrain and humid conditions. Therefore, different regions often have different diseases. In addition, there are differences between the north and the south in the treatment methods, medicines used, and dosage for general diseases, which is what is meant by "adapting to the times, adapting to the individual, and adapting to the local conditions".

4. Other factors

TCM also attaches great importance to factors such as the strength of natural endowment, the fatness or thinness of the body, the mood (pleasant, melancholy, irritable), and mental stimulation, believing that they are closely related to the occurrence and development of diseases and must be taken into account during treatment. For example, people with a strong constitution can tolerate heavy medicines, while those with a weak constitution should not use strong doses; people who are plump are prone to excessive dampness and phlegm, and those who are thin are prone to yin deficiency and internal heat. Although these are not rigid rules, they have very practical reference value when dealing with specific diseases.

The theoretical system of TCM is established on the basis of holism. Starting from the holistic concept, TCM has two prominent points in clinical practice: First, it does not merely focus on the local symptoms of a disease while ignoring the impact on other parts; nor does it attach importance to a certain pathogenic factor while neglecting other factors caused by it. At the same time, in addition to timely treatment, it also takes advantage of seasons for prevention and treatment. For example, cough is a lung disorder. If it persists for a long time, it can affect the heart, accompanied by heart pain, a sensation of something stuck in the throat, swollen and painful throat; or affect the liver, accompanied by pain under the two ribs, inability to turn around, and distension in the two ribs when turning; it can also affect the stomach, causing vomiting, or affect the bladder, causing enuresis when coughing, which are called heart cough, liver cough, stomach cough, and bladder cough respectively, with different treatment methods for each. Another example is stagnation of qi, which may cause gastrointestinal disorders, or abdominal pain in women during menstruation, so both the gastrointestinal tract and menstruation regulation must be taken into account. Also, such as rheumatic arthralgia treated in dog days, and pulmonary tuberculosis treated in cool autumn, the curative effect is better than in winter or summer, which is due to the fact that the nature of the disease and the nature of visceral qi are suitable for heat and cool autumn. Second, it is recognized that the disease and the patient cannot be viewed separately. For each disease, one should think from two aspects: One is the pathogenic factors, and the other is the healthy qi, that is, the patient's resistance and recovery ability. Therefore, on the one hand, it is necessary to eliminate pathogenic factors and improve the condition; on the other hand, it is necessary to regulate the patient's physiological functions, enhance their natural resistance, and help them recover health. This puts forward two treatment methods: "strengthening healthy qi" and "eliminating pathogenic factors", as well as two tactical approaches: "When pathogenic factors are eliminated, healthy qi will recover naturally; when healthy qi is sufficient, pathogenic factors will retreat naturally". It is not difficult to understand that the process of a disease is a process of contradictory struggle between healthy qi and pathogenic factors. Only when pathogenic factors retreat and healthy qi enters the recovery stage does this struggle end. The struggle between healthy qi and pathogenic factors can be acute or slow, long or short. Although it varies according to the disease and the individual, it mainly depends on the comparison of the strength of both sides during the development of the disease. If healthy qi defeats pathogenic factors, the patient will recover; if pathogenic factors defeat healthy qi, the condition will worsen. Therefore, TCM attaches importance to avoiding pathogenic factors when not ill, and is eager to eliminate pathogenic factors when affected by them, but at the same time does not neglect strengthening healthy qi. In some cases, strengthening healthy qi is taken as the main approach. This is an overview of the holistic concept of TCM, indicating that this concept runs through physiology, pathology, diagnosis, and treatment. To further understand these principles, one must study *Huangdi Neijing* (The Yellow Emperor's Inner Canon), which is the source of TCM theory and has been guiding the practice of TCM.

II. Syndrome Differentiation and Treatment

Syndrome differentiation and treatment is a diagnostic and therapeutic rule commonly applied in TCM. From the recognition of diseases to the administration of treatment, it all relies on this rule. Syndrome differentiation and treatment is based on the integration of theory, method, prescription, and medicine, without which it cannot be carried out. It has theories and principles, and combines theory with practice.

The meaning of syndrome differentiation and treatment: "Bian" (differentiation) refers to analysis and discrimination; "zheng" (syndrome) refers to evidence and essence; "*lun*" (discussion) refers to deliberation and consideration; "*zhi*" (treatment) refers to the guiding principle of treatment. Syndrome and treatment are concrete realities; differentiation and discussion are flexible processes that require analysis and thinking. Our predecessors told us: for a specific syndrome, apply a specific method and use specific medicines. To figure out on what basis we recognize a syndrome and on what basis we use such methods and medicines, we need to make great efforts in differentiation and discussion. The occurrence of a disease must be due to certain factors, and such factors will manifest as certain symptoms. Without symptoms, it is impossible to distinguish the nature of the disease. At the same time, merely focusing on symptoms cannot lead to a comprehensive understanding of the condition. Sometimes, the manifestation of symptoms may not reflect the true state, which TCM calls "false appearance". This requires meticulous syndrome differentiation. In general, syndrome differentiation is the process of identifying the objective laws of a disease from its course, ensuring that symptoms and etiology are unified. To use dialectical terms, it is "essence determines phenomenon, and phenomenon manifests essence". Therefore, TCM follows certain steps in treating diseases: observing symptoms, determining etiology, discussing treatment methods, and then prescribing medicines. Hence, in TCM, for any disease, before clarifying the syndrome, it is impossible to determine the treatment method, let alone prescribe medicines. This is where the importance of syndrome differentiation and treatment lies.

Symptoms are the reactions of the human body to pathogenic factors, reflecting the nature of pathogenic factors and the strength of physiological functions. In terms of symptom manifestations, from trivial to obvious, from superficial to deep, we can identify pathogenic factors and physiological and pathological conditions. We can also detect the advancement or retreat of pathogenic factors and their development direction as symptoms disappear or emerge.

Etiologies are mainly the six pathogenic factors and seven emotions, which are the main factors of the two major categories of diseases: external contractions and internal injuries. For example, *Huangdi Neijing* (The Yellow Emperor's Inner Canon) points out that wind pathogen causes dizziness and convulsions; heat pathogen causes carbuncles and swellings; dryness pathogen causes thirst and dry, cracked skin; cold pathogen causes edema; dampness pathogen causes diarrhea. It also points out that anger causes qi to rebel upward; joy causes qi to relax; grief causes qi to dissipate; fear causes qi to sink; shock causes qi to become disordered; overthinking causes qi to stagnate. All these are observations of changes in the six excesses and seven emotions through symptoms. No disease is without a cause. Etiology is the root of disease, which can directly harm the human body and trigger various symptoms. The etiology in TCM mainly includes two aspects: the body's healthy qi and pathogenic factors, that is, from an overall observation of the patient's body. Although pathogenic factors are indeed etiological factors, the body's own hypofunction or hyperfunction is also considered an etiological factor.

Symptoms are the main objects of syndrome differentiation. To identify these objects, accurate diagnosis is required. TCM diagnosis includes observing complexion, listening to sounds, feeling the pulse, and inquiring, with the aim of observing and analyzing symptoms. That is, connecting symptoms and distinguishing the main symptoms and main pulse conditions, so as to correctly grasp the condition and not be confused by possible false appearances. Therefore, the key points of diagnosis, in addition to listening to the patient's main complaints, should also objectively observe other related symptoms from various aspects to infer the cause of the disease. Because symptoms are a reflection of the cause, but one cannot only look at superficial phenomena; one must see the hidden side and also the development trend of the next stage. In short, one must see the real side and not be confused by false appearances. This means that diagnosis cannot be determined solely based on the patient's subjective symptoms, and further syndrome differentiation is needed. For example, some diseases can form a preliminary impression based on general symptoms, but after in-depth analysis, this preliminary impression is often negated. For instance, if a patient complains of internal heat, dry mouth, along with fever, headache and other symptoms, it can generally be regarded as a warm-heat disease. However, if a careful examination reveals that although the patient is thirsty, they do not want to drink, feel bloated after drinking, and prefer hot water, it can be determined that thirst is a false appearance and not true internal heat. This shows the importance of syndrome differentiation in confirming a diagnosis. The symptoms of a disease can be simple or complex. Complexity does not mean disorder; as long as one understands the interrelationships of symptoms, analyzes and summarizes them, one can discover their causes and effects, origins and developments, thereby achieving a comprehensive and correct understanding.

TCM syndrome differentiation objectively identifies internal contradictions based on the occurrence and development of the disease. It includes both positive and negative aspects, points out the universality and particularity of contradictions in each disease, and becomes a cognitive method with substantial content. As for treatment, it is to formulate a policy based on the results of syndrome differentiation and prescribe medications according to the policy.

In treatment, three aspects should be mastered: etiology, disease symptoms, and the location of the disease. For example, if syndrome differentiation confirms that the etiology is food retention, the symptoms are abdominal distension, and the disease location is in the intestines and stomach, then the treatment policy is to soothe the middle jiao and promote digestion, and drugs that induce vomiting, resolve stagnation, or promote bowel movements are selected for treatment. Another example: After syndrome differentiation, it is confirmed that the etiology is blood deficiency, the symptoms are dizziness, palpitations, and restlessness, and the disease location is in the heart and liver meridians. Then, the treatment focuses on nourishing the heart and liver blood, combined with methods such as calming yang and tranquilizing the mind. Here, it can be seen that "syndrome differentiation" and "treatment" are connected, and the basic requirement is to apply them flexibly according to specific conditions.

The above discussion concerns the significance and methods of syndrome differentiation and treatment. As for the principles of syndrome differentiation, there are those based on the six meridians, those based on the triple energizer, and most importantly, those based on the eight principles: yin, yang, exterior, interior, deficiency, excess, cold, and heat. The meaning of the eight principles is to first divide yin and yang into opposing aspects, then determine the location of the disease using exterior and interior, assess the severity of the disease using deficiency and excess, and identify the nature of the disease using cold and heat. By integrating the results determined from these aspects, different disease patterns such as exterior-cold-excess syndrome, interior-heat-deficiency syndrome, etc., can be identified, which also encompass the aforementioned etiology, symptoms, and location of the disease. Clinical syndrome differentiation is an extremely meticulous task; variations in symptoms indicate changes in the condition. Sometimes, what appears to be a minor change may actually signal a shift in the disease's trend. For example, fever is a common symptom, but in clinical practice, a series of questions must be clarified: Is there aversion to cold? Is there sweating? How high is the fever? Does the aversion to cold subside and the fever decrease after sweating? Does the pulse calm down as the fever decreases? Are there cases where the aversion to cold disappears after sweating but the fever increases instead, or the fever gradually decreases but sweating persists, or sudden chills and sudden fever alternate throughout the day? It is also necessary to observe if there is clouding of consciousness? Is there thirst, and is it true or false thirst? Is there constipation or diarrhea? Are there symptoms such as headache, body pain, or cough? Additionally, what is the timing of the rise and fall of the fever throughout the day, and what is the pulse condition and tongue coating like? The reason for such a detailed understanding of a single fever symptom is that if other different symptoms accompany the fever, the diagnosis and treatment will differ. On the other hand, through the above differentiations, the condition in terms of exterior-interior, deficiency-excess, and cold-heat can be determined, thereby formulating the treatment strategy. For instance, fever with aversion to cold, headache, body pain, and absence of sweating indicates the initial stage of cold damage, treated with the acrid-warm diaphoresis method; if accompanied by cough, with or without sweating, it is a wind-cold syndrome, treated with the method of diffusing the lung to dispel pathogens; if there is sweating and thirst, it is the initial stage of wind-warm disease, treated with the acrid-cool clearing and resolving method; if there is no aversion to cold and high fever persists, it is a yangming heat syndrome, treated with the acrid-cold heat-clearing method; if the fever intensifies in the late afternoon and there is constipation, it is a stomach excess syndrome, treated with the bitter-cold purging method; if there is alternating chills and fever,occurring several times a day, it is a shaoyang disease, treated with the harmonizing method to reduce fever; if the tongue is red and consciousness is clouded, it is a syndrome of heat invading the pericardium, treated with the method of clearing the heart and cooling the nutrient-blood aspect. Other conditions, such as fever subsiding but sweating persisting without cease, require prevention of yang depletion and collapse, etc. These examples illustrate that syndrome differentiation aims to distinguish the nature of the disease, and only by clarifying the nature can treatment be formulated; otherwise, a slight error in the beginning can lead to a huge mistake in the end. However, syndrome differentiation does not end here, because the struggle between pathogenic factors and healthy qi is often a complex pathological process. In this process, due to the ebb and flow of pathogenic factors and healthy qi and the mutual influence among various parts of the body, the syndrome can change at any time, forming stages in the development of the disease.

Thus, syndrome differentiation is needed not only at the onset of the disease but also at each stage of its development. In summary, treatment must first be based on syndrome differentiation; without syndrome differentiation, there can be no basis for treatment. Therefore, when someone asks what medicine to use for treating cough, even though it is known to be a lung disorder, without knowing the specific symptoms, it is impossible to answer. Similarly, if someone asks whether dendrobium can be used for dry mouth, even though it is known that dendrobium can treat dry mouth, it cannot be answered until it is clarified what kind of dry mouth it is. Hence, syndrome differentiation and treatment is the fundamental principle of TCM diagnosis and treatment, and its essence lies in a treatment system that integrates theory, method, prescription, and medicine.

Section 2 Basic Theorie

I. Yin and Yang

The theory of yin and yang is a way of thinking summarized by ancient people from observing natural phenomena to explain them. Our predecessors discovered that all things and phenomena have two opposing attributes, which are contradictory yet unified and universally present in all things. Thus, they established the theory of yin and yang, using the terms "yin" and "yang" to represent the contradictory unity existing in all things. For example, heaven is yang, earth is yin; the sun is yang, the moon is yin; day is yang, night is yin; fire is yang, water is yin, etc. They used the principle of opposition and complementarity, contradiction and unity to explain all changes in the universe. TCM uses the theory of yin and yang to explain basic medical issues, thereby forming the ideological system of TCM theory. It runs through all aspects of TCM, such as physiology, pathology, diagnosis, treatment, and medicinals, constituting a complete set of medical methods that conform to objective reality and flexibly guide

TCM clinical practice.

1. In physiology

TCM holds that human physiology can also be explained by the theory of yin and yang. Generally speaking, yang is characterized by movement, and yin by stillness; yang has the ability to protect the body surface, and yin has the function of preserving internal essence. Therefore, in physiology, yang represents the body surface, such as the skin, hair, muscles, tendons, and bones, while yin represents the internal *zang-fu* organs. The five *zang* organs, which are mainly responsible for storing essence, are yin, and the six *fu*-organs, which are mainly responsible for digestion and transportation, are yang. In terms of location: the upper jiao is yang, the lower jiao is yin; the outer side is yang, the inner side is yin. In terms of substances and functions: Blood is yin, qi is yang; the body (form) is yin, the function (activity) is yang. Every part has the attributes of yin and yang, which are used to explain the specific nature and special functions of physiology.

2.In pathology

Based on the location and nature of the disease, exterior syndromes are classified as yang, and interior syndromes as yin; heat syndromes as yang, and cold syndromes as yin. All cases of functional weakness, such as shortness of breath, reluctance to speak, fear of cold, fatigue, and inability to withstand labor, are mostly due to yang deficiency; losses of substances, such as anemia, sallow complexion, spermatorrhea, and emaciation, are mostly due to yin deficiency. Therefore, general symptoms are divided into four types: yang deficiency, yin deficiency, yang excess, and yin excess. It is pointed out that yang deficiency should be accompanied by cold manifestations externally, and yin deficiency should be accompanied by heat manifestations internally; conversely, yang excess should present with heat externally, and yin excess with cold internally. For example, symptoms of yang excess include fever, dry mouth, rapid breathing, and chest oppression; symptoms of yin excess include fear of cold, cold limbs, and even shivering. However, sometimes yin deficiency can also cause symptoms similar to heat syndromes, such as rapid pulse and mania; yang deficiency can present with symptoms similar to cold syndromes, such as abdominal distension. In summary, all hyperactive, excited, and heat - inclined conditions are classified as yang syndromes, while weak, latent, and cold - inclined ones are classified as yin syndromes. Extending this to surgery, yang syndromes are mostly characterized by redness, swelling, and heat, while yin syndromes are mostly pale, sunken, and without heat.

3. In diagnosis

Take pulse diagnosis, for example, there are six key aspects. In terms of pulse rate, there are slow (chi) and rapid (shu); in terms of pulse quality, floating (fu) and deep (chen); in terms of pulse movement, smooth (hua) and rough (se). Rapid, floating, and smooth pulses belong to yang, while slow, deep, and rough pulses belong to yin; yin pulses are mostly seen in yin syndromes, and yang pulses in yang syndromes. In tongue diagnosis, changes in the tongue proper are related to blood disorders. A red or crimson color indicates blood heat, which belongs to yang; a pale or blue color indicates blood deficiency or blood cold, which belongs to yin. Changes in the tongue coating are mostly related to disorders of the intestines and stomach. A dry, yellow coating belongs to yang, and a moist, white coating belongs to yin. Therefore, *Huangdi Neijing* states: “A good diagnostician, when observing the complexion and feeling the pulse, first distinguishes between yin and yang.”

4. In treatment

Using diaphoresis for exterior syndromes, purgation for interior syndromes, warming methods for cold syndromes, and cooling methods for heat syndromes all contain the meaning of yin and yang. The main idea is that when yang prevails, yin is diseased; when yin prevails, yang is diseased.

When yang prevails, there is heat; when yin prevails, there is cold. Severe cold can present with heat - like signs, and severe heat can present with cold - like signs. Therefore, *Huangdi Neijing* puts forward major principles such as "treating yin for yang diseases, treating yang for yin diseases; guiding yang from yin, guiding yin from yang".

5. In medication

The properties of Chinese medicinal herbs are mainly distinguished by their qi (odor) and flavor. Generally, qi is yang, and flavor is yin. Qi is divided into four types: cold and cool belong to yin, warm and hot belong to yang. Flavors are divided into five types: Acrid and sweet belong to yang, sour, bitter, and salty belong to yin. Therefore, those with acrid and hot properties, such as aconite, cinnamon, and dried ginger, are called yang herbs, which can ascend and disperse; those with bitter and cold properties, such as coptis, honeysuckle, and gentian, are called yin herbs, which can descend and purge. In addition, those with aromatic stomachic effects, such as amomum and cardamom, are also called yang herbs; those with the effect of nourishing the liver and kidney, such as polygonum multiflorum and rehmannia, are also called yin herbs.

Incidentally, since the pharmacology of Chinese medicinal herbs is the application of basic TCM theories in Chinese materia medica, to have a thorough understanding of the qi and flavor of Chinese medicinal herbs, one must first understand the TCM theory of yin and yang, and then can use medicines appropriately in combination with syndrome differentiation.

Huangdi Neijing says: "Yin and yang can be counted as ten, and extended to a hundred; counted as a thousand, and extended to ten thousand... Yet their essence is one."This explains that regardless of the size of things, as long as there exists a relationship of unity of opposites, yin and yang can be used to explain them. Therefore, in TCM, there is a further analysis of yang within yin, yin within yin, yang within yang, and yin within yang, that is, distinguishing yin and yang within yin and yang themselves. For example, within a day, daytime is yang and night is yin; during daytime, the first half of the day is yang within yang, the second half of the day is yin within yang; the first half of the night is yin within yin, and the second half of the night is yang within yin. Taking *zang-fu* organs as another example, the six *fu*-organs are yang and the five *zang*-organs are yin; among the five *zang*-organs, the heart and lung are yang, while the liver, spleen, and kidney are yin; further, the heart is yang within yang, the lung is yin within yang, the liver is yang within yin, the kidney is yin within yin, and the spleen is the extreme yin within yin. The same applies to the qi and flavor of medicines: qi is yang and flavor is yin; a strong flavor is yin within yin, a mild flavor is yang within yin; a strong qi is yang within yang, a mild qi is yin within yang. Such analysis is summarized from objective reality and verified in objective practice. Take the example of spontaneous sweating: Daytime is the time when yang is exuberant; if spontaneous sweating occurs during the day, it is regarded as yang deficiency, because daytime belongs to yang, and medicines such as milkvetch and prepared common monkshood that tonify qi and yang are used to stop it; spontaneous sweating at night is regarded as yin deficiency, because night belongs to yin, and medicines such as rehmannia root and asiatic cornelian cherry that tonify blood and nourish yin are used to stop it. Another example is fever of unknown cause that occurs at a fixed time: If it occurs at night, tonifying yin medicines are mostly used, which is called the method of nourishing yin to reduce fever; if it occurs during the day, tonifying yang medicines are mostly used, which is called the method of using sweet-warm medicines to eliminate heat. It can thus be seen that the theory of yin and yang in TCM is an accessible classification method and a summarizing principle that simplifies complexity.

Yin and yang are general terms for the unity of opposites in things, thus encompassing opposites in substances, functions, and locations. However, it should be clear that TCM applies yin and yang extensively in various aspects, each with specific references. Therefore, to thoroughly understand the principles of TCM's use of yin and yang, one must go through clinical practice, as only through clinical practice can one comprehend the actual role of yin and yang. For example, heat belongs to yang, but heat varies in terms of exterior-interior and deficiency-excess. Hence, fever caused by wind-cold (common cold) should be treated with diaphoresis, called dispersing and releasing the exterior; fever caused by suppurative swellings should be treated with internal (resolving) methods, called dissipating and clearing; fever caused by liver fire should be treated with clearing and descending methods, called calming the liver and clearing heat; fever caused by consumptive diseases should be treated with tonifying methods, called nourishing yin to reduce steaming heat. Thus, while heat belonging to yang is the general case, whether heat pertains to the exterior, interior, deficiency, or excess is flexible.

Furthermore, clinically, there are often distinctions such as yin excess with yang deficiency, yang excess with yin deficiency, yang deficiency with yin excess, and yin deficiency with yang excess. This means that for the same yin and yang syndromes, there are cases where yin excess causes yang deficiency, yang excess causes yin deficiency, yang deficiency causes yin excess, or yin deficiency causes yang excess. These differ from the general syndromes of yang deficiency, yin deficiency, yang excess, and yin excess. If it is simple yin deficiency or yang deficiency, the treatment method is relatively straightforward; if yin deficiency or yang deficiency is caused by yang excess or yin excess, then both the root and branch must be addressed. For instance, ascites is treated with the method of warming and moving to expel and transform: warming and moving nourishes yang, while expelling and transforming eliminates water-dampness generated due to yang deficiency. Thirst is treated with the method of clearing the stomach and generating fluid: Clearing the stomach reduces heat, while generating fluid replenishes the body fluids consumed due to yang excess. Here, yin and yang may refer to functions or substances, and their locations also differ, but they all have specific references.

Finally, it should be noted that yin and yang are a prominent focus in TCM theory. In the application of yin and yang in TCM, there are two most important concepts: First, "yang generates and yin grows; yang restrains and yin stores." Generation and growth, restraint and storage, mean mutual dependence and mutual restriction. Yin and yang are opposite in function and manifestation, yet they are compatible and mutually promoting, and can never be separated. Hence, *Huangdi Neijing* states: "Yin is inside, acting as the guardian of yang; yang is outside, acting as the messenger of yin." It also says: "If the two are disharmonious, it is like spring without autumn, or winter without summer." Second, yin-yang harmony. Yin and yang must be harmonious, that is, contradictions must be unified. Not only must the opposites of yin excess, yang excess, yin deficiency, and yang deficiency within the human body be unified, but the internal and external environments must also be unified, so that internal and external harmony maintains bodily health. Thus, *Huangdi Neijing* states: "When yin and yang are harmonious, qi and blood are fluid and smooth." It also says: "When yin is stable and yang is secure, the spirit is balanced."

II. Five Elements

In addition to using the theory of yin and yang to explain the unity of opposites within the human body, TCM also employs the five elements theory to illustrate the internal connections within the human body.

The five elements are wood, fire, earth, metal, and water. The relationships between these five mainly include two aspects: "mutual generation" and "mutual restriction." Mutual generation refers to the relationship of mutual nurturing and promotion.

The mutual generation relationship among the five elements is as follows: wood generates fire, fire generates earth, earth generates metal, metal generates water, and water generates wood. From the mutual generation relationship of the five elements, it can be seen that any one element has two aspects: that which generates it and that which it generates. Taking wood as an example, water generates wood, and wood generates fire. Thus, using the parent-child relationship as a metaphor, water is the mother of wood, and fire is the child of wood. The same logic applies to the other four elements.

Mutual restriction refers to the relationship of mutual restraint and overcoming. The mutual restriction relationship among the five elements is: metal restricts wood, wood restricts earth, earth restricts water, water restricts fire, and fire restricts metal. In this mutual restriction relationship of the five elements, it can also be seen that any one element has two aspects: that which restricts it and that which it restricts. Taking wood again as an example, metal restricts wood, and wood restricts earth. That is to say, metal is that which wood "cannot overcome," and earth is that which wood "can overcome."

The above two aspects of mutual generation and mutual restriction among the five elements are not independent of each other but interact with each other. That is, there is a close connection between generation and restriction—generation contains restriction, and restriction contains generation. This interactive relationship is called the "restriction and transformation" relationship. For example: wood restricts earth, earth generates metal, and metal restricts wood.

The restriction and transformation relationship is a necessary condition for maintaining balance. Otherwise, if there is generation without restriction, the strong will become stronger; if there is restriction without generation, the weak will become weaker.

There is also an abnormal phenomenon in generation and restriction: that which I restrict may sometimes restrict me in return, and that which restricts me may sometimes be restricted by me. For example, water normally restricts fire, but under certain circumstances, fire can also restrict water in return, which is called "counter-restriction."

Generation, restriction, and counter-restriction all have a condition: If one's own qi is sufficient, generation can occur; otherwise, it cannot. If one's own qi is excessive, it can restrict that which it can overcome and counter-restrict that which restricts it. If one's own qi is insufficient, not only can it not restrict that which it can overcome, but it will also be taken advantage of and counter-restricted by that which restricts it. Hence, *Huangdi Neijing* states: "When qi is excessive, it restricts that which it can overcome and counter-restricts that which restricts it; when qi is insufficient, that which restricts it will take advantage and counter-restrict it, and that which it can overcome will lightly counter-restrict it."

The application of the five elements in TCM mainly involves classifying natural phenomena and human body tissues under certain circumstances according to the attributes of the five elements, and explaining the interrelationships between *zang-fu* organs through the relationships of generation and restriction. In terms of nature, directions (east, south, center, west, north), seasons (spring, summer, late summer, autumn, winter), climates (wind, summer heat, dampness, dryness, cold), life processes (birth, growth, transformation, harvest, storage), five colors (green, red, yellow, white, black), and five flavors (sour, bitter, sweet, acrid, salty) can all be subordinated in the order of wood, fire, earth, metal, and water. In terms of the human body, with the liver, heart, spleen, lung, and kidney as the center, it is connected to the seven orifices (eyes, tongue, mouth, nose, ears), the five body tissues (tendon, vessel, muscle, skin and hair, bone), and the five emotions (anger, joy, thinking, worry, fear), etc. After understanding this classification method, when encountering things belonging to the nature of a certain element, they can be combined and analyzed through direct or indirect relationships to understand the nature of the thing. The attached table is as follows.

Five Elements	Direction	Season	Climate	Animal	Plant	Qi	Flavor	Color	Tone	Number	Internal Organ	Seven Orifices	Body Tissue	Emotion	Sound	Disease Location	Pathological State
Wood	East	Spring	Wind	Chicken	Wheat	Dry	Sour	Green	Jiao	Eight	Liver	Eye	Tendon	Anger	Shout	Neck	Clenching
Fire	South	Summer	Heat	Sheep	Millet	Scorched	Bitter	Red	Zheng	Seven	Heart	Tongue	Vessel	Joy	Laugh	Chest and Hypochondrium	Anxiety
Earth	Center	Late Summer	Dampness	Ox	Millet	Fragrant	Sweet	Yellow	Gong	Five	Spleen	Mouth	Muscle	Thought	Sing	Spine	Hiccup
Metal	West	Autumn	Dryness	Horse	Grain	Fishy	Pungent	White	Shang	Nine	Lung	Nose	Skin and Hair	Worry	Cry	Shoulder and Back	Cough
Water	North	Winter	Cold	Pig	Bean	Rotten	Salty	Black	Yu	Six	Kidney	Ear	Bone	Fear	Groan	Lumbar and Thigh	Tremor

Like the theory of yin and yang, the five elements theory in TCM also guides TCM clinical practice. For example, wood has the nature of being unobstructed and smooth, so liver qi should also be unobstructed; if it is stagnated, it causes disease, and the treatment is to soothe the liver and regulate qi. Wood can restrict earth, so liver disease can affect the spleen; before it affects the spleen, prevention should be taken in advance; when spleen disease is found, it is appropriate to soothe the liver and strengthen the spleen. Water can generate wood, so for symptoms of liver deficiency, the method of nourishing the kidney can be used to soften the liver. Metal can restrict wood, so for symptoms of liver hyperactivity, the method of assisting metal and calming the liver can be used. For other visceral diseases, such as treating pulmonary consumption with the method of nourishing earth to generate metal, and treating spleen diarrhea with the method of benefiting fire to nourish earth, all are handled according to the principles of mutual generation and mutual restriction of the five elements. From the application of these treatment methods, it can also explain that TCM not only does not isolate the internal organs but also attaches great importance to the close connections between them. When organ A is diseased, treatment is often carried out from organ B or C, thus there are methods such as "moxibustion with ginger", "moxibustion withgarlic" and "when deficient, tonify its mother; when excessive, reduce its child".

Furthermore, from the connection between the five elements and the human viscera and superficial organs, for example, the eye belongs to the liver; for red eyes and photophobia caused by internal heat, the method of clearing the liver is often used. Muscles belong to the spleen; for emaciation and weakness, the method of tonifying the spleen is often used. Another example is that the liver governs wind; for symptoms such as dizziness and vertigo due to liver wind rising, the method of softening the liver and extinguishing wind is often used. The spleen governs dampness; for symptoms such as chest and abdominal distension, scanty urine and other stagnation symptoms, the method of strengthening the spleen and regulating dampness is often used. These are all analyzed and summarized using the five elements. Of course, this does not mean that all treatment methods cannot be separated from the five elements, nor is it allowed to mechanically apply the five elements to any disease. Instead, they should be flexibly applied according to specific circumstances.

Although TCM's five elements theory is based on five substances and deduced in conjunction with the internal organs, it does not mean that the organ is composed of that element, but is only used to explain its nature. Previous generations pointed out that the nature of the five elements is: Wood qi is upright, its nature is gentle, its function is bending and straightening, and its transformation is prosperity; fire qi rises and disperses, its nature is rapid, its function is burning, and its transformation is luxuriance; earth qi is flat and thick, its nature is harmonious, its function is high and low, and its transformation is plumpness; metal qi is bright, its nature is firm and strong, its function is scattering, and its transformation is solid contraction; water qi is internally bright, its nature is flowing downward, its function is overflowing, and its transformation is solid condensation. The "qi" mentioned here refers to instinct, "nature" refers to temperament, "function" refers to role, and "transformation" refers to change. The temperament, function and transformation of each element are based on instinct. For example, the instinct of wood is upright, so its temperament is gentle and compliant, its function is to seek straightness in bending, and its transformation is vigorous growth. Therefore, in combination with the five *zang*-organs, in terms of pathological changes, it is advocated that stagnated wood should be freed, stagnated fire should be dispersed, stagnated earth should be purged, stagnated metal should be drained, and stagnated water should be checked. All are based on five different natures to make them unobstructed, developed, dredged, descended and unblocked, so as to restore their instincts.

Yin and yang need to be balanced, and the five elements must also seek balance. Therefore, *Huangdi Neijing* also points out the normal qi, excess, and deficiency phenomena of the five elements, stating: "What is the normal qi? For wood, it is 'fuhe' (spreading harmony); for fire, it is 'shengming' (rising brightness); for earth, it is 'beihua' (comprehensive transformation); for metal, it is 'shenping' (prudent peace); for water, it is 'jingshun' (calm smoothness). In excess: For wood, it is 'fasheng' (germination); for fire, it is 'hexi' (blazing brightness); for earth, it is 'dunfu' (abundant prosperity); for metal, it is 'jiancheng' (firm formation); for water, it is 'liuyan' (overflowing flow). In deficiency: For wood, it is 'weihe' (diminished harmony); for fire, it is 'fuming' (hidden brightness); for earth, it is 'beijian' (humble supervision); for metal, it is 'congge' (following transformation); for water, it is 'helliu' (dried-up flow)." These terms are all used to describe the normal and abnormal phenomena of the five elements. For example, when wood attains its normal state, it spreads harmonious qi, hence called "fuhe"; when wood qi is deficient, yang harmony is constrained, called "weihe"; when there is excess, germination is unrestrained, hence called "fasheng". When studying the five elements, careful understanding of this aspect makes it easier to grasp their application rules.

III. Meridians and Collaterals

The theory of meridians and collaterals is also an important part of the theoretical system of TCM. *Huangdi Neijing* states: "Meridians are that by which life and death are determined, diseases are managed, and deficiency and excess are regulated; their pathways must not be obstructed." It also says: "The twelve meridians are the basis of human life, the cause of disease formation, the means by which humans are treated, and the origin of disease resolution. They are the starting point of learning and the ultimate goal of medical practice; what the unskilled find easy, the superior find difficult." It solemnly points out the importance of meridians, which is a compulsory course for physicians. Like the theories of yin and yang and the five elements, it runs through all aspects of TCM, including physiology, pathology, diagnosis, treatment methods, and medicinals, and plays a significant role.

Meridians and collaterals: The straight ones are meridians, the transverse ones are collaterals, which network the entire body and connect in a complex manner. Their functions are to internally belong to the *zang-fu* organs, externally connect to the body form, circulate qi and blood, nourish yin and yang, moisten the tendons and bones, and facilitate the joints. The main meridians and collaterals of the whole body include the twelve regular meridians, the twelve divergent meridians, the twelve muscle meridians, and the eight extraordinary meridians. Among them, the twelve regular meridians are divided into six yang meridians and six yin meridians, which connect sequentially and circulate through the *zang-fu* organs, head and face, and limbs; the divergent meridians are branches of the twelve regular meridians, forming interior-exterior combinations between yang and yin meridians, focusing on deep connections; the muscle meridians start from the extremities, run on the body surface, focusing on superficial connections; the eight extraordinary meridians regulate the twelve regular meridians. Therefore, meridians are the necessary pathways for the circulation of qi and blood, running through the interior and exterior, upper and lower, left and right, front and back of the human body, thereby connecting all parts of the body, including the five *zang*-organs, six*fu*-organs, head and face, trunk, limbs, and nine orifices, into an organic unified whole. Moreover, due to the mutual connection of meridians, moving from yin to yang, from yang to yin, from interior to exterior, from exterior to interior, from top to bottom, from bottom to top, qi and blood flow in an endless cycle, so-called yin and yang following each other, interior and exterior connecting, like a ring without end.

The physiological functions of the human body are mainly centered on the five *zang*-organs and six *fu*-organs, but it is the meridians and collaterals that play an important role in maintaining the balanced coordination between the internal and external, upper and lower parts of the body and enabling organic overall activities. The theory of meridians and collaterals was formed by predecessors through the analysis and research of the therapeutic effects of countless cases in long-term clinical practice. Therefore, using meridians and collaterals to analyze syndromes can also serve as one of the criteria for syndrome differentiation and treatment. Most of the transmission of external pathogens occurs from the exterior to the interior and from shallow to deep through the meridians and collaterals. Take apoplexy as an example: Mild cases affect the collaterals, with symptoms such as numbness of the skin and deviation of the mouth and eyes; more severe cases affect the meridians, with symptoms such as hemiplegia and inability to bear the body weight; even more severe cases affect the *fu*-organs and *zang*-organs, with symptoms such as lockjaw, stiff tongue, unconsciousness, and retention or incontinence of urine and feces. Also, diseases originating from the internal organs will similarly be reflected in their affiliated meridians and collaterals. For example, if there is pathogenic qi in the lung and heart, it remains in the two elbows; if there is pathogenic qi in the liver, it remains in the two hypochondria; if there is pathogenic qi in the spleen, it remains in the two thighs; if there is pathogenic qi in the kidney, it remains in the two popliteal fossa. The retention of qi causes pain, which is often encountered in clinical practice.

In clinical treatment, meridians and collaterals are also one of the important bases. It is well-known that needling the Hegu point on the hand can treat swollen gums and toothache; needling the Zusanli point can treat stomach diseases, and these all work through the meridians and collaterals. In addition, meridians and collaterals are also related to prescription and medication. For example, in Chinese materia medica, the main therapeutic functions of medicines are classified into the twelve meridians, and medicines of a certain type are used for diseases of a certain meridian. Like ephedra entering the Taiyang meridian, pueraria entering the Yangming meridian, and bupleurum entering the Shaoyang meridian. The above three medicines can all treat wind-cold headache. If the pain is in the back of the head and nape, it belongs to the Taiyang meridian, and ephedra is used; if the pain is in the forehead and superciliary ridge, it belongs to the Yangming meridian, and pueraria is used; if the pain is on both sides or one side of the head, it belongs to the Shaoyang meridian, and bupleurum is used. There are also some other medicines that are often used for certain diseases and become the main medicines for such diseases, such as magnolia flower for nasal congestion, lychee seed for hernia, turmeric for arm pain, cibotium for spinal pain, etc., all of which are based on the meridian classification.

It is incomplete to think that the theory of meridians and collaterals is specifically the theoretical basis for guiding acupuncture and moxibustion treatment. TCM, whether internal medicine, surgery, gynecology, pediatrics, tuina, or orthopedics, has never been separated from the scope guided by the theory of meridians and collaterals. The importance of the theory of meridians and collaterals has proven its practical value in long-term practice, and recently, through close cooperation between traditional Chinese and Western medicine, some issues have been initially confirmed in experimental research. For example, after needling points such as Weizhong, Neiting, and Zusanli, significant changes occur in gastric peristalsis, wave speed, wave amplitude, gastric tension, and emptying time;

needling points such as Hegu and Sanyinjiao can strengthen uterine contractions and shorten the interval; needling points such as Danzhong, Tiantu, Hegu, and Juque, under X-ray observation, can enhance esophageal wall peristalsis, increase the esophageal lumen, and relieve the pain of dysphagia, etc. These not only illustrate the impact of acupuncture on visceral activities but also the relationship between meridians and collaterals and organs, which is worthy of attention.

IV. Prevention

The purpose of prevention is to eliminate diseases and ensure health. *Huangdi Neijing* mentioned a long time ago: "A sage does not treat a disease that has already occurred but treats a disease that has not yet occurred. To administer medicine after a disease has developed is like digging a well when one is thirsty or casting weapons when a battle has begun, which is too late." Under the guidance of the preventive thought in *Huangdi Neijing*, knowledge about personal hygiene and public health has long been recorded in books such as *Qianjin Fang* (Prescriptions Worth a Thousand Gold). Now, let's focus on the basic spirit of TCM prevention.

First, predecessors believed that the occurrence of diseases, in addition to improper daily diet and living habits, is closely related to climate changes in nature, and the strength of one's own physical strength is an especially major factor. Therefore, to maintain health, one must first replenish energy, and second, avoid the invasion of external pathogens. *Huangdi Neijing* once said: "Where pathogenic factors gather, the qi (referring to the essence qi of the human body) must be deficient." It also said: "Avoid pathogenic factors and evil winds in a timely manner; keep the mind calm and free from desires, so that true qi follows, and spirit is retained internally—how can diseases occur?" It also indicated methods to exercise in adaptation to the normal climate of the four seasons, such as nourishing yang qi in spring and summer, nourishing yin qi in autumn and winter, as well as the ways of nurturing life in spring, nurturing growth in summer, nurturing harvest in autumn, and nurturing storage in winter. The goal is to make the internal and external environments adapt to each other, prevent diseases, and thus achieve health and longevity. This is the basic theory of TCM prevention.

Second, early treatment. It is recognized that treating a disease as soon as it occurs yields twice the result with half the effort. For example, *Huangdi Neijing* pointed out: "When pathogenic wind arrives, it is as rapid as wind and rain. Therefore, a good physician treats diseases at the skin, the next best at the muscles, then at the tendons and vessels, then at the six *fu*-organs, and then at the five *zang*-organs. Treating diseases of the five *zang*-organs results in a fifty-fifty chance of survival." This means that external pathogens invading the human body mostly enter from the exterior to the interior. When the disease is at the skin, it should be treated promptly; if delayed, it will gradually penetrate deeper. When it spreads to the *zang-fu* organs, the disease becomes severe and difficult to treat. Therefore, providing medical treatment in advance to prevent the deterioration of the disease is extremely important for clinical work.

Third, the occurrence and development of diseases have their own laws. To grasp the condition, one must be foresighted. For example, *Synopsis of the Golden Chamber* states: "When seeing a liver disease, know that the liver transmits to the spleen, and first strengthen the spleen." Because liver disease often affects the spleen; if, when treating liver disease, attention is paid to the spleen to prevent it from being damaged, then the transmission of liver disease can be prevented, and recovery becomes easier. TCM attaches great importance to the development of pathogenic factors in clinical work and emphasizes the need to timely control their changes. There are many discussions on these issues in *Treatise on Febrile Diseases* and the study of warm diseases. In addition, in diagnosis such as pulse-taking and tongue inspection, the signs of pathogenic transmission are often pointed out, which are worthy of reference.

It can thus be seen that TCM prevention includes two aspects: Prevention of diseases before they occur and prevention and treatment after diseases have occurred. Preventing the occurrence of diseases is the main focus; if one has already fallen ill, the spirit of prevention should be carried through to treatment, that is, efforts should be made during treatment to prevent the disease from developing for the worse. This medical method that integrates prevention into treatment is also one of the characteristics of TCM, and rich experience has been accumulated in this regard.

Section 3 Physiology

I. The Five *Zang*-Organs and Six *Fu*-Organs (Including the Extraordinary *Fu*- Organs)

TCM attaches importance to the physiological functions of the internal organs, the reflections of their pathological changes, and the connections between the internal organs and between the internal organs and various body tissues. According to the nature and functions of the internal organs, they are divided into five *zang*-organs and six *fu*-organs; another part is called the extraordinary *fu*-organs and the transmitting and transforming *fu*-organs.

The five *zang*-organs are the heart, liver, spleen, lung, and kidney; the six *fu*-organs are the gallbladder, stomach, small intestine, large intestine, bladder, and triple energizer. Among the five *zang*-organs, there is also the pericardium, which is the outer protector of the heart. It is sometimes considered independent and listed alongside the five *zang*-organs, making them six *zang*-organs. However, the functions and pathological changes of the pericardium are always consistent with those of the heart. Both *zang-fu*organs are internal organs, and their difference lies in that the five *zang*-organs store essence and do not excrete, while the six *fu*-organs transmit and transform substances and do not store. Organs with the functions of receiving, transporting, and transforming water and grains belong to the *fu*-organs; those that do not directly transmit and transform water and grains but have the function of storing essence belong to the *zang*-organs.

1. Heart

The heart generates blood and is in charge of storing the spirit. It is the master of human life activities. If the heart itself is unhealthy, or affected by emotional stimulation, or invaded by pathogenic factors, symptoms such as palpitations, fear, insomnia, or poor memory, abnormal laughter, or delirium, loss of consciousness may appear. When the heart is diseased, not only can it not control itself, but it can also affect the activities of other *zang-fu* organs, causing them to be disordered.

2. Liver

The liver stores blood and is in charge of planning. The liver has a strong nature, so it is also called the "general". When stimulated mentally, it often affects its normal function, leading to symptoms such as anger, headache and distension, and even upward reversal of fire qi causing hematemesis. The liver is also the "congenital foundation" of women (meaning it includes reproductive functions), so regulating menstruation and promoting conception must attach importance to the treatment of the liver.

3. Spleen

The spleen controls blood and is in charge of transportation and transformation. The power to maintain life is mainly nutrition. The spleen can digest water and grains and transport the essence of food to the whole body, so it is called the "acquired foundation". If the spleen's transportation and transformation ability is insufficient, there will be distension after eating, which may cause muscle emaciation and mental fatigue. The spleen also controls the transportation and transformation of water dampness. Symptoms of water dampness retention, such as chest tightness, nausea and vomiting, diarrhea, and skin edema, are mostly caused by spleen weakness. Therefore, methods of strengthening the spleen are often used to resolve dampness.

4. Lung

The lung is in charge of qi and governs purification and descent. If lung qi fails to descend, it is most likely to cause cough and asthma. In cases of deficiency, symptoms such as shortness of breath and weak speech are common. The lung has a regulatory effect on the blood circulation dominated by the heart. To describe the close relationship between the two, predecessors called the heart the "monarch" and the lung the "assistant minister".

5. Kidney

The kidney stores essence and is in charge of strength. The kidney plays a positive role in maintaining people's energy. Kidney deficiency can lead to symptoms such as dizziness, tinnitus, blurred vision, lumbago, leg soreness, and listlessness with a desire to lie down. The kidney is the "congenital foundation" of men, which has the same meaning as the liver being the congenital foundation of women, referring to reproductive functions. Therefore, symptoms such as decreased sexual desire, spermatorrhea, cold semen, and premature ejaculation are all treated from the kidney. The kidney has a different characteristic from other internal organs: there are two kidneys, the left one is the kidney, and the right one is the life gate. The kidney governs yin, and the life gate governs yang, so the kidney is also called the "*zang* of water and fire". In clinical practice, what is generally referred to as true yin and true yang also refers to this.

6. Gallbladder

The gallbladder is a pure *fu*-organ and is in charge of decision-making. The gallbladder and the liver are interior-exterior related. Although liver qi is strong, it cannot make decisions without the gallbladder. The liver and gallbladder complement each other, and courage is thus formed. In the human body, the heart is the "monarch fire", and the gallbladder and life gate are the "ministerial fire". If gallbladder fire is hyperactive, symptoms such as irritability, easy anger, headache and distension, chest tightness, hypochondriac pain, bitter taste in the mouth, and vomiting of bitter water will appear.

7. Stomach

The stomach is the sea of water and grains and is in charge of reception. The stomach and the spleen are interior-exterior related. Although predecessors distinguished that the stomach is in charge of reception and the spleen is in charge of digestion, the basic function of the stomach is not only to receive but also to digest. Therefore, the spleen and stomach are often mentioned together. It is also believed that without reception, there can be no digestion. Hence, it is said that "those who can take in grains thrive, those who cannot perish; those with stomach qi live, those without die", emphasizing the great importance of the stomach's function.

8. Small Intestine

The small intestine is the *fu*-organ that receives and contains, and is in charge of transforming substances. The small intestine receives the digested water and grains from the stomach, further separates the clear from the turbid: The essence is stored in the five *zang*-organs, the waste is excreted through the six *fu*-organs, the water in the waste is sent to the bladder, and the dregs are sent to the large intestine. These are all the tasks of the small intestine in transforming substances.

9. Large Intestine

The large intestine is the *fu*-organ that conducts and is in charge of excretion. The large intestine receives the waste from the small intestine and is responsible for transporting and excreting it, being the final stage of the entire digestive process. Since the function of the large intestine is to conduct waste and manage defecation, issues such as constipation, diarrhea, dysentery, and bloody stool are all addressed starting from the large intestine, with different treatments such as unblocking, moistening, and astringing.

10.Bladder

The bladder is the official of the region and is in charge of qi transformation. The bladder is where water and fluid are stored. If qi transformation is impaired, there will be urinary retention; if qi transformation is uncontrolled, there will be enuresis or urinary incontinence. However, the qi transformation of the bladder is related to the kidney: sufficient kidney qi enables transformation, while deficient kidney qi impairs it. Therefore, in treating difficulty in urination or incontinence, methods to warm the kidney are sometimes used.

11.Triple Energizer

The triple energizer is the official in charge of waterways and is in charge of water circulation. The triple energizer consists of the upper energizer, middle energizer, and lower energizer. Its main function is to dredge the waterways. For example, in treating water retention with abdominal distension, regulating qi is often used to assist water circulation, and the so-called qi-regulating medicines mostly include those that smooth the triple energizer.

Each *zang* or *fu*-organ has its main function and operates in mutual cooperation. Therefore, there is a "mutual domination" relationship between *zang*-organs: The kidney dominates the heart, the heart dominates the lung, the lung dominates the liver, and the liver dominates the spleen. "Domination" here means management, i.e., mutual restriction to maintain balance. There is also a "mutual combination" relationship between *zang* and *fu* organs: The lung combines with the large intestine, the heart combines with the small intestine, the liver combines with the gallbladder, the spleen combines with the stomach, and the kidney combines with the bladder. "Combination" means coordination, indicating that the *zang*-organ is the substance and the *fu*-organ is the function, and together they complete their comprehensive functions. *Zang*-organs belong to yin and the interior, while *fu*-organs belong to yang and the exterior, so this combination is also called "interior-exterior".

Although the *zang-fu* organs are located inside the body, they are closely connected with various body tissues and organs. Therefore, observing the manifestations of body tissues and organs can help determine the condition of the *zang-fu* organs, which is of great significance in diagnosis. The commonly used relationships between internal organs and body tissues/organs in clinical practice are as follows: The liver opens into the eyes, its filling is in the tendons, and its luster is in the nails; the heart opens into the tongue, its filling is in the vessels, and its luster is in the face; the spleen opens into the mouth, its filling is in the muscles, and its luster is in the lips; the lung opens into the nose, its filling is in the skin, and its luster is in the hair; the kidney opens into the ears, its filling is in the bones, and its luster is in the hair. Additionally, the spleen governs the limbs; the elbows are associated with the heart and lung, the armpits with the liver, the thighs with the spleen, the popliteal fossae with the kidney, and so on.

Beyond the *zang* and *fu* organs, there are the extraordinary *fu*-organs, namely the brain, marrow, bones, vessels, gallbladder, and the uterus (female's womb). The meaning of "extraordinary" is that they are like *zang*-organs yet not *zang*-organs, like *fu*-organs yet not *fu*-organs; in form, they resemble *fu*-organs, but in function, they are similar to *zang*-organs. They are a type of internal organ that is out of the ordinary. They are also extremely important parts of the human body. These extraordinary *fu*-organs are not isolated; they are all connected to the *zang* and *fu*-organs. For example, the brain is related to the heart and liver. Moreover, since the brain is related to the marrow, and the marrow is related to the bones, and the bones belong to the kidney, the brain is also related to the kidney. The female's womb (uterus) belongs to the liver, and because menstruation, nurturing the fetus, etc., are related to blood, it is also related to the heart and spleen. Corresponding to the extraordinary *fu*-organs are the transmitting and transforming *fu*-organs, namely the stomach, large intestine, small intestine, triple energizer, and bladder. These five*fu*-organs, among the six *fu*-organs, all belong to the digestive system. As mentioned above, all tissues of the body are organically connected, forming an integral and indivisible whole.

In addition to being familiar with the functions of the five*zang*-organs, one must also understand their natures. These natures are like a person's character. Adjusting the pathological changes caused by their loss of balance based on their natures has proven to be completely correct. For example: the liver likes to be unobstructed and free; the heart likes to be open and bright; the spleen likes to be healthy and transporting; the lung likes to be pure and descending; the kidney likes to be moist and downward. In treatment, there is a rule: The liver desires to be dispersed, so acrid foods should be eaten to disperse it; the liver dislikes urgency, so sweet foods should be eaten to soothe it. The heart desires to be softened, so salty foods should be eaten to soften it; the heart dislikes laxity, so sour foods should be eaten to astringe it. The spleen desires to be soothed, so sweet foods should be eaten to soothe it; the spleen dislikes dampness, so bitter foods should be eaten to dry it. The lung desires to be astringed, so sour foods should be eaten to astringe it; the lung dislikes upward reversal of qi, so bitter foods should be eaten to descend it. The kidney desires to be firm, so bitter foods should be eaten to firm it; the kidney dislikes dryness, so acrid foods should be eaten to moisten it.

By combining the normal physiological activities of the five *zang*-organs with certain abnormal conditions, one can detect their pathological changes. Predecessors have accumulated a lot of experience in this regard. As mentioned above, the heart stores the spirit: Excessive laughter indicates excessive spirit, while grief and crying indicate insufficient spirit. The lung governs qi: Cough and asthma indicate excessive qi, while shortness of breath and difficulty in breathing indicate insufficient qi. The liver governs blood: Proneness to anger indicates excessive blood, while fearfulness indicates insufficient blood. The spleen governs the body form: Abdominal distension and difficulty in urination indicate excessive superficiality, while inability to use the limbs indicates insufficient form. The kidney governs will: Diarrhea and abdominal distension indicate excessive will, while cold limbs indicate insufficient will. Another example: Chest and abdominal distension with a heavy and unclear voice indicates accumulated dampness in the middle jiao; a low and faint voice that cannot be sustained indicates extreme deficiency in qi; speaking without regard to intimacy or distance, and not covering oneself with clothes and quilts indicates disordered spirit; incessant diarrhea indicates insecurity of the large intestine; urinary incontinence indicates inability of the bladder to restrain. There are also such cases: The head is the residence of clarity and brightness; a drooping head that cannot be raised and sunken eyes with no luster indicate extreme mental exhaustion; the back is the residence of the chest; a hunchback with drooping shoulders indicates weakness of visceral qi; the waist is the residence of the kidney; low back pain with inability to turn indicates deficiency of the kidney; the knees are the residence of the tendons; difficulty in flexing and extending joints, and walking with a stoop indicate weakness of the tendons; the bones are the residence of the marrow; inability to stand for long, and trembling when walking or standing indicate weak bones. All such phenomena show that what is inside is manifested outside. Therefore, the internal condition can be detected from the outside, which is of great help in clinical practice.

II. The Twelve Regular Meridians (Including the Eight Extraordinary Meridians)

There is a close connection with the *zang-fu* organs, and the *zang-fu* organs also need them to establish close links with various tissues—these are the meridians and collaterals. Meridians and collaterals are the abbreviations of meridians and collaterals. Meridians run straight up and down, and collaterals run horizontally left and right. To understand with a simple analogy, meridians are like the Yangtze River and Yellow River on the ground, and collaterals are like the streams and ditches between the rivers, connecting up and down, linking left and right, like a ring, flowing ceaselessly and circulating endlessly.

The meridians and collaterals are quite complex, with twelve main ones called the regular meridians, namely: the Lung Meridian of Hand-Taiyin, the Heart Meridian of Hand-Shaoyin, and the Pericardium Meridian of Hand-Jueyin, which are the three Yin meridians of the hand; the Small Intestine Meridian of Hand-Taiyang, the Triple Energizer Meridian of Hand-Shaoyang, and the Large Intestine Meridian of

Hand-Yangming, which are the three Yang meridians of the hand; the Spleen Meridian of Foot-Taiyin, the Kidney Meridian of Foot-Shaoyin, and the Liver Meridian of Foot-Jueyin, which are the three Yin meridians of the foot; the Bladder Meridian of Foot-Taiyang, the Gallbladder Meridian of Foot-Shaoyang, and the Stomach Meridian of Foot-Yangming, which are the three Yang meridians of the foot. There is a simple mnemonic for the circulation routes of these twelve meridians: "The three Yin meridians of the hand go from the *zang*-organs to the hands; the three Yang meridians of the hand go from the hands to the head; the three Yang meridians of the foot go from the head to the feet; the three Yin meridians of the foot go from the feet to the *zang*-organs." That is, the Yin meridians of the hand go from the chest to the hands and connect with the Yang meridians of the hand, then the Yang meridians of the hand go from the hands to the head and connect with the Yang meridians of the foot, then the Yang meridians of the foot go from the head to the feet and connect with the Yin meridians of the foot, and then the Yin meridians of the foot go from the feet to the internal *zang*-organs and connect with the Yin meridians of the hand, forming a cycle. To separate the twelve meridians: Starting from the Lung Meridian of Hand-Taiyin, then the Large Intestine Meridian of Hand-Yangming, then the Stomach Meridian of Foot-Yangming, then the Spleen Meridian of Foot-Taiyin, then the Heart Meridian of Hand-Shaoyin, then the Small Intestine Meridian of Hand-Taiyang, then the Bladder Meridian of Foot-Taiyang, then the Kidney Meridian of Foot-Shaoyin, then the Pericardium Meridian of Hand-Jueyin, then the Triple Energizer Meridian of Hand-Shaoyang, then the Gallbladder Meridian of Foot-Shaoyang, then the Liver Meridian of Foot-Jueyin, and back to the Lung Meridian of Hand-Taiyin. In this way, it circulates endlessly, moving from Yin to Yang, from Yang to Yin, from the exterior to the interior, from the interior to the exterior, from top to bottom, and from bottom to top.

It is generally thought that meridians and collaterals are applicable only to acupuncture and moxibustion. Little do people know that since meridians and collaterals circulate throughout the body, they naturally divide the whole body into several regions and establish the exterior-interior relationship between the body surface and internal organs. Therefore, from the symptoms occurring in a certain region, we can detect the affected meridian and *zang-fu* organs, and treat according to this meridian and *zang-fu* organs. Hence, they also occupy an important position in clinical internal medicine. For example, the onset of the twelve meridians: The onset of the Lung Meridian of Hand-Taiyin commonly presents with asthma and cough, pain in the supraclavicular fossa, pain and coldness in the anterior medial border of the arm, and heat in the palm; The onset of the Large Intestine Meridian of Hand-Yangming commonly presents with toothache, sore throat, pain in the anterior part of the shoulder and arm, and pain and immobility of the index finger; The onset of the Stomach Meridian of Foot-Yangming commonly presents with nosebleed, deviated mouth, sores inside the lips, swelling and pain of the kneecap, pain along the lateral side of the chest, breast, thigh, dorsum of the foot, and inability to flex and extend the middle toe; The onset of the Spleen Meridian of Foot-Taiyin commonly presents with stiffness of the root of the tongue, epigastric pain, swelling and coldness in the medial side of the thigh and knee, and inability to move the big toe; The onset of the Heart Meridian of Hand-Shaoyin commonly presents with heart pain, hypochondriac pain, pain and coldness in the posterior medial border of the arm, and heat in the palm; The onset of the Small Intestine Meridian of Hand-Taiyang commonly presents with sore throat, swelling of the cheek, pain in the posterior lateral border of the shoulder, arm and elbow; The onset of the Bladder Meridian of Foot-Taiyang commonly presents with headache, stiff neck, pain in the lumbar spine, pain in the sacrum, popliteal fossa, calf and foot, and inability to use the little toe; The onset of the Kidney Meridian of Foot-Shaoyin commonly presents with swollen throat, restlessness, pain and flaccidity with coldness in the posterior medial border of the spine and thigh, and heat pain in the sole; The onset of the Pericardium Meridian of Hand-Jueyin commonly presents with heat in the palm, contracture of the elbow and arm, swelling in the armpit, and chest and hypochondriac fullness; The onset of the Triple Energizer Meridian of Hand-Shaoyang commonly presents with deafness, sore throat, pain in the cheek, pain in the posterior ear, shoulder, arm and lateral side of the elbow, and inability to use the ring finger; The onset of the Gallbladder Meridian of Foot-Shaoyang commonly presents with headache, pain in the outer corner of the eye, swelling in the armpit, pain from the chest and hypochondrium, thigh, knee, lateral side down to the anterior part of the lateral malleolus of the tibia; The onset of the Liver Meridian of Foot-Jueyin commonly presents with dry throat, chest fullness, hernia, enuresis, or difficulty in urination. For the above twelve meridian symptoms, we can treat the respective meridians and *zang-fu* organs based on where the pain or hot swelling occurs, which is as clear as day.

A separate part of the twelve meridians, which travels in and out between yin and yang meridians, serving as a connecting passage midway, is deeper and longer than the collaterals, called "divergent meridians". In addition to the divergent meridians, there are those that circulate on the body surface without entering the internal organs, starting from the tips of the limbs, running between the wrists, elbows, armpits, ankles, knees, and thighs of the limbs, which is just the opposite of the divergent meridians that go deep into the body, called "muscle meridians". There are also fifteen collaterals that act as links for the transmission of meridians, and the collaterals and sub-collaterals are intricately distributed among the meridians.

The twelve meridians are called regular meridians, and in contrast to them are the "extraordinary meridians", including the Du Meridian, Ren

Meridian, Chong Meridian, Dai Meridian, Yangqiao Meridian, Yinqiao Meridian, Yangwei Meridian, and Yinwei Meridian, known as the eight extraordinary meridians, which can supplement the deficiencies of the regular meridians. Among the eight meridians, the Du Meridian runs along the spine inside the back, governing the yang of the whole body; the Ren Meridian runs along the abdomen inside the front, governing the yin of the whole body; the Chong Meridian runs inside the abdomen and spreads in the chest, being the vital passage of the twelve meridians, all originating from the perineum, so-called "one source with three branches"; the Dai Meridian encircles below the hypochondria, like a girdle, governing and constraining all meridians; "qiao" has the meaning of agility, with the meridian running on the lateral side of the limbs called Yangqiao, and on the medial side called Yinqiao; "wei" has the meaning of connection, with Yangwei connecting all yang meridians and Yinwei connecting all yin meridians. Among the eight meridians, the Du Meridian, Ren Meridian and the twelve regular meridians are combined, called the fourteen meridians, which are the most important.

Each of the Fourteen Meridians has acupoints. The term "xue" (acupoint) implies a hole or aperture, so they are also called "kongxue" (acupoints). These acupoints are connected to specific meridians and are the sites where visceral qi is transmitted and accumulates on the body surface, hence also referred to as "shuxue" (acupuncture points) – "shu" meaning transportation, which is sometimes written as "shuxue" (shu stream points) and abbreviated as "yuxue" (back-shu points). There are over 360 acupoints in the Fourteen Meridians, each with a specific name. A brief introduction to the starting and ending acupoints of each meridian and the total number of acupoints is as follows:

1. Lung Meridian of Hand-Taiyin: Starts at Zhongfu (Middle Residence) in the middle jiao and ends at Shaoshang (Lesser Shang) on the thumb, with a total of 11 acupoints.

2.Large Intestine Meridian of Hand-Yangming: Starts at Shangyang (Shang Yang) on the index finger and ends at Yingxiang (Welcome Fragrance) beside the nose, with a total of 20 acupoints.

3.Stomach Meridian of Foot-Yangming: Starts at Chengqi (Receive Qi) below the eye and ends at Lidui (Strict Exchange) on the second toe, with a total of 45 acupoints.

4.Spleen Meridian of Foot-Taiyin: Starts at Yinbai (Hidden White) on the big toe and ends at Dabao (Great Wrapper) in the chest and hypochondrium, with a total of 21 acupoints.

5.Heart Meridian of Hand-Shaoyin: Starts at Jiquan (Extreme Spring) in the chest and ends at Shaochong (Lesser Rushing) on the little finger, with a total of 9 acupoints.

6.Small Intestine Meridian of Hand-Taiyang: Starts at Shaoze (Lesser Marsh) on the little finger and ends at Tinggong (Palace of Hearing) in front of the ear, with a total of 19 acupoints.

7.Bladder Meridian of Foot-Taiyang: Starts at Jingming (Bright Eyes) at the inner corner of the eye and ends at Zhiyin (Reaching Yin) on the little toe, with a total of 67 acupoints.

8.Kidney Meridian of Foot-Shaoyin: Starts at Yongquan (Gushing Spring) on the sole of the foot and ends at Shufu (Transport Residence) below the great bone, with a total of 27 acupoints.

9.Pericardium Meridian of Hand-Jueyin: Starts at Tianchi (Heavenly Pool) in the chest and ends at Zhongchong (Middle Rushing) on the ring finger, with a total of 9 acupoints.

10.Triple Energizer Meridian of Hand-Shaoyang: Starts at Guanchong (Pass Rushing) on the ring finger and ends at Sizhukong (Silken

Bamboo Hollow) at the outer corner of the eye, with a total of 23 acupoints.

11.Foot-Shaoyang: Starts at Tongziliao (Pupil Seam) at the outer corner of the eye and ends at Jiaoyin (Orifice Yin) on the little toe and second toe, with a total of 44 acupoints.

12.Liver Meridian of Foot-Jueyin: Starts at Dadun (Great Thickness) on the big toe and ends at Qimen (Cycle Gate) in the chest, with a total of 14 acupoints.

13.Du Meridian: Starts at Changqiang (Long Strength) at the coccyx and ends at Yinjiao (Gum Intersection) on the upper gum inside the lip, with a total of 28 acupoints.

14.Ren Meridian: Starts at Huiyin (Meeting Yin) at the perineum and ends at Chengjiang (Receive Fluid) below the lip, with a total of 24 acupoints.

Visceral organs and meridians have an indivisible relationship in terms of physiology. Yu Jiayan once said, "He who treats diseases without understanding the viscera and meridians will make mistakes as soon as he opens his mouth or acts." But after understanding the viscera and meridians, how exactly are they applied in clinical practice? Let us take the liver as an example to illustrate. From the physiological and pathological aspects of the viscera and meridians, the understanding of liver diseases can be divided into the following points:

1. Based on the idea that "the liver stores blood" and "its transformation is flourishing," it is recognized that anemia is closely related to the liver.

2. Based on the notions that "the liver is the root of endurance" and "the abode of the ethereal soul," and that "planning emanates from it," it is recognized that liver diseases are highly related to fatigue and emotions.

3. Based on the descriptions of the liver as "the general official" and that "its emotion is anger," it is recognized that liver qi tends to rebel violently.

4. Based on the characteristics that "its nature is mild warmth" and "it is the lesser yang within yin," it is recognized that liver diseases can give rise to symptoms of "fire."

5. Based on the connections that "wind qi communicates with the liver" and "its function is movement," it is recognized that liver diseases can also produce symptoms of "wind."

6. Based on the principles that "the third month of spring is the time of sprouting and unfolding, and going against this harms the liver," and that "its order is to disperse," it is recognized that liver diseases may involve stagnation and failure of qi and blood to flow freely.

7. Based on the observations that "the liver opens into the eyes," "its luster is in the nails," and "its filling is in the tendons," it is recognized that liver diseases can affect the eyes and fascia.

8. Based on the description that "the Liver Meridian of Foot-Jueyin runs along the medial aspect of the thigh, enters the pubic hair region, passes through the external genitalia, reaches the lower abdomen, ascends through the diaphragm, spreads over the hypochondria, follows behind the throat, ascends to the back of the nose, connects with the eye system, rises to the forehead, and meets the Du Meridian at the top of the head," it is recognized that liver diseases can also affect the head and face, the top of the head, the hypochondria, the lower abdomen, the external genitalia, and the lower limbs.

In addition, according to the laws of generation and restriction in the five elements, "water generates wood, and wood restricts earth," it is recognized that deficiency of kidney yin can lead to liver diseases, and liver diseases can easily harm the spleen and stomach, thus giving rise to terms such as yin deficiency with liver hyperactivity and disharmony between the liver and stomach. In this way, understanding liver diseases based on the physiological functions and pathological changes of the liver and the Liver Meridian forms a set of theories for treating liver diseases. Using this as a basis to analyze symptoms and consider treatment methods can make everything clear and logical.

III. Qi and Blood

Emphasizing both qi and blood, and regarding qi as the commander of blood, this is a cognitive method in TCM physiology. There are quite a few names for qi, such as yuanqi (primordial qi), zhenqi (true qi), and jingqi (essential qi). These all refer to qi and blood, other substances, and abilities within the entire human body; although the names are different, they are essentially the same. There are also the terms yangqi (yang qi) and yinqi (yin qi), which distinguish two major functions within yuanqi: one that can protect the body surface, and the other that can preserve energy to prevent its depletion, so they are also called zhenyang (true yang) and zhenyin (true yin). There are also zongqi (pectoral qi) and zhongqi (middle qi), referring to parts of yuanqi that belong to the upper jiao (lung) and the middle jiao (spleen and stomach) respectively, so they are also called feiqi (lung qi) and weiqi (stomach qi). Generally speaking, they are all yuanqi.

The qi in qi and blood represents ability in some contexts and substance in others, hence the saying that qi is formless and blood is formless. Our understanding is that predecessors put qi and blood on an equal footing; since blood is a substance, qi should also be a substance, and the function exerted by qi is "ability." Blood circulates within the vessels to nourish the entire body, and qi can improve the function of blood and assist in its normal circulation. Both are important factors constituting the normal physiological activities of the human body. *Huangdi Neijing* states: "Blood is mainly responsible for nourishing, and qi is mainly responsible for warming." This indicates that the two are absolutely inseparable. If qi is stimulated psychologically or environmentally—whether it is emotions such as joy, anger, sorrow, or pleasure, climatic factors such as cold or heat, or work-related factors such as overwork or leisure—it will affect blood. Therefore, predecessors attached special importance to qi, calling it "qi is the commander of blood" and also saying "all diseases arise from qi."

Generally speaking, although diseases of the blood system should be treated with blood-nourishing medicines, there are also treatment methods such as regulating qi to harmonize blood, promoting qi to expel blood stasis, and replenishing qi for blood loss. This is because when qi moves, blood moves; when qi stagnates, blood stagnates. To ensure the normal circulation of blood, qi movement must first be smooth; to eliminate blood stasis, qi must first be unblocked. In cases of incessant bleeding, qi-tonifying medicines can be used to help contain it; for severe anemia, according to the principle that yang generates yin,qi-tonifying medicines are also needed to accelerate recovery. These methods are all very effective in clinical practice.

In clinical practice, TCM often refers to qi as the gas produced due to disorders of *zang-fu*functions or indigestion. Common manifestations include chest and diaphragmatic stuffiness, hypochondriac and epigastric obstruction, uncomfortable tendons and vessels, and internal abdominal gurgling and rushing. Terms such as qi stagnation, qi congestion, qi depression, qi accumulation, qi gathering, and qi blockage are used as pathological explanations. Diseases with these symptoms are often named with the character "qi", such as qi syncope, qi diaphragmatic disorder, qi distension, qi tympany, qi hiccup, qi stranguria, qi constipation, qi goiter, qi hernia, and liver qi pain, stomach qi pain, etc. For example, clinically seen syncope, diaphragmatic disorders, tympanites, etc., have various causes; among them, those caused by qi disorders can be relieved by regulating qi movement, thus there are various treatment methods such as soothing qi, dispersing qi, regulating qi, promoting qi, diffusing qi, harmonizing qi, descending qi, and breaking qi. Therefore, the meaning of qi in physiology is different from that in pathology, and they should be distinguished.

Regarding the function of blood, *Huangdi Neijing* points out: "The eyes receive blood and can see; the feet receive blood and can walk; the palms receive blood and can grasp; the fingers receive blood and can pick up." This indicates that the entire body relies on blood for nutrition, hence it also says: "To sustain life, nothing is more precious than this." In terms of physiology, it specifically states: "The heart generates blood, the liver stores blood, the spleen controls blood." If the heart is weak or blood is deficient, and circulation is disturbed, symptoms such as palpitations, fear, and intermittent pulse may appear; when excessive mental stimulation affects the liver's duty of storing blood, it can easily cause vomiting of blood or nosebleeds; when the spleen's function is disordered, it loses its controlling effect, leading to symptoms such as bloody stool, menorrhagia, and metrorrhagia in women. Commonly used treatment methods such as harmonizing blood, nourishing blood, and guiding blood back to the meridians are mostly targeted at the heart, liver, and spleen. When treating consumptive diseases with methods targeting the heart, liver, and spleen fails to achieve results, the focus shifts to the kidney, emphasizing the "congenital foundation". As *General Treatise on the Etiology and Pathogenesis of Diseases* states: "Excessive desires and overstrain damage kidney qi, deplete essence and blood, cause *zang-fu* deficiency, and prevent qi and blood from nourishing the body."

Blood congeals when encountering cold and moves recklessly when encountering heat. This cold and heat include external cold and heat pathogens, cold and pungent-hot foods, as well as constitutional tendencies to cold, heat, and excessive liver fire. Therefore, blood diseases are mainly divided into blood stasis and bleeding, which are certainly closely related to qi. Blood deficiency mostly arises from excessive fatigue, excessive traumatic bleeding, post-illness, and postpartum in women. When blood deficiency syndrome occurs, treatment must target the heart, liver, and spleen, and if necessary, further target the kidney.

IV. Essence, Qi, and Spirit

Essence, qi, and spirit are called the "three treasures" in TCM, indicating their extreme importance to the human body. Qi has been discussed above; now let's first talk about essence. Essence is the material basis for human growth, development, and reproductive capacity. TCM attributes essence to the kidney. *Huangdi Neijing* states: "The kidney governs water and receives and stores the essence of the five *zang*-organs and six *fu*-organs." It also says: "The kidney is responsible for hibernation, the root of storage, and the place of essence." Moreover, "the combination of the two essences forms the body" and "at the beginning of human life, essence is formed first", after which body tissues such as the brain, marrow, bones, tendons, vessels, skin, muscles, and hair gradually develop. Since essence is the foundation of life, the kidney is called the "congenital foundation". After birth, the body relies on food for nourishment, which is the function of the spleen and stomach, hence the spleen and stomach are called the "acquired foundation". Clinically, it is believed that insufficient congenital foundation can be nourished through the acquired foundation.

Essence is closely related to physical strength. Therefore, people suffering from spermatorrhea often experience symptoms such as soreness in the waist, pain in the back, weakness in the feet and legs; in severe cases, they may suffer from extreme fatigue, shortness of breath, dull skin, tinnitus, dull eyesight, and inability to stand for a long time, which is called "essence exhaustion". Since the kidney is in charge of storing essence, the above symptoms are generally referred to as kidney deficiency, and treatment mainly focuses on tonifying the kidney.

It must be pointed out that in many places in TCM books, "essence" refers to the generalized essence, that is, the essential qi of the human body. For example, *Huangdi Neijing* says: "When essential qi is depleted, there is deficiency." It also says: "When essential qi is exhausted, the body is destroyed." In terms of diseases, it is said that "if one does not store essence in winter, they will surely suffer from warm diseases in spring" and "those who were once rich and then poor are said to have lost essence", etc. There are also references to a single substance, such as: "Heat is pathogenic qi, and sweat is essential qi." These should not be confused with the narrow sense of essence.

Next, let's talk about spirit. Predecessors believed that all tissues of the human body are tangible, and there is a high-level, intangible ability that presides over activities, called "spirit". If the spirit is vigorous, the internal organs and the body will be active; once the spirit is scattered, everything will cease to function. Regarding the activities of the spirit in the internal organs, *The Classic of Difficult Issues* pointed out: "*Zang* organs are where the human spirit resides. The liver stores the ethereal soul, the lung stores the corporeal soul, the heart stores the spirit, the spleen stores intention and wisdom, and the kidney stores essence and will." It can be seen that the ethereal soul, corporeal soul, intention, will, etc., mentioned in TCM used to distinguish the activity phenomena of each *zang*-organ. Although the names are different, they generally refer to the same spirit. Since the heart commands the internal organs, the spirit of the heart is generally used to summarize the spirits of the other four *zang* organs, and there is a close relationship between them. *Huangdi Neijing* says: "That which comes with birth is called essence; the combination of the two essences is called spirit; that which follows the spirit in coming and going is called the ethereal soul; that which comes and goes with essence is called the corporeal soul. That which is responsible for dealing with things is called the heart; that which the heart remembers is called intention; that which intention retains is called will; that which changes based on will is called thinking; that which longs for distant things based on thinking is called consideration; that which deals with things based on consideration is called wisdom." This series of ideological and conscious activities are all functions of the spirit.

When the spirit is diseased, a series of symptoms will occur, such as chest oppression with dysphoria, discomfort in both hypochondria, loss of mental control, weakness in hands and feet, mania and disorientation, memory loss, atrophy of the external genitalia, soreness and pain in the waist and spine with inability to bend, stretch, or turn. Prepared formulas such as Cinnabar Sedative Pill and Amber Mind-Stabilizing Pill are used to treat such diseases. However, the spirit is not empty; it needs substances for nourishment. *Huangdi Neijing* states: "The five flavors enter the mouth and are stored in the intestines and stomach. The stored flavors nourish the fiveqi. When qi is harmonious, they generate, body fluids are formed, and the spirit is naturally produced." Therefore, in treating mental diseases, one cannot rely solely on calming the spirit and stabilizing the will, but must combine methods such as nourishing blood and tonifying qi.

Essence, qi, and spirit have a chain relationship. Qi is generated from essence, and essence is transformed into qi. When essence and qi are abundant, the spirit is naturally active; conversely, if the spirit is not vigorous, it is certain that essence and qi are insufficient. At the same time, excessive activity of the spirit can also affect essence and qi, thereby weakening the body. Therefore, in health preservation and treatment, they must be taken care of mutually.

V. Body Fluids

Jin (jin, fluid) and ye (ye, humor) are two liquid substances of different natures, but they are not equivalent to the commonly referred to water. *Huangdi Neijing* points out: "The triple energizer emits qi, which warms the muscles and fills the skin as jin; that which remains and does not circulate is ye." Therefore, when body fluids are depleted, in the case of jin, the interstices are opened and there is profuse sweating; in the case of ye, the body withers, the hair is haggard, tinnitus, joint soreness, and the bones and joints have difficulty in flexing and extending.

Body fluids can be transformed into blood, so *Huangdi Neijing* states: "Those who have lost blood should not sweat; those who have lost sweat should not lose blood." Hence, TCM has the saying that body fluids and blood share the same origin. The reason is that blood loss presents four major symptoms: Vomiting blood, nosebleed, bloody stool, and bloody urine; while loss of body fluids also presents four major symptoms: vomiting, regurgitation, consumption, and sweating. Hematemesis arises from the cardiac orifice, similar to vomiting; nosebleed is called "red sweat," similar to sweating; bloody stool comes from the large intestine, similar to diarrhea; bloody urine originates from the bladder, similar to lower consumption. Comparing the two, their natures are similar. Therefore, preserving body fluids is equivalent to preserving blood, and nourishing blood can also generate body fluids. In clinical practice, blood loss and loss of body fluids are often mentioned together. *Treatise on Febrile Diseases* advocates that those with a history of blood loss should not be induced to sweat, and in the study of warm diseases, it is advocated that "retaining one portion of body fluids means retaining one portion of vitality." The views of both are consistent.

Body fluids can also be transformed into sweat, nasal mucus, tears, saliva, and spittle, which are mainly associated with the kidney, hence the kidney is said to govern the five fluids. In people with spleen yang deficiency, body fluids fail to transform and can condense into phlegm and fluid retention. When phlegm and fluid retention block the interior, body fluids cannot rise upward, resulting in dry mouth without a desire to drink, which should be treated with warm medicines to harmonize.

A common symptom of insufficient body fluids in clinical practice is thirst, mostly caused by febrile diseases. Commonly used body fluid-generating medicines include dendrobium, ophiopogon, polygonatum, and trichosanthes root. However, mild thirst does not necessarily require body fluid-generating medicines; clearing heat will allow body fluids to return naturally. Body fluid-generating medicines are mostly sticky and greasy, so their potential drawbacks should be considered when used. Severe thirst cannot be treated solely by generating body fluids; further combination with blood-nourishing and yin-nourishing methods is needed.

Section 4 Etiology

I. External Causes

Etiological factors are pathogenic factors, divided into internal causes, external causes, and neither internal nor external causes. Diseases arising from external sources are external causes; those arising from internal sources are internal causes; those not belonging to the above categories, such as accidental trauma and injuries from insects or beasts, are neither internal nor external causes.

External causes are mainly the six excesses, namely wind, cold, summer heat, dampness, dryness, and fire. Cold, summer heat, dryness, dampness, and wind are originally the normal qi of the four seasons: Spring is dominated by wind, summer by summer heat, late summer by dampness, autumn by dryness, and winter by cold. Under normal circumstances, they are called the fiveqi. Moreover, since summer heat is heat, extreme heat can transform into fire, and the other factors—wind, dampness, dryness, and cold—can also transform into fire under certain conditions. Thus, "fire" is added, and they are generally referred to as the "six qi." The six qi are normal climatic conditions, also called "healthy qi." If a qi appears at an inappropriate time, it becomes abnormal climate, called "pathogenic qi," such as wind pathogen, summer heat pathogen, damp pathogen, etc. Since such phenomena are abnormal, they are also called the "six excesses."

The six excesses are the main factors of exogenous diseases. When the internal and external environment of the human body is imbalanced, exposure to the six excesses can cause disease. Among them, except for summer heat and dryness, which occur in summer and autumn, wind, cold, dampness, and fire can be found in all four seasons. Therefore, exogenous etiological factors are most commonly these four qi.

1. Wind

Wind is characterized by mobility and variability, and is widely prevalent. It often transforms with the climate due to different seasons, resulting in differences such as wind-warmth, wind-heat, and wind-cold. It also often combines with other pathogens to form wind-summer heat, wind-dampness, wind-dryness, wind-fire, etc. Hence, predecessors called wind "the leader of all diseases."

Diseases caused by invasion of wind pathogen: Mild cases affect the upper jiao qi level, known as wind damage, presenting symptoms such as aversion to wind, fever, headache, nasal congestion, runny nose, cough, and a heavy voice. Severe cases involving the meridians and *zang-fu* organs are called "wind stroke," manifesting as deviation of the mouth and eyes, slurred speech, hemiplegia, sudden collapse; mild cases may regain consciousness after a short time, while severe cases result in loss of consciousness. However, this kind of "wind stroke" (referred to in TCM as "true wind stroke") differs from that caused by internal factors, as it must present exterior symptoms such as "fever or no fever, sweating or no sweating" for differentiation.

Endogenous wind, mostly caused by deficiency of yin and blood or excessive phlegm-fire heat, leads to syncope, convulsions, dizziness, numbness, opisthotonos, etc. Though resembling wind symptoms, it is completely different from external wind and is called "internal wind."

2. Cold

Cold is a yin pathogen with a contracting nature. When it injures the body surface, it is called cold damage, showing symptoms such as aversion to cold, fever, headache, body pain, floating and tight pulse, and white greasy tongue coating. Direct injury to the interior is called "cold stroke," presenting with vomiting clear water, abdominal pain, borborygmus, diarrhea, along with severe cold limbs and hidden pulse.

Dispelling cold pathogen can only be done with acrid-warm methods, but for cold damage, the main approach is to release the exterior, while for cold stroke, warming the middle jiao and restoring yang is appropriate. Cold damage can transform into heat during transmission, so one cannot stubbornly adhere to warming and dispersing; cold stroke rarely transforms into heat and often causes yang qi to decline gradually.

Cold pathogen is most likely to injure yang, and yang deficiency can also produce cold signs, such as vomiting, abdominal pain, diarrhea, cold limbs, etc. This is cold arising internally, hence called "internal cold." Since this cold is fundamentally caused by yang deficiency, treatment focuses on supporting yang, differing from the warming method for cold stroke.

3. Summer heat

Summer heat is the dominant qi of summer. According to *Huangdi*

Neijing: "In the heavens, it is heat; on the earth, it is fire; its nature is summer heat." It also says: "Diseases before the Summer Solstice are warm diseases; diseases after the Summer Solstice are summer heat diseases." It can be known that summer heat diseases are heat diseases, differing only in season. Therefore, exposure to summer heat often shows heat symptoms such as high fever, thirst, restlessness, spontaneous sweating, etc. Due to summer heat injuring qi and affecting the heart, symptoms like panting, loud breathing, and a surging yet deficient pulse are often concurrent.

Summer heat with wind injuring the exterior, affecting the upper jiao, is similar to the initial stage of wind-warmth, with symptoms such as aversion to wind, body heat, thirst, spontaneous sweating, etc. If one travels long distances under the scorching sun or works in the fields, exposed to summer heat, symptoms like body heat, thirst, headache, rapid breathing, heavy body and weak limbs, mental fatigue, scanty dark urine occur, which is called heat stroke, also known as sunstroke. Those with inherently weak constitution, overexertion, excessive sweating and weak heart may also experience dizziness, restlessness, collapse and loss of consciousness, with incessant cold sweating.

Heat stroke is a heat syndrome, mostly caused by activity (such as working or traveling under the scorching sun). Yang is associated with activity, so it is also called yang summer heat; on the contrary, in summer, diseases caused by inactivity, i.e., seeking cool in pavilions by water, or sleeping outdoors to enjoy the cool, lying exposed to wind, resulting in aversion to cold, fever, headache, absence of sweating, etc., or due to indulging in cold raw foods, accompanied by abdominal pain and diarrhea, are called yin summer heat. Yin summer heat is actually a cold pathogen syndrome.

Summer heat qi is most likely to injure qi and yin; if it lingers, it can consume yin fluid, cause mental fatigue, resembling consumption, known as summer heat consumption.

Summer heat often carries dampness, resulting from the steaming of heat and dampness in the environment, or excessive consumption of melons and fruits leading to internal accumulation of dampness, which, combined with exposure to summer heat pathogen, exacerbates summer heat-dampness. Hence, summer heat syndrome often has concurrent symptoms such as chest tightness and nausea, and predecessors held the view that treating summer heat must also treat dampness.

4. Dampness

Dampness is a turbid and heavy pathogen, sticky and difficult to resolve. Among external causes, it mostly refers to fog, dew, or rainy dampness. Those affected may develop chills and fever, nasal congestion, a heavy and wrapped sensation in the head, and aching joints. It can also occur due to sitting or lying on damp ground, living in a humid environment, working in water, or sweat-soaked clothing, allowing dampness to penetrate from the skin into the muscles and meridians, leading to symptoms such as edema and heavy, painful joints.

Indulging in rich, greasy foods, or overeating cold raw fruits, melons, and sweet, greasy foods can impair spleen yang's transportation, causing dampness to arise internally, known as internal dampness. Internal dampness in the upper part manifests as chest tightness, unsmooth qi, and excessive phlegm; in the middle part as epigastric stuffiness, vomiting, poor appetite, and indigestion; in the lower part as abdominal fullness, scanty urine, and diarrhea; it can also rise to the head causing facial edema, descend to the feet causing swelling, and spread to the muscles and meridians causing aching limbs.

Dampness is of a yin nature. When combined with wind pathogen, it becomes wind-dampness; when combined with cold pathogen, it becomes cold-dampness, both of which are relatively easy to treat. If combined with heat pathogen to form damp-heat, it is like oil mixed with flour, difficult to resolve quickly. Dampness and heat have different natures, and the symptoms of damp-heat diseases are often contradictory. For example, in damp-warm disease, there is body heat with cold feet, thirst with a preference for hot drinks, and a thick, greasy, yellow tongue coating. Treatment must address both aspects.

5. Dryness

Dryness is the dominant qi of autumn, also called autumn dryness. Exogenous autumn dryness pathogen mostly affects the upper jiao, similar to wind damage, presenting with slight chills and fever, headache, dry mouth, dry lips, dry nose, dry throat, dry cough without phlegm, or scanty, sticky phlegm with blood, and dry, hard stools.

Dryness is also the residual qi of fire; dryness often occurs after febrile diseases. Dryness is closely related to body fluids and blood; deficiency of body fluids and blood makes one prone to dryness syndrome. These are all internal injuries, different from the external invasion of autumn dryness qi. Therefore, autumn dryness should be treated with sweet-cool formulas supplemented with slightly acrid, clearing and draining agents, while internal injury dryness is suitable only for sweet-cool, clearing and moistening methods. Internal injury dryness involves a wider range: Externally, there is dry, rough skin, chapped lips, dry eyes, and a hot sensation in the nostrils; internally, there are symptoms such as excessive drinking, polyphagia, dry throat with dysphagia, constipation, and dark, scanty urine.

Excessive use of warm-hot medicines, or excessive depletion through diaphoresis, emesis, or purgation, can damage fluids and cause dryness, which can develop into severe conditions such as flaccidity, convulsions, and consumptive cough.

6. Fire

In terms of external causes, fire is a heat pathogen, transformed from the fiveqi of wind, cold, summer heat, dryness, and dampness. When it blazes, it pervades the triple jiao, manifesting as bad breath, swollen and painful throat, a tongue with prickles, chest tightness, irritability, intense thirst with a desire for cold drinks, abdominal fullness, dark urine, and even rashes, delirium, mania, and reckless blood flow, like a wildfire spreading.

The five *zang*-organs can also generate fire, called the five emotions' fire. Among them, liver-gallbladder fire (also called "ministerial fire") is the most common, presenting with red eyes, bitter taste in the mouth, dizzy, distending headache, flushed face, tinnitus, restlessness, disordered dreams, chest tightness, hypochondriac distension, as well as nocturnal emission and stranguria. Whether fire transformed from the fiveqi or fire from the five emotions, most are excess fire, which should be treated with bitter-cold medicines to directly reduce it, not by ordinary heat-clearing formulas.

Yin deficiency with internal heat presents with tidal fever, night sweats, a flushed cheeks, restlessness with insomnia, and a red, glossy, peeled tongue. Or yang deficiency in the lower part with fire floating upward, presenting with toothache, restlessness, head sweats, tinnitus, etc., called "deficient fire." Deficient fire is relative to excess fire: Excess fire can be purged, while deficient fire should be tonified; excess fire can be descended, while deficient fire should be guided back to its origin. Both excess fire and deficient fire involve water deficiency, but excess fire often has excessive fire first followed by water deficiency, with acute heat; deficient fire has water deficiency first followed by excessive fire, with mild heat.

Exogenous syndromes caused by the six excesses refer to symptoms resulting from the invasion of wind, cold, summer heat, dampness, dryness, and fire pathogens into the body surface. There are also those that directly attack the internal organs, such as cold stroke, which, although belonging to external pathogens, cannot be regarded as exogenous diseases. Meanwhile, internal wind, internal cold, internal dampness, as well as dryness due to internal deficiency of body fluids and blood, and fire from internal stagnation of the five emotions, although sharing the same names as the six excesses, differ in nature and must be strictly distinguished. Particularly for syndromes where external and internal causes are mixed, such as concurrent external cold and internal dampness, and concurrent external cold and external dampness, both involving cold and damp pathogens, the treatment methods are different and must be clearly differentiated.

Epidemic pathogens are also one of the external pathogenic factors. “Yi” (epidemic) refers to mutual infection, regardless of age, with similar symptoms, i.e., contagious; “li” (pestilence) refers to a toxic and perverse qi in nature that is most harmful to health, different from the ordinary six excesses. Pestilential qi often arises from the brewing of excessive rain, extreme drought, or the death of livestock from plague,decomposition of filth, etc. It is divided into cold epidemic and warm epidemic in nature, mostly inhaled through the mouth and nose, directly entering the intestines and stomach, with extremely rapid onset.

Infection by the six excesses does not cause immediate illness; symptoms appear after a certain period. For example, cold pathogens contracted in winter may cause warm diseases in summer; summer heat pathogens contracted in summer may cause summer heat diseases in autumn. This is called “latent pathogen.” Latent pathogens, as opposed to new infections, are mainly differentiated based on the exterior-interior nature, severity of symptoms, and speed of transmission. Taking warm diseases as an example: New warm diseases often start with exterior symptoms, have a mild onset, gradually transform into heat, progress from exterior to interior, and transmit relatively slowly. Latent warm diseases have no exterior symptoms at the beginning; once they occur, they show severe internal heat with a tendency to consume yin and fluids. Even if triggered by a new infection stirring up the latent pathogen, although there may be exterior symptoms at the beginning, their transmission is particularly rapid.

II. Internal Causes

Internal causes are mainly the seven emotions, along with phlegm, blood stasis, parasites, etc., all of which are important factors.

1. Seven Emotions

The seven emotions are worry, thought, joy, anger, sorrow, fear, and shock. *Huangdi Neijing* points out: "Anger causes qi to rise; joy causes qi to relax; sorrow causes qi to dissipate; fear causes qi to sink; shock causes qi to become disordered; thought causes qi to stagnate." It also states: "Joy injures the heart; anger injures the liver; thought injures the spleen; worry injures the lung; fear injures the kidney." Accordingly, diseases caused by the seven emotions are emotional diseases, resulting from mental changes due to external stimuli. Due to different external stimuli, there are different mental responses. Common symptoms include depression, moodiness, restlessness, fearfulness and suspicion, insomnia and dreaminess, sadness and crying, loss of appetite, chest tightness and sighing, and in severe cases, mental confusion, disordered speech, like madness or idiocy.

Diseases caused by the seven emotions mainly involve changes in qi. *Huangdi Neijing* mentions qi rising, qi relaxing, qi dissipating, qi sinking, qi disorder, and qi stagnation. Later scholars, based on these theories, have also used terms such as qi stagnation, qi congestion, qi depression, and qi blockage. Generally speaking, the seven emotions first affect qi, and qi and blood are inseparable, so the condition further affects blood. Diseases of qi and blood caused by the seven emotions can be either deficient or excessive, but in the initial stage, excess is more common than deficiency. Therefore, regulating qi and blood to make them smooth and balanced is indeed an important step.

Changes in the seven emotions are caused by external stimuli, which may seem like external factors, but they are ultimately different from the onset of diseases due to general external causes. For diseases caused by external factors, the illness can be cured as long as the external factors are removed. However, the seven emotions have already caused mental changes and altered internal living conditions, so even if the stimuli no longer exist, recovery cannot be immediate.

For the same seven emotions-related diseases, there are significant differences in symptoms due to the varying intensity of stimuli. Meanwhile, the patient's constitution and sensitivity also have a great impact on the onset of the disease, which requires careful observation.

2. Phlegm

Weakness of spleen yang leads to failure in transforming water dampness, which condenses into phlegm; heat in the lung can also scorch body fluids into phlegm. In terms of the relationship between phlegm and internal organs, the lung and spleen are the most closely related.

The main symptom of phlegm is cough; if it blocks the downward purification of qi movement, it causes asthma. It can also flow through the meridians, leading to symptoms such as numbness of hands and feet, stiffness and slurred speech of the tongue, scrofula, goiter, etc. If combined with other factors, there are cold phlegm, heat phlegm, dry phlegm, damp phlegm, wind phlegm, etc., and the symptoms become more complex.

Phlegm occupies an important position in the causes of diseases. In addition to diseases caused by phlegm, many diseases can also lead to phlegm, and if there is phlegm turbidity, it must be taken into account. It is obvious that diseases such as wind damage and cold damage are often accompanied by cough with phlegm, and phlegm-resolving drugs are often added to wind-cold-dispersing formulas. For wind stroke, eliminating phlegm to open the orifices is particularly an important treatment method.

3. Diet

Diet is the source of nutrition, but indulging in food without moderation, resulting in failure to digest and transport, can also cause diseases. For example, symptoms such as chest and diaphragmatic stuffiness, epigastric and abdominal distension and pain, vomiting and acid regurgitation, or causing chills, fever, headache, diarrhea are called food injury.

Food injury mostly leads to gastrointestinal diseases, which is what *Huangdi Neijing* says: "When diet is doubled, the intestines and stomach are injured." There are also people with weak digestive function who cannot eat much, feel full after eating, and have loose stools when taking a little greasy food, which TCM calls spleen deficiency. Moreover, being able to eat but not digest is called stomach excess and spleen deficiency, and feeling hungry but unable to eat is called spleen excess and stomach deficiency.

4. Worms

Intestinal parasites such as roundworms, pinworms, and tapeworms are common. They are mostly caused by excessive dampness and heat, unclean diet, mixed consumption of raw vegetables, fruits, and pungent, dry, fatty, and sweet foods.

Symptoms of intestinal parasitic diseases include sallow complexion and emaciation, dark circles under the eyes and below the nose, itching of the nostrils or anus, white spots like millet grains inside the lips, decreased or abnormally increased appetite, some even having a craving for raw rice and tea leaves, paroxysmal abdominal pain, and changes in facial complexion. In children, it is particularly easy to cause malnutrition, with a large and hard abdomen, commonly known as malnutrition with abdominal distension and food accumulation.

Consumptive disease, also called "transmitted corpse consumption", is transmitted by consumptive worms and affects the lung. Symptoms include cough and hemoptysis, loss of voice and shortness of breath, bone steaming and night sweats, pale complexion with bright red cheeks like makeup, which is most harmful to people.

Although the causes of diseases are divided into external and internal causes, they cannot be viewed in isolation. TCM classifies diseases into two categories: Exogenous and internal injuries, with the six excesses and seven emotions as the main causes of the two categories. In fact, external causes are not easy to invade the human body without going through internal causes, and similarly, internal causes are often triggered by external causes. At the same time, in addition to the main causes of the disease, attention should also be paid to other predisposing factors, such as living conditions, nutrition, and living environment, which are all greatly related.

III. Neither Internal nor External Causes

The occurrence of diseases can be due to accidental injuries, which belong to neither internal nor external causes, thus called neither internal nor external causes.

1. Sexual overstrain

It refers to excessive sexual desire that injures essence and qi. It not only leads to physical weakness but also makes one susceptible to pathogenic factors. Its symptoms are mostly haggard complexion, melancholy expression, soreness in the lower back and waist, cold limbs, nocturnal emission and spermatorrhea, impotence and premature ejaculation, which can thus cause palpitations, night sweats, tidal fever, etc.

2. Metal and blade injuries

It refers to injuries from swords, knives, or falls and knocks. They mainly involve swelling, pain, and bleeding on the body surface, or injuries to tendons, fractures, skin lacerations, or stagnation of blood stasis, etc.

3. Scalds and burns

It refers to injuries from hot liquids or fire.

4. Insect and beast injuries

It refers to bites from venomous snakes, fierce beasts, etc. In addition to direct damage to the body surface, they can also cause poisoning of varying degrees.

5. Poisoning

Generally, it refers to food poisoning or drug poisoning, as stated in *Huangdi Neijing*: "When diagnosing a disease, if one does not inquire about its origin—such as worries, grief, improper diet, excessive daily activities, or injury from poison—and rushes to feel the pulse at the wrist, what disease can be accurately diagnosed?"

Neither internal nor external causes are also related to internal and external causes. For example, after a knife wound, external pathogens can invade through the wound, leading to severe tetanus. Therefore, none of the three causes can be viewed in isolation.

The theory of the three causes first appeared in *Synopsis of the Golden Chamber*: "All kinds of diseases and hardships do not exceed three categories: First, pathogenic factors invading the meridians and entering the *zang-fu* organs, which is caused by internal factors; second, pathogens spreading through the limbs, nine orifices, and blood vessels, causing obstruction, which is caused by external invasion of the skin; third, injuries from sexual activities, metal blades, insects, and beasts. With these details, all causes of diseases are covered." Later, Chen Wuze wrote *Three Causes and One Disease Syndrome Formula Discussion* (abbreviated as *Three Causes Formula*), pointing out: "First, internal causes are the seven emotions, originating from the *zang-fu* organs and manifesting in the limbs; second, external causes are the six excesses, starting from the meridians and lodging in the *zang-fu* organs; third, neither internal nor external causes include diet, hunger and satiety, injury to qi from shouting, as well as injuries from tigers, wolves, venomous insects, metal wounds, crushing, drowning, etc." Although both theories are divided into three causes, their meanings are different. *Synopsis of the Golden Chamber* focuses on external pathogens, considering injuries to the skin and blood vessels as superficial, i.e., external causes; and invasion from meridians into the *zang-fu* organs as deep, i.e., internal causes. It classifies internal and external based on the depth of the disease location, not from the perspective of pathogenic factors. *Three Causes Formula* 立论 based on the relationship between heaven, human body, exterior and interior, regarding the six excesses that invade from outside as external causes; the seven emotions that injure from inside as internal causes; and factors such as diet, hunger and satiety that are unrelated to the six excesses and seven emotions as neither internal nor external causes. In terms of pathogenic factors, the classification in *Three Causes Formula* is clearer. After each category, there are discussions and formulas, which can be used as reference materials.

IV. Summary of the Three Causes

Every disease has a cause. One cause can lead to many different diseases, and the same disease can be caused by various different reasons. Hence, TCM has the characteristic of "treating different diseases with the same method and different methods for the same disease". One formula can treat several different diseases, and sometimes several formulas are needed to treat one disease. For example, the same heat pathogen can manifest as fever, cough, or bleeding. As long as it is confirmed to be heat pathogen, different diseases can be treated with cooling formulas. Another example is the same symptom of fever, which can be caused by heat pathogen, cold pathogen, or blood disorders. Although the fever is the same, the causes are different, so one cannot rely solely on cooling formulas to reduce the fever. This illustrates the importance of pathogenic factors in treatment. Therefore, when treating any disease, the cause must first be clarified.

To facilitate a preliminary grasp of etiological factors, I intend to merge, supplement, and present thirteen key points encompassing internal causes, external causes, and neither internal nor external causes, namely: wind, cold, summer heat, dampness, dryness, fire, pestilence, phlegm, food, worms, qi, blood, and deficiency. These are explained below in conjunction with general treatment methods. Admittedly, this is not yet fully refined and can only be applied after understanding the three causes, but it is still of some help in clinical practice.

1. Wind

Mild cases affect the exterior, presenting symptoms such as nasal congestion with a heavy voice, frequent clear nasal discharge, and cough; slightly severe cases involve fever, headache, spontaneous sweating or absence of sweating. Severe cases attack the interior: In the meridians, there are symptoms like deviation of the mouth and eyes, numbness of the arms, muscle insensitivity, and a heavy sensation in the body; in the *zang-fu* organs, there are symptoms such as drooling, stiff tongue with slurred speech, and loss of consciousness.

Wind pathogen invades from outside and must be dispelled externally; treatment methods involve acrid dispersion. For exterior conditions, dispersing wind by ventilating the lung is appropriate; for interior conditions, expelling wind to eliminate pathogens is suitable. As for the use of methods such as nourishing yin to calm wind, eliminating phlegm, or reducing fire in treating wind stroke, these belong to the treatments for apoplectic-like syndrome, which should be sought among the causes of deficiency, phlegm, and fire.

2. Cold

When injuring the exterior, symptoms include aversion to cold with fever, severe pain in the head and neck, body aches, and absence of sweating; when attacking the interior, symptoms are vomiting, diarrhea, abdominal pain, and cold limbs.

Cold pathogen is also an external pathogen, but its cold nature easily injures yang qi. Hence, for exterior conditions, acrid-warm dispersion is used; for interior conditions, warming the middle jiao is appropriate. If there is simultaneous illness in both the exterior and interior, both warming the interior and dispersing the exterior should be used together.

3. Summer heat

Mild cases present with fever, profuse sweating, irritable thirst, and lassitude with shortness of breath; severe cases involve fainting, high fever, body weakness, sweating, and rapid breathing.

Although summer heat is an external pathogen, its hot nature consumes qi, so sweating should not be induced. Mild cases are suitable for dissipating heat to repel summer heat; severe cases are suitable for clearing the heart and eliminating summer heat. The differences between summer heat and heat lie in summer heat being accompanied by dampness, so aromatic substances are often used as auxiliary. If yin summer heat is caused by seeking excessive coolness and consuming cold drinks, it is fundamentally a cold syndrome and can be treated with reference to cold pathogen.

4. Dampness

Exterior dampness presents with chills and fever, a heavy and wrapped sensation in the head, chest tightness, and a heavy body; internal dampness in the middle jiao manifests as chest tightness, a greasy tongue coating, and disharmony between the spleen and stomach; in the lower jiao, it manifests as diarrhea, swollen feet, and difficulty in urination. Accumulated dampness turning into water leads to abdominal swelling, or overflowing to the skin causing general edema.

Dampness is a turbid, tangible pathogen. Aromatic substances can transform dampness, bitter-warm medicines can dry dampness, wind medicines can overcome dampness, diuretics can guide dampness, and purgatives can expel dampness. Therefore, for exterior conditions, inducing sweating to dispel dampness is appropriate; in the middle jiao, mild cases are suitable for aromatic transformation of dampness, severe cases for warming and drying damp turbidity; in the lower jiao, promoting diuresis through the bladder or attacking and expelling accumulated water is appropriate. When dampness combines with heat to form damp-heat syndrome, the treatment method involves clearing heat and transforming dampness, and it is necessary to assess whether dampness is heavier than heat or heat is heavier than dampness and adjust the treatment accordingly.

5. Dryness

Autumn dryness injuring the exterior presents with slight fever, dry cough, dry nose, and dry mouth. Dryness of body fluids injuring the interior leads to dry mouth, excessive thirst, chapped lips, and constipation.

For exterior conditions, acrid-sweet and slightly cool medicines that gently ventilate the upper jiao are appropriate; for interior conditions, sweet-cool and moistening medicines that nourish the lung and stomach are suitable. If yin and blood dryness manifests with wind symptoms, it should be included in the scope of deficiency syndrome for treatment.

6. Fire

Pathogenic heat blazing presents with high fever, bad breath, abdominal fullness, and constipation; stagnated pathogenic fire failing to erupt leads to symptoms such as irritability, headache and distension, swollen throat, and toothache; hyperactivity of monarch fire manifests as restlessness and insomnia with a red and crimson tip of the tongue; restless ministerial fire presents with headache and distension, tinnitus, and nocturnal emission; deficient fire blazing internally shows symptoms such as tidal fever, night sweats, and a flushed face.

Fire has a flaming and upward nature, and its function is heat, so treatment is mainly based on clearing and descending. Excessive fire should be controlled, stagnated fire should be dispersed, monarch fire should be calmed, ministerial fire should be drained with bitterness, and deficient fire should be lurked and nourished. Fire causes heat, and heat causes dryness; understanding fire and dryness, heat is already included.

7. Pestilence

Cold pestilence is characterized by back cold, head distension, chest tightness, and hand numbness; warm pestilence is marked by high fever, delirium, sore throat, and rash.

Pestilential diseases do not transmit along meridians. Although they have stages of exterior and interior, most pathogens lurk in the middle jiao. Treatment should focus on eliminating filth and warming transformation, or clearing pestilence and detoxifying.

8. Phlegm

Wind-phlegm is often accompanied by cough and aversion to wind; phlegm-heat is often seen with cough and dry mouth; damp-phlegm is often accompanied by cough and nausea; phlegm-fluid is often marked by cough and shortness of breath; accumulated phlegm-fluid is often accompanied by cough and chest or hypochondriac pain; phlegm-qi coagulation often leads to scrofula, etc.

The formation of phlegm is nothing more than accumulation of dampness and condensation by heat. For dampness, invigorating the spleen to resolve phlegm is appropriate; for heat, clearing the lung to resolve phlegm is suitable. Then, according to specific conditions, treatment is differentiated: For exogenous diseases, dispersion is used; for phlegm-fluid, warming transformation is applied; for accumulated phlegm-fluid, purgation is used; for phlegm nodules and scrofula, resolving, dispersing, and softening hardness are adopted. Phlegm symptoms often appear in exogenous and internal injury diseases, either treated as the main symptom or as a concomitant symptom, depending on the condition.

9. Food

Food injury in the stomach is characterized by chest fullness, acid regurgitation, and belching of rotten qi; in the intestines, it causes abdominal pain and diarrhea.

For internal obstruction due to food stagnation, elimination and promotion are the main treatments: For the stomach, promoting digestion and transportation is appropriate; for the intestines, guiding stagnation is suitable. The treatment of other diseases caused by food injury, such as dysentery, is no exception.

10. Worms

Worm diseases are often characterized by heart upset, paroxysmal abdominal pain, sallow complexion, and even abdominal distension like a drum.

When there are worms, insecticides should be used for treatment.

Generally, insecticidal drugs are mostly used, and sometimes a mixture of acrid, sour, bitter, and descending medicines is used to weaken and kill the worms.

11. Qi

Qi stagnation is marked by depression, anger, chest and hypochondriac discomfort, epigastric and abdominal fullness; qi rebellion is characterized by chest tightness, blockage, and shortness of breath; floating qi is seen with palpitations, fear, and restlessness; qi sinking is manifested by lassitude, fatigue, weakness of limbs, and a constant feeling of downward sagging in the abdomen.

TCM attaches great importance to qi system diseases. *Huangdi Neijing* says: "All diseases arise from qi." Qi stagnation should be dispersed and unblocked; qi rebellion should be settled and descended; qi floating should be calmed and anchored; qi collapse should be raised and lifted. All blood diseases are often caused by qi system disorders, or even if not caused by qi system, they need to be treated from the qi system, which should be paid close attention to.

12. Blood

Blood heat is characterized by reckless bleeding; blood cold is often marked by stagnation; blood stasis is often seen with abdominal masses and amenorrhea. Failure of blood to be contained is often accompanied by vomiting blood, nosebleed, and incessant metrorrhagia.

Blood should circulate smoothly. Blood diseases either involve reckless bleeding or stagnation. For bleeding, stopping is needed, with cooling and astringing methods appropriate; for stagnation, unblocking is required, with warming and stasis-dispersing methods suitable. For cases of qi deficiency failing to contain blood or qi stagnation causing blood stasis, methods of benefiting qi to contain blood or regulating qi to dispel stasis should be used in combination.

13. Deficiency

Essence deficiency is characterized by tinnitus in the brain, back pain, lumbar soreness, weak feet, impotence, and premature ejaculation; spirit deficiency is marked by palpitations, insomnia, trance, amnesia, and inability to think; qi deficiency is manifested by low voice, shortness of breath, frequent chest tightness, fatigue, spontaneous sweating, and slow digestion; blood deficiency is seen with dizziness, hair loss, dull nails, pale complexion, emaciation, dry skin, scanty and pale menstrual flow, or amenorrhea.

Deficiency syndromes should be treated with tonification: Essence deficiency requires tonifying the kidney; spirit deficiency requires tonifying the heart; blood deficiency requires tonifying the liver; qi deficiency requires tonifying the lung and spleen. They can also be simply divided into yang deficiency and yin deficiency. Yang deficiency is characterized by fear of cold, shortness of breath, spontaneous sweating, reduced appetite, and loose stools; yin deficiency presents with bone steaming, palpitations, night sweats, spermatorrhea, amenorrhea, etc. Tonifying yang is suitable with sweet-warm medicines to benefit fire, and tonifying yin is mainly with sweet-cool medicines to nourish water.

In the thirteen key points, we have dispersed the seven emotions into various aspects and added qi and blood. Although qi and blood are not etiological factors, and disorders of qi and blood are often caused by multiple reasons, once they lead to disorders of qi or blood, they can often become important etiological factors. For example, qi stagnation caused by the seven emotions can affect other internal organs and produce a series of symptoms, and treatment mainly focuses on regulating qi.

Therefore, *Huangdi Neijing* points out that wind is the leader of all diseases for exogenous diseases, and for internal injury syndromes, it also points out that all diseases arise from qi. It is obvious that qi is also one of the etiological factors in pathology. In addition, deficiency is added as a cause. Deficiency is the consequence of other factors, but once it becomes deficiency, it can also cause other pathological changes. For example, excessive sweating due to wind damage can cause yang deficiency, with symptoms such as incessant sweating, which should be treated from the perspective of deficiency; persistent diarrhea leading to deficiency of both the spleen and kidney, at this time, the cause of the disease can be ignored, and treatment can be focused on deficiency; other conditions of weakness caused by excessive fatigue, excessive sexual activity, as well as general weakness after illness and women's postpartum weakness, should also be treated from the perspective of deficiency. In short, disease can lead to deficiency, and deficiency can also cause disease. Once it reaches the state of deficiency, it becomes an etiological factor.

The symptoms caused by each etiological factor are quite complex, and sometimes etiological factors and symptoms can be mutually causal. Although there are many changes in clinical practice, if we can grasp several main key points, distinguish the main causes and main symptoms according to the syndrome differentiation methods of exterior-interior, deficiency-excess, cold-heat, and then modify the treatment according to the main treatment, we will not be at a loss.

Chapter Two The Section of Principles

Section 1 Syndrome Differentiation

I. Exterior, Interior, Cold, Heat, Deficiency, Excess

Every disease has intricate symptoms. To find its key and grasp its main aspects, one must know how to use the eight principles. The eight principles are yin-yang, exterior-interior, cold-heat, deficiency-excess, which are the guidelines for syndrome differentiation, among which yin-yang is particularly the guideline of guidelines. Exterior-interior, cold-heat, deficiency-excess are actually deductions of yin-yang, also known as the six changes, which indicate the location of the pathological changes, the manifestations of the disease condition, and the changes in the waxing and waning of pathogenic factors and healthy qi. Therefore, by observing the entire situation of the syndrome according to the eight principles, analyzing and summarizing, it is not difficult to draw a diagnostic conclusion. The aspect of yin-yang has been described in Chapter One, and the meaning of the six changes is further explained as follows.

1. Exterior and Interior

Exterior refers to the outside, and interior refers to the inside. In terms of the inside and outside of the human body, the exterior refers to the body surface, including tissues such as the skin and muscles; the interior refers to the internal organs, including organs such as the *zang-fu* organs and the brain. Therefore, symptoms caused by pathogenic factors invading the human body, such as aversion to cold, fever, headache, stiff neck, body pain, soreness and weakness of the limbs, as well as sweating or absence of sweating, which belong to the body surface, are all exterior syndromes; symptoms such as delirium, restlessness, thirst, chest tightness, vomiting, diarrhea, abdominal pain and distension, which belong to the internal body, are all interior syndromes.

When pathogenic factors such as wind and cold invade the human body, they first damage the skin, hair, and meridians, which are generally referred to as exterior syndromes. Diseases caused by the seven emotions (joy, anger, etc.) or improper diet and overstrain mostly arise internally, so they are generally called interior syndromes. This is a general overview of distinguishing exterior and interior. However, exterior pathogens can transmit inward to the *zang-fu* organs, and the symptoms thus manifested become interior syndromes. There are also cases where exterior pathogens have transmitted inward but not yet reached the interior, which is called half-exterior and half-interior syndrome. When exterior pathogens transmit inward while exterior symptoms still remain, it is called concurrent exterior and interior syndromes. The transmission of pathogenic factors from the exterior to the interior, i.e., from outside to inside, indicates that the disease is severe and adverse. For example, at the initial stage of cold damage, symptoms such as chills, fever, severe headache and stiff neck are all signs of pathogens being in the exterior; if the fever persists, accompanied by symptoms like bitter taste in the mouth, nausea, or chest tightness, or scanty dark urine, it indicates that the pathogen tends to invade the interior; if there are symptoms such as high fever, thirst, restlessness, delirium, or abdominal pain with constipation, or diarrhea, it clearly indicates that the pathogen has invaded the interior. Conversely, interior syndromes can also transmit from the interior to the exterior, which indicates that the disease is mild and favorable. For example, in measles and rashes, at the initial stage, there are fever, restlessness, cough, and chest tightness; when red rashes appear on the skin, the condition gradually relieves. Therefore, in clinical practice, when distinguishing exterior and interior syndromes, it is more important to pay attention to their transmission tendency.

2. Cold and Heat

Symptoms of cold syndromes include no thirst, preference for hot drinks, cold limbs, aversion to wind and cold, clear and profuse urine, loose stools, pale complexion, white and slippery tongue coating, and slow pulse. Symptoms of heat syndromes include thirst with preference for cold drinks, tidal fever, restlessness, scanty and yellow urine, constipation, red face and eyes, yellow and dry tongue coating, rapid pulse, etc. It can be seen here that the manifestations of the disease have two different phenomena: Cold and heat. Distinguishing cold and heat is a key to determining whether to use warm or cool medicines.

Cold and heat syndromes are sometimes not entirely systemic symptoms. For example, fever is systemic, while yellowish urine may be related to fever, or it may only be due to heat in the bladder. Therefore, when differentiating cold and heat syndromes, in addition to general cases, it is necessary to further distinguish between upper and lower parts. Generally, cold in the upper part is mostly characterized by acid regurgitation, vomiting clear water, indigestion, or a feeling of cold in the chest; heat in the upper part is mostly characterized by headache and distension, red eyes, sore throat, swollen and painful gums, dry mouth with preference for cold drinks. Cold in the lower part is mostly marked by abdominal pain with preference for pressure, loose stools or diarrhea, cold shins and feet; heat in the lower part is mostly characterized by difficult and dry stools, turbid yellow urine, or scanty, painful urination. These symptoms may only appear in the upper part, or only in the lower part, or both upper and lower parts may be hot or cold, or there may be heat in the upper part and cold in the lower part, or cold in the upper part and heat in the lower part. There can also be phenomena such as heat in the stomach and cold in the intestines, or cold in the stomach and heat in the intestines in a gastrointestinal disease, which must be clearly analyzed.

3. Deficiency and Excess

Deficiency and excess refer to both healthy qi and pathogenic factors. From the perspective of the human body, they refer to the strength of healthy qi; from the perspective of the disease condition, they refer to the prosperity and decline of pathogenic factors. However, in general clinical practice, deficiency mostly refers to healthy qi, and excess mostly refers to pathogenic factors. Because abundant healthy qi is not called excess, and retreated pathogenic factors are not called deficiency. Therefore, *Huangdi Neijing* states: "When pathogenic factors are exuberant, it is excess; when essential qi is depleted, it is deficiency." Manifestations of deficiency syndromes include fatigue, weak voice, shortness of breath, spontaneous and night sweats, dizziness, palpitations, and thready, weak pulse. Manifestations of excess syndromes include profuse phlegm and qi congestion, chest tightness and abdominal distension, constipation or loose and foul stools, and full, slippery, large pulse, etc. Generally, for strong individuals with new diseases, the syndrome is mostly excessive; for weak individuals with chronic diseases, the syndrome is mostly deficiency. When a patient's constitution and pathological mechanism show abundance, solidity, and strength, it is called excess syndrome; conversely, when they show insufficiency, decline, and relaxation, it is called deficiency syndrome.

Distinguishing deficiency and excess is the basis for attacking pathogens and tonifying healthy qi. Diseases that are purely deficient or purely excessive are easier to distinguish and simpler to treat; there are cases of intermingled deficiency and excess, such as when healthy qi is strong and pathogens are excessive, even severe conditions can be saved, but when healthy qi is deficient and pathogens are excessive, even mild conditions can be dangerous. During the course of any disease, the waxing and waning of pathogens and healthy qi often occur, and attention must be paid to changes such as deficiency within excess, excess within deficiency, more deficiency and less excess, less deficiency and more excess, etc. For example, exogenous wind-cold with aversion to cold, fever, and a floating and tight pulse is an exterior excess syndrome; if after sweating, sweating persists, the body temperature drops suddenly, and instead, the aversion to cold becomes more severe, this is a sign of transformation into a deficiency syndrome; or if the aversion to cold subsides, the body heat increases, and there is thirst with a desire to drink, this is a sign of transformation into an interior syndrome. If a febrile disease presents with a dry and rough tongue coating, it indicates that body fluids are deficient; or if the tongue is shiny, red, and crimson, it indicates that yin has been consumed by pathogenic heat, and treatment cannot rely solely on methods to reduce fever.

Exterior-interior, cold-heat, and deficiency-excess are methods of summarizing symptoms; looking at a single symptom in isolation is meaningless. Because each symptom can appear in two aspects: For example, exterior syndromes can have aversion to cold, interior syndromes can also have aversion to cold; deficiency syndromes can have aversion to cold, excess syndromes can also have aversion to cold; cold syndromes can have aversion to cold, and heat syndromes can also have aversion to cold. To determine which type it belongs to, it is necessary to combine multiple symptoms. Therefore, by analyzing many symptoms and connecting those with similar natures, forming a syndrome complex, we can diagnose whether it is exterior or interior, deficiency or excess, cold or heat. Symptoms are superficial, and many of them are hidden and false, called false manifestations. Taking cold and heat as an example: True cold should present with a deep, thready, or slow, weak pulse, symptoms such as cold limbs, vomiting, abdominal pain, diarrhea, clear and frequent urine; even if there is fever, the patient does not want to remove clothing and bedding, which is a sign of floating heat on the exterior and deep cold in the interior.

True heat should present with a rapid, forceful, slippery, large, and solid pulse, symptoms such as restlessness, rapid breathing, chest tightness, thirst, abdominal distension, constipation, scanty dark urine, and fever with no desire to cover with bedding. False cold syndrome is cold on the exterior but hot in the interior, with a rapid pulse; the body feels cold but the patient does not want to wear clothing, or the stool is foul, or there is severe thirst with a desire to drink. This kind of coldness is not a cold manifestation but a heat syndrome, which is called extreme heat with concomitant cold transformation, or yang excess repelling yin. False heat syndrome is hot on the exterior but cold in the interior, with a weak pulse, or a deficient, rapid, floating, large, and rootless pulse; the body has fever but the mind is calm, there is delirium but the voice is low; or there is mania but it stops when restrained; or there are false rashes that are light red and fragmented; or there is a preference for cold drinks but only a small amount is consumed; or urine is profuse; or there is no constipation. This kind of heat manifestation is not true heat but a cold syndrome, which is called extreme cold with concomitant heat transformation, or yin excess separating yang. Regarding deficiency and excess, extreme deficiency can present with excess manifestations, which are false excess; extreme excess can present with deficiency manifestations, which are false deficiency. Therefore, Zhang Jingyue said: "External symptoms resembling excess but with a weak, spiritless pulse are all deficiency syndromes that should be tonified; external symptoms resembling deficiency but with a vigorous pulse are all excess syndromes that should be attacked. Between deficiency and excess, there are many similarities and doubts, and one must distinguish their true nature." This explains that the purpose of syndrome differentiation is to understand the essence of the disease; to grasp the truth, one must observe from multiple aspects.

The six changes are categorized using yin and yang: The exterior is yang; the interior is yin; heat is yang; cold is yin; excess is yang; deficiency is yin. Therefore, sometimes the movement or stillness of a disease condition and the progression or regression of the illness is referred to as yin syndrome and yang syndrome, or as disease in yang and disease in yin. Hence, yin and yang are considered the overarching principles of the eight principles. However, in clinical practice, terms such as true yang deficiency, true yin deficiency, yang exhaustion, and yin exhaustion are used, which are not broad terms. Previous scholars explained that true yang and true yin both pertain to the kidney: True yang is the true fire. In cases of true fire deficiency, the right cubit pulse is necessarily weak, and one should greatly tonify the original yang, avoiding damage to its yin qi. Cold and moistening medicines are forbidden, as they may assist yin pathogens; acrid and dispersing medicines are particularly forbidden, as they may injure yin qi. Only sweet-warm medicines that benefit fire, tonifying yang to match yin, are appropriate. True yin is the true water. In cases of true water deficiency, the pulse is necessarily thready and rapid, and one should greatly tonify true yin, avoiding damage to its yang qi. Acrid and drying medicines are forbidden, as they may assist yang pathogens; bitter-cold medicines are particularly forbidden, as they may damage original yang. Only purely sweet medicines that strengthen water, tonifying yin to match yang, are appropriate. As for distinguishing between yang exhaustion and yin exhaustion, careful observation of symptoms is required: For example, sweating with an aversion to cold, cold hands and feet, cool skin and cold sweat with a faint, sticky taste, weak breathing, and a floating, rapid, and empty pulse indicate yang exhaustion. Aversion to heat, warm hands and feet, hot skin, hot sweat with a salty taste, rapid breathing, and a surging, large, and rootless pulse indicate yin exhaustion. Yang exhaustion and yin exhaustion are severe conditions, mostly occurring in situations such as high fever fumigation, excessive sweating, excessive vomiting and diarrhea, or incessant bleeding, and are often critical signs.

The content of eight-principle syndrome differentiation includes the relationship between the body surface and the interior, indicating the nature and development of the disease. The final stage of syndrome differentiation is for treatment: Distinguishing exterior and interior can determine whether to use diaphoresis or purgation; distinguishing cold and heat can determine whether to use warm or cool medicines; distinguishing deficiency and excess can determine whether to use tonification or purgation. However, diaphoresis includes acrid-warm diaphoresis and acrid-cool diaphoresis; purgation includes cool purgation and warm purgation; other methods such as warming, cooling, tonifying, and purging also have different applications. Determining specific treatment strategies requires combining exterior-interior, cold-heat, and deficiency-excess. For example, combining exterior syndrome with cold syndrome and excess syndrome results in an exterior cold excess syndrome, which is an excess syndrome caused by external cold pathogen invading the body surface, and can be treated with acrid-warm diaphoresis. Or combining interior syndrome with cold syndrome and deficiency syndrome results in an interior cold deficiency syndrome, which is a cold syndrome caused by internal yang deficiency, and can be treated with warm tonification. Similarly, the combination of exterior-interior, cold-heat, and deficiency-excess in clinical practice results in eight basic types: Exterior cold excess syndrome, exterior cold deficiency syndrome, exterior heat excess syndrome, exterior heat deficiency syndrome, interior cold excess syndrome, interior cold deficiency syndrome, interior heat excess syndrome, and interior heat deficiency syndrome. On this basis, eight mixed types can also be derived: exterior cold and interior heat syndrome, exterior heat and interior cold syndrome, exterior deficiency and interior excess syndrome, exterior excess and interior deficiency syndrome, simultaneous exterior and interior cold syndrome, simultaneous exterior and interior heat syndrome, simultaneous exterior and interior deficiency syndrome, and simultaneous exterior and interior excess syndrome. Within the scope of interior syndromes, there are several complex types: upper heat and lower cold syndrome, upper cold and lower heat syndrome, upper deficiency and lower excess syndrome, upper excess and lower deficiency syndrome, true cold with false heat syndrome, true heat with false cold syndrome, true deficiency with false excess syndrome, true excess with false deficiency syndrome, as well as half-exterior and half-interior syndrome, intermingled cold and heat syndrome, and deficiency with excess syndrome. Despite the many changes in diseases, they are clearly within the scope of exterior-interior, cold-heat, and deficiency-excess. Therefore, as long as one can grasp these eight principles, they can be clearly understood.

Of the aforementioned changes, some are common, some are relatively rare, some have little difference from each other, and some, though similar, must be distinguished. Since syndrome differentiation is a complex and meticulous task, it is worthwhile to elaborate further for the sake of drawing inferences by analogy and flexible application.

(1) Exterior cold excess syndrome: Invasion of wind-cold on the body surface. Main symptoms include aversion to cold, headache, body pain, floating and tight pulse, with or without fever.

(2) Exterior cold deficiency syndrome: Insufficiency of defensive qi. Main symptoms include aversion to wind and cold, easy sweating, and increased coldness after sweating.

(3) Exterior heat excess syndrome: Initial stage of exogenous warm disease. Main symptoms include aversion to wind or no aversion to wind, fever, headache, with or without spontaneous sweating.

(4) Exterior heat deficiency syndrome: Similar to yin deficiency with tidal fever. Main symptoms include afternoon heat in the muscles, heat in the palms, and spontaneous sweating.

(5) Interior cold excess syndrome: Direct attack of cold pathogen on the internal organs. Main symptoms include abdominal pain, diarrhea, severe cold limbs, and deep, hidden pulse.

(6) Interior cold deficiency syndrome: Mostly caused by spleen and kidney yang deficiency. Main symptoms include timidness, fatigue, cold limbs, loose stools, weak pulse, and the wollen and delicate tongue that is not ruddy.

(7) Interior heat excess syndrome: External pathogens transforming into heat and transmitting inward. Main symptoms include high fever, thirst, restlessness, constipation, dark urine, and severe delirium.

(8) Interior heat deficiency syndrome: Mostly caused by liver and kidney yin deficiency. Main symptoms include heat in the palms, dizziness, thirst, restlessness, and insomnia. If tidal fever occurs, refer to exterior heat deficiency syndrome.

(9) Exterior cold and interior heat syndrome: Exogenous cold pathogen with internal stagnated heat. Main symptoms include chills, fever, absence of sweating, and restlessness. Also, false cold syndrome with fear of cold, reluctance to wear clothing, and severe thirst with desire to drink belongs to this category.

(10) Exterior heat and interior cold syndrome: Cold accumulated internally with heat escaping externally; the heat is false heat, and the cold is true cold. Main symptoms include body heat without desire to remove clothing, aversion to wind, diarrhea, and clear, profuse urine.

(11) Exterior deficiency and interior excess syndrome: Mostly caused by injury to the exterior due to sweating, with pathogens transmitting inward. Main symptoms include sweating with aversion to wind, chest fullness and hardness, belching, nausea, and vomiting.

(12) Exterior excess and interior deficiency syndrome: A body with internal injury affected by external pathogens again; or improper purgation in exterior syndrome, which injures the interior, though the exterior pathogens have not yet inwardly sunk. Main symptoms include chills, fever, body pain, timidness, and deep, weak pulse.

(13) Simultaneous exterior and interior cold syndrome: Cold pathogen injuring the exterior and further attacking the interior. Main symptoms include chills, fever, abdominal pain, and diarrhea.

(14) Simultaneous exterior and interior heat syndrome: Exterior pathogens transforming into heat and transmitting inward, with fever persisting and even worsening; refer to interior heat excess syndrome.

(15) Simultaneous exterior and interior deficiency syndrome: Deficiency of both yin and yang. Main symptoms include excessive sweating, aversion to cold, timidness, palpitations, and irregularly intermittent pulse.

(16) Simultaneous exterior and interior excess syndrome: Exogenous cold pathogen with internal retention of phlegm-fluid or undigested food. Main symptoms include chills, fever, cough, asthma, or belching of foul gas, abdominal distension. Also, simultaneous exterior and interior cold or heat syndromes caused by cold or heat pathogens belong to this category.

(17) Upper heat and lower cold syndrome: Cold in the lower jiao and heat in the upper jiao. Main symptoms include abdominal fullness, cold feet, dry mouth, and heat sensation in the chest. Also, fire failing to return to its source and floating upward, with symptoms such as cold feet, red face, dry mouth, and dry throat, belongs to this category.

(18) Upper cold and lower heat syndrome: Heat in the lower abdomen and cold-fluid in the diaphragm. Main symptoms include scanty dark urine, profuse phlegm, and cold sensation in the chest.

(19) Upper deficiency and lower excess syndrome: Turbid yin in the lower part with failure of clear yang to rise. Main symptoms include abdominal fullness, diarrhea, dizziness, and blurred vision.

(20) Upper excess and lower deficiency syndrome: Yang deficiency in the lower part with obstruction of phlegm-fluid in the upper part. Main symptoms include cold body and cold feet, frequent urination, expectoration, and dyspnea.

(21) True cold with false heat syndrome: Refer to exterior heat and interior cold syndrome.

(22) True heat with false cold syndrome: Refer to exterior cold and interior heat syndrome.

(23) Half-exterior and half-interior syndrome: Exterior pathogens transmitting inward without forming an interior syndrome. Main symptoms include alternating chills and fever, bitter taste in the mouth, and dry throat.

(24) Intermingled cold and heat syndrome: Internal obstruction of damp-heat, or internal phlegm-fluid with exterior heat sinking inward. Main symptoms include chest tightness, dry mouth without desire to drink, scanty dark urine, or restlessness with stuffiness and fullness, nausea, and vomiting.

(25) Deficiency with excess syndrome: A weak body with pathogens, or pathogens lingering as healthy qi gradually declines, all belong to this category. Refer to exterior deficiency and interior excess, exterior excess and interior deficiency, upper deficiency and lower excess, upper excess and lower deficiency, etc.

For any acute febrile disease or internal injury syndrome during its development, the above methods can be used for diagnosis. In terms of acute febrile diseases, for example, the initial stage of cold damage is an exterior cold excess syndrome; if excessive sweating damages yang qi, it becomes an exterior cold deficiency syndrome; if cold pathogens transform into heat and transmit inward, it becomes an interior heat excess syndrome; if they transmit to the half-exterior and half-interior stage, it is a half-exterior and half-interior syndrome; when physical strength fails, with symptoms such as diarrhea, cold limbs, and restlessness, it is an interior cold deficiency syndrome or exterior heat and interior cold syndrome. Another example: Kidney diarrhea (i.e., dawn diarrhea) is an interior cold deficiency syndrome; lung consumption is an interior heat deficiency syndrome; phlegm-fluid cough is an upper excess and lower deficiency syndrome. The above is the comprehensive application of the eight principles. In clinical practice, syndrome differentiation and treatment can be carried out based on these to achieve therapeutic effects.

II. Six Channels

The meaning of the six channels is to divide the human body into six regions, and the syndromes appearing in these six regions are regarded as six types. This method first appeared in *Huangdi Neijing* and was more systematically analyzed and summarized in *Treatise on Febrile Diseases*. The names of the six channels are Taiyang, Yangming, and Shaoyang, called the three yang; and Taiyin, Shaoyin, and Jueyin, called the three yin. When analyzing and summarizing symptoms, according to their different natures, those showing excited phenomena are classified into the three yang, and those showing declining phenomena into the three yin. Six-channel syndrome differentiation is not only widely used in exogenous diseases but also in many aspects of internal injury syndromes.

1. Taiyang Pulse Syndrome

The disease presents with fever, aversion to cold, severe headache and stiff neck, body pain, lumbar soreness, absence of sweating, and a floating and tight pulse. This is the initial stage of cold pathogen invading the exterior, generally called Taiyang disease. In Taiyang disease, cases with spontaneous sweating and a floating and slow pulse are called wind stroke (i.e., wind damage); those accompanied by thirst without aversion to cold, or slight aversion to cold, belong to warm disease.

2. Yangming Pulse Syndrome

External pathogens in the Taiyang channel that cannot be relieved in time, and the pathogenic factors develop inward. The disease presents with high fever, profuse sweating, no aversion to cold but rather aversion to heat, thirst, and a slippery and large pulse. At this time, the formless heat pathogen pervades the intestines and stomach, but the waste in the intestines has not yet become dry feces, with heat but no excess, called Yangming channel syndrome. If there are dry feces in the intestines, with additional symptoms such as constipation, abdominal fullness, abdominal pain, restlessness, delirium, and even confusion, with heat and excess, it is called Yangming fu syndrome. This is the second stage of exogenous disease, where the pathogen has transformed into fire, showing a series of heat manifestations, hence called Yangming disease.

3. Shaoyang Pulse Syndrome

Pathogens transmitting from the exterior to the interior belong neither to Taiyang (Initial Yang) Syndrome nor to Yangming (Greater Yang) Syndrome, but are in the intermediate shaoyang (Lesser Yang) stage, characterized as a half-exterior and half-interior syndrome. Symptoms include alternating chills and fever, recurring several times a day, bitter taste in the mouth, dry throat, dizziness, restlessness, vomiting with loss of appetite, and a wiry and rapid pulse. Since it is in the half-exterior and half-interior stage, it is called half-exterior and half-interior syndrome.

4. Taiyin Pulse Syndrome

The three yin diseases are mainly deficiency syndromes, generally without fever; on the contrary, they mostly present cold manifestations. Symptoms of Taiyin disease include abdominal fullness with spontaneous diarrhea, or abdominal pain with a preference for pressure, no thirst, warm hands and feet, vomiting, inability to eat, and a slow and weak pulse.

5. Shaoyin Pulse Syndrome

Symptoms include aversion to cold, cold limbs, diarrhea with undigested food, fatigue with a desire to sleep, and a thready and weak pulse. This is a systemic deficiency-cold syndrome due to yang qi weakness. Therefore, Shaoyin disease is more severe than Taiyin disease. However, Shaoyin governs water and fire; yang deficiency leads to cold transformation, while yin deficiency leads to fire transformation. Hence, in addition to the above deficiency-cold syndrome, there can also be internal heat symptoms such as restlessness, inability to sleep, heat diarrhea, and sore throat.

6. Jueyin Pulse Syndrome

Jueyin disease is the late stage of exogenous diseases, the final stage of struggle between pathogens and healthy qi. Symptoms are mostly a mixture of yin and yang, with cold and heat syndromes appearing together, such as unquenchable thirst, qi rushing upward to the chest, a burning pain in the chest, and hunger without desire to eat. It is particularly characterized by alternating cold limbs and heat. Alternating cold limbs and heat means that the cold limbs can warm up spontaneously, then become cold again after warming, and warm up again after being cold. If the duration of cold limbs is longer than that of heat, or if the cold limbs do not recover, the prognosis is poor; if heat lasts longer than cold limbs, and the cold limbs subside with the return of heat, it indicates the recovery of healthy qi, with hope for improvement.

The occurrence of six-channel symptoms is due to the transmission of pathogenic factors. This phenomenon of transmission from one channel to another is called "channel transmission". The key to whether channel transmission occurs depends on the comparison between pathogenic factors and physical strength. For example, when pathogens are exuberant and healthy qi is weak, there are more chances of transmission; when healthy qi is exuberant and pathogens are mild, there are fewer chances of transmission. Additionally, those with strong physical strength tend to have transmission within the three yang channels, while those with weak physical strength are prone to transmission to the three yin channels. Therefore, channel transmission does not mean all six channels are affected; some stop at Taiyang without transmission, some only transmit to Yangming, and some recover after affecting all three yang channels.

Channel transmission follows a certain order, i.e., proceeding from Taiyang to Yangming, then to Shaoyang, Taiyin, Shaoyin, and finally Jueyin, which is called "sequential channel transmission". There is also transmission without following the order, skipping one or two channels, such as Taiyang transmitting to Shaoyang instead of Yangming, or directly transmitting to yin channels without passing through Shaoyang, which is called "trans-channel transmission". Trans-channel transmission is mostly caused by exuberant pathogens and deficient healthy qi, with pathogens invading through deficiency. In addition, when three yin diseases do not transmit from yang channels but present Taiyin or Shaoyin symptoms from the onset, it is called "direct attack". Direct attack means pathogens invade directly; all three yin channels can be affected by direct attack, but Taiyin and Shaoyin are more common.

Each of the six channels has main symptoms and main pulses, and in clinical practice, they often appearintricatel. For example, there may be both Taiyang exterior syndrome and Yangming interior syndrome; or

Taiyang exterior syndrome has not fully resolved when Yangming interior syndrome appears. The former is called "combined disease", and the latter "concurrent disease". The difference is that combined disease refers to two or three channels being affected simultaneously, not due to transmission, such as Taiyang-Yangming combined disease, three yang combined disease, etc.; concurrent disease refers to one channel not subsiding before transmitting to another, with symptoms of the previous channel still present along with symptoms of the subsequent channel, such as Taiyang-Yangming concurrent disease, Yangming-Shaoyang concurrent disease, etc.

The basic essence of syndrome differentiation using the six channels is as described above. It not only illustrates the general conditions in the developmental process of exogenous diseases but also shows that the six channels form an interconnected whole that influences each other. In this way, one can observe the occurrence and changes of exogenous diseases from a comprehensive perspective, thereby grasping the laws of treatment, making it a fundamental method in syndrome differentiation. To learn six-channel syndrome differentiation, one must delve into *Treatise on Febrile Diseases*. There are hundreds of annotations on *Treatise on Febrile Diseases*, each with its own strengths. A relatively concise and outlining one is You Zaijing's *Collected Pearls on Febrile Diseases*. In addition, Ke Yunbo's *Laisu Collection on Febrile Diseases* classifies formulas and syndromes, along with their modifications and changes, in a clear manner, which can also serve as a reference.

III. Triple Jiao (Including Defense, Qi, Nutrient, and Blood)

The triple jiao syndrome differentiation method is a development of the six-channel syndrome differentiation method. The book *Systematic Differentiation of Warm Diseases* was compiled using this method. Its main essence lies in distinguishing the severity, depth, and mildness of febrile diseases throughout their developmental process. For example, exogenous warm diseases initially occur in the upper jiao, where the disease is shallow and mild; then they sequentially spread to the middle jiao and lower jiao, gradually becoming deeper and more severe. Therefore, although the term "triple jiao" has the same name as the triple jiao in the *zang-fu* organs, its meaning and function are different.

1. Upper Jiao Symptoms

The upper jiao refers to the two meridians and zang organs: the Lung Meridian of Hand-Taiyin and the Pericardium Meridian of Hand-Jueyin. The lung governs qi and controls the skin and hair; the pericardium governs blood and connects to the spirit. Warm pathogens first invade the lung, with symptoms including slight aversion to wind and cold, body heat, spontaneous sweating, headache, thirst or no thirst, cough, and a floating, slippery, and rapid pulse. If heat transmits to the pericardium, symptoms such as restlessness, thirst, delirium, restless sleep at night, and a crimson tongue will appear. Generally, warm pathogens transmit from the lung to the stomach, i.e., from the upper jiao to the middle jiao, which is called "normal transmission". If they rapidly transmit from the lung to the pericardium, i.e., from qi to blood, it is called "abnormal transmission".

2. Middle Jiao Symptoms

The middle jiao refers to the two meridians and zang organs: the Stomach Meridian of Foot-Yangming and the Spleen Meridian of Foot-Taiyin. Yangming governs dryness, and Taiyin governs dampness. When upper jiao warm pathogens transmit to Yangming, symptoms include high fever, profuse sweating, worsening in the afternoon, red face and eyes, rapid breathing, constipation, scanty dark urine, dry mouth with desire to drink, a yellow, dry tongue coating, or black with prickles. If they transmit to Taiyin, symptoms include mild body heat, worsening in the afternoon, headache and distension, heavy body, chest tightness with loss of appetite, nausea and desire to vomit, difficult urination, and a white, greasy or slightly yellow tongue coating. During this period, if heat is excessive or damp-heat steams, rashes or white papules may appear on the skin, along with mania, delirium, or a state of consciousness that is neither fully clear nor confused.

3. Lower Jiao Symptoms

The lower jiao refers to the two meridians and zang organs: the Kidney Meridian of Foot-Shaoyin and the Liver Meridian of Foot-Jueyin. The kidney governs yin, and the liver governs blood. When warm pathogens reach this stage, they often further damage blood and consume yin after depleting body fluids. In the kidney, symptoms include relative calm during the day, restlessness at night, dry mouth without desire to drink much, sore throat, or sores making it impossible to speak, diarrhea, and scanty dark urine. In the liver, symptoms include alternating cold limbs and heat, burning pain in the chest, extreme restlessness and irritancy, occasional retching, or headache with salivation, discomfort in the stomach and inability to eat. In the upper part, there may be dry, eroded mouth; in the lower part, diarrhea with tenesmus. There may also be wind stirring with convulsions, scrotal contraction, abdominal pain, etc.

By comparing triple jiao syndrome differentiation with six-channel syndrome differentiation, it is not difficult to realize that the triple jiao, from top to bottom, represents a vertical relationship, while the six channels, from exterior to interior, represent a horizontal relationship. If these two methods are combined, the intersection point of the vertical and horizontal axes is the middle jiao in the triple jiao system, which corresponds to Yangming and Taiyin in the six-channel system, essentially the same location. Therefore, there is no fundamental difference between the Yangming syndrome in warm diseases and that in cold damage, nor between the Taiyin syndrome in warm diseases and that in cold damage. In particular, the Yangming syndrome after cold pathogens transform into heat is fundamentally the same as that in warm diseases. The only difference is that the Taiyin syndrome in warm diseases is related to damp-heat, while the Taiyin syndrome in cold damage is related to cold-damp, with different pathogenic factors. Furthermore, the Taiyang in the six channels cannot be separated from the upper jiao lung; similarly, the Shaoyin and Jueyin in the six channels correspond to the lower jiao liver and kidney. Precisely because of this, although the triple jiao and six channels are two different syndrome differentiation methods with their own emphases, they also share common ground and are often used in combination in clinical practice.

While using the triple jiao for syndrome differentiation, distinguishing between defense (wei), qi, nutrient (ying), and blood is also an extremely important part. Defense, qi, nutrient, and blood are associated with the triple jiao and represent four levels of pathological depth, thus customarily referred to as the defense level, qi level, nutrient level, and blood level. The shallowest is the defense level, followed by the qi level, then the deeper nutrient level, and the deepest is the blood level. The entry and exit of pathogenic factors in the defense, qi, nutrient, and blood levels are closely related to the transmission of the triple jiao.

1. Defense Level Symptoms

Pathogens invading the exterior and affecting the lung internally present with fever, slight aversion to wind and cold, nasal congestion, cough, thin white tongue-coating, etc. The initial stage of upper jiao diseases belongs to the defense level, which is the exterior syndrome.

2. Qi Level Symptoms

Exterior pathogens entering the interior, presenting with high fever, thirst, slippery and rapid or surging pulse, and the tongue coating turning from white to yellow. The Yangming symptoms of the middle jiao all belong to the qi level, which is the interior syndrome.

3. Nutrient Level Symptoms

Pathogens in the upper energizer undergo reversed transmission to the pericardium, manifesting as agitation and delirium; or pathogens in the middle energizer cause skin rashes with delirium due to damp-heat effusion. These symptoms indicate transmission to the nutrient level. At this stage, the most reliable diagnostic sign is a crimson tongue.

4. Blood Level Symptoms

Heat pathogens invading the blood level (heat penetrating the blood) manifest as mania, delirium, convulsions, skin rashes, and internal bleeding including hematemesis, epistaxis, and bloody stool, with a thready or wiry rapid pulse and a deep crimson tongue devoid of moisture. These symptoms, in terms of triple jiao differentiation, belong to lower jiao diseases.

The syndrome differentiation methods of the triple jiao and defense, qi, nutrient, and blood originated from Ye Tianshi, who clearly stated: "Warm pathogens attack from above, first invading the lung." He also said: "After the defense comes the qi; after the nutrient comes the blood." In terms of treatment, he concisely pointed out: "For pathogens in the defense, diaphoresis is appropriate; when reaching the qi, clearing the qi is permissible; when entering the nutrient, it is still possible to disperse heat and transform it back to the qi; when entering the blood, fearing consumption and agitation of blood, it is necessary to clear and disperse the blood directly." From this, it can be understood that the triple jiao and defense, qi, nutrient, and blood are closely connected, forming a set of diagnostic and therapeutic methods in TCM. To clarify their meaning and facilitate mastery and application, a comprehensive explanation is provided as follows.The entire course of exogenous warm diseases can be divided into four stages.

First, the aversion to cold stage: This is the earliest stage of warm disease. One first feels chilly and afraid of wind, with slight body heat or higher temperature in the afternoon, accompanied by headache, cough, soreness in the limbs, spontaneous sweating or absence of sweating, dry mouth or not, and a thin white tongue coating. Since the pathogen is in the upper jiao, which pertains to the lung, and the lung governs the defense (wei), it is called upper jiao disease, i.e., the pathogen is in the defense level, which is the same as the generally referred to exterior syndrome. Since the pathogen is in the exterior, it should be dispersed. Therefore, as long as there is a trace of feeling chilly and afraid of wind, there is a trace of exterior syndrome; even if the feeling of being chilly and afraid of wind has diminished, and the body heat lingers without other pathological changes, it still belongs to the upper jiao defense level.

Second, the heat transformation stage: The main symptoms are that after the disappearance of feeling chilly and afraid of wind, the body heat increases, accompanied by dryness of the mouth, irritability, dark yellow urine, or worsening cough. This is the beginning of heat transformation. Generally speaking, the heat pathogen is still in the upper jiao defense level. Then, the body heat becomes intense, with aversion to heat, profuse sweating, thirst with desire to drink cold drinks, a slippery and large pulse, and the tongue coating turning yellow. At this point, the heat pathogen has transferred from the upper jiao to the middle jiao, and from the defense level to the qi level. The middle jiao pertains to the stomach, and the stomach belongs to Yangming. Treatment should focus on clearing heat and expelling pathogens. For constipation, purgation can be used.

Third, the nutrient invasion stage: Heat stagnates in the middle jiao, moving from qi to nutrient. The tongue starts to become crimson, and there is restlessness at night. There are three characteristics: delirium, rashes, or bleeding from the mouth and nose. At this time, although the warm pathogen is still based in the middle jiao, it has affected the pericardium, which is related to blood, hence called the nutrient level. When warm disease reaches this stage, it gradually deteriorates, which is actually a critical juncture for the progression or regression of the disease. Treatment should involve adding blood-cooling medicines to heat-clearing ones, still hoping to reverse it back to the qi level.

Fourth, the yin injury stage: Prolonged warm pathogens will inevitably damage body fluids and yin. Damage to body fluids is more common in the middle jiao and is relatively mild; damage to yin is more common in the lower jiao and is the most severe. Kidney yin and liver blood are damaged, with a shiny, dry, crimson tongue, leading to reckless movement of deficient yang, causing convulsions, limb twitching, etc. This stage is also called pathogen entering the blood level. The blood level does not solely refer to blood but includes true yin, so large doses of yin-nourishing and yang-subduing medicines are necessary. Most deaths from warm diseases occur at this stage.

As described above, it can be understood that the triple jiao refers to the location of the disease, and defense, qi, nutrient, and blood refer to the severity and depth of the pathological changes. Discussion of the triple jiao cannot be separated from defense, qi, nutrient, and blood, and discussion of defense, qi, nutrient, and blood cannot be separated from the triple jiao; however, the locations of the upper, middle, and lower jiao and the four stages of defense, qi, nutrient, and blood themselves should be clearly distinguished to avoid ambiguity in treatment.

Regarding the triple jiao syndrome differentiation method, one can read Ye Tianshi's "On Exogenous Warm Heat" (included in *Compilation of Warm Heat Classics*) and Wu Jutong's *Systematic Differentiation of Warm Diseases*.

IV. Pathogenesis

The term "pathogenesis" is found in *Huangdi Neijing* and refers to a method of symptom classification. While emphasizing diagnostic methods such as observation of complexion and pulse, *Huangdi Neijing* also attaches great importance to symptoms. Pathogenesis puts forward guidelines from complex symptoms, serving as the basis for syndrome differentiation to identify causes. Hence, it is said: "Carefully adhere to pathogenesis, each governing its category; for those present, investigate them; for those absent, investigate them."

The *Huangdi Neijing* puts forward only nineteen articles on pathogenesis, all referring to general symptoms rather than fixed diseases. Although the etiological factors it points out are mainly the six excesses, they can also be applied to other miscellaneous syndromes. For example, it states: General wind syndromes with tremors and dizziness all belong to the Liver Meridian; general damp syndromes with edema and distension all belong to the Spleen Meridian; general pain, itching, sores, and ulcers all belong to the Heart Meridian; general qi syndromes with dyspnea, counterflow, stuffiness, as well as general lung atrophy, asthma, vomiting, etc., all belong to the upper jiao Lung Meridian; general cold syndromes with contraction and spasm, as well as general cold limbs, abnormal urination and defecation (either retention or incontinence), etc., all belong to the lower jiao Kidney Meridian; general acute tendons and vessels rigidity, etc., all belong to wind pathogen; general clear urine without heat sensation or sediment, etc., all belong to cold pathogen; general convulsive diseases with stiff neck, etc., all belong to damp pathogen; general abdominal gurgling sounds, hollow and drum-like abdomen, etc.; general severe abdominal distension, as well as general acid regurgitation, urgent diarrhea, etc., all belong to heat pathogen; general heat syndromes with dizziness, 闷 ness and convulsions; general lockjaw, teeth chattering, trembling, involuntary movements, etc.; general upward counterflow, etc.; general restlessness, mania, mental disorders, etc.; general edema, soreness, fear, etc., as well as general muscle spasms, opisthotonos, turbid urine, etc., all belong to fire pathogen. Later, Liu Wansu added one more: general dryness and lack of moisture, dry and stiff tendons and vessels, chapped skin, etc., all belong to dryness pathogen.

The nineteen articles are certainly not comprehensive, but they play a great role in inspiring and guiding clinical practice. The main thing is that with such a concept, one can repeatedly explore the causes of diseases within this scope. For example, when encountering a patient whose main complaints are dizziness, blurred vision, and hand tremors, the initial impression is a Liver Meridian disease, and then the four diagnostic methods are used to diagnose whether it conforms to a Liver Meridian disease, then further analyze its deficiency, excess, cold, and heat, and observe whether there are other factors mixed in. Therefore, *Huangdi Neijing* says: "For those present, investigate them; for those absent, investigate them." It also says: "For excess, blame it; for deficiency, blame it." One must understand the spirit of *Huangdi Neijing* and consider each symptom from both positive and negative aspects. If one thinks that the pathogenesis of all diseases is only those few articles and makes one-sided affirmations, it becomes meaningless dogma.

After studying the eight principles, six channels, triple jiao, and even pathogenesis, we believe it is also necessary to learn about the comparison and classification of syndromes in TCM. TCM diagnosis focuses on syndrome differentiation, but a single symptom alone is meaningless. It is essential to compare and distinguish several similar symptoms. For example, regarding fever, there are fever with aversion to cold, fever without aversion to cold, alternating chills and fever, tidal fever, bone steaming, oppressive heat, fever during the day, fever at night, fever with spontaneous sweating, and fever without sweating. Similarly, regarding sweating, there are spontaneous sweating, night sweating, sweating only on the head, sweating on the palms and soles, sweating with aversion to cold, sweating with a salty taste, and incessant sweating. Analyzing the nature of these symptoms leads to distinctions such as exterior deficiency syndrome, exterior excess syndrome, cold syndrome, heat syndrome, yang syndrome, yin syndrome, etc. Without careful differentiation, a diagnosis cannot be made. Syndromes are built upon symptoms; only by analyzing symptoms can syndromes be determined. Xu Lingtai once said: The general term for symptoms is a disease; a disease must have changing symptoms. For instance, Taiyang wind strike is a disease, with symptoms such as aversion to wind, body heat, spontaneous sweating, and headache—these are the primary symptoms of Taiyang disease, which together constitute Taiyang disease. If Taiyang disease is accompanied by diarrhea, insomnia, restlessness, and stuffiness, these become associated symptoms of Taiyang disease. Another example: Malaria is a disease, with symptoms of alternating chills and fever, vomiting, and bitter taste in the mouth, which together form malaria. If malaria is accompanied by headache, distension, cough with counterflow, and constipation, these are associated symptoms of malaria; if malaria is also accompanied by diarrhea dozens of times a day, this is not an associated symptom but a concurrent disease, because malaria is one disease and diarrhea is another, each with its own primary symptoms. And so on, there are countless examples. For diseases and symptoms, one must seek their origins and distinguish their sequences. This explains that to understand a disease or a syndrome, one must first clarify similar symptoms and connect the symptoms of each disease and syndrome. For reference materials on these aspects, one can consult Cheng Wuji's *Explicit Theories on Cold Damage*, which differentiates symptoms of cold damage and integrates them with six-channel syndrome differentiation.

Section 2 Diagnostic Methods

I. Inspection

TCM diagnostic methods are divided into inspection, auscultation and olfaction, inquiry, and palpation, known as the four diagnostics.

Inspection relies on the doctor's vision to observe the patient's spirit, complexion, tongue coating, as well as physical form and overall condition.

1. Spirit

The strength of spirit is based on the abundance or decline of healthy qi. When healthy qi is sufficient, the spirit is not fatigued, the eyes are bright, speech is clear, the mind is unconfused, and breathing is calm. Even with an acute temporary condition, the prognosis is often good. Conversely, when healthy qi is deficient, the spirit is listless, the eyes are dull, speech is weak, the mind is restless, and breathing is rapid. Even if the temporary condition is not severe, one must be vigilant against deterioration.

Patients with abundant spirit have high confidence, strong autonomy, fewer worries, tolerance for pain, and can struggle resolutely against the disease—this is a favorable condition for treatment.

2. Complexion

Observing complexion includes the face and the skin of the whole body, divided into green, red, yellow, white, and black. According to the five elements theory, these correspond to the five *zang* organs, with internal organs assigned to different parts of the face. For example, red, the color of fire, indicates heat; it is believed that in liver heat disease, the left cheek reddens first; in lung heat disease, the right cheek reddens first; in heart heat disease, the forehead reddens first; in kidney heat disease, the cheeks redden first; in spleen heat disease, the nose reddens first. These have some accuracy but cannot be used in isolation to make a diagnosis.

Clinically common observations: A greenish facial complexion indicates acute infantile convulsions or severe phlegm-induced asthma; a greenish-black complexion indicates cold-induced pain; a pale complexion indicates qi deficiency or blood loss; a yellow complexion indicates dampness, and when accompanied by yellow eyes, it indicates jaundice; a red complexion indicates upward counterflow of liver fire or excessive heat in Yangming; a red complexion appearing solely on the cheeks indicates yin deficiency with hyperactive fire; a black complexion indicates water retention, or female labor jaundice; a blackish hue around the eye sockets in women indicates leukorrheal disease.

While observing the complexion, it is essential to observe the qi, which is categorized into five types: floating or sinking, clear or turbid, faint or intense, scattered or aggregated, lustrous or withered. A complexion appearing on the surface of the skin is floating, indicating a disease in the exterior; one hidden beneath the skin is sinking, indicating a disease in the interior; a bright complexion is clear, indicating a disease in yang; a heavy and stagnant complexion is turbid, indicating a disease in yin; a pale complexion is faint, indicating a mild disease; a deep and intense complexion is severe, indicating a serious disease; a dispersed complexion is scattered, indicating the disease is about to heal; an aggregated complexion is concentrated, indicating the disease is ongoing; a bright complexion is lustrous, indicating a favorable prognosis; a withered complexion is morbid, indicating an unfavorable prognosis. Through observing the qi, one can gain a deeper understanding of the diagnosis based on complexion. For example, in wind-warm disease, the facial complexion is mostly clear, and any redness appears floating on the surface; in damp-warm disease, the facial complexion is dull and turbid, yellowish with a blackish tinge. Another example is jaundice: A bright yellow like an orange is yang jaundice; a yellow like that from smoke is yin jaundice.

Observing the complexion is not only useful for diagnosing pathogenic factors but also highly relevant to healthy qi. Patients with nutritional deficiencies will not have a radiant complexion; those who are overly fatigued or weak from chronic illness will not have a glowing appearance. Therefore, combining the observation of complexion and qi allows for distinguishing diseases and assessing the patient's physical strength.

In addition to combining complexion and qi to differentiate diseases, one can also combine them with syndromes to verify the prognosis (favorable or unfavorable) of the complexion. For example, rib pain or infantile convulsions with spasms are all liver diseases; a greenish-yellow and lustrous complexion is favorable, while a purely white complexion is unfavorable. Cough and asthma, night sweats and spermatorrhea, or consumptive heat with bone steaming are all deficiency syndromes of the lung and kidney; a yellowish-white complexion is favorable, while a purely red complexion is unfavorable.

3. Tongue Coating

Observing the tongue is an important part of inspection. The definitions of the tongue body and coating: The tongue body refers to the tongue quality, and the coating is a thin layer of dirty coating on the tongue quality, similar to moss growing on the ground, hence called tongue coating. Observing the tongue quality helps distinguish the deficiency or excess of zang qi; observing the tongue coating helps distinguish the clarity or turbidity of stomach qi and the nature of exogenous pathogenic factors. In general, observing changes in thetongue quality and tongue coating can reveal the nature of the disease and the waxing and waning of healthy qi and pathogenic factors.

Next, one should know the division of the tongue coating. According to the five *zang* organs, the tip of the tongue belongs to the heart, the root of the tongue belongs to the kidney, the center belongs to the lung and stomach, and the sides belong to the liver and gallbladder. According to the triple jiao, the tip of the tongue belongs to the upper jiao, the middle of the tongue belongs to the middle jiao, and the root of the tongue belongs to the lower jiao.

Before discussing pathological tongue coatings, one should first mention the normal tongue coating. In healthy individuals, except for variations in some people due to constitution and habits, the standard is a ruddiness tongue body covered with a thin white coating, neither dry nor wet. However, people with excessive phlegm and dampness often have a thicker tongue coating; those with a constitution of yin deficiency and internal heat often have a slightly yellowish tongue coating; those who drink alcohol or smoke often have a yellow and greasy tongue coating, or with a grayish-black tinge; infants who are breastfed often have a white, greasy, and slippery coating. There are also congenital conditions such as a smooth, coating-less tongue, a patchy tongue coating, or a tongue with many cracks. These must be clarified through inquiry; as long as they are usual conditions without disease symptoms, they are within the normal range.

Observing the tongue requires careful attention; the tongue body and coating must be observed separately and then together. For the sake of clarity, they are described separately as follows.

(1) Tongue quality: Divided into five colors: pale, red, crimson, purple, and blue. A pale tongue texture indicates a deficient cold syndrome or a state of extreme anemia after severe blood loss. Bright red indicates a warm-heat syndrome or yin deficiency with excessive fire; a red tongue tip indicates excessive heat in the upper jiao or blazing heart fire; red tongue edges indicate liver heat. An extremely red tongue is crimson, i.e., deep red, mostly indicating pathogenic heat entering the nutrient level. Purple-red

indicates extreme heat in all three jiaos; a dark purple tongue indicates accumulated blood stasis; a pale purple with a bluish tinge and relatively moist texture indicates a yin syndrome of cold pathogens directly attacking the liver and kidney. A blue tongue is also called a green tongue; a blue and slippery tongue indicates a yin cold syndrome, while a dry one indicates static heat syndrome, both being dangerous signs.

(2) Tongue coating: Divided into white, yellow, gray, and black. ① White coating: Thin, white, and slippery indicates the initial stage of a cold; white, slippery, and sticky indicates internal phlegm-dampness; white and thickly greasy indicates extremely severe damp turbidity; white like accumulated powder indicates severe filthy turbidity in pestilential diseases; white and greasy like alkali indicates food stagnation with stagnated damp turbidity. White coating in exogenous diseases mostly indicates an exterior syndrome. ② Yellow coating: Light yellow and not dry indicates pathogens initially transmitting inward; yellow and greasy indicates damp-heat; yellow and filthy greasy indicates dampness exceeding heat; dark yellow with scorched cracks indicates heat exceeding dampness. ③ Gray-black coating: A thin, greasy, smooth, and moist gray coating indicates retained fluid or direct attack of yin cold; an extremely gray coating turns black; a dry black coating indicates intense heat damaging body fluids, with fire extreme appearing like water; a smooth and moist one indicates yang deficiency with excessive cold, where water restrains fire.

Diet can discolor the tongue coating, such as initial consumption of soy milk or milk often resulting in a white and greasy coating; drinking orange juice often turning it light yellow; eating Chinese olives or pickles often turning it gray-black. Such discoloration mostly floats on the tongue coating, unrelated to the tongue quality, called "stained tongue," which is not a reliable basis for diagnosis.

In addition to observing the colors of the tongue quality and coating, one must distinguish between old and tender, dry and moist, soft and hard, trembling and flaccid, thick and thin, loose and greasy, radiant and withered, swollen and shrunken. A firm, contracted, and old tongue indicates excess; a puffy obesity, and tender tongue indicates deficiency; dryness indicates depleted fluids; moistness indicates uninjured fluids; softness indicates self-nourishment of qi and fluids; hardness indicates loss of nourishment in the collaterals; trembling indicates wind or deficiency; flaccidity (inability to move) indicates deficient healthy qi; a thin coating indicates initially contracted exterior pathogens; a thick coating indicates deeply entrenched interior pathogens; loose coating with no substance indicates sufficient healthy qi to transform pathogens; greasy coating with a base indicates the entrenchment of filthy turbidity; radiance (luster) in disease is auspicious; withered (lifelessness) in disease is mostly ominous; swelling (puffiness) indicates water-dampness; shrinkage indicates heart deficiency or consumption by internal heat.

A tongue entirely without coating is called a smooth tongue, mostly indicating yin deficiency; a smooth tongue like a membrane-removed pig kidney indicates extremely damaged liver and kidney yin. A missing patch in the middle of the tongue coating is called a peeled coating; a red peeled coating indicates yin deficiency with heat; an eroded and patchy peeled coating is called a spotted peeled coating, mostly indicating damage to yin by pestilential damp-heat. A smooth tongue with cracks or a dry, cracked coating both indicate damaged fluids; red prickles or red dots on the tongue indicate extremely severe internal heat. White spots like blisters on the tongue with stinging pain during eating are called gan (canker sores), indicating stomach heat; white membranous growths like mold spreading gradually are called mi (erosions), mostly seen in syndromes of heat lingering with yin damage.

After observing changes in the tongue quality and coating separately, the two must be considered together for comprehensiveness. For example, a crimson tongue indicates pathogenic heat entering the nutrient level, but if accompanied by a yellow-white coating, it means pathogenic factors in the qi level are not exhausted; a white coating with a red base indicates dampness suppressing and stagnating heat, and one must not solely clear the nutrient level. Another example: A greasy tongue indicates dampness, and yellow indicates transformation into heat in the stomach; if the coating is thick, greasy, and yellow but the tongue quality is not red, transforming dampness remains the key; conversely, if the greasy coating is not moist and the tongue quality shows a delicate redness, one must prevent transformation into heat and damage to fluids, and even with a thick coating, acrid-drying substances to transform dampness cannot be used. Such variations are numerous, and one cannot focus on only one aspect.

4. Physical Form and Posture

Observing the patient's physical build, posture, and movements is also of great help in diagnosis. For example, obese individuals are prone to phlegm-dampness, while thin individuals are prone to internal heat; inability to lift one arm indicates impediment (bi) syndrome; hemiplegia indicates wind stroke; difficulty in flexing and extending the knees with a stooped posture when walking indicates a disorder of the sinews; inability to stand for long with shaking when walking indicates a disorder of the bones; being able to turn over easily due to a light body sensation indicates a yang disease; being unable to turn over due to a heavy body sensation indicates a yin disease; often lying with one leg bent or curled up mostly indicates abdominal pain; picking at clothes, touching the bed, or making aimless hand movements (like arranging threads) indicates scattered spirit; limb spasms and opisthotonos indicate convulsive disease or infantile convulsions, etc.

5. Other Parts

Red eyes indicate heat; yellow eyes indicate jaundice; squinting eyes mostly indicate liver wind. Nasal congestion with discharge indicates a cold; dry nostrils with a black, smoke-like appearance indicate deep heat in yang toxicity; flaring nostrils indicates lung wind or impending lung failure. Lockjaw with inability to speak indicates convulsion; deviated mouth corner indicates wind stroke.

All parts observable by the eye fall within the scope of inspection, which is the first step in diagnosis.

II. Auscultation and Oifaction

Auscultation and olfaction involve two aspects: on the one hand, using hearing to listen to the patient's speech, breathing, coughing, and other sounds, noting their pitch, clarity, etc.; on the other hand, using smell to distinguish the odors of the breath, disease-related odors, and excreta.

1. Sounds

A low and weak tone indicates internal injury and deficiency syndrome; whispering and repetition indicate insufficient mental vitality; delirious speech indicates excessive heat with clouded consciousness; loud shouting and cursing without regard for relatives or strangers indicates mania.

Weak breathing indicates healthy qi deficiency; rough breathing indicates heat in the lung and stomach; more exhalation than inhalation indicates phlegm obstruction; a sawing sound in the throat indicates phlegm-induced asthma; difficulty in inhaling, as if about to stop, but feeling relieved by taking a long breath indicates kidney deficiency with inability to grasp qi; frequent sighing mostly indicates emotional distress; chest and diaphragm stuffiness is common in qi stagnation syndrome caused by grief, depression, worry, or anxiety.

In cough diseases, a sudden cough with a hoarse voice indicates excess in the lung; a prolonged cough with a weak voice indicates deficiency in the lung; a strenuous cough with less sputum indicates lung heat; a cough with phlegm and shortness of breath indicates phlegm-fluid; a sudden, non-stop cough with a red face and nausea indicates whooping cough.

Continuous hiccups indicate cold in the stomach; loud and forceful hiccups indicate excess heat; weak hiccups that fail to reach the throat indicate deficient cold; intermittent hiccups, with one hiccup after a long pause, mostly indicate a declining stomach qi in chronic diseases or the late stage of acute diseases.

Patients may make a special sound, often from the nose, a continuous groaning, mostly indicating pain; groaning with a furrowed brow indicates headache; pressing the chest with the hand indicates chest or epigastric pain; hands on the waist with difficulty in turning indicates lower back pain.

2. Odors

Foul breath indicates damp-heat in the stomach; belching with a sour and rotten odor indicates retained food in the stomach; phlegm with a fishy and foul odor indicates lung heat; extremely foul-smelling phlegm with pus indicates lung abscess.

Sour-smelling, loose stools indicate accumulated heat and food stagnation in the intestines; foul-smelling, turbid urine indicates damp-heat in the bladder; extremely foul flatulence mostly indicates indigestion.

Disease-related odor refers to a specific sour and foul smell emitted by patients, commonly seen in acute febrile diseases and pestilential diseases. Weak individuals are easily infected upon smelling it. For example, in warm diseases, after sweating, if the fever persists, the sweat first has a sour odor; during the eruption of rashes or macules, the odor becomes stronger. In pestilential diseases, the disease-related odor is noticeable from the onset.

III. Inquiry

To diagnose a disease, it is necessary to understand the patient's living habits, mental state, as well as the onset and progression of the illness. When necessary, their family history and personal past medical history should also be understood. Generally, in clinical practice, the course of the disease and subjective symptoms are the main contents of inquiry. There is a certain procedure for inquiry. Zhang Jingyue once composed the "Ten Inquiries Song": "First inquire about cold and heat, second about sweat; third about the head and body, fourth about bowel and bladder; fifth about diet, sixth about the chest; seventh about deafness, eighth about thirst, all to be distinguished; ninth, observe yin and yang through pulse and complexion; tenth, discern the spirit through odor and sound." The ten inquiries include the differentiation between exogenous and internal injuries, explained as follows.

1. Cold and Heat

Presence of cold and heat is mostly an exterior syndrome or exogenous syndrome; absence of cold and heat is mostly an interior syndrome or internal injury miscellaneous syndrome. Fever with aversion to cold indicates a disease in yang; absence of fever with aversion to cold indicates a disease in yin. Further analysis can be made by combining other symptoms: for example, fever with aversion to cold accompanied by headache and body pain is Taiyang disease; fever without aversion to cold accompanied by thirst is Yangming disease; alternating cold and heat accompanied by bitter taste in the mouth, dry throat, and dizziness is Shaoyang disease. There are also cases of deficiency-cold syndrome with no fever but only aversion to cold and constant cold hands and feet;

deficiency-heat syndrome with tidal fever or bouts of hot flushes and burning sensation in the palms and soles. In addition, the timing of fever should be distinguished: reduction in the morning and exacerbation in the evening indicates seasonal pathogens; subsiding early and rising in the evening or rising early and subsiding in the evening indicates consumptive disease; periodic onset at fixed intervals, once a day, once every two days, or once every three days indicates malaria.

2. Sweat

Sweat is closely related to cold and heat. For example, exogenous fever without sweat is cold damage; with sweat is wind damage; reduction of fever after sweating indicates the disease is gradually subsiding; increased fever after sweating indicates pathogens are gradually entering the interior. In deficiency syndromes, yin deficiency with night sweats is accompanied by fatigue after sweating; yang deficiency with spontaneous sweating is accompanied by a feeling of cold after sweating. Furthermore, in exterior syndrome, excessive sweating after diaphoresis, a sudden drop in fever, and exacerbated aversion to cold is called yang exhaustion, with the risk of collapse; there is also sweating with shivering, similar to collapse but with peaceful sleeping and calm pulse, called battle sweat, which is a sign of disease transformation and need not cause alarm. If sweat comes like beads or oil, with cold limbs and hidden pulse, it is a sign of impending death, called extinction sweat.

3. Head

Headache without cessation, accompanied by cold and heat, is mostly exogenous. Pain in the head and nape belongs to Taiyang; pain in the forehead belongs to Yangming; pain in thebilateral sides of the head belongs to Shaoyang; pain in the vertex of the head belongs to Jueyin. Intermittent pain accompanied by dizziness and heavy distension is mostly internal injury miscellaneous syndrome. Pain with distension and heat sensation belongs to liver fire; dizziness with photophobia belongs to liver yang; severe pain with a blue complexion belongs to liver cold; heavy, muddled head with ringing belongs to brain deficiency. Internal obstruction of phlegm-dampness and failure of clear yang to rise can also cause dizziness, often accompanied by a greasy tongue and nausea.

4. Body

General soreness with exterior syndrome is mostly exogenous, relieved after sweating. Soreness without cold and heat, located in the joints or migrating to the limbs, is wind-cold-damp impediment, often related to the climate. Numbness of the hands and feet, or numbness in one part of the body, is qi deficiency. Numbness only in the thumb or index finger, extending to the elbow and arm, is a precursor to wind stroke. Body pain and discomfort that occur when lying down for extended periods and are relieved after activity indicate a disharmony of qi and blood. Heavy body pain with difficulty in movement is dampness obstructing the meridians.

5. Bowel Movements

Constipation with ability to eat is yang binding; constipation with inability to eat is yin binding. Abdominal fullness and pain is excess syndrome; absence of fullness and pain is deficiency syndrome. Chronic constipation in patients with long-term illness, the olderly, or postpartum women is blood depletion and fluid dryness. Dry stool followed by loose stool is middle qi deficiency. Persistently loose stools are spleen deficiency. Diarrhea at dawn (cockcrow) is kidney deficiency. Diarrhea with abdominal pain and foul-smelling stools is food injury. Pain followed by diarrhea, with sticky, foul-smelling, red and white stools and tenesmus, is dysentery. Sudden vomiting, incessant watery diarrhea, numb limbs, and sweating on the head is cholera.

6. Urine

Clear white urine indicates cold; yellowish-red urine indicates heat; turbid and unsmooth urine indicates damp-heat. Frequent and uncontrollable urination indicates a deficiency syndrome; frequent urination with excessive thirst and drinking indicates wasting-thirst (xiao-ke). Dribbling during urination with stabbing pain in the urethra indicates strangury syndrome. Inability to urinate with severe abdominal distension indicates retention of urine (long-bi). In patients with diarrhea, urine is necessarily scanty; if urine gradually increases, the diarrhea is about to heal.

7. Diet

The stomach governs reception, and the spleen governs digestion. Being able to eat and easily hungry indicates a strong stomach; difficulty in digesting food after eating indicates a weak spleen. Preference for cold food indicates stomach heat; preference for warm food indicates stomach cold. Vomiting immediately after eating indicates a heat syndrome; vomiting in the evening what was eaten in the morning indicates a cold syndrome. In children, excessive eating, abdominal pain, and emaciation are mostly due to intestinal parasites. Nausea at the sight of food in pregnant women is morning sickness, a physiological phenomenon. A bitter taste in the mouth indicates fire in the liver and gallbladder; a sweet taste indicates damp-heat in the spleen; a sour taste indicates disharmony between the liver and stomach; a salty taste indicates kidney deficiency with water overflowing; a bland taste with much clear fluid indicates stomach cold.

8. Chest

Fullness and stuffiness in the chest and diaphragm are mostly due to qi stagnation; restlessness and discomfort are mostly due to heat stagnation; chest fullness with pain indicates bound chest (jie-xiong); distension without pain extending to the epigastrium indicates focal qi (pi-qi); chest pain radiating to the back and back pain radiating to the chest indicates chest impediment (xiong-bi) syndrome. When inquiring about chest symptoms, it is necessary to relate them to the epigastrium, abdomen, and hypochondria. For example, epigastric pain belongs to the stomach: Pain worsening after eating indicates excess; pain alleviating after eating indicates deficiency. Abdominal pain belongs to the intestines: Pain with refusal to be pressed indicates excess; pain with a preference for pressure indicates deficiency. Hypochondriac pain belongs to the liver: Sudden pain is in the qi; Long-term pain enters the collaterals.

9. Deafness

Sudden deafness is mostly excessive, due to upward counterflow of liver and gallbladder fire; long-term deafness is deficiency, due to internal depletion of liver and kidney yin. Deafness often starts with tinnitus: Tinnitus like the tide or wind indicates wind-heat; tinnitus like continuous cicada chirping indicates yin deficiency; there is also purulent discharge with swelling, with both ringing and deafness, which is damp-heat in the liver meridian.

10.Thirst

Dry mouth with a desire to drink is true thirst, due to fire in the stomach; inability to drink, or drinking little even if thirsty, is false thirst, due to dampness in the stomach. A preference for cold drinks when thirsty indicates stomach heat; conversely, a preference for hot drinks indicates internal cold.

In inquiry, the quality of sleep should also be noted. For example, insomnia is mostly a deficiency syndrome; short sleep with easy awakening is due to restless spirit; excessive dreaming while sleep is due to hyperactive ministerial fire; crying out in dreams is due to deficient gallbladder qi; chest and diaphragm stuffiness with inability to sleep peacefully is due to internal obstruction of damp-phlegm.

In addition, whether memory has declined, whether sexual desire is normal, whether there is spermatorrhea, etc., should all be asked about as long as they are related to the illness, without being weary of seeking details.

For female patients, during inquiry, it is important to ask whether menstruation is regular. For example, menstruation occurring earlier with bright red color is mostly due to heat; menstruation occurring later with purplish stasis is mostly due to excess; scanty and pale menstruation is mostly due to deficiency; abdominal pain before menstruation with scanty, stagnant flow mixed with stasis is mostly due to qi stagnation. If menstruation occurs with cold, fever, or menstrual flow starts during fever with clouded consciousness, it is heat entering the blood chamber. In general, if menstruation stops, married women should be considered for possible pregnancy.

Pediatrics was traditionally called the "mute department" because it is generally impossible to directly hear the sick child's complaints. However, inquiry cannot be neglected, and detailed questions must be asked of the child's caregiver. In addition to asking about the onset time and course of the illness, attention should also be paid to whether the child has been vaccinated against smallpox or has had measles.

IV. Palpation

Palpation mainly involves pulse-taking and includes other forms of touch examination.

1. Pulse Palpation

Pulse palpation is performed at the cun kou (the radial artery behind the palm) on both hands, using the index, middle, and ring fingers with light pressure, heavy pressure, or single-finger pressure, combined pressure, to detect the pulse condition. Each hand is divided into three positions, with the bony prominence behind the palm as the marker, named "guan" (pass). The position before guan is called "cun" (inch), and the position after guan is called "chi" (foot). The cun, guan, and chi on both hands form six positions in total, namely left cun, left guan, left chi, right cun, right guan, and right chi. These six positions correspond to the internal organs: the left cun corresponds to the heart and pericardium; the left guan corresponds to the liver and gallbladder; the left chi corresponds to the kidney, bladder, and small intestine; the right cun corresponds to the lung; the right guan corresponds to the spleen and stomach; the right chi corresponds to the kidney, life gate, and large intestine.

Generally speaking, there are twenty-eight pulse conditions, named as follows: floating, sinking, slow, rapid, slippery, rough, empty, full, long, short, surging, minute, tight, moderate, hollow, string-like, leathery, firm, soft, weak, thin, scattered, hidden, moving, hurried, knotted, intermittent, and swift. Most of these pulses are relative. For example, floating and sinking distinguish exterior and interior; slow and rapid distinguish cold and heat; rough and slippery distinguish deficiency and excess. The other pulses are derived from these six. For instance: An extremely forceful floating pulse, like pressing on a drum skin, is leathery; an extremely weak floating pulse, like cotton in water, is soft. A sinking pulse that can only be felt when pressed against the bone is hidden; a solid sinking pulse is firm; a weak sinking pulse that can only be felt with light pressure is weak. A pulse that is forceful in floating, middle, and sinking positions, responding to the fingers with a full sensation, is full; a pulse that is weak in all three positions, responding with an empty sensation, is empty; a pulse that is large on floating but hollow when pressed, like a green onion stalk, is hollow. A slow, thin, short pulse with sluggish movement is rough; a pulse with four beats per breath, smooth and even, is moderate; a moderate pulse with occasional pauses is knotted; a rapid pulse at the guan position, with no beginning or end, is moving; a rapid pulse with occasional pauses is hurried; seven to eight beats per breath is swift; a pulse with irregular slow and rapid beats but regular pauses is intermittent; a pulse with irregular beats, floating and chaotic when pressed, is scattered. A slippery pulse like pressing on a string is string-like; a forceful, twisting pulse like a rope is tight; a pulse that is neither small nor large, like following a long pole, is long; a pulse that is strong on arrival and weak on departure, large on arrival and long on departure, is surging; an extremely soft, thin rough pulse that seems about to disappear when pressed is minute; a pulse that is minute and thin is thin; a pulse that feels like a bean and retreats as soon as it responds to the finger is short. Therefore, floating-sinking, slow-rapid, and rough-slippery are the key principles of the twenty-eight pulses. Learning pulse palpation should start with these six principles, as they are easier to understand and comprehend. Specific information is as follows:

Floating pulse (superficial, weakens on pressure):
- leather pulse (floating and extremely forceful, taut like a drumhead)
- Soft pulse (floating and extremely forceless, like cotton floating on water)
- Replete pulse (forceful at all levels: superficial, middle, deep)
- Feeble pulse (forceless at all levels: superficial, middle, deep)
- Hollow pulse (large on light pressure, empty at the middle level)

Deep pulse (palpable only with heavy pressure):
- Hidden pulse (palpable only by pressing to the bone, indicating deep concealment of pulse)
- Firm pulse (deep, replete, large, wiry, and long)
- Weak pulse (deep, thread, and forceless)

Slow pulse (less than 3 beats per respiration or <60 bpm):
- Moderate pulse (four beats per respiration: 60-70 bpm)
- Knotted pulse (slow with irregular pauses: no fixed interval)
- Regularly intermittent pulse (weak with regular pauses: fixed interval)
- Scattered pulse (floating, disordered, and rootless)

Rapid pulse（more than 5 beats per respiration or >90 bpm）:
- Throbbing pulse (throbbing rapidly at the guan position, bean-sized without clear head or tail)
- Abrupt pulse (rapid with irregular pauses)
- Swift pulse (7-8 beats per breath: >140 bpm, extremely rapid)

Slippery pulse（smooth and flowing movement）:
- Wiry pulse (straight and tense like a tightened string)
- Tense pulse (forceful and urgent, like a twisted rope)
- Long pulse (straight and extended, exceeding the three pulse positions)
- surging pulse (large and flooding, strong on arrival but fading on retreat like tidal waves)

Uneven pulse（rough and hesitant movement）:
- Short pulse (abrupt withdrawal after palpation, failing to fill the pulse positions)
- Faint pulse (extremely thin and soft, almost imperceptible on heavy pressure)
- Thready pulse (thin but clearly palpable, softer than faint pulse)

The twenty-eight pulses rarely appear alone; common combined pulses include the following: floating-tight, floating-moderate, floating-slippery, floating-rapid, floating-slow, floating-large; sinking-tight, sinking-slippery, sinking-string-like, sinking-thin, sinking-rapid, sinking-slow, sinking-minute; slow-rough; slippery-rapid, string-like-rapid, surging-rapid, thin-rapid; soft-rapid, soft-thin, soft-slippery, soft-rough, soft-moderate; empty-thin, empty-rapid, empty-string-like; minute-thin, minute-weak; string-like-tight, string-like-thin; thin-tight, thin-slow; and combinations of three pulses such as floating-tight-rapid, floating-slippery-rapid, sinking-thin-minute, etc.

Diagnosing diseases based on pulse conditions is mainly as follows:

-A floating pulse indicates an exterior syndrome; forceful is exterior excess, weak is exterior deficiency.

-A sinking pulse indicates an interior syndrome; forceful is interior excess, weak is interior deficiency.

-A slow pulse indicates a cold syndrome; forceful is accumulated cold, weak is deficient cold.

-A rapid pulse indicates a heat syndrome; forceful is excess heat, weak is deficient heat.

-A slippery pulse indicates phlegm syndrome or heat syndrome.

-A rough pulse indicates blood deficiency or blood cold.

-An empty pulse indicates deficiency syndrome or summerheat injury.

-A full pulse indicates excess syndrome or fire pathogen.

-A short pulse indicates deficient primordial qi.

-A surging pulse indicates heat syndrome or yang excess with yin decline.

-A minute pulse indicates yang exhaustion or dual deficiency of qi and blood.

-A tight pulse indicates cold syndrome or pain syndrome.

-A moderate pulse indicates health or dampness.

-A hollow pulse indicates severe blood loss.

-A string-like pulse indicates liver qi or phlegm-fluid.

-A leathery pulse indicates exterior cold or middle deficiency.

-A firm pulse indicates persistent accumulation.

-A soft pulse indicates yang deficiency or damp disease.

-A weak pulse indicates yin deficiency.

-A thin pulse indicates blood deficiency or qi decline.

-A scattered pulse indicates decline of kidney qi.

-A hidden pulse indicates deep-lying pathogenic factors.

-A moving pulse indicates fright syndrome or pain syndrome.

-A hurried pulse indicates hyperactive fire.

-A knotted pulse indicates cold accumulation.

-An intermittent pulse indicates decline of zang qi.

-A swift pulse indicates hyperactive yang pathogen or exhaustion of true yin.

Each pulse has its own characteristics and corresponding main symptoms. Since they often appear in combinations, further exploration is necessary for clinical application. For example: Floating-tight pulse indicates cold damage; floating-moderate pulse indicates wind stroke; floating-empty pulse indicates summerheat injury; floating-hollow pulse indicates blood loss; floating-rapid pulse indicates wind-heat. Sinking-thin pulse indicates deficient cold; sinking-rapid pulse indicates internal heat; sinking-tight pulse indicates cold pain; sinking-string-like pulse indicates latent fluid retention; sinking-slow pulse indicates chronic cold. Floating-slow pulse indicates exterior cold; sinking-slow pulse indicates interior cold; slow-rough pulse indicates blood deficiency; slow-moderate pulse indicates cold-dampness. Slippery-rapid pulse indicates excess heat; string-like-slippery pulse indicates liver fire; thin-slippery pulse indicates yin deficiency with internal heat; floating-slippery pulse indicates wind-phlegm; sinking-slippery pulse indicates retained food; slippery-large pulse indicates stomach heat. Thin-moderate pulse indicates damp impediment; moderate-weak pulse indicates qi deficiency. These all reflect the waxing and waning of healthy qi and pathogenic factors, the nature of pathogenic factors, and the location of the disease. Therefore, it is essential to closely combine them with syndromes and observe whether the pulse and symptoms are consistent.

Distinguishing the twenty-eight pulses is not a simple task and must be gradually understood through clinical practice. The following is a summary of the twenty-eight pulses by predecessors for memorization: "Floating pulse travels at the skin; sinking pulse travels at the muscles and bones. Once floating and sinking are clear, slow and rapid should be perceived: Three beats per breath is slow; six beats per breath is rapid. Floating, sinking, slow, and rapid each have deficiency and excess: Weak is deficiency; forceful is excess. Once slow and rapid are clear, positions must be recognized: Soft pulse is floating and weak; weak pulse is sinking and weak (i.e., floating and weak is soft; sinking and weak is weak). Extremely sinking is firm; extremely floating is leathery. All three positions being small, the minute pulse can be identified. All three positions being large, the scattered pulse can be understood. The one called hidden does not appear in floating; only the middle position being weak, it is called hollow. Once positions are clear, the number of beats should be distinct: Four beats per breath is moderate; seven beats per breath is swift. Rapid with pauses is called hurried; moderate with pauses is called knotted. Once the number of beats is recognized, shapes should be distinguished: Tight is rough and bouncing; string-like is thin and straight; long is stretched out; short is contracted. What is called surging comes forcefully and fades weakly. What is called moving shakes without shifting. What is called slippery flows smoothly. What is called rough advances and retreats with difficulty. What is called thin is like a thread. What is called intermittent is like having regular pauses. Intermittent is not a type of thin; its beats are irregular. Large is associated with surging; small is the same as thin."

Beyond the twenty-eight pulses, there are seven strange pulses: (1) Sparrow pecking: repeatedly tapping the finger, suddenly present and suddenly absent, like a sparrow pecking food; (2) Roof leaking: like drops from a broken roof, one drop after a long time, splashing weakly; (3) Stone flicking: coming firmly and hurriedly, slow to arrive and quick to depart, like flicking a stone with the finger; (4) Cable unraveling: pulse coming rapid and moving, then immediately scattered and disorderly; (5) Fish gliding: pulse with a fixed head and wagging tail, floating and drifting; (6) Shrimp swimming: pulse in the skin, like a shrimp swimming on the water surface, disappearing suddenly, then returning after a moment; (7) Cauldron boiling: having an outward flow but no inward, like boiling soup, with neither pulse beats nor breathing. These pulses all indicate extreme heart failure, signifying that vitality is exhausted, mostly being fatal signs. In *Huangdi Neijing*, they are called "true *zang* pulses," meaning they have no harmonious qi, indicating that stomach qi is exhausted.

2. Palpation

Generally, it involves palpating the chest, abdomen, hands, and feet. For example, in cases of epigastric fullness, if it is hard and painful when pressed, it is bound chest; if soft and painless when pressed, it is focal qi. Another example: abdominal fullness with refusal to be pressed, painful when pressed, indicates excess or heat; preference for pressure, painless when pressed, indicates deficiency or cold; abdominal distension that sounds like a drum when tapped is qi distension; thin skin that feels like a bag of chaff when pressed is water distension.

Warmth in the back of the hands indicates exogenous pathogenic factors; heat in the palms indicates yin deficiency. Warm hands and feet suggest a mild illness; cold hands and feet indicate a severe illness. Swollen feet that remain indented when pressed indicate water retention. A faint and thin dorsalis pedis pulse indicates weakness in the acquired vitality.

The art of pulse palpation is rather subtle, and it is not easy to distinguish without deep comprehension. When starting to practice pulse palpation clinically, two points should be noted. Firstly, one must calm the mind and avoid impetuosity. First, lift, then press, and then search.Lifting means taking the pulse with a light touch, pressing with a heavy touch to determine if it is floating or sinking, and then searching for its characteristics with neither too light nor too heavy pressure. Secondly, combine the pulse condition with the syndrome to see if they are consistent. For example, a yang syndrome should present a yang pulse, and a yin syndrome a yin pulse—this is a consistency between pulse and syndrome. If an exogenous syndrome presents a thin and weak pulse, or a deficiency syndrome presents a slippery and large pulse, indicating inconsistency between pulse and syndrome, the prognosis is generally poor, which must be paid attention to in clinical practice.

The four diagnostic methods must be integrated, and they must also be closely combined with syndromes. Predecessors sometimes disregarded the pulse and followed the symptoms, and sometimes disregarded the symptoms and followed the pulse, as emergency measures for treatment. In fact, such measures are decisions made after overall consideration based on the results of the four diagnoses. Among the four diagnoses, pulse palpation and tongue inspection are the most important. For further study, one can generally refer to books such as *Essentials of the Four Diagnoses*, *Binhu's Pulse Rhymes*, and *Tongue Inspection in Cold Damage*.

Section 3 Therapeutic Methods

I. Regular Treatment and Contrary Treatment

TCM treats diseases from a holistic perspective, attaching great importance to the patient's physical strength—healthy qi, and the cause of the disease—pathogenic factors, regarding the disease as a process of struggle between pathogenic factors and healthy qi. This struggle ends only when pathogenic factors recede and healthy qi enters a stage of recovery. That is, when healthy qi prevails, the disease is cured; when pathogenic factors prevail, it leads to severe illness or death. Therefore, *Huangdi Neijing* put forward a guiding principle: "Tonify for deficiency, purge for excess." Tonification is to support insufficient healthy qi, and purgation is to expel invading pathogenic factors. There are various methods within tonification and purgation, but the only goal is to restore health.

Targeting deficiency, tonification is used; for excess, purgation is used. When both deficiency and excess exist, one considers tonifying first then purging, purging first then tonifying, or combining tonification and purgation. Any treatment conducted directly, using methods opposite to the nature of the disease, whether tonification or purgation, is called "regular treatment." Conversely, using methods consistent with the nature of the disease is called "contrary treatment."

To be specific, regular treatment means using hot medicines for cold syndromes and cold medicines for heat syndromes; for example, using moistening methods for dryness manifestations, soothing methods for spasms, and astringent methods for dissipation. Contrary treatment is used relatively rarely. In fact, contrary treatment does not truly follow the condition of the disease. On the surface, the purpose of the treatment seems to be in the same direction as the disease, but upon careful examination, it is still opposite to the cause of the disease. For instance, in cases of deficient distension caused by sluggish digestive function, tonics are administered instead of qi-regulating and stagnation-resolving medicines. This is because the disease arises from deficiency, and the symptoms cannot be improved without enhancing the function. Another example: For diarrhea caused by internal stagnation, purgatives are given instead of astringent anti-diarrheal medicines. This is also because the diarrhea is caused by stagnation; it cannot be stopped without removing the stagnation, and even if it is temporarily stopped, it will recur in the future. Moreover, when a disease is severe, false manifestations often appear. For example, in cases of extreme cold with yang repelled to the exterior, symptoms of restlessness may occur. If cold medicines are used to treat the restlessness, it will worsen the root cause; but if extremely hot medicines are used directly, they will be repelled and not absorbed. At this time, methods such as taking hot medicines cold or adding a small amount of cold medicines to hot medicines can be used. These all fall into the category of contrary treatment, but in essence, they are still regular treatment.

It can be seen from this that regular treatment and contrary treatment are consistent in nature, differing only in tactics. Before applying these two different tactics, understanding the cause and symptoms of the disease is the most important key issue. Many therapeutic principles established by later generations are mostly promoted and applied based on *Huangdi Neijing*. As for the specific application of regular treatment and contrary treatment, *Huangdi Neijing* already has relatively detailed instructions: In terms of etiology, such as "Treat cold with heat; treat heat with cold; eliminate exogenous pathogens; warm for exhaustion; disperse and purge for excess", these are all regular treatments; and such as "For heat that persists after using cold, treat the yin; for cold that persists after using heat, treat the yang", these are all contrary treatments. In terms of symptoms, such as "Reduce hardness; disperse stagnation; attack retention; moisten dryness; relieve spasm; astringe dissipation; calm fright; suppress and astringe hyperactivity", these are all regular treatments; and such as "Treat obstruction with tonification; treat diarrhea with purgation", these are all contrary treatments. These treatment methods are included in the "Principles of Treatment" chapter of *Essentials of Huangdi Neijing*, which can be referred to.

II. Treating the Root and Treating the Branch

Treating the root and treating the branch are also commonly used therapeutic principles. One must understand the root and the branch to determine measures such as priority, urgency, sequence, etc., in treatment.

The meaning of root and branch has two aspects: (1) In terms of the human body and the disease, the human body is the root, and the disease is the branch. The purpose of treating diseases is to restore the patient's health. If one only focuses on the disease and ignores the human body, it will inevitably lead to the disease being cured but the vital qi being severely damaged, or the vital qi being damaged while the disease remains, or leaving sequelae resulting in disability, or even the disease being eliminated but the person dying along with it. This is the first thing that should be noted. (2) In terms of the cause and symptoms of the disease, the cause is the root, and the symptoms are the branch. The occurrence of symptoms must have a cause; if the cause can be removed, the symptoms will naturally disappear. TCM often says, "In treating diseases, one must seek the root", which refers to this.

The root refers to the fundamental cause. In treating diseases, it is essential to attach importance to the root, seek out the source, and understand the underlying reasons. That is to say, in treating diseases, one must grasp the main issue; once the main issue is resolved, the secondary ones will naturally be easily addressed. Hence, there are two sayings: "dispelling pathogens to support healthy qi" and "supporting healthy qi to dispel pathogens," holding that supporting healthy qi will naturally drive away pathogens, and driving away pathogens will naturally restore healthy qi. These two sayings may seem contradictory on the surface, but in fact, they both start from the root. For diseases caused by deficiency, supporting healthy qi is the main focus; for diseases caused by pathogens, dispelling pathogens takes precedence. Wang Yinghuan once wrote a poem about treating the root cause of diseases: "When seeing phlegm, do not rush to treat phlegm; when seeing blood, do not rush to treat blood; when there is no sweat, do not induce sweating; when there is heat, do not rush to clear heat; when there is asthma, do not consume qi; when there is spermatorrhea, do not astringe and stop it. Only when you understand the essence of this can you be an outstanding doctor." The meaning is that phlegm, blood loss, absence of sweat, fever, asthma, spermatorrhea, etc., are all superficial phenomena. Each of these conditions has a main cause. Without exploring the root cause and finding a solution, merely using conventional methods such as resolving phlegm, stopping bleeding, inducing sweating, clearing heat, relieving asthma, and securing essence will not work.

Although treating diseases must aim at the root, one cannot ignore the branch. We realize that seeking the cause is certainly necessary, and syndrome differentiation is equally important, as syndrome differentiation is for the purpose of finding the cause. However, on the other hand, besides identifying the main cause, it is also necessary to identify the main symptom, because quickly alleviating symptoms is an important part of relieving the patient's suffering. For example, in a wind-cold cold, there are symptoms such as fever, headache, general soreness, and restlessness. Wind-cold is the main cause, and other symptoms are caused by wind-cold. Among the symptoms, fever is a main symptom, and the degree of fever can aggravate or alleviate other symptoms. Therefore, using diaphoresis to disperse wind-cold is the main treatment method, but adding some heat-clearing medicines to help reduce fever and alleviate other symptoms is also reasonable. Previous doctors either prescribed medicines based solely on the cause or took symptoms into account. In ancient prescriptions, it is often noted what medicine to add for thirst, what medicine to add for cough, which shows that while treating the root, the branch was not neglected. But it should also be said that treating the root is the main thing, and treating the branch is secondary.

If one fails to distinguish between primary and secondary, and adds a certain medicine upon seeing a certain symptom, it will be chaotic and violate the principles of prescription formulation.

Clinically, if the branch symptoms are considered to have taken an important position, the method of treating the branch first should be adopted. For example, in ascites caused by liver disease, the liver disease is the root, and ascites is the branch. But when it reaches the point of abdominal distension, difficulty in breathing, and difficulty in urination and defecation, it is like a flood, and without dredging, the critical situation cannot be relieved. At this time, one can no longer use methods to soothe the liver; only strong medicines to purge water can be used, and after the water subsides, then consider treating the root. Another example: Difficulty in urination can quickly worsen the condition. Whenever difficulty in urination is found in any disease, promoting urination should be treated as an emergency. In addition, if a patient with phlegm asthma is choking and about to die, Chenxiang (agarwood) can be used temporarily to break qi; in laryngeal wind with swollen and blocked throat, unable to take soup and water, acupuncture can be used first to expel bad blood, and then medicines can be administered accordingly. Previous doctors said, "In acute cases, treat the branch." Treating the branch is originally an expedient measure, and it should not be continued after achieving the goal, which is the biggest difference from treating the root.

When a person suffers from two diseases at the same time, the root and branch must also be distinguished. Generally, the prior disease is the root, and the subsequent disease is the branch. The prior disease mostly refers to intractable chronic diseases, while the subsequent disease is often an acute illness such as a cold. In such cases, the cold should be treated first, followed by the chronic disease. This is because chronic diseases cannot be eliminated in a short time, while acute illnesses like colds are easy to resolve and can otherwise develop into severe conditions, exacerbating the chronic disease. There are also cases where a cold suddenly complicates with gastrointestinal disease, leading to diarrhea with undigested food and a pulse turning from floating to sinking. In such instances, fearing that external pathogens may invade internally taking advantage of deficiency, it is necessary to urgently treat the interior first, then resolve the exterior. These examples illustrate that treating the root is the principle in treatment, but under this principle, one should also grasp the order of priority and urgency, applying methods flexibly. *Huangdi Neijing* points out: "For those who first have cold and then develop illness, treat the root; for those who first have illness and then develop cold, treat the root; for those who first have heat and then develop illness, treat the root; for those who first have heat and then develop abdominal fullness, treat the branch; for those who first have illness and then develop diarrhea, treat the root; for those who first have diarrhea and then develop other illnesses, treat the root; for those who first have illness and then develop abdominal fullness, treat the branch; for those who first have abdominal fullness and then develop vexation, treat the root; for difficulty in urination and defecation, treat the branch; for normal urination and defecation, treat the root; for those who first have difficulty in urination and defecation and then develop illness, treat the root. When a disease occurs with excess, root first then branch, treating the root first, then the branch; when a disease occurs with deficiency, branch first then root, treating the branch first, then the root." The above statements are very specific about the methods of treating root and branch. Therefore, *Huangdi Neijing* also summarized: "Those who understand root and branch will succeed in all endeavors; those who do not understand root and branch act blindly."

III. The Eight Methods

After identifying the condition, the next step is to select the treatment method. Treatment methods include diaphoresis, emesis, purgation, harmonization, clearing, warming, resolving, and tonification, which are abbreviated as the eight methods: sweat, vomit, purge, harmonize, clear, warm, resolve, and tonify. These eight methods point out the direction of treatment based on the cause, symptoms, and location of the disease. When flexibly applied in clinical practice, more methods can be derived.

1. Diaphoresis

Aimed at dispelling wind and cold, it is often used when external pathogens invade the muscular superficies, as stated in *Huangdi Neijing*: "For pathogens in the skin, dispel them with diaphoresis." Hence, it is also called relieving the exterior, resolving the muscles, or dispersing. For example, in the initial stage of exogenous disease, with aversion to cold, fever, headache, and joint pain, after sweating, the fever subsides, the body cools down, and all symptoms disappear.

Diaphoresis can be divided into two types: pungent-warm diaphoresis, suitable for exterior cold syndromes caused by exogenous wind-cold; and pungent-cool diaphoresis, suitable for exterior heat syndromes caused by exogenous wind-warm or wind-heat. For cases where cold and heat are not obvious, a pungent-mild diaphoresis can be used.

The main purpose of diaphoresis is to induce sweating. If a patient has an exterior syndrome with spontaneous sweating or has already been given a diaphoretic, can diaphoresis be applied again? This must be determined based on specific circumstances. Generally, exterior syndrome is characterized by aversion to cold and fever as the main symptoms. If after sweating the fever does not subside and aversion to cold remains, it indicates that the exterior pathogens are not eliminated, and diaphoresis is still appropriate. If there is no aversion to cold, but the fever does not subside, or the fever increases, suggesting that the pathogen tends to transmit inward, diaphoresis should not be applied again.

Diaphoresis can dispel external pathogens but can also consume fluids. It should be used cautiously in patients with blood deficiency, heart weakness, or ulcers to avoid complications such as convulsions. Excessive sweating, with unceasing perspiration, can also lead to the risk of collapse.

Diaphoresis includes the method of diffusing the lung. For example, in wind-cold cough, nasal congestion, and hoarseness, medicines that lightly disperse the upper jiao are used. The purpose is not to induce sweating but to promote the diffusion of lung qi.

2. Emesis

Often used for blockage of phlegm and food in the throat and chest diaphragm. For example, in laryngeal conditions such as tangling throat wind and lockjaw throat wind, which are caused by obstruction of wind-phlegm and stagnant fire, resulting in unbearable swelling and blockage; another example is stagnation of accumulated food with fullness and pain in the chest diaphragm. As long as the contents are vomited out, relief can be achieved. Hence, it is also called vomiting induction, which is what *Huangdi Neijing* refers to as "for those in the upper part, let them rise and escape."

Emesis methods all use emetic medicines, but sometimes medicines are chosen based on the syndrome. After taking the medicine, a chicken feather or finger is used to stimulate the throat to induce vomiting, so it is also called inducing vomiting method.

Emesis is mostly used for tangible excess pathogens in the upper part of the stomach. Generally, one episode of vomiting brings relief, and repeated use is not necessary. For patients who have vomiting initially, not only should emesis not be applied again, but also care should be taken to prevent damage to the stomach, and methods to harmonize the middle jiao should be given. In other cases, emesis is inappropriate for weak patients, those who have just given birth, or those with cold limbs.

Using emesis for acute diseases, which contains a meaning of dispersion, can also relieve the exterior and reduce fever. In miscellaneous diseases or women's diseases, emesis can replace the lifting method; for example, predecessors also used emesis to treat urinary retention or pregnancy-related uterine obstruction.

3. Purgation

Generally refers to promoting bowel movements to eliminate accumulated feces in the intestines, so it is also called purgation therapy or cathartic method, which is what *Huangdi Neijing* refers to as "for those in the lower part, guide and exhaust them."

Purgative formulas are divided into two categories: One is drastic purgation, using powerful laxatives, mostly used in excess heat syndromes with a tendency of fluid depletion and yin exhaustion, namely the so-called "urgent purgation to preserve yin." The other is mild purgation, which is further divided into two types: One using relatively mild laxatives, and the other using oily and moist agents to assist in downward movement. However, whether drastic or mild purgation, they are all suitable for excess syndromes, which is consistent.

Due to different causes of interior excess, there are two types: cool purgation and warm purgation. Cool purgation refers to bitter-cold laxatives, and warm purgation refers to acrid-heat laxatives. Generally, bitter-cold ones are used more often because most cases of constipation or diarrhea are caused by heat accumulation or damp-heat.

Besides promoting bowel movements, purgation is also used for untransformed phlegm-fluid, coagulated blood stasis, and ascites with abdominal distension, etc. The medicines used in these cases are different from those for bowel movements.

When using purgation, the patient's constitution must be considered, and contraindications must be understood. In general, it cannot be used for exterior syndromes without interior syndromes, for interior syndromes that are not excess syndromes, or for constipation due to fluid deficiency in post-illness or post-partum periods. Misusing purgation in deficiency syndromes can easily damage the acquired foundation (spleen and stomach), causing hiccups or even collapse.

4. Harmonization

Harmonization means reconciling. Pathogens in the exterior can be treated with diaphoresis, and those in the interior with purgation. If pathogens are in the half-exterior and half-interior, where neither diaphoresis nor purgation is applicable, and the condition is progressing, a relatively mild method is needed to eliminate pathogens. Hence, the harmonization method is used in exogenous diseases, with the main purpose still being to expel pathogens.

In miscellaneous diseases, the use of harmonization has a slightly different meaning. For example, in cases of blood deficiency with consumptive heat, reduced appetite, and irregular menstruation in women, methods to harmonize the liver and spleen can be used. Another example: chest fullness without pain, epigastric upset with nausea, and intermingled phlegm and heat can be treated with methods of acrid opening and bitter descending to harmonize the stomach. Additionally, for those affected by summerheat-dampness, with internal injury from diet, indistinct cold and heat, head distension, chest tightness, and stagnation in the abdomen, aromatic transformation and harmonizing the middle jiao can be used. Such cases all fall within the scope of harmonization.

Therefore, the application of harmonization is quite extensive, including reconciling shaoyang, calming the interior and repelling the exterior, regulating qi and blood, smoothing qi movement, aromatic transformation and harmonizing the middle jiao, etc. Although the purposes are the same, the methods vary.

5. Clearing Method

Any treatment using cooling and refreshing agents to treat warm-heat conditions is called the clearing method, which is what *Huangdi Neijing* refers to as "treating heat with cold," also known as the clearing and resolving method.

Warm-heat syndromes include exterior heat, interior heat, deficiency heat, excess heat, heat in the qi level, and heat in the blood level. When using cooling agents, it is necessary to distinguish the nature of the heat and its location. For example, exterior heat syndromes should use acrid-cool medicines; for interior heat with deficiency syndromes, sweet-cold medicines are adopted; for excess syndromes, bitter-cold medicines are used. Clear heat in the qi level for qi-level heat, and clear heat in the blood level for blood-level heat.

The clearing method includes sedation and detoxification. For instance, when liver yang or liver fire disturbs upward, causing dizziness and head distension, liver-clearing formulas can calm wind and relieve pain; in cases of warm toxicity, using heat-clearing and nutrient-cooling methods has a detoxifying effect.

Clinically, the clearing and resolving method is used relatively frequently, but it should not be overused or used for a long time, especially bitter-cold medicines, which can damage the spleen and stomach and affect digestion. It should be used with caution in those with inherently weak constitutions, inherently cold *zang-fu* organs, poor appetite, loose stools, as well as post-illness or post-partum conditions.

6. Warming Method

Often used for cold diseases, which is what *Huangdi Neijing* refers to as "treating cold with heat."

Cold diseases can be distinguished into exterior cold, interior cold, etc. However, in terms of the warming method, it generally refers to interior cold, so warming the middle jiao is the main treatment. For example, vomiting clear water, loose stools with diarrhea, abdominal pain with a preference for pressure, cold limbs, a deep, hidden, slow, and faint pulse are all targets of the warming method.

Cold diseases can be caused by cold pathogens directly attacking the internal organs, or gradually forming due to yang deficiency. Therefore, the use of the warming method either focuses on expelling cold or on supporting yang. But the purpose of expelling cold is to prevent damage to yang, also called restoring yang; supporting yang is also to dispel deep-seated and chronic cold. There is an interrelationship between the two.

The warming method includes an excitatory effect. Some syndromes caused by yang deficiency, such as spontaneous sweating with coldness, poor digestion, shortness of breath with a weak voice, limp limbs with fatigue, urinary incontinence, and decreased sexual desire, all require conditioning with the warming method.

The warming method is often used in combination with other methods. For example, the diaphoresis method is divided into acrid-warm and acrid-cool; the purgation method is divided into warm purgation and cool purgation; the tonification method is divided into warm tonification and cool tonification.

7. Reducing Method

Mainly refers to promoting digestion to eliminate stagnation in the intestines and stomach. For example, internal obstruction due to food accumulation with abdominal fullness is treated with digestion and conduction. Secondly, it is reducing hardness, mostly used for syndromes with condensed and formed masses, such as abdominal masses and scrofula. Because such syndromes are mostly caused by stagnation of qi, blood, phlegm, and stasis, they develop gradually and resolve slowly, which cannot be completely eliminated by aggressive purgation. They require grinding, moving, and dissipating methods to achieve results gradually. Thirdly, it is reducing phlegm. Phlegm turbidity has various causes, including cold phlegm, damp phlegm, phlegm-heat, and stubborn phlegm, so methods such as warming transformation, clearing transformation, purging phlegm, and resolving phlegm are used respectively, collectively called reducing phlegm.

Promoting diuresis is also within the reducing method. It is normal for water-dampness to be excreted through urine. If water-dampness accumulates internally, with oliguria, or is excreted through the intestines causing diarrhea, it should be guided to be discharged through urine, generally called diuresis, also known as bland diffusion. This method can disperse and eliminate water-dampness, so it is also called separate drainage or separate reduction.

In some aspects, the reducing method is close to the harmonization method and the purgation method, but the harmonization method focuses on reconciling, while the reducing method has a nature of reducing and eliminating; the purgation method focuses on aggressive purging, while the reducing method has the meaning of assisting movement. Therefore, the reducing method is not suitable for extremely deficient people nor for acute conditions; it is a method of eliminating pathogens and grinding accumulations between the two.

8. Tonifying Method

It is to supplement insufficient physical strength, thereby eliminating all debilitating syndromes. Hence, *Huangdi Neijing* says "tonify for deficiency." The medicines used are mostly nourishing, so it is also called nourishing or supplementing.

In clinical practice, the tonifying method is divided into replenishing qi, nourishing blood, benefiting essence, calming the spirit, promoting the production of body fluids, filling the marrow, etc. In short, its purpose is to strengthen the body.

Tonics can be divided into three natures: One is warm tonification, used for yang deficiency syndromes; another is clear tonification, used for yin deficiency syndromes; and the third is mild tonification, used for general deficiency syndromes.

Due to the varying severity of the condition, it is further divided into drastic tonification and gentle tonification. Drastic tonification is often used for extremely weak and deficient bodies, or to rescue collapse for emergency purposes; gentle tonification is used for those who are deficient but cannot tolerate strong tonics, or who are deficient without extreme cold or heat symptoms, and only suitable for mild formulations to nourish gradually.

When using the tonifying method, attention must be paid to the spleen and stomach, because most tonics are stagnant and difficult to digest. On the one hand, those with weak spleen and stomach cannot properly circulate the medicinal effects; on the other hand, they will also affect digestion and absorption.

The tonifying method includes the astringent method. For example, in cases of incessant heavy sweating, incessant severe hematemesis, long-term unhealed spermatorrhea and slipping of sperm in men, metrorrhagia and excessive leukorrhea in women, astringent medicines mostly rely on the assistance of the tonifying method.

Failing to tonify when there is deficiency will inevitably lead to damage over time, making it more difficult to treat; however, tonifying when it is not needed can also cause pathological changes, especially when residual pathogens are not completely eliminated, using tonics early will have the disadvantage of "closing the door and retaining the thief".

The above is an overview of the eight methods, from which we can see that each of the eight methods has its unique function, but they are not used in isolation but are interrelated. Therefore, after understanding the meaning of the eight methods, we must further understand the connections between them and how to comprehensively apply them, so as to flexibly adapt to changes in the condition and achieve better therapeutic effects.

First of all, it should be pointed out that most of the eight methods are relative. For example, the diaphoresis method is used for exterior syndromes, and the purgation method is used for interior syndromes; since exterior and interior are relative, the diaphoresis and purgation methods are naturally relative. Moreover, the purgation method is to expel pathogenic factors, and the tonifying method is to support healthy qi; clearing can reduce heat, with a sedative effect, and warming can dispel cold, with an excitatory effect. Purgation and tonification, clearing and warming are also relative. However, diaphoresis and purgation, purgation and tonification, clearing and warming can all be used in combination, which is what is called in clinical practice "relieving both exterior and interior", "simultaneously attacking and tonifying", "using both cold and warm", etc. In short, a disease can have multiple causes and can occur in several parts. Especially in the course of a disease's development, the situation is often complex, so multiple methods must be used flexibly for treatment.

Examples are as follows:

(1) Combined use of diaphoresis and purgation: When there are both exterior and interior syndromes, the usual method is to first relieve the exterior and then attack the interior. But when both exterior and interior are acute, one cannot stick to the routine, but can use diaphoresis and purgation together, working on both aspects. For example, Guizhi Decoction, which relieves the exterior, can be added with rhubarb to attack the interior, treating exterior-interior syndromes with cold, heat, headache accompanied by abdominal fullness and pain.

(2) Combined use of purgation and tonification: When a person with an inherently weak constitution is affected by excess pathogens, or when pathogens persist and healthy qi gradually declines, resulting in a situation of deficient healthy qi and excess pathogens, expelling pathogens may worry about the inability of healthy qi to sustain, and tonifying healthy qi may fear the consolidation of pathogens. Only by combining purgation and tonification can both aspects be taken into account. For example, Huanglong Decoction uses rhubarb and mirabilite to unblock the bowels, and also uses ginseng and angelica to nourish qi and blood.

(3) Combined use of cold and warm: When a disease presents with upper heat and lower cold, or upper cold and lower heat, one cannot focus on only one aspect. For example, Huanglian Decoction uses Huanglian (Coptis) and Ganjiang (Dried Ginger) to treat heat in the chest, pathogenic factors in the stomach, and abdominal pain, which is the meaning of combining cold and warm. There are many such examples. Clinically, conditions such as the condensation of dampness and heat pathogens, or the binding of fluid retention and heat pathogens, are mostly treated with Sanren Decoction and Xiexin Decoction. The former uses Houpo (Magnolia Bark) together with Huashi (Talc), and the latter uses Banxia (Pinellia) together with Huanglian (Coptis), both of which are methods of combining

cold and warm.

In addition, one reducing and one tonifying method can also be used together. For example, in cases of weak spleen and stomach, indigestion, and stagnation of food accumulation, Baizhu (Atractylodes Macrocephala) is used to tonify the middle jiao and strengthen the spleen, while Zhishi (Immature Bitter Orange) is used to reduce distension and widen the diaphragm, combined to form Zhizhu Pills. Furthermore, the harmonization method is designed for conditions where diaphoresis and purgation are inappropriate, with Xiaochaihu Decoction as its representative formula. However, it must also be modified in combination with other methods according to different syndromes: For example, if there is a tendency to cold, Huangqin (Scutellaria) is removed; if there is a tendency to heat, Huangqin is increased; if there is a tendency to deficiency, Renshen (Ginseng) is used in larger amounts; if there is a tendency to excess, Renshen is reduced; if there is a tendency to dryness, Tianhuafen (Trichosanthes Root) is added; if there is a tendency to dampness, Shengjiang (Fresh Ginger) and Banxia are used in larger amounts; if there is a tendency to exterior syndrome, Guizhi (Cinnamon Twig) is added; if there is a tendency to interior syndrome, Mangxiao (Mirabilite) is added. In this way, the same harmonization method also includes clearing, warming, diaphoresis, purgation, tonification, and other methods.

Therefore, to further explain the application of the eight methods, in fact, it is rare to use a single method alone. The reason is that the eight methods are formulated based on the three factors (endogenous, exogenous, and non-endogenous non-exogenous causes), the four diagnostic methods, and the eight principles. Each disease has its cause and location, and the eight methods are established to address these aspects. However, among the eight methods, diaphoresis, emesis, purgation, and harmonization only indicate the location of the disease without explaining the cause, while warming, clearing, reducing, and tonification only indicate the cause without explaining the location. Meanwhile, the same cause can present different symptoms when affecting different locations. Therefore, after understanding the eight methods, it is still insufficient if one does not know how to combine them. As mentioned above, diaphoresis includes acrid-warm diaphoresis, acrid-cool diaphoresis, and acrid-mild diaphoresis; purgation includes warm purgation, cool purgation, and moist purgation, etc. These are all specific measures formulated based on the cause, location, and symptoms. To put it more clearly, for example, in tonification, one must ask: In which aspect is the deficiency? What components are lacking? What is its nature? What symptoms does it present? Assuming the answer is: deficiency in the liver, insufficient blood, with symptoms such as internal heat and dizziness. Then, methods of nourishing yin and blood, supplemented by sedation, can be adopted. Otherwise, with an unclear target and blind tonification, even if some parts are correct, the effect will not be significant.

While applying the eight methods appropriately, one must also understand their contraindications. *Treatise on Cold Damage* puts forward the pulse and symptoms of diseases that can or cannot be treated with diaphoresis, emesis, or purgation. Later, Cheng Zhongling wrote "On the Eight Methods" (*Medical Insights*), which is more detailed. He explained the indications for each treatment method, and also pointed out various drawbacks such as not using when it should be used, using when it should not be used, situations where it should not be used but cannot be avoided, and using when it should be used but knowing how to start but not how to stop, all confirmed with specific examples, which are extremely helpful in clinical practice and can be referred to.

IV. Treatment Methods Used Commonly

There are quite a few commonly used treatment methods in prescriptions, and they are quite detailed. These methods are the results of flexibly applying the eight methods in combination with the cause and syndrome to specific problems, serving as a good model for further research. Here are some examples with additional explanations as follows.

1. **Acrid-warm diaphoresis:** Used for exterior syndrome due to exogenous wind-cold, with absence of sweating and a floating-tight pulse. Medicinal herbs include Mahuang (Ephedra), Guizhi (Cinnamon Twig), Zisu (Perilla), and Congbai (Welsh Onion).
2. **Acrid-cool exterior-relieving:** Used for the initial stage of wind-warm syndrome. Medicinal herbs include Douchi (Fermented Soybean), Fangfeng (Saposhnikovia), Bohe (Mentha), Sangye (Mulberry Leaf), and Juhua (Chrysanthemum).
3. **Lightly diffusing lung qi:** Used for hoarseness due to wind invasion, where the lung (metal) is excess and fails to sound. Medicinal herbs include Mahuang (Ephedra), Chantui (Cicada Slough), Jiegeng (Platycodon). If there is nasal congestion and discharge, Xinyi (Magnolia Flower) and Cang'erzi (Xanthium) are used.
4. **Clearing and dispersing summer wind:** Used for summer colds. Medicinal herbs include Xiangru (Elsholtzia), Huoxiang (Agastache), Qinghao (Artemisia Annua), and Peilan (Eupatorium).
5. **Dispersing and transforming exterior dampness:** Used for exogenous dampness from mist, dew, rain. Medicinal herbs include Cangzhu (Atractylodes), Baizhi (Angelica Dahurica), Fangfeng (Saposhnikovia).
6. **Clearing qi and moistening dryness:** Used for affection by autumn dryness, with impaired clear orifices. Medicinal herbs include Bohe (Mentha), Jiaoshanzhi (Charred Gardenia), Lianqiao (Forsythia),

Sangye (Mulberry Leaf), Xingren (Apricot Kernel).

7. **Relieving both aspects of Taiyang:** Used for wind-dampness, dispersing wind to relieve Taiyang channel, and draining dampness to infiltrate Taiyang fu (i.e., bladder). Medicinal herbs include Qianghuo (Notopterygium), Fangfeng (Saposhnikovia), Zexie (Alisma), Fuling (Poria).
8. **Removing impediment pain:** Used for wind-cold-damp impediment, with joint pain. Medicinal herbs include Guizhi (Cinnamon Twig), Qianghuo (Notopterygium), Duhuo (Angelica Pubescens), Chuanwu (Aconitum), Caowu (Aconitum Kusnezoffii), Haifengteng (Piper Kadsura).
9. **Harmonizing nutrient and defense:** Used for wind damage, relieving the muscles and dispersing pathogens by harmonizing qi and blood, different from direct exterior dispersion. Medicinal herbs include Guizhi (Cinnamon Twig), Baishao (White Peony Root), Shengjiang (Fresh Ginger), Hongzao (Jujube).
10. **Securing the exterior and dispelling pathogens:** Used for frail constitution prone to colds, or lingering colds. Medicinal herbs include Huangqi (Astragalus), Baizhu (Atractylodes Macrocephala), Fangfeng (Saposhnikovia).
11. **Cooling and expelling pathogens:** Used for exogenous disease with unresolved sweating, where pathogens tend to transform into heat and transmit inward. Medicinal herbs include Gegen (Pueraria), Jinyinhua (Honeysuckle), Lianqiao (Forsythia), Bohe (Mentha), Lugen (Reed Rhizome).
12. **Acrid-cold clearing the stomach:** Used for stomach heat syndrome, with a slippery, large, and rapid pulse. Medicinal herbs include Shigao (Gypsum), Zhimu (Anemarrhena), Huashi (Talc), Zhuru (Bamboo Shavings).
13. **Bitter-cold purging fire:** Used for warm pathogens transforming into

fire, blazing in the triple jiao. Medicinal herbs include Huanglian (Coptis), Huangqin (Scutellaria), Dahuang (Rhubarb), Jiaoshanzhi (Charred Gardenia).

14. **Clearing and transforming damp-heat:** Used for warm pathogens with dampness, or intermingled spleen dampness and stomach heat. Medicinal herbs include Huangqin (Scutellaria), Houpo (Magnolia Bark), Huashi (Talc), Banxia (Pinellia), Tongcao (Tetrapanax).
15. **Dispelling summerheat and regulating primordial qi:** Used for summerheat damaging qi. Medicinal herbs include Renshen (Ginseng), Maidong (Ophiopogon), Wuweizi (Schisandra), Zhuye (Bamboo Leaf).
16. **Clearing pestilence and detoxifying:** Used for warm-toxin syndrome. Medicinal herbs include Daqingye (Isatis Leaf), Banlangen (Isatis Root), Xuanshen (Scrophularia), Mabo (Lasiosphaera).
17. **Clearing the nutrient level and expelling macules:** Used for heat in the nutrient level with eruption of macules and rashes. Medicinal herbs include Shengdi (Rehmannia), Doujuan (Germinated Soybean), Shigao (Gypsum), Chishao (Red Peony Root), Danpi (Moutan Bark).
18. **Clearing and purging the pericardium:** Used for warm pathogens invading the pericardium, with clouded consciousness and delirium. Medicinal preparations include Zixuedan (Purple Snow Pill), Niuhuang Qingxin Wan (Bezoar Heart-Clearing Pill); for cases with dampness, Shenxidan (Divine Rhinoceros Pill) is used.
19. **Purging interior excess heat:** Used for heat accumulation in the intestines and stomach, constipation. Medicinal herbs include Dahuang (Rhubarb), Zhishi (Immature Bitter Orange), Xuanmingfen (Sodium Sulfate).
20. **Clearing, transforming, and eliminating accumulation:** Used for damp-heat with food stagnation, abdominal pain and diarrhea. Medicinal herbs include Muxiang (Costus), Zhishi (Immature Bitter

Orange), Huanglian (Coptis), Qingpi (Green Tangerine Peel), Binglang (Areca Nut).

21. **Clearing and descending ministerial fire:** Used for hyperactivity of liver and gallbladder fire. Medicinal herbs include Longdancao (Gentiana), Chishao (Red Peony Root), Huangqin (Scutellaria), Jiaoshanzhi (Charred Gardenia), Mutong (Akebia).
22. **Acrid-hot expelling cold:** Used for cold pathogens directly attacking the three yin channels. Medicinal herbs include Fuzi (Aconite), Ganjiang (Dried Ginger), Rougui (Cinnamon Bark).
23. **Sweet-warm tonifying yang:** Used for kidney yang deficiency. Medicinal herbs include Lurong (Deer Antler), Gouqizi (Lycium), Bajitian (Morinda).
24. **Warming and activating spleen yang:** Used for spleen cold deficiency. Medicinal herbs include Baizhu (Atractylodes Macrocephala), Paojiang (Roasted Ginger), Rouguo (Myristica).
25. **Acrid-slippery unblocking yang:** Used for chest impediment, where yang is obstructed by cold. Medicinal herbs include Xiebai (Allium Macrostemon), Guizhi (Cinnamon Twig), Gualou (Trichosanthes).
26. **Supplementing Fire to Nourish Earth:** Used for decline of life-gate fire with prolonged spleen-deficiency diarrhea. Medicinal herbs include Buguzhi (Psoralea), Yizhiren (Alpinia Oxyphylla), Paojiang (Roasted Ginger).
27. **Guiding Fire Back to Its Source:** Used for floating yang rising upward, with upper heat and lower cold. Medicinal herbs include Shudi (Processed Rehmannia), Fuzi (Aconite), Rougui (Cinnamon Bark), Wuweizi (Schisandra).
28. **Calming the Liver and Regulating Qi:** Used for rebellious rising of liver qi with chest and abdominal distension and pain. Medicinal herbs include Qingpi (Green Tangerine Peel), Zhiqiao (Bitter Orange), Chuanlianzi (Melia Toosendan), Yanhusuo (Corydalis).

29. **Soothing the Liver and Harmonizing Collaterals:** Used for hypochondriac pain with long-standing disorder entering the collaterals. Medicinal herbs include Danshen (Salvia), Taoren (Peach Kernel), Yujin (Curcuma), Juluo (Tangerine Pith).
30. **Dispersing Qi and Relieving Middle Distension:** Used for chest tightness, belching, and frequent flatulence. Medicinal herbs include Xiangfu (Cyperus), Chenpi (Tangerine Peel), Zhiqiao (Bitter Orange), Foshou (Citrus Medica).
31. **Lowering Qi and Calming Rebellion:** Used for excess syndrome of asthma. Medicinal herbs include Chenxiang (Agarwood), Tanxiang (Sandalwood), Wuyao (Lindera), Zhishi (Immature Bitter Orange).
32. **Heavy Sedation to Lower Rebellion:** Used for deficient stomach with hiccups and upward rushing qi. Medicinal herbs include Daizheshi (Hematite), Cishi (Magnetite).
33. **Regulating Liver and Spleen:** Used for liver-spleen qi stagnation. Medicinal herbs include Danggui (Angelica), Baishao (White Peony Root), Chaihu (Bupleurum), Baizhu (Atractylodes Macrocephala), Fuling (Poria).
34. **Promoting Qi and Expelling Stasis:** Used for dysmenorrhea in women with scanty menstruation and blood stasis. Medicinal herbs include Chuanxiong (Ligusticum), Honghua (Safflower), Yimucao (Motherwort), Xiangfu (Cyperus).
35. **Warming the Channels and Harmonizing Nutrient:** Used for cold in the blood with delayed menstruation. Medicinal herbs include Danggui (Angelica), Airong (Moxa Wool), Rougui (Cinnamon Bark).
36. **Clearing Heat and Cooling Blood:** Used for bleeding due to heat in the blood, or advanced menstruation. Medicinal herbs include Shengdi (Rehmannia), Danpi (Moutan Bark), Cebaiye (Platycladus Leaf), Oujie (Lotus Node), Huangqin (Scutellaria).
37. **Warming and Unblocking Liver Channel:** Used for cold pain in the

lower abdomen, or hernia with swelling and sagging. Medicinal herbs include Wuyao (Lindera), Xiaohuixiang (Fennel), Lizihou (Lychee Seed), Yanhusuo (Corydalis).

38. **Activating Blood and Relieving Pain:** Used for stagnant blood retention and traumatic injuries. Medicinal herbs include Honghua (Safflower), Shensanqi (Notoginseng), Tubiechong (Eupolyphaga), Luodedda (Centella), Ruxiang (Frankincense), Moyao (Myrrh).
39. **Resolving Masses and Eliminating Accumulation:** Used for abdominal masses and hepatosplenomegaly. Medicinal herbs include Sanleng (Sparganium), Peng'ezhu (Curcuma Zedoaria), Chuanshanjia (Pangolin).
40. **Diffusing Lung and Resolving Phlegm:** Used for wind-cold cough. Medicinal herbs include Niubangzi (Arctium), Jiegeng (Platycodon), Xingren (Apricot Kernel), Xiangbei (Fritillaria Thunbergii).
41. **Warming and Transforming Damp-Phlegm:** Used for cough with profuse thin white phlegm. Medicinal herbs include Banxia (Pinellia), Chenpi (Tangerine Peel), Fuling (Poria).
42. **Clearing and Resolving Phlegm-Heat:** Used for cough with sticky phlegm and latent heat in the lung. Medicinal herbs include Tianzhuhuang (Bamboo Mushroom), Chuanbei (Fritillaria Cirrhosa), Haizhe (Jellyfish), Biji (Water Chestnut).
43. **Purifying Lung and Expelling Phlegm:** Used for profuse phlegm with cough and asthma. Medicinal herbs include Suzi (Perilla Seed), Xuanfuhua (Inula), Baiguo (Ginkgo).
44. **Warming and Resolving Phlegm-Fluid:** Used for cough with phlegm-fluid retention. Medicinal herbs include Guizhi (Cinnamon Twig), Baizhu (Atractylodes Macrocephala), Banxia (Pinellia), Wuweizi (Schisandra), Ganjiang (Dried Ginger).
45. **Opening Orifices and Expelling Phlegm:** Used for apoplexy with coma and excessive phlegm. Medicinal herbs include Yuanzhi

(Polygala), Changpu (Acorus), Zhuli (Bamboo Juice), Zaojiaotan (Gleditsia 炭).

46. **Resolving Phlegm Nodules:** Used for scrofula. Medicinal herbs include Kunbu (Kelp), Haizao (Sargassum), Shancigu (Iphigenia), Jiangcan (Bombyx Batryticatus).
47. **Aromatic Transformation of Damp-Turbidity:** Used for dampness obstructing the middle jiao. Medicinal herbs include Cangzhu (Atractylodes), Houpo (Magnolia Bark), Chenpi (Tangerine Peel).
48. **Acrid-Aromatic Tonifying Stomach:** Used for qi obstruction with damp stagnation and poor appetite. Medicinal herbs include Doukou (Amomum), Sharen (Amomum Villosum), Foshou (Citrus Medica).
49. **Draining and Resolving Water-Dampness:** Used for retained dampness with dysuria. Medicinal herbs include Zexie (Alisma), Cheqianzi (Plantago Seed), Fuling(Poria). For jaundice with scanty reddish urine, Yinchenhao (Artemisia Capillaris) is used.
50. **Clearing and Relieving Strangury and Turbidity:** Used for stranguria with turbid urine and painful dysuria. Medicinal herbs include Qumai (Dianthus), Shiwei (Pyrrosia), Haijinsha (Lygodium), Bianxu (Polygonum Aviculare).
51. **Attacking and Expelling Water-Fluid:** Used for ascites or fluid retention in the chest and hypochondrium. Medicinal herbs include Tinglizi (Lepidium), Daji (Euphorbia Pekinensis), Gansui (Euphorbia Kansui), Qianniuzi (Pharbitis), Shanglu (Phytolacca).
52. **Resolving Edema by Differentiation:** Used for general edema. For edema in the upper body, diaphoresis is appropriate; for the lower body, diuresis is suitable, the so-called "opening the ghost gate" (referring to pores) and "purifying the bladder" (referring to the bladder). Medicinal herbs include Fuping (Duckweed), Fangfeng (Saposhnikovia), Dongguapi (Wax Gourd Peel), Shengjiangpi (Fresh Ginger Peel), Fangji (Stephania).

53. **Resolving Food Stagnation and Harmonizing the Middle Jiao:** Used for food retention syndrome. Medicinal herbs include Shenqu (Massa Fermentata), Shanzha (Hawthorn), Laifuzi (Raphanus Seed).

54. **Expelling Intestinal Parasites:** Used for parasitic accumulation with abdominal distension and emaciation. Medicinal herbs include Shijunzi (Quisqualis), Leiwan (Omphalia), Binglang (Areca Nut), Wuguchong (Gryllotalpa).

55. **Nourishing Blood and Tonifying the Liver:** Used for blood deficiency syndrome. Medicinal herbs include Heshouwu (Polygonum Multiflorum), Danggui Shen (Angelica Body), Baishao (White Peony Root), Tongshayuan (Astragalus Complanatus), Ejiao (Donkey-Hide Gelatin).

56. **Nourishing Kidney Yin:** Used for yin deficiency syndrome. Medicinal herbs include Shengdi (Rehmannia), Yurou (Cornus), Nvzhenzi (Ligustrum Lucidum).

57. **Softening the Liver and Subduing Yang:** Used for liver yang disturbing upward. Medicinal herbs include Baishao (White Peony Root), Juhua (Chrysanthemum), Tianma (Gastrodia), Gouteng (Uncaria).

58. **Nourishing Yin and Calming Wind:** Used for yin deficiency stirring internal wind. Medicinal herbs include Guiban (Turtle Shell), Muli (Oyster), Biejia (Soft-Shelled Turtle Shell), Daimao (Hawksbill Turtle Shell).

59. **Nourishing the Heart and Calming the Spirit:** Used for palpitations and insomnia. Medicinal herbs include Ejiao (Donkey-Hide Gelatin), Zaoren (Jujube Seed), Yejiaoteng (Polygonum Multiflorum Vine), Baiziren (Platycladus Seed).

60. **Nourishing Yin and Relieving Steaming Heat:** Used for yin deficiency with tidal fever. Medicinal herbs include Biejia (Soft-Shelled Turtle Shell), Digupi (Lycium Bark), Yinchaihu

(Stellaria), Danpi (Moutan Bark).

61. **Clearing and Nourishing the Lung:** Used for lung heat with qi and yin deficiency. Medicinal herbs include Shashen (Adenophora), Maidong (Ophiopogon), Yuzhu (Polygonatum).
62. **Sweet-Cool Promoting Fluid Production:** Used for consumption of stomach yin. Medicinal herbs include Shihu (Dendrobium), Tianhuafen (Trichosanthes Root), Lugen (Reed Rhizome).
63. **Tonifying Middle Qi:** Used for spleen and stomach qi deficiency. Medicinal herbs include Huangqi (Astragalus), Dangshen (Codonopsis), Baizhu (Atractylodes Macrocephala), Shanyao (Yam). For sinking of middle qi, Shengma (Cimicifuga) and Chaihu (Bupleurum) are used.
64. **Securing the Sperm Gate:** Used for spermatorrhea and involuntary emission. Medicinal herbs include Jinyingzi (Rosa Laevigata), Lianxu (Lotus Stamen), Lianrou (Lotus Seed), Duanshilong (Calcined Dragon Bone).
65. **Tonifying the Intestines and Astringing Prolapse:** Used for persistent diarrhea. Medicinal herbs include Biandou (Hyacinth Bean), Hezi (Chebula), Chishizhi (Red Halloysite), Mikel (Poppy Shell).
66. **Moistening the Intestines and Unblocking Bowels:** Used for dryness of the large intestine with hard, difficult stools. Medicinal herbs include Maren (Hemp Seed), Yuliren (Prunus Humilis Seed), Gualouren (Trichosanthes Seed).
67. **Raising Clear Qi and Lowering Turbid Qi:** Used for sinking of clear yang and obstruction of turbid qi in the middle. Medicinal herbs include Gegen (Pueraria), Shanyao (Yam), Biandou (Hyacinth Bean), Chenpi (Tangerine Peel).
68. **Communicating the Heart and Kidney:** Used for disharmony between fire and water with insomnia. Medicinal herbs include Huanglian (Coptis), Rougui (Cinnamon Bark).

69. **Promoting Mutual Generation of Metal and Water:** Used for deficiency of both lung and kidney with tidal fever and red cheeks. Medicinal herbs include Shengdi (Rehmannia), Tiandong (Asparagus), Maidong (Ophiopogon), Baihe (Lily).
70. **Cultivating Earth to Generate Metal:** Used for lung deficiency and spleen weakness where clear tonification is difficult. Medicinal herbs include Shanyao (Yam), Qianshi (Euryale), Biandou (Hyacinth Bean), Guya (Rice Sprout).
71. **Supporting Earth to Restrain Wood:** Used for liver hyperactivity and spleen weakness with abdominal pain and diarrhea. Medicinal herbs include Baizhu (Atractylodes Macrocephala), Fangfeng (Saposhnikovia), Baishao (White Peony Root), Chenpi (Tangerine Peel), Gancao (Licorice).

The above treatment methods: 1-10 are mostly used for exogenous syndromes; 11-28 are mostly used for cold and heat syndromes; 29-40 are mostly used for diseases of qi and blood levels; 41-55 are mostly used for phlegm, food, and water-damp syndromes; 56 onwards are mostly used for deficiency syndromes. In terms of the eight methods, many more principles have been derived, but they are still not comprehensive. There are more detailed treatment methods when dealing with specific syndromes. From these methods, it can be seen that the eight methods are therapeutic principles that must be selected after repeated research based on the cause, symptoms, and location of the disease. It can also be seen that several herbs have similar effects but different applications, which should be appropriately selected.

Chapter Three Formulas

Section 1 Formulation of Prescriptions

I. Monarch, Minister, Assistant, and Guide

A prescription composed of multiple medicinal herbs is called a formula. The composition of a formula follows certain rules, known as formulation principles. Therefore, a formula is a further development of treatment using single herbs. Its characteristics are: having a comprehensive effect, a broader therapeutic range, and being able to moderate the toxicity of herbs, reducing or avoiding adverse reactions.

The composition of a formula is divided into four aspects: monarch, minister, assistant, and guide. Generally, most prescriptions contain more than four kinds of herbs, all compatibilities according to these four aspects. Even if there are fewer than four herbs or as many as dozens, they cannot deviate from this principle. Otherwise, it would be disorganized with an unclear direction, which the predecessors referred to as "having herbs but no formula."

1. **Monarch:** The monarch is the main herb of a formula, a herb that can play a major role in targeting the main cause and main symptoms of a disease, which is what *Huangdi Neijing* says: "That which addresses the main disease is called the monarch." The monarch herb is not necessarily only one in a formula, nor is it necessary that only potent herbs can serve as the monarch. It is mainly determined based on specific circumstances and needs. Li Dongyuan once said: "For example, in treating wind, windproof is used as the monarch; in treating cold, monkshood is used as the monarch; in treating dampness, stephania is used as the monarch; in clearing the upper jiao, coptis is used as the monarch; in clearing the middle jiao, scutellaria is used as

the monarch." By analogy, even herbs with relatively mild properties such as mulberry leaf, chrysanthemum, dried tangerine peel, bamboo shavings, etc., are qualified to be monarch herbs.

2. **Minister:** *Huangdi Neijing* states: "That which assists the monarch is called the minister." The minister refers to herbs that assist and enhance the efficacy of the monarch herb. For example, cinnamon twig in Mahuang Decoction helps ephedra induce sweating to relieve the exterior, so it is the minister herb in Mahuang Decoction. The number of minister herbs in a formula is not limited to one; one monarch herb can be paired with several minister herbs; if there are two monarch herbs in a formula, more minister herbs can be used for compatibility.
3. **Assistant:** Below the minister is the assistant. The assistant herb is a compatible herb similar to the minister herb. In addition to assisting the monarch herb like the minister herb, it can also help the monarch herb relieve certain secondary symptoms. For example, almond is used as the assistant in Mahuang Decoction, and its effect is to diffuse the lung and calm cough, helping the monarch herb relieve the secondary symptoms of Mahuang Decoction syndrome. On the other hand, if the monarch herb is toxic or has an overly biased nature, the assistant herb can be used to moderate it.
4. **Guide:** From the meaning of the word "guide," the guide herb is the relatively least important herb in a formula. *Huangdi Neijing* says: "That which responds to the minister is called the guide." It can be seen that the guide herb is an auxiliary herb to the minister herb. In clinical practice, the guide herb is generally understood as a channel-guiding herb, which means leading the medicinal power to the disease location, so it is also called a guiding herb, commonly known as a medicine guide.

Although the terms such as monarch, minister, assistant, and guide have feudal connotations, they essentially represent the main herbs and auxiliary herbs to explain the organizational form of a formula. For thousands of years, TCM has accumulated extremely rich experience in the compatibility of formulas. Both classical formulas and contemporary formulas are formulated in accordance with this principle.

Incidentally, let me mention the issue of "classical formulas" and "contemporary formulas". The development of TCM from the use of single herbs to formulas happened a long time ago. In *Huangdi Neijing*, there are formulas such as the blood depletion formula composed of cuttlebone, rush, and sparrow eggs, the insomnia formula composed of prepared pinellia and glutinous rice, and the alcohol wind formula composed of alisma, atractylodes macrocephala, and piricularia. When Zhang Zhongjing extensively collected various formulas and wrote *Treatise on Cold Damage* and *Synopsis of the Golden Chamber*, formulas became more complete. Later generations valued his works as classics and called his formulas classical formulas, while referring to later formulas as contemporary formulas. We believe that the efficacy of classical formulas is confirmed, but the value of contemporary formulas is also undeniable. The formation of contemporary formulas is also one of the examples of the continuous development of TCM. For the same reason, as mentioned above, the six-channel syndrome differentiation method is mainly based on *Treatise on Cold Damage*, and the triple-jiao syndrome differentiation method is mainly based on *Systematic Differentiation of Warm Diseases*. One was in the Han Dynasty, and the other in the Qing Dynasty. They not only do not conflict but also complement each other. The formulas in *Systematic Differentiation of Warm Diseases* have many developments and supplements based on those in *Treatise on Cold Damage*. Therefore, under the goal of making the past serve the present, we should attach importance to classical formulas, contemporary formulas, and also effective modern formulas.

II. Seven Formulas

In application, formulas are divided into seven categories according to the number of herbs used and the speed of producing efficacy, referred to as the seven formulas for short, namely large formulas, small formulas, slow formulas, rapid formulas, odd formulas, even formulas, and compound formulas.

1. **Large formulas:** When pathogenic factors are strong and cannot be overcome without great strength, large formulas must be used. For example, Dachengqi Decoction in the purgation method is a large formula. When using large formulas, one should first consider whether the healthy qi can withstand it, because severe purgation can damage yin, and excessive sweating can cause yang exhaustion. If the pathogen is removed but the healthy qi is damaged accordingly, the significance of using a large formula is lost.
2. **Small formulas:** Small formulas are relative to large formulas. For mild and superficial pathogenic factors, only mild formulas are needed, or the dosage of a large formula is reduced, which is called a small formula. For example, Xiaochengqi Decoction in the purgation method is a small formula.
3. **Slow formulas:** For general chronic and debilitating diseases, which cannot be expected to take effect quickly, formulas with mild medicinal effects should be used for long-term conditioning. For example, Sijunzi Decoction in the tonification method belongs to slow formulas.
4. **Rapid formulas:** Rapid formulas are relative to slow formulas. They are used for emergency treatment when the disease condition is critical.

For example, in cases of incessant diarrhea, cold limbs, and a faint pulse on the verge of extinction, Sini Decoction is used to restore yang. For acute diseases, rapid formulas require not only specific medicinal effects but also large dosages, so they are often used in combination with large formulas.

5. **Odd formulas:** "Odd" refers to an odd number, and an odd formula means having a single focus. If there is only one cause of the disease, one monarch herb is used to treat the main symptom to ensure the specificity of the medicinal effect, so it is called an odd formula. However, an odd formula is not equivalent to a single herb; it also has minister herbs, assistant herbs, etc., for compatibility.
6. **Even formulas:** "Even" refers to an even number, implying considering both aspects. If there are two causes at the same time, requiring two monarch herbs for treatment, it is called an even formula. In clinical practice, what is called simultaneous application of diaphoresis and purgation, or combined use of attack and tonification, all belong to even formulas.
7. **Compound formulas:** "Compound" means complex or repeated. For conditions with multiple causes or complex pathogenesis, compound formulas are needed for treatment. For example, Wuji Powder is composed of formulas such as Mahuang Decoction, Guizhi Decoction, Pingwei Powder, and Erchen Decoction, using a single formula to dispel wind, cold, phlegm, dampness, as well as resolve focal distension and eliminate accumulation. Another meaning refers to cases where one method is ineffective, then another method is used; if that is also ineffective, yet another method is employed, as stated in *Huangdi Neijing*: "If the odd formula fails, use the even formula; if the even formula fails, use counter-assistance to eliminate it." Therefore, in certain situations, compound formulas are also called repeated formulas, differing from the general compound formulas that

are relative to single herbs.

The seven formulas are one of the principles for formulating prescriptions. In addition, there are classifications based on therapeutic effects. For example, Zhang Jingyue divided formulas into "eight arrays": tonifying array, harmonizing array, attacking array, dispersing array, cold array, hot array, securing array, and adaptive array. Formulas in the tonifying array are used for conditions of primordial qi deficiency and physical weakness; those in the harmonizing array are used to regulate the excess of pathogenic factors; those in the attacking array are used for internal excess syndromes; those in the dispersing array are used for exogenous syndromes; those in the cold array are used for heat syndromes; those in the hot array are used for cold syndromes; those in the securing array are used for syndromes of unchecked diarrhea; those in the adaptive array are formulated according to specific symptoms. Currently, the classification of formulas generally follows that in Wang Ang's *Collected Explanations of Medical Formulas*, which divides them into 22 categories:

(1) Tonifying and nourishing formulas: Nourish deficiencies of yin, yang, qi, and blood in the human body, eliminating all debilitating conditions, such as Liuwei Dihuang Pills, Sijunzi Decoction, etc.

(2) Exterior-releasing formulas: Disperse external pathogens, relieving exterior syndromes, such as Mahuang Decoction, Guizhi Decoction, etc.

(3) Emetic formulas: Guide pathogens upward, inducing vomiting, such as Gualou 蒂 Powder, Shenlu Powder, etc.

(4) Interior-attacking formulas: Mainly promote bowel movements and guide out stagnation, clearing excess pathogens in the intestines and stomach, such as Dachengqi Decoction, Daxianxiong Decoction, etc.

(5) Exterior-interior formulas: Both disperse exterior pathogens and eliminate interior pathogens, relieving both exterior and interior, such as

Dachaihu Decoction, Guizhi plus Dahuang Decoction, etc.

(6) Harmonizing formulas: Achieve the purpose of eliminating pathogens through harmonizing methods, such as Xiaochaihu Decoction, Xiaoyao Powder, etc.

(7) Qi-regulating formulas: Soothe qi movement, relieve stagnation and descend rebellion, such as Siqi Decoction, Xuanfu Daizhe Decoction, etc.

(8) Blood-regulating formulas: Harmonize blood and dispel stasis, nourish the nutrient system and stop bleeding, such as Siwu Decoction, Jiaoai Decoction, etc.

(9) Wind-dispelling formulas: Unblock yang and disperse wind, nourish yin and calm wind, such as Xiaoxuming Decoction, Dihuang Yinzi, etc.

(10) Cold-dispelling formulas: Support yang and warm the middle, expel internal cold, such as Zhenwu Decoction, Sini Decoction, etc.

(11) Summerheat-clearing formulas: Clear summerheat pathogens, such as Xiangru Drink, Liuyi Powder, etc.

(12) Dampness-draining formulas: Eliminate water-dampness, such as Wucha Powder, Wupi Drink, etc.

(13) Dryness-moistening formulas: Moisten dryness of fluids and blood, such as Qiongyu Ointment, Xiaoke Formula, etc.

(14) Fire-purging formulas: Clear heat and detoxify, such as Baihu Decoction, Huanglian Jiedu Decoction, etc.

(15) Phlegm-removing formulas: Resolve and expel phlegm, such as Erchen Decoction, Mengshi Guntan Pills, etc.

(16) Food-dispersing formulas: Eliminate accumulation and promote

qi, strengthen the spleen and stomach, such as Zhizhu Pills, Baohe Pills, etc.

(17) Astringent formulas: Astringe essence and qi, secure and stop leakage, such as Zhenren Yangzang Decoction, Jinsuo Gujing Pills, etc.

(18) Anthelmintic formulas: Expel intestinal parasites, such as Jixiao Pills, Huachong Pills, etc.

(19) Eye-benefiting formulas: Specifically treat eye diseases, such as Yanggan Pills, Boyun Tuiyi Pills, etc.

(20) Carbuncle and ulcer formulas: Specifically treat surgical swollen ulcers and open ulcers, such as Zhenren Huoming Yin (Nobleman's Life-Preserving Drink), Sanzhong Kuijian Tang (Swelling-Reducing and Hardness-Breaking Decoction), etc.

(21) Menstrual and obstetric formulas: Specifically treat gynecological menstrual diseases, as well as pre-natal and post-natal conditions, such as Liuhe Decoction (Six-Harmony Decoction), Dasheng Yin (Fetal Delivery Drink), etc.

(22) Emergency formulas: Including formulas for first aid in cases of death from freezing, drowning, and venomous insect bites, etc.

TCM formulas are generally difficult to classify because a single formula often has multiple effects and thus cannot be confined to a single category. Even if several formulas have the same therapeutic purpose, their applications can differ greatly. For example, tonifying and nourishing formulas are not only used for deficiency syndromes but also for other conditions; moreover, tonifying formulas are not suitable for all deficiency syndromes. In addition, the addition or subtraction of herbs in a formula and the amount of dosage can change its nature and effects. For instance, Mahuang Decoction, composed of ephedra, cinnamon twig, almond, and licorice, is a diaphoretic and exterior-releasing formula. If cinnamon twig is replaced with gypsum, it becomes Maxing Shigan Decoction, which treats heat in the lung with asthma. If cinnamon twig is removed, it becomes San'ao Decoction, which treats wind-cold colds, nasal congestion, cough, etc. Another example: Xiaochengqi Decoction and Houpo Sanwu Decoction are both composed of rhubarb, immature bitter orange, and magnolia bark. However, in Xiaochengqi Decoction, rhubarb is the monarch herb, and magnolia bark is the assistant, with the dosage of magnolia bark being half that of rhubarb; in Houpo Sanwu Decoction, magnolia bark is the monarch herb, and rhubarb is the assistant, with the dosage of magnolia bark being double that of rhubarb. Thus, Xiaochengqi Decoction is suitable for purging heat and unblocking the bowels, while Houpo Sanwu Decoction is a formula for promoting qi and relieving fullness. This indicates that classification based on therapeutic effects refers to their main effects, which must be considered during application.

III. Dosage Forms

There are various dosage forms of TCM formulas, each with different properties and effects. Commonly used ones include pills, powders, ointments, pellets, wines, decoctions, etc.

1. **Pills:** Pills are commonly known as boluses or medicinal pills. They are round preparations made by grinding herbs into fine powder and adding cold boiled water, honey, rice paste, flour paste, or other binders. According to therapeutic requirements, pills vary in size and weight, ranging from as small as mustard seeds to as large as bullets, or the size of mung beans or phoenix tree seeds. Generally, large pills weigh 3 grams, 6 grams, or 9 grams each; small pills are 200-400 pills per 30 grams; very small pills are 600-1500 pills per 30 grams; extremely small pills are 5000-10000 pills per 30 grams.

   Pills are absorbed slowly in the stomach and are mostly used for chronic diseases that require long-term administration. Hence, the saying of the predecessors, "Pills are for slow action," conveys this meaning. Pills are also often used for diseases in the lower jiao, as they are absorbed slowly and take effect when reaching the intestines. In addition, pills can be used for acute and severe cases because they can be prepared in advance for convenient use.

2. **Powders:** Powders are fine medicinal powders. There are procedures such as separate grinding, combined grinding, and sequential blending. Generally, combined grinding is mostly used, but drugs with viscosity such as frankincense, myrrh, dragon's blood, and catechu; or drugs with strong volatility such as musk, borneol, and camphor; or more precious drugs such as rhinoceros horn, antelope horn, pearl, bear bile, and toad venom are all ground separately. Sequential blending is used when the prescription contains a small amount of precious drugs or other drugs that must be ground separately. The method is: After separately grinding the drugs that need to be blended, place one kind in a mortar, then add an equal amount of other medicinal powder, grind evenly, then add an equal amount of other medicinal powder and grind together, continuously doubling the amount until all are mixed uniformly.

   Powders used for internal administration have a faster medicinal effect than pills; they are also used for insufflation into the nose or as external application.

3. **Ointments:** Ointments are made by decocting drugs with water, concentrating the decoction into a thick semi-solid state. An appropriate amount is taken and infused with boiling water for administration. The general preparation method is: soak the drugs in water overnight, decoct 2-4 times, filter the decoction in separate portions, combine them and continue to simmer until it no longer soaks through paper. In addition, those decocted with vegetable oil are

plasters for external application.

Ointments are mostly tonic, used for chronic deficiency syndromes, and the nourishing ointments taken in winter also belong to this category.

4. **Pellets (Dan):** Pellets are made by methods such as sublimation or fusion, mainly using mineral drugs. There are also those made by mixing ordinary drugs, which derives from the meaning of "sincere and without falseness is called Dan". Pellets come in various dosage forms, including pills, powders, and lozenges.

   Their usage is the same as that of pills and powders.

5. **Medicinal Wines:** Medicinal wines are the extracts obtained by soaking drugs in white wine as a solvent, so they are commonly called medicinal liquors. The preparation methods are divided into cold soaking and hot soaking. Cold soaking involves soaking the drugs in wine, which can be taken after a period of time; hot soaking involves sealing the drugs and wine in an altar, heating slowly over a water bath with a gentle fire, maintaining a low temperature, and after 3-7 days, removing the fire and letting it cool.

   Medicinal wines are mostly used for wind-damp impediment pain, relying on the power of wine to help circulate qi and blood, enhancing the efficacy of relaxing tendons and activating collaterals.

6. **Decoctions:** Decoctions are water decoctions. The appropriate amount of water is used to decoct the drugs to obtain the medicinal juice, which is poured out, and then water is added for re-decoction. The first decoction is called the first boil, and the second is called the second boil. Generally, each dose is decocted twice. The administration methods include taking the first and second boils separately, or combining the first and second decoctions and then dividing them into two doses.

   In clinical practice, decoctions are the most widely used, not only because they are absorbed quickly and have strong effects, but also because they are convenient for modification according to symptoms.

Pills, powders, ointments, pellets, and medicinal wines are mostly proprietary medicines, but they can also be prescribed and combined according to the needs of the condition. Some pills, powders, ointments, and pellets, in addition to being used alone, can also be wrapped and decocted in decoctions or taken with medicinal juice.

Section 2 Basic Formulas and Prescriptions

I. Basic Formulas

Xu Lingtai said: "Those who wish to treat diseases must first recognize the name of the disease; only after recognizing the disease name can they seek the cause of the disease. Knowing the cause, they should then distinguish the different factors leading to it and the resulting variations in symptoms, and thereafter examine the methods of treatment. Each disease has its main formula, and each formula has its main herb. Sometimes the disease name is the same but the causes differ, or the causes are the same but the symptoms vary—yet in such cases, there are still respective main formulas and main herbs. Amidst the myriad changes, there exists an unchanging principle; even with additions or subtractions, there is an orderly discipline." Indeed, in treating each disease, one must differentiate syndromes to identify the cause before determining the treatment strategy. Meanwhile, each disease has its primary treatment method, and inevitably its main formula and main herb—this is the fundamental principle of treating diseases. On this basis, only by making appropriate additions or subtractions according to specific conditions and applying them flexibly can good results be achieved.

The established formulas passed down by predecessors are all derived from practice and must be valued, especially several basic formulas, which must be familiarized. A selection of these is now briefly explained to give a general idea:

1. **Sijunzi Decoction:** Ginseng, Atractylodes macrocephala, Poria, Licorice. It is the main formula for replenishing qi, used for symptoms such as weak spleen and stomach, poor appetite, and diarrhea. For qi stagnation, dried tangerine peel can be added, known as Yigong Powder; for stomach cold, costus and amomum can be added, known as Xiangsha Liujunzi Decoction.
2. **Siwu Decoction:** Rehmannia, Angelica, White peony root, Ligusticum. It is the main formula for nourishing blood, used for liver blood deficiency and stagnation, and irregular menstruation in women. For deficiency of both qi and blood, it can be used together with Sijunzi Decoction, known as Bazhen Decoction; removing rehmannia and white peony root, it is called Foshou Powder, which can promote blood circulation.
3. **Liuwei Dihuang Pills:** Prepared rehmannia, Cornus, Yam, Poria, Moutan bark, Alisma. It is the main formula for nourishing yin, used for symptoms such as deficiency of kidney fluid, lumbago, and spermatorrhea. For deficient cold, monkshood and cinnamon can be added, known as Guifu Bawei Pills; for internal heat, phellodendron and anemarrhena can be added, known as Zhibai Bawei Pills; adding only cinnamon, it is called Qiwei Dihuang Pills, which can guide fire back to its source; adding schisandra, it is called Qiwei Duqi Pills, which can treat consumptive cough.
4. **Sini Decoction:** Monk shood, Dried ginger, Roasted licorice. It is the main formula for restoring yang, used for excessive cold with deficient yang, cold limbs, and incessant watery diarrhea. For cold damaging the blood aspect with a faint, thready pulse, angelica and akebia can be

added, known as Danggui Sini Decoction; for wind-dampness struggling against each other with general aching and pain, atractylodes and jujube can be added, known as Zhufu Decoction.

5. **Guizhi Decoction:** Cinnamon twig, White peony root, Roasted licorice, Fresh ginger, Jujube. It is the main formula for harmonizing nutrient and defense, and also treats wind damage. For incessant sweating, monkshood can be added, known as Guizhi plus Fuzi Decoction; for insecure sperm gate, dragon bone and oyster can be added, known as Guizhi plus Longgu Muli Decoction; doubling white peony root and adding maltose, it is called Xiaojianzhong Decoction; adding astragalus, it is called Huangqi Jianzhong Decoction, which treats abdominal pain due to deficiency cold of middle qi.
6. **Mahuang Decoction:** Ephedra, Cinnamon twig, Almond, Roasted licorice. It is the main formula for dispelling wind-cold, used for cold and heat, absence of sweating, and a floating-tight pulse. For external dampness, atractylodes can be added, known as Mahuang plus Zhuyu Decoction; removing cinnamon twig and adding gypsum, it is called Maxing Shigan Decoction, which treats exterior pathogens inwardly trapped with heat in the lung and asthma.
7. **Yinqiao Powder:** Honeysuckle, Forsythia, Fermented soybean, Schizonepeta, Mentha, Arctium, Platycodon, Licorice, Bamboo leaf, Reed rhizome. It is the main formula for the initial stage of wind-warm syndrome, used for fever, thirst, and a floating-rapid pulse. For cough, almond and fritillaria thunbergii can be added to diffuse the lung and resolve phlegm; for severe heat, gardenia and scutellaria can be added to clear qi.
8. **Liuyi Powder:** Talc, Licorice. It is the main formula for clearing summerheat, used for symptoms such as body heat, restlessness, thirst, and scanty reddish urine. To clear the heart, cinnabar can be added, known as Yiyuan Powder; to dispel wind, mint can be added, known

as Jisu Powder.

9. **Pingwei Powder:** Atractylodes lancea, Magnolia bark, Dried tangerine peel, Roasted licorice, Fresh ginger, Jujube. It is the main formula for transforming dampness, used for stuffiness, nausea, vomiting, and white greasy tongue coating. For those with profuse phlegm, it can be used together with Erchen Decoction, known as Pingchen Decoction; for diarrhea with scanty urine, it can be used together with Wuling Powder, known as Weiling Decoction.
10. **Wuling Powder:** Poria, Alisma, Polyporus, Atractylodes macrocephala, Cinnamon twig. It is the main formula for draining dampness, used for dysuria and vomiting after drinking water. For cases with thirst but no cold, cinnamon twig can be removed, known as Siling Powder.
11. **Shizao Decoction:** Genkwa flower, Kansui, Euphorbia pekinensis, Jujube. It is the main formula for purging water, used for internal retention of fluid, with fullness and pain in the chest and hypochondrium.
12. **Qiongyu Ointment:** Rehmannia, Ginseng, Poria, White honey. It is the main formula for moistening dryness, used for depletion of body fluids and qi deficiency with dry cough.
13. **Wuren Pills:** Peach kernel, Almond, Platycladus seed, Pine nut, Prunus humilis seed, Dried tangerine peel. It is the main formula for moistening the intestines, used for difficult defecation due to fluid depletion.
14. **Baihu Decoction:** Gypsum, Anemarrhena, Licorice, Japonica rice. It is the main formula for clearing heat, used for high fever, thirst, sweating, and a surging pulse. For qi and yin deficiency, ginseng can be added, known as Renshen Baihu Decoction; for cases with dampness, atractylodes lancea can be added, known as Cangzhu Baihu Decoction.

15. **Huanglian Jiedu Decoction:** Coptis, Scutellaria, Phellodendron, Gardenia. It is the main formula for purging fire, used for accumulated heat in the triple jiao, mania, restlessness, and reckless blood flow.
16. **Puji Xiaodu Yin:** Scrophularia, Coptis, Scutellaria, Forsythia, Isatis root, Lasiosphaera, Arctium, Mint, Bombyx batryticatus, Cimicifuga, Bupleurum, Platycodon, Licorice, Dried tangerine peel. It is the main formula for clearing warm-toxin, used for “swollen head plague”, sore throat, thirst, etc.
17. **Qinggu Powder:** Starwort root, Picrorhiza, Gentiana macrophylla, Turtle shell, Wolfberry bark, Artemisia annua, Anemarrhena, Licorice. It is the main formula for clearing deficiency heat, used for steaming bone consumptive heat, yin deficiency, afternoon tidal fever, or night fever.
18. **Sanren Decoction:** Almond, Amomum fruit, Coix seed, Magnolia bark, Pinellia, Tetrapanax, Talc, Bamboo leaf. It is the main formula for clearing and transforming damp-heat, used for damp-warm syndrome with body heat, chest tightness, and thirst without desire to drink.
19. **Dayuan Yin:** Magnolia bark, Dichroa, Amomum tsao-ko, Areca nut, Scutellaria, Anemarrhena, Acorus, Green tangerine peel, Licorice. It is the main formula for treating damp-heat pestilence, used for damp-turbidity with heat blocking the middle jiao, cold-heat, chest tightness, thick greasy tongue coating, etc.
20. **Erchen Decoction:** Ginger-processed pinellia, Dried tangerine peel, Poria, Licorice, Fresh ginger. It is the main formula for eliminating phlegm, and can also regulate qi, dispel dampness, and harmonize the middle. For stubborn phlegm, bile arisaema and immature bitter orange can be added, known as Daotan Decoction; for gallbladder deficiency with insomnia, bamboo shavings and immature bitter orange can be added, known as Wendan Decoction.

21. **Qingqi Huatan Pills:** Ginger-processed pinellia, Bile arisaema, Tangerine red, Immature bitter orange, Almond, Trichosanthes seed, Scutellaria, Poria. It is the main formula for clearing phlegm-heat, used for excessive qi-fire condensing body fluids into phlegm.
22. **Sanzi Yangqin Decoction:** Perilla seed, White mustard seed, Raphani seed. It is the main formula for calming phlegm asthma, used for excessive qi with profuse phlegm, asthma, fullness, and chest tightness.
23. **Baohe Pills:** Hawthorn, Medicated leaven, Poria, Pinellia, Dried tangerine peel, Raphani seed, Forsythia, Malt. It is the main formula for promoting digestion, used for symptoms such as belching with foul odor, acid regurgitation, abdominal pain, and diarrhea. For qi stagnation, it can be used together with Yueju Pills, known as Yueju Baohe Pills.
24. **Xiaohuoluo Dan (Minor Collateral-Activating Pellet):** Aconitum carmichaelii, Aconitum kusnezoffii, Ligusticum chuanxiong, Lumbricus, Arisaema cum bile, Olibanum, Myrrha. It is the main formula for activating collaterals, used for symptoms such as phlegm-dampness invading the collaterals and numbness of hands and feet.
25. **Tianwang Buxin Dan (Heavenly King Heart-Tonifying Pellet):** Ziziphus jujuba var. spinosa, Angelica sinensis, Rehmannia glutinosa, Platycladus orientalis, Asparagus cochinchinensis, Ophiopogon japonicus, Polygala tenuifolia, Schisandra chinensis, Ginseng, Salvia miltiorrhiza, Scrophularia ningpoensis, Platycodon grandiflorus. It is the main formula for tranquilizing the mind, used for amnesia, palpitations, insomnia, and deficiency-fire flaring upward, etc.
26. **Niuhuang Qingxin Wan (Bezoar Heart-Clearing Pill):** Calculus bovis, Coptis chinensis, Scutellaria baicalensis, Gardenia jasminoides, Curcuma aromatica, Cinnabaris. It is the main formula for opening the

orifices, used for pathogenic factors invading the pericardium with clouded consciousness.

27. **Jinsuo Gujing Wan (Golden Lock Essence-Securing Pill):** Astragalus complanatus, Euryale ferox, Nelumbo nucifera stamen, Os draconis, Concha ostreae. It is the main formula for securing essence, used for insecure essence gate with involuntary emission.
28. **Muli San (Oyster Powder):** Calcined Concha ostreae, Astragalus membranaceus, Ephedra root, Triticum aestivum var. germinatum. It is the main formula for securing the exterior, used for yang deficiency with spontaneous sweating.
29. **Hezi San (Chebula Powder):** Papaver somniferum shell, Terminalia chebula, Roasted Zingiber officinale, Citrus reticulata red peel. It is the main formula for astringing the intestines, used for incessant diarrhea and prolapse of the rectum.
30. **Buzhong Yiqi Decoction (Middle-Jiao Tonifying and Qi-Boosting Decoction):** Astragalus membranaceus, Ginseng, Glycyrrhiza uralensis, Atractylodes macrocephala, Citrus reticulata, Angelica sinensis, Cimicifuga foetida, Bupleurum chinense, Ginger, Jujube. It is the main formula for lifting and raising, used for middle qi sinking or qi deficiency failing to contain blood.
31. **Qiqi Decoction (Seven-Qi Decoction):** Magnolia officinalis, Pinellia ternata, Poria cocos, Perilla frutescens, Ginger, Jujube. It is the main formula for promoting qi movement, used for qi stagnation with chest fullness and dyspnea.
32. **Yueju Wan (Depression-Relieving Pill):** Cyperus rotundus, Atractylodes lancea, Ligusticum chuanxiong, Massa medicata fermentata, Gardenia jasminoides. It is the main formula for relieving stagnation, used for chest and diaphragm stuffiness, acid regurgitation, vomiting, and indigestion, etc.
33. **Shihui San (Ten-Ash Powder):** Cirsium japonicum, Cephalanoplos

segetum, Platycladus orientalis leaf, Nelumbo nucifera leaf, Imperata cylindrica root, Rubia cordifolia, Rheum palmatum, Gardenia jasminoides, Trachycarpus fortunei bark, Paeonia suffruticosa root bark. It is the main formula for stopping bleeding, used for hematemesis due to physical overstrain.

34. **Taoren Chengqi Decoction (Peach Kernel Qi-Ordering Decoction):** Prunus persica seed, Rheum palmatum, Cinnamomum cassia twig, Glycyrrhiza uralensis, Sodium sulfate. It is the main formula for dispelling stasis, used for blood accumulation and amenorrhea in women.

35. **Xiaochaihu Decoction (Minor Bupleurum Decoction):** Bupleurum chinense, Scutellaria baicalensis, Ginseng, Pinellia ternata, Roasted Glycyrrhiza uralensis, Ginger, Jujube. It is the main formula for harmonizing, used for alternating cold and heat, fullness and discomfort in the chest and hypochondria, bitter taste in the mouth, dizziness, etc.

36. **Xiaoyao San (Free and Easy Wanderer Powder):** Bupleurum chinense, Angelica sinensis, Paeonia lactiflora, Atractylodes macrocephala, Poria cocos, Glycyrrhiza uralensis, Mentha haplocalyx, Zingiber officinale. It is the main formula for soothing the liver, used for headache, dizziness, depression, and irregular menstruation in women. For excessive fire, Paeonia suffruticosa root bark and Gardenia jasminoides can be added, known as Jiawei Xiaoyao San (Modified Free and Easy Wanderer Powder).

37. **Guadi San (Melon Stalk Powder):** Cucumis melo stalk, Vigna umbellata, Fermented Glycine max. It is the main formula for inducing vomiting, used for phlegm accumulation in the upper epigastrium.

38. **Dachengqi Decoction (Major Qi-Ordering Decoction):** Rheum palmatum, Magnolia officinalis, Citrus aurantium, Sodium sulfate. It is the main formula for purging, used for excess heat with constipation,

abdominal pain with refusal to press; for insufficient body fluids, sodium sulfate can be removed, and Cannabis sativa seed, Prunus armeniaca seed, and Oryza sativa can be added, known as Piyao Maren Wan (Spleen-Constrained Hemp Seed Pill).

39. **Muxiang Binlang Wan (Costus and Areca Pill):** Aucklandia lappa, Areca catechu, Citrus reticulata green peel, Citrus reticulata peel, Curcuma zedoaria, Coptis chinensis, Phellodendron chinense, Rheum palmatum, Cyperus rotundus, Pharbitis nil. It is the main formula for guiding out stagnation, used for chest stuffiness, abdominal distension, constipation, or diarrhea with tenesmus, etc.
40. **Huachong Wan (Parasite-Expelling Pill):** Quisqualis indica, Carpesium abrotanoides, Areca catechu, Melia toosendan, Ulmus pumila, Plumbum rubrum, Dried alum. It is the main formula for killing parasites, used for paroxysmal abdominal pain caused by intestinal parasites.

The above formulas are only examples of general treatments from the aspects of etiology and symptoms. Lei Futing once said:"I once studied how Danxi treated diseases. Whenever encountering qi deficiency, he used Sijunzi Decoction; for blood deficiency, Siwu Decoction; for phlegm-fluid retention, Erchen Decoction; for dampness and food stagnation, Pingwei Powder. He mainly used these four formulas, and further referred to methods of relieving stagnation. The herbs used were not numerous, yet they often hit the mark." It can be seen that mastering general treatment formulas is essential in clinical practice. However, general formulas should also be in line with the disease condition and are not equivalent to vague application. In general, each disease has its main formula, and one disease with several symptoms also has respective main formulas. The general treatment formulas mentioned here are those that can treat multiple diseases.

Therefore, after understanding general treatment formulas, one should further study the main formulas for each disease and various symptoms to make more detailed modifications according to symptoms. For reference books in this regard, *Lantai Guifan* (Standards of the Imperial Library) can be used, and *Yifang Jijie* (Collected Explanations of Medical Formulas) is the most commonly used for general situations.

II. Examples of Prescriptions

TCM prescriptions actually include a set of knowledge involving principles, methods, formulas, and herbs, which is the specific manifestation of combining theory and practice. A characteristic of TCM prescriptions is that there are both medical records and formulas. The record refers to the pulse record; when writing a prescription, the pulse record is written first, followed by the formulation of the formula. The content of the pulse record includes four items: symptoms, causes, pulses, and treatments, with pulses encompassing the four diagnostic methods. Generally, symptoms are described first, followed by causes, then pulse, tongue, complexion, and finally the treatment principle. Of course, this is not rigid; one can first describe symptoms and pulses, then causes and treatments, or first put forward the cause, then describe pulses and symptoms, but generally within this scope. For example, Ye Tianshi's pulse records for treating cough: "The right pulse is floating and rapid; wind-warm invades the lung and transforms into dryness, with itching in the throat and uncomfortable cough; using the acrid-sweet-cool-moistening method." Another: "Chronic overstrain combined with wind-warm, dry throat, heat cough, insufficient physique and pulse; using a sweet-moderating and gentle formula." Another: "White tongue coating, cough, ear distension, dry mouth; these are caused by upward stagnation of dryness-heat and failure of lung qi to disperse. Acrid-cool should be used, and light diet is advisable." Another: "The pulse is weak; long-term cough, emaciation, reduced appetite, sweating, shortness of breath. Long-term deficiency failing to recover is called impairment; following *Huangdi Neijing*, for insufficient physique, nourish and warm qi." The above records, although differing in the order of describing symptoms, causes, pulses, and treatments, are written truthfully and flexibly without being constrained, yet still within the scope of symptoms, causes, pulses, and treatments.

After a comprehensive understanding of the disease and symptoms, the formula is then written. When writing the formula, one should have a clear idea of which are the main herbs and which are the auxiliary ones. Generally, main herbs are written first, followed by auxiliary herbs, with the auxiliary herbs also ordered by their importance, which contains the meaning of monarch, minister, assistant, and guide. In the past, prescriptions were written vertically, customarily divided into three rows, sometimes two or four rows, depending on the number of herbs. The first row is written first, then the second and third rows. Therefore, TCM prescriptions should be read row by row; reading them line by line makes it impossible to distinguish primary and secondary herbs. Now, most are written horizontally, which is clearer than before.

For ease of understanding, several recent medical records are appended, including the handling of decoctions, pills, powders, and ointments. They are not demonstrations but for reference only.

Case 1: The patient complained of an enlarged liver for nearly a year, with pulling pain in the right hypochondrium, most obvious at the hypochondriac region, sometimes radiating to the back and lower abdomen, easy fatigue, poor appetite, and a long-standing condition of dysmenorrhea, feeling particularly mentally fatigued during menstruation. The pulse is thready and string-like, the tongue is clean, and bowel and bladder movements are normal. The hypochondrium is the territory of the liver. Predecessors said that long-term pain enters the collaterals, so the method of soothing qi and harmonizing blood is intended.

Danggui Xu (Radix Angelicae Sinensis, fibrous part) 6g, Sheng Baishao (Radix Paeoniae Alba, raw) 6g, Ruan Chaihu (Radix Bupleuri, processed) 3g (stir-fried), Danshen (Radix Salviae Miltiorrhizae) 6g, Taoren Ni (Semen Persicae, mashed) 5g (wrapped), Guang Yujin (Radix Curcumae) 5g, Chuanlianzi (Fructus Toosendan) 5g, Lulutong (Fructus Liquidambaris) 5g, Juluo (Pericarpium Citri Reticulatae, vascular bundle) 3g, Chenxiang Qu (Massa Medicata Fermentata with Lignum Aquilariae Resinatum) 5g, Foshou (Fructus Citri Sarcodactylis) 2g

Case 2: Stomach pain occurs when fasting, relieved by food intake, slight acid regurgitation, inability to tolerate cold foods, stool either yellow or black, and emaciation. The syndrome is attributed to deficiency-cold of middle qi; Huangqi Jianzhong Decoction with modifications is intended.

Zhi Huangqi (Radix Astragali, honey-fried) 9g, Chao Guizhi (Ramulus Cinnamomi, stir-fried) 2g, Chao Baishao (Radix Paeoniae Alba, stir-fried) 5g, Zhi Gancao (Radix Glycyrrhizae, honey-fried) 3g, Ejiao (Colla Corii Asini) 5g, Paojiangtan (Rhizoma Zingiberis, charred) 2g, Hongzao (Fructus Jujubae) 4 pieces, Yitang (Maltose) 30g (to be taken with medicinal juice in 2 divided doses)

Case 3: For half a year, there has been frequent gum bleeding, accompanied by weakness in limbs, gradually increasing dizziness, blurred vision, tinnitus, palpitations, and flusteredness. Hospital examination showed pancytopenia, diagnosed as aplastic anemia. Current diagnosis: sallow complexion, excessive sweating of hands and feet, pale tongue, floating-large and rapid pulse. Due to the root of overstrain, the treatment is intended to warm and nourish the liver and kidney, focusing on the life gate.

Shudi (Radix Rehmanniae Preparata) 12g, Shufupian (Radix Aconiti Lateralis Preparata) 6g, Sheng Huangqi (Radix Astragali, raw) 9g,

Lujiaojiao (Colla Cornu Cervi) 6g, Shanyurou (Fructus Corni) 6g, Gouqizi (Fructus Lycii) 9g, Chao Baishao (Radix Paeoniae Alba, stir-fried) 9g, Tongshayuan (Semen Astragali Complanati) 9g, Duanmuli (Concha Ostreae, calcined) 15g, Longyanrou (Arillus Longan) 15g, Hongzao (Fructus Jujubae) 10 pieces

Case 4: From autumn to winter, diarrhea has persisted, 2-3 times a day, borborygmus without abdominal pain, but the abdomen cannot tolerate wind and cold; even a slight feeling of coolness increases the frequency of bowel movements and worsens borborygmus. The pulse is deep and weak, and appetite is still acceptable. The disease is in the lower jiao; warming the kidney and tonifying the intestines, with slight reference to lifting the clear, a pill formula is intended for long-term administration.

Shufupian (Radix Aconiti Lateralis Preparata) 60g, Paojiangtan (Rhizoma Zingiberis, charred) 30g, Chao Baizhu (Rhizoma Atractylodis Macrocephalae, stir-fried) 60g, Wei Yizhi (Fructus Alpiniae Oxyphyllae, simmered) 60g, Wei Rouguo (Semen Myristicae, simmered) 60g, Hezipi (Pericarpium Terminaliae Chebulae) 45g, Yun Fuling (Poria, Yun) 90g, Chao Shanyao (Rhizoma Dioscoreae, stir-fried) 90g, Wei Gegen (Radix Puerariae Lobatae, simmered) 30g

All herbs are ground into fine powder, made into pills with water, as large as mung beans. Take 3g each time, twice a day, in the morning and before bedtime, with warm boiled water.

Case 5: Suffering from paragonimiasis for nearly two years, expectorating phlegm mixed with blood, slightly fishy in smell; recently, palpitations and insomnia, physical strength not as good as before. There is no such disease name in TCM; tentatively, a formula is made according to the lung worm syndrome and corpse stagnation syndrome recorded in Q*ianjin Yaofang* (Essential Prescriptions Worth a Thousand Gold) and *Wai Tai Mi Yao* (Secret Recipes from the Imperial Library).

Maidong (Radix Ophiopogonis) 45g, Shexiang (Moschus) 0.5g, Huanglian (Rhizoma Coptidis) 30g, Zhusha (Cinnabaris) 6g, Xionghuang (Realgar) 3g, Chuanjiao (Pericarpium Zanthoxyli) 30g, Taoren (Semen Persicae) 60g, Tagan (Liver of Lutra lutra) 60g

The above herbs are mixed and ground into fine powder. Take 4.5g each time, three times a day, after breakfast, lunch, and dinner, with warm boiled water.

Case 6: Spermatorrhea for many years, sometimes with dreams, sometimes without dreams; the effect of medication is inconsistent. Recently, impotence has developed, accompanied by weak limbs, soreness of the waist, weight loss, anxiety and fear, unable to relieve oneself. The pulse is deep and thready; in winter, the four extremities are cold, frequent and urgent urination. Yin deficiency affecting yang, extreme deficiency of the lower origin, and timidity of heart qi failing to communicate with the kidney is also one of the causes. Taking advantage of the winter season when the body tends to store essence, an ointment formula is intended for nourishment.

Zhi Huangqi (Radix Astragali, honey-fried) 90g, Yetai Shen (Radix Ginseng, wild) 90g, Shanyao (Rhizoma Dioscoreae) 90g, Shudi (Radix Rehmanniae Preparata) 120g, Shanyurou (Fructus Corni) 45g, Zhi Huangjing (Rhizoma Polygonati, processed) 90g, Danggui Shen (Radix Angelicae Sinensis, body) 45g, Chao Baishao (Radix Paeoniae Alba, stir-fried) 45g, Zhi Shouwu (Radix Polygoni Multiflori, processed) 90g, Tongshayuan (Semen Astragali Complanati) 90g, Tusizi Bing (Semen Cuscutae, cake) 90g, Gouqizi (Fructus Lycii) 90g, Yinyanghuo (Herba Epimedii) 90g, Buguzhi (Fructus Psoraleae) 90g, Shechuangzi (Fructus Cnidii) 45g, Jiucaizi (Semen Allii Tuberosi) 60g, Fupenzi (Fructus Rubi)

60g, Jinyingzi (Fructus Rosae Laevigatae) 90g, Zhi Gouji (Rhizoma Cibotii, honey-fried) 60g, Chao Duzhong (Cortex Eucommiae, stir-fried) 90g, Bei Wuwei (Fructus Schisandrae Chinensis) 30g, Jie Changpu (Rhizoma Acori Tatarinowii, nodal part) 15g, Zhi Yuanzhi (Radix Polygalae, honey-fried) 45g, Yun Fushen (Poria cum Radice Pini, Yun) 90g, Duan Longmu (Os Draconis and Concha Ostreae, calcined) 90g each, Xiang Lianrou (Semen Nelumbinis, Hunan) 240g, Hongzao (Fructus Jujubae) 240g

Soak in plenty of water overnight, decoct thoroughly 3 times, filter to get clear juice, then add: Guilu Erxian Jiao (Colla Carapacis et Plastri Testudinis and Colla Cornu Cervi) 240g (first melted with aged wine), 2 Huanggou Shen (Penis et Testis Canis) (first simmered and melted), 500g Bingtang (Rock Sugar). Stir and condense into an ointment. Take one spoonful each time on an empty stomach in the morning and afternoon, with boiled water. In case of catching a cold, suspend activities for several days.

To study prescriptions, one must read many medical records. Medical records are TCM clinical records; for example, *Linzheng Zhinan* (Guide to Clinical Practice) is Ye Tianshi's medical records, which are his daily treatment plans. Since TCM prescriptions not only record the medications used but also comprehensively document the patient's causes of illness, symptoms, four diagnostic findings, treatment methods, prescriptions, as well as detailed analyses and diagnoses, they are the product of combining theory and practice, and are of great help and inspiration for learning. Meanwhile, one's own insights and experience are after all limited, so it is necessary to read extensively the medical records of various schools. Although not all may be beneficial, they must have their own strengths. We believe that only by absorbing the essence of various sources like bees making honey can one enrich their own knowledge and experience. Therefore, it can also be said that the medical records of various schools are a doctor's lifelong good teachers.

Chapter Four Drugs

Section 1 Collection and Processing

I. Collection

According to Li Shizhen's *Compendium of Materia Medica*, there are 1892 types of TCM. Later, Zhao Xuemin's *Supplements to the Compendium of Materia Medica* added 760 more types. Since then, folk medicinal herbs have continued to emerge in various regions, and it is generally estimated that there are about 3000 types. These traditional Chinese medicines include three categories: animals, plants, and minerals, with plants accounting for the majority. Hence, books on TCM drugs are called "bencao" (materia medica).

The origin and collection time of drugs are closely related to their efficacy. Therefore, Li Dongyuan once said: "All herbs, trees, insects, and worms have their producing regions; roots, leaves, flowers, and fruits are collected at specific times. If the region is incorrect, their nature and flavor will differ slightly; if the time is improper, their qi and flavor will be incomplete." For example, Fritillaria produced in Sichuan and Zhejiang have different effects; Notopterygium and Angelica pubescens, Carthamus tinctorius and Crocus sativus are also different. Thus, many names of traditional Chinese medicines are based on their producing regions, such as Dangshen (Codonopsis) named after Shangdang, and Chuanxiong (Ligusticum chuanxiong) named after Sichuan. In general prescriptions, the producing regions are specifically indicated, such as Chuanbeimu (Sichuan Fritillaria), Zhebeimu (Zhejiang Fritillaria), as well as Chuan Guizhi (Sichuan Cinnamon twig), Chuan Huangbai (Sichuan Phellodendron),

Guang Muxiang (Guangdong Aucklandia), Qin Danggui (Gansu Angelica), Hang Juhua (Hangzhou Chrysanthemum), Yun Fuling (Yunnan Poria), Jian Zexie (Fujian Alisma), etc. Currently, some of these are no longer necessary, but some should still be specified.

Since plants have specific growth and maturity periods, and the parts used as medicine include roots, stems, flowers, and leaves, the preservation or loss of the drug's qi and flavor depends entirely on whether the collection season is appropriate. Timely collection not only improves efficacy but also ensures a good harvest. A brief introduction is as follows.

1. **Roots:** Drugs using roots, which take their ascending qi, such as Cimicifugae Rhizoma (Shengma) and Puerariae Lobatae Radix (Gegen), should be collected when they have not yet sprouted or have withered, as the essence is stored in the lower part, making their medicinal power stronger.
2. **Stems:** They can ascend and descend, taking their qi-regulating property, such as Perillae Caulis (Sugeng) and Pogostemonis Caulis (Huogeng). They should be collected when growing most vigorously.
3. **Leaves:** Taking their dispersing property, such as Mori Folium (Sangye) and Nelumbinis Folium (Heye), they are also best collected when growing luxuriantly, but should not be picked after rain to prevent mildew and deterioration.
4. **Branches:** Taking their property of spreading horizontally to the limbs, such as Mori Ramulus (Sangzhi), the collection method is the same as that for stems and leaves.
5. **Flowers:** Taking their aromatic and dispersing property, such as Chrysanthemi Flos (Juhua) and Magnoliae Flos (Xinyihua), they should be collected when in bud or just blooming, as their aroma is the strongest.
6. **Fruits:** Taking their descending qi, such as Aurantii Fructus

Immaturus (Zhishi) and Citri Reticulatae Viride Pericarpium (Qingpi). They should be collected when newly ripe or not fully ripe.

7. **Seeds:** Taking their descending qi, such as Perillae Fructus (Suzi) and Plantaginis Semen (Cheqianzi), they should be collected when fully ripe.
8. *Kernels:* Taking their moistening and descending property, such as Armeniacae Semen Amarum (Xingren) and Platycladi Semen (Baiziren), they are suitable to be collected when fully ripe.
9. **Nodes:** Taking their property of benefiting joints, such as Pinaceae Lignum Nodi (Songjie), those that are solid are preferred.
10. **Sprouts:** Taking their dispersing property, such as Oryzae Fructus Germinatus (Guya) and Hordei Fructus Germinatus (Maiya), they can be artificially germinated at any time.
11. **Thorns:** Taking their breaking and attacking property, such as Gleditsiae Spina (Zaojiaoci).
12. **Barks:** Barks acting on the skin, taking the meaning of reaching the skin, such as Zingiberis Rhizomatis Cortex (Shengjiangpi) and Poriae Cutis (Fulingpi).
13. **Hearts:** Taking the meaning of acting on internal organs, such as Bambusae Folium Cum Spica (Zhuyexin) and Nelumbinis Plumula (Lianzixin).
14. **Veins:** Taking the meaning of being able to enter the meridians and collaterals, such as Citri Reticulatae Pericarpium Viride Vena (Juluo) and Luffae Fructus Retinervus (Sigualuo), they should be collected when mature.
15. **Vines:** Taking their property of moving through the meridians and limbs, such as Trachelospermi Caulis et Folium (Luoshiteng) and Piperis Kadsurae Caulis (Haifengteng), they should be collected when luxuriant.

The above are general guidelines, and there are differences in specific applications. For example, Puerariae Lobatae Radix (Gegen) is solid, ascending body fluids but not qi; Cimicifugae Rhizoma (Shengma) is hollow, ascending qi but not body fluids; Achyranthis Bidentatae Radix (Niuxi) has a solid root with no hollow shape, a bitter taste and no dispersedqi, so it has no ascending and dispersed power. Therefore, to determine the effect of a drug, it is necessary to comprehensively consider its shape, color, smell and taste, and not draw conclusions based on only one aspect. Even the collection time is affected by the earlier or later solar terms and climate changes, which impact the growth and maturity of drugs, so it must be determined according to the actual situation.

II. Processing

Some raw medicines are toxic or have intense properties and cannot be taken directly; some have an unpleasant smell, which is not conducive to taking; some must have inapplicable parts removed; and some have different effects when raw and processed. Therefore, many traditional Chinese medicines are processed. The significance of drug processing is nothing more than eliminating or reducing the toxicity of drugs and appropriately improving their properties. For the former, such as Pinelliae Rhizoma (Banxia), raw Pinelliae Rhizoma will irritate the throat, causing hoarseness or poisoning, and must be processed with ginger juice; for the latter, such as Rehmanniae Radix (Shengdi), raw Rehmanniae Radix is cold in nature and can cool blood, while processed into Rehmanniae Radix Praeparata (Shudi), its nature becomes warm and it can tonify blood; or stir-frying Rehmanniae Radix into carbonisata makes it stop bleeding, and stir-frying Rehmanniae Radix Praeparata until loose can reduce the drawback of stickiness and greasiness. The processing of Chinese herbal medicinals is called Paozhi, also known as Xiuzhi.

1. Calcinating (Duan): Burn the drug directly in fire until red-hot, or put it in a fire-resistant vessel and burn it thoroughly. This method is mostly used for mineral and shell drugs, such as Os Draconis (Longgu) and Concha Ostreae (Muli).

2. Roasting (Pao): Put the drug in a high-temperature iron pot and stir-fry quickly until it is brown and cracked on all sides, such as Zingiberis Rhizoma Praeparatum (Paojiang).

3.Simmering (Wei): Wrap the drug with wet paper or batter, bury it in appropriate fire ash, or roast it over a low fire until the surface of the paper or batter is charred, such as simmered ginger (Weijiang) and simmered aucklandia (Weimuxiang).

4.Stir-frying (Chao): Put the drug in a pot and stir-fry, either until yellow, charred, or turned into charcoal, such as stir-fried atractylodes macrocephala (Chao Baizhu), stir-fried rice sprout (Chao Guya), charred gardenia (Jiaoshanzhi), charred hawthorn (Jiaozhatan), etc.

5.Stir-frying with honey (Zhi): When stir-frying the drug, mix in honey, yak ghee, etc., until it turns yellow, such as honey-fried astragalus (Zhi Huangqi), honey-fried licorice (Zhi Gancao), etc.

6.Roasting (Bei): Dry the drug over a gentle fire, such as processed leeches (Zhi Shuizhi), processed horseflies (Zhi Mengchong), etc.

7.Drying (Hong): Dry the drug by roasting over a gentle fire, but the fire is weaker than that used in roasting, such as processed chrysanthemum (Zhi Juhua), processed honeysuckle (Zhi Jinyinhua), etc.

8.Washing (Xi): Wash the drug with water to remove soil and impurities.

9.Soaking and rinsing (Piao): Soak the drug in water to remove saltiness or fishy smell; the time is longer than washing, and the water must be changed frequently, such as processed cistanche (Zhi Congrong), processed kelp (Zhi Kunbu), etc.

10.Soaking (Pao): Put the drug in clear water or boiling water to facilitate peeling off the outer skin, such as processed almonds (Zhi Xingren), processed peach kernels (Zhi Taoren), etc.

11.Steeping (Zi): Gradually moisten the drug with water to make it soft for slicing.

12.Levigating (Fei): Grind the drug powder together with water to make it finer and cleaner, such as processed talc (Zhi Huashi), processed cinnabar (Zhi Zhusha), etc.

13.Steaming (Zheng): Steam the drug in a barrel over water, such as processed rhubarb (Zhi Dahuang), processed polygonum multiflorum (Zhi Shouwu), etc.

14.Boiling (Zhu): Boil the drug in water or other liquids, such as processed genkwa flower (Zhi Yuanhua), etc.

15.Quenching (Cui): Heat the drug in fire until red-hot, take it out and put it into water or vinegar, such as processed magnetite (Zhi Cishi), processed pyrite (Zhi Ziran tong), etc.

In summary, processing is inseparable from water and fire. Among the above methods, 1-7 are fire-processing methods, 8-12 are water-processing methods, and 13-15 are combined water and fire processing methods.

During processing, wine, vinegar, salt water, etc., are used as needed for treatment. For example, processing with wine is to promote ascending and lifting; processing with ginger juice is to promote dispersion; processing with salt water is to direct the drug to the kidney and soften hardness; processing with vinegar is to direct the drug to the liver and promote astringency; processing with boy's urine is to clear fire and promote descending; processing with rice water is to moisten dryness and harmonize the middle; processing with milk is to moisten dryness and generate blood; processing with honey is to exert a sweet and moderate effect and tonify the spleen. There are also processing with earth-frying to direct the drug to the middle jiao; processing with bran-frying to invigorate the intestines and stomach; soaking with black bean and licorice decoction to detoxify; smearing and roasting with sheep butter and lard to facilitate penetration into bones. These are the experiences of predecessors and are still used today.

In TCM shops, most drugs that should be processed are pre-processed. Even if not specified in the prescription, they are processed when dispensing. However, situations vary slightly in different regions, and many drugs are used both raw and processed with different processing methods. Therefore, it is better to specify them in the prescription, such as raw coix seed (Sheng Yiyiren), stir-fried coix seed (Chao Yiyiren), fresh polygonum multiflorum (Xian Shouwu), dried polygonum multiflorum (Gan Shouwu), processed polygonum multiflorum (Zhi Shouwu), as well as ginger-processed pinellia (Jiang Banxia), fa-processed pinellia (Fa Banxia), water-roasted polygala (Shui Zhi Yuanzhi), honey-roasted polygala (Mi Zhi Yuanzhi), etc.

Section 2 Properties of Drugs

I. Qi and Flavor

In studying drugs, emphasis should be placed on their efficacy; however, a more important aspect is the study of their pharmacological actions. TCM uses the theories of Yin-Yang and the Five Elements to differentiate the properties of drugs, categorizing them into Qi and flavor. The occurrence of diseases, whether caused by external or internal factors, leads to an imbalance (excess or deficiency) of visceral Qi within the body.

Since drugs have their own tendencies in terms of Qi and flavor, they can be used to correct such imbalances in the diseased body. For example, heat diseases are treated with cold-natured drugs, cold diseases with hot-natured drugs, deficiency conditions with tonics, and excess conditions with purgatives. All these utilize the inherent tendencies of drugs to adjust the imbalance in the diseased body, that is, using one tendency to counteract another, aiming to restore balance. This aligns with the statement in *The Inner Canon of Huangdi*: "Treat cold with heat, treat heat with cold, regulate their Qi to bring them to balance."

1.Qi

The Qi of medicinal properties is divided into four categories: cold, hot, warm, and cool. Beyond these four, there is also neutral Qi. In reality, so-called neutral Qi still leans slightly toward warmth or coolness, but its nature is relatively mild and less pronounced. Hence, they are generally referred to as the four Qi.

The four distinct medicinal properties—cold, hot, warm, and cool—can be viewed from two perspectives. Hot and cold are two extremes; warm is less intense than hot, and cool is less intense than cold. Specifically, there are cold-natured, cool-natured, hot-natured, and warm-natured drugs, which can also be simply categorized as cold-cool drugs and warm-hot drugs. The classification of drugs into the four Qi is a generalization of their properties, derived from the various reactions they induce in the human body. For instance, since gypsum and anemarrhena can treat heat diseases, they are known to have cold-cool properties; since aconite and cinnamon can treat cold diseases, they are known to have warm-hot properties. In other words, cold and cool-natured drugs have the effects of clearing heat and purging fire, while hot and warm-natured drugs have the effects of dispelling cold and restoring Yang.

A clear understanding of the four Qi is essential before using drugs.

When classified using Yin-Yang, cold-cool drugs belong to Yin, and warm-hot drugs belong to Yang. It is known that Yin-Yang is the guiding principle of syndrome differentiation: excess Yang leads to Yin diseases, excess Yin leads to Yang diseases; excess Yang generates heat, excess Yin generates cold; Yin deficiency gives rise to internal heat, and Yang deficiency gives rise to external cold. For this series of syndromes, the fundamental treatment principles are: treat Yin diseases with Yang drugs, treat Yang diseases with Yin drugs; treat heat with cold drugs, treat cold with hot drugs; nourish Yin for Yin deficiency, and support Yang for Yang deficiency. If one only focuses on efficacy while ignoring the four Qi, treating heat with hot drugs would be like adding fuel to the fire, and treating cold with cold drugs would be like adding frost to snow. As predecessors once said: "If Cinnamon Twig Decoction is taken, those with excess Yang will perish; if Chengqi Decoction enters the stomach, those with excess Yin will surely die." This is not the fault of Cinnamon Twig Decoction or Chengqi Decoction, but the adverse consequence of failing to understand the medicinal properties of these formulas.

2.Flavor

Flavors are divided into five tastes: sour, bitter, sweet, pungent, and salty. Our predecessors identified the flavors of medicines by personally tasting them. Through long-term practice, they gradually realized that medicines have various tastes and thus possess different properties. The *Huangdi Neijing* states that "pungent disperses, sour astringes, sweet moderates, bitter can firm, salty softens", which summarizes the functions of the five flavors. On this basis, predecessors further supplemented: Pungent flavors can disperse and promote circulation; sour flavors can astringe and secure; sweet flavors can tonify and harmonize; bitter flavors can dry and purge; salty flavors can soften and descend. Specifically, all pungent medicines such as perilla and ephedra can dispel exterior pathogens, and cyperus and amomum can promote qi and relax the chest; sour medicines such as pomegranate rind and gallnut can astringe and secure the intestines, and dogwood and schisandra can stop prolapse and secure essence; sweet medicines such as astragalus and prepared rehmannia can tonify qi and yin, and licorice and jujube can tonify deficiency and moderate the middle; bitter medicines such as coptis and phellodendron can purge fire and dry dampness, and rhubarb and aloe can purge heat and promote bowel movements; salty medicines such as seaweed and kelp can resolve phlegm and soften hardness, and mirabilite can moisten the intestines and purge. In addition, there are bland-flavored medicines such as poria and tetrapanax, which have the effect of draining dampness and promoting diuresis, making it six flavors in total. However, since bland is not a distinct taste, they are generally still called the five flavors.

The correspondence between the five flavors and the five elements is: Sour belongs to wood, bitter to fire, sweet to earth, pungent to metal, and salty to water. Therefore, the relationship between the five flavors and the five *zang*-organs is: Sour enters the liver, bitter enters the heart, sweet enters the spleen, pungent enters the lung, and salty enters the kidney. However, like the four qi mentioned above, the five flavors are all biased in nature. They can adjust the imbalance of *zang*-qi, and can also damage *zang*-qi and cause diseases. For example, pungent travels to qi, so qi diseases cannot use too many pungent flavors; salty travels to blood, so blood diseases cannot use too many salty flavors; bitter travels to bones, so bone diseases cannot use too many bitter flavors; sweet travels to muscles, so muscle diseases cannot use too many sweet flavors; sour travels to tendons, so tendon diseases cannot use too many sour flavors. Another example: Excessive use of salty flavors leads to blood vessel stasis and discoloration; excessive use of bitter flavors leads to withered skin and hair; excessive use of pungent flavors leads to tense tendons and withered nails;

excessive use of sour flavors leads to rough and thickened muscles; excessive use of sweet flavors leads to bone pain and hair loss. This is the impact of the five flavors on the physiology of the five *zang*-organs, which not only applies to treatment with medicines but also serves as a criterion for dietary maintenance.

Like the four qi, the five flavors can also be classified into yin and yang categories: Pungent, sweet, and bland belong to yang; sour, bitter, and salty belong to yin. More importantly, the properties of a medicine are a combination of its qi and flavor. Each medicine has both qi and flavor; some have the same qi but different flavors, and some have different qi but the same flavor. For example, with the same warm nature, there are the pungent-warm of ginger, the bitter-warm of magnolia bark, the sweet-warm of astragalus, the sour-warm of papaya, and the salty-warm of gecko. Another example, with the same pungent flavor, there are the pungent-cold of gypsum, the pungent-cool of mint, the pungent-hot of aconite, and the pungent-warm of pinellia. There are also those with one qi and multiple flavors, such as the bitter-pungent-warm of ephedra, the pungent-sweet-warm of cinnamon twig, and the sweet-pungent-slightly bitter-slightly cold of cimicifuga. These intricate combinations of qi and flavor precisely indicate that the properties of medicines are diverse.

There are many medicines with the same qi and flavor but completely different effects. The reason is that qi and flavor have varying degrees of thickness: those with thick qiare floating, those with thick flavor are sinking, those with thin flavor are ascending, and those with thin qi are descending. Ascent, descent, floating, and sinking are the tendencies of medicinal actions; different tendencies lead to differences in efficacy. "Ascent" means rising upward, "descent" means falling downward, "floating" means dispersing outward, and "sinking" means purging and draining. Ascending-floating medicines mostly rise upward and act on the exterior, with effects such as lifting yang, inducing sweating, and clearing the head and eyes. Descending-sinking medicines mostly go downward and act on the interior, with effects such as subduing yang, lowering rebellious qi, and promoting the smooth flow of urine and bowel movements. It is easy to understand that diseases can occur on the exterior, interior, upper body, or lower body, and the disease tendency can be upward rebellion or downward collapse. Therefore, to use medicines appropriately, in addition to paying attention to qi and flavor, one must also understand ascent, descent, floating, and sinking, and know that these tendencies can be transformed through processing. For example, stir-frying with wine makes a medicine ascend; stir-frying with ginger juice makes it disperse; stir-frying with vinegar makes it astringe; stir-frying with salt water makes it descend. Hence, Li Shizhen said: "An ascending medicine, guided by a salty-cold substance, will sink and reach the lower jiao directly; a sinking medicine, guided by wine, will float and reach the top of the head."

Studying the qi, flavor, ascent, descent, floating, and sinking of medicines is, in general, to understand their properties. We believe that when researching Chinese medicines, this aspect must be emphasized. If one only pays attention to efficacy while ignoring properties, they cannot truly master the efficacy of medicines. For instance, pinellia, Sichuan fritillary, and seaweed can all resolve phlegm, but pinellia, being pungent and warm, can transform damp-phlegm; Sichuan fritillary, being sweet, bitter, and slightly cold, can transform heat-phlegm; seaweed, being bitter, salty, and cold, can dissipate phlegm nodules. Another example: Astragalus, Chinese yam, and adenophora are all tonics, but astragalus, being sweet and warm, is used to tonify qi deficiency; Chinese yam, being sweet and neutral, is used to tonify spleen deficiency; adenophora, being sweet, slightly bitter, and slightly cold, is used to tonify insufficient lung yin. These medicines have similar efficacy but different effects, mainly due to differences in their properties. If one does not consider this aspect, they may likely use a variety of phlegm-resolving medicines indiscriminately for phlegm syndromes, or a variety of tonic medicines for deficiency syndromes, which clearly does not conform to the principle of treating the root cause in medication.

A supplementary explanation here is that the composition of formulas also attaches importance to qi and flavor. The book *Systematic Differentiation of Warm Diseases* mostly specifies the qi and flavor of the formulas used. For example, Yinqiao Powder is a mild acrid-cool formula, Sangju Yin is a light acrid-cool formula, and Baihu decoction is a heavy acrid-cool formula. It also points out that Qingluo Yin follows the acrid-cool and aromatic method, Qingying decoction follows the salty-cold, bitter, and sweet method, Xinjia Xiangru Yin follows the combined acrid-warm and acrid-cool method, and Qingshu Yiqi decoction follows the combined method of acrid-sweet transforming yang and sour-sweet transforming yin, etc. When learning formulas, one must pay attention to this, as it not only clarifies the treatment guidelines but also helps understand the changes in efficacy after medicines are composed into formulas.

II. Efficacy

Xu Zhicai of the Northern Qi Dynasty once classified the efficacy of drugs into ten types, saying: "Drugs have ten major categories: Xuan (dispersing), Tong (unblocking), Bu (tonifying), Xie (purging), Qing (light), Zhong (heavy), Hua (slippery), Se (astringent), Zao (drying), Shi (moistening), which are the main aspects of drugs." The contents are: Xuan can eliminate congestion, such as ginger and orange peel, which are qi-regulating and stomach-harmonizing drugs; Tong can remove stagnation, such as tetrapanax and stephania, which are diuretics; Bu can alleviate weakness, such as ginseng and mutton, which are tonic and nutritious drugs; Xie can relieve obstruction, such as Lepidium and rhubarb, which are water-purging and bowel-relaxing drugs; Qing can reduce excess, such as ephedra and pueraria, which are muscle-relaxing and diaphoretic drugs; Zhong can dispel fear, such as magnetite and iron powder, which are tranquilizing and sedative drugs; Hua can remove adhesion, such as winter mallow seeds and elm bark, which are diuretic and intestine-moistening drugs; Se can prevent prolapse, such as oyster and dragon bone, which are astringent and consolidating drugs; Zao can eliminate dampness, such as mulberry bark and adzuki beans, which are dampness-regulating and phlegm-resolving drugs; Shi can relieve dryness, such as white quartz and purple quartz, which are moistening drugs. Kou Zongshi of the Song Dynasty added two types: Han (cold) can remove heat, i.e., cooling drugs; Re (hot) can remove cold, i.e., warm-hot drugs. Jia Jiuru of the Qing Dynasty put forward: Xiong (powerful) can disperse externally, Rui (sharp) can descend, He (harmonizing) can soothe the middle, Huan (mild) can control urgency, Ping (mild) can nourish, Jing (calm) can control movement, etc. Each has its own insights and can be used for reference.

The current general classification is clearer, roughly as follows:

(1) Exterior-releasing drugs: Having a dispersing effect, including relieving external pathogens such as wind-cold, wind-heat, wind-dampness, and summer heat invading the exterior. Acrid-warm exterior-releasing drugs such as ephedra, cinnamon twig, perilla, notopterygium, angelica pubescens, schizonepeta, saposhnikovia, asarum, elsholtzia, angelica dahurica, gentiana macrophylla; acrid-cool exterior-releasing drugs such as pueraria, bupleurum, mint, fermented soybean, soybean sprout, mulberry leaf, chrysanthemum, duckweed, cimicifuga; wind-dampness-dispelling drugs such as clematis, angelica dahurica, trachelospermum, acanthopanax bark, kadsura pepper stem, etc.

(2) Purgative drugs: Having the effect of relaxing the bowels (including expelling water). Cold-purging drugs such as rhubarb, mirabilite; hot-purging drugs such as croton; moist-purging drugs such as hemp seed, trichosanthes seed, bunge cherry seed; water-expelling drugs such as euphorbia, genkwa, kansui, morning glory seed, pokeweed, lepidium, etc.

(3) Dampness-regulating drugs: Having the effect of eliminating dampness and promoting diuresis. Aromatic dampness-transforming drugs such as agastache, eupatorium, finger citron, atractylodes, magnolia bark, amomum tsao-ko; bland-dispersing drugs such as poria, tetrapanax, coix seed; diuretic drugs such as plantain, alisma, akebia, stephania, dianthus superbus, polyporus, dioscorea collettii, polygonum aviculare, etc.

(4) Cold-dispelling drugs: Having the effect of warming the middle (including restoring yang). Middle-warming and cold-dispelling drugs such as evodia, clove, dried ginger, fennel, aconite; yang-supporting and fire-strengthening drugs such as monkshood, cinnamon, alpinia oxyphylla, nutmeg, morinda officinalis, etc.

(5) Heat-clearing drugs: Having the effect of clearing internal heat (including detoxifying). Bitter-cold heat-clearing drugs such as coptis, scutellaria, phellodendron, anemarrhena, gardenia, gentian, forsythia, artemisia annua, prunella vulgaris, moutan bark, honeysuckle; sweet-cold heat-clearing drugs such as fresh rehmannia, gypsum, bamboo leaf, bamboo shavings, trichosanthes root, wolfberry bark, reed rhizome, cogongrass rhizome; heat-clearing and detoxifying drugs such as scrophularia, rhinoceros horn, indigo naturalis, isatis leaf, lasiosphaera, belamcanda, sophora tonkinensis, viola yedoensis, isatis root, etc.

(6) Emetic drugs: Having the effect of inducing vomiting. Such as melon pedicel, veratrum, copper sulfate, etc.

(7) Digestive drugs: Having the effect of promoting digestion and

invigorating the stomach. Such as medicated leaven, hawthorn, malt, amomum, coix seed, radish seed, chicken's gizzard membrane, etc.

(8) Antitussive drugs: Having the effect of clearing the lung (including resolving phlegm and relieving asthma). Clearing the lung to stop cough such as peucedanum, arctium, almond, fritillary, platycodon, mulberry bark, loquat leaf, aristolochia, lily, stemona, boat-fruited sterculia; warming the lung to stop cough such as cynanchum, inula, aster, coltsfoot flower; resolving phlegm and relieving asthma such as bile arisaema, pinellia, white mustard seed, perilla seed, bamboo yellow, pumice, stalactite, bamboo juice, seaweed, kelp, sea loquat, etc.

(9) Qi-regulating drugs: Having the effect of smoothing qi movement. Promoting qi circulation such as dried tangerine peel, lindera, aucklandia, cyperus, curcuma, toosendan fruit, citrus medica; breakingqi stagnation such as immature bitter orange, green tangerine peel, agarwood, magnolia bark, etc.

(10) Blood-regulating drugs: Having the effect of harmonizing blood, including breaking blood stasis and stopping bleeding. Activating blood circulation such as angelica, ligusticum, safflower, spatholobus, trogopterus dung, corydalis, frankincense, myrrh; breaking blood stasis such as peach kernel, patrinia, motherwort, turmeric, artemisia anomala, ground beetle, leech, horsefly; stopping bleeding such as agrimony, pseudo-ginseng, typha pollen, bletilla, sophora flower, sanguisorba, arborvitae leaf, rubia, carbonized hair, thistle, small thistle, palm, lotus node, etc.

(11) Tonic drugs: Having the effect of nourishing and strengthening (including tonifying qi, blood, warming tonification, and cooling tonification). Tonifying qi such as ginseng, codonopsis, astragalus, atractylodes, yam, licorice; tonifying blood such as prepared rehmannia, polygonum multiflorum, donkey-hide gelatin, longan aril, angelica body,

white peony root; warming and tonifying such as pilose antler, cistanche, dodder, gecko, schisandra, psoralea, cibotium, eucommia, dipsacus, seal penis, antler gelatin, tiger bone gelatin; cooling and tonifying such as adenophora, ophiopogon, dendrobium, privet fruit, turtle shell, turtle carapace, wolfberry, privet fruit, asparagus, etc.

(12) Orifice-opening drugs: Having the effect of refreshing the mind and dispelling filth. Such as musk, bezoar, toad venom, borneol, storax, benzoin, acorus, etc.

(13) Sedative drugs: Having the effect of heavy settling, including calming wind and tranquilizing the mind. Heavy settling such as magnetite, haematite; calming wind and subduing yang such as gastrodia, uncaria, abalone shell, oyster, antelope horn, hawksbill shell, centipede, scorpion; tranquilizing the mind such as polygala, jujube seed, platycladus seed, dragon's tooth, cinnabar, poria with hostwood, pearl powder, etc.

(14) Astringent drugs: Having the astringent effect (including stopping sweating, securing essence, and controlling diarrhea). Stopping sweating such as ephedra root, floating wheat, glutinous rice root, schisandra; securing essence such as cherokee rose, gorgon fruit, lotus stamen, lotus seed, dragon bone; controlling diarrhea such as poppy shell, red halloysite, pomegranate rind, terminalia, etc.

(15) Anthelmintic drugs: Having the effect of killing parasites. Such as quisqualis, ulmus pumila, omphalia, carpesium, torreya, areca nut, realgar, chinaberry root, etc.

From the above, we can see the richness of traditional Chinese medicines and their diverse functions in treatment. We understand that the action of drugs on the human body mainly involves two aspects: One is to restore and strengthen physical strength, and the other is to eliminate pathogenic factors. In simple terms, it is to strengthen the healthy qi and eliminate pathogenic factors, which is also the principle stated in *The Inner Canon of Huangdi*: "Tonify in deficiency, purge in excess". For the convenience of learning and clinical application, the most commonly used drugs are further described below in combination with common symptoms, with notes on whether they should be used raw or processed.

1.Healthy qi-strengthening category

(1) Those pertaining to the lung: divided into lung qi deficiency and lung yin deficiency.

Tonifying lung qi - sun-dried ginseng, raw astragalus, cordyceps, yam.

Tonifying lung yin - northern adenophora, ophiopogon, Sichuan lily.

(2) Those pertaining to the heart: divided into heart blood deficiency and restless spirit.

Tonifying heart blood - fine Rehmannia, Ophiopogon japonicus, Ziziphus jujuba var. spinosa, Platycladus orientalis seed, longan aril, jujube, Schisandra chinensis, floating wheat.

Tranquilizing the mind - dragon's tooth, Yun Poria cum Radice Pini (when mixed with cinnabar, it is called Zhu Fushen), pearl powder.

(3) Those pertaining to the liver: divided into liver blood deficiency and liver yang ascending.

Tonifying liver blood - Angelica sinensis body, Paeonia lactiflora, processed Polygonum multiflorum, donkey-hide gelatin, Astragalus complanatus.

Subduing yang and calming wind - raw oyster, raw abalone shell, Uncaria rhynchophylla, Gastrodia elata, Hangzhou Chrysanthemum morifolium, antelope horn tip, stir-fried scorpion.

(4) Those pertaining to the spleen: divided into middle qi deficiency

and middle qi sinking.

Tonifying middle qi - Codonopsis pilosula, Atractylodes macrocephala, Dioscorea opposita, honey-fried Glycyrrhiza uralensis, Dolichos lablab, maltose.

Raising middle qi - honey-fried Cimicifuga foetida, soft Bupleurum chinense, simmered Pueraria lobata.

(5) Those pertaining to the kidney: divided into yin deficiency, yang deficiency, insecure essence gate, and weak muscles and bones.

Tonifying yin - Rehmannia glutinosa preparata, Cornus officinalis, Asparagus cochinchinensis, Cuscutae semen cake, Morus alba fruit, ripe Ligustrum lucidum, honey-fried Trionyx sinensis shell, turtle shell, processed Polygonatum sibiricum, placenta hominis, walnut meat.

Tonifying yang - Lycium barbarum, Cervus elaphus velvet, Callorhinus ursinus kidney, Alpinia oxyphylla, Cervus elaphus antler glue, Cinnamomum cassia, prepared Aconitum carmichaeli, Morinda officinalis flesh, Cynomorium songaricum, Trigonella foenum-graecum.

Securing essence - Rosa laevigata, calcined Os draconis, calcined Concha ostreae, Nelumbo nucifera stamen, Euryale ferox, Mantidis ootheca.

Strengthening muscles and bones - stir-fried Eucommia ulmoides, Dipsacus asperoides, honey-fried Panthera tigris bone, Achyranthes bidentata, honey-fried Cibotium barometz, Psoralea corylifolia, Chaenomeles sinensis.

(6) Those pertaining to the intestines and stomach: divided into fluid deficiency, weak digestion, loose bowels, and constipation.

Nourishing fluids - Dendrobium nobile (fresh one is called fresh Dendrobium), Trichosanthes kirilowii root, Polygonatum odoratum.

Aiding digestion - Gallus gallus domesticus gizzard lining, Amomum villosum, Amomum kravanh, stir-fried Oryza sativa germ.

Astringing the large intestine - Terminalia chebula, Papaver somniferum shell, Halloysitum rubrum, simmered Myristica fragrans.

Relieving constipation - raw Rheum palmatum (stir-fried Rheum palmatum can also be used), Natrii sulfas exsiccatus, Aloe vera, Citrus aurantium.

Moistening the intestines - Cannabis sativa seed, Trichosanthes kirilowii seed, Prunus japonicus seed, light Cynomorium songaricum, honey.

(7) Those pertaining to the bladder: divided into scanty and painful urination, and enuresis or incontinence.

Diuresis - Yun Poria cocos, Polyporus umbellatus, red Poria cocos, Plantago asiatica seed, Alisma plantago-aquatica, Benincasa hispida skin, Tetrapanax papyrifer, Akebia quinata, Areca catechu skin.

Relieving stranguria - Pyrrosia lingua, Dianthus superbus spike, Polygonum aviculare, Lygodium japonicum, Smilax glabra.

Stopping enuresis - Rubus idaeus, Schisandra chinensis, Bombyx mori cocoon.

2.Pathogen-expelling category

(1) Those pertaining to external pathogens: divided into wind-heat, wind-cold, summer-heat pathogen, internal cold, and wind-damp pain.

Dispelling wind-heat - Morus alba leaf, Hangzhou Chrysanthemum morifolium, Mentha haplocalyx, clear Glycine max sprout, light fermented soybean, Schizonepeta tenuifolia, Saposhnikovia divaricata, Pueraria lobata, soft Bupleurum chinense, Cicadae periostracum, Vitex trifolia, Platycodon grandiflorus.

Dispelling wind-cold - raw Ephedra sinica (honey-fried Ephedra sinica can also be used), Cinnamomum cassia twig, Perilla frutescens, Notopterygium incisum, Angelica pubescens, Allium fistulosum white, Zingiber officinale, Angelica dahurica, Asarum sieboldii, Ligusticum sinense, Magnolia biondii flower.

Clearing summer-heat pathogen - Elsholtzia ciliata, Agastache rugosa, Eupatorium fortunei, Nelumbo nucifera leaf (from after Dragon Boat Festival to before Mid-Autumn Festival, fresh Agastache rugosa, fresh Eupatorium fortunei, fresh Nelumbo nucifera leaf are generally used), Artemisia annua.

Warming the middle to dispel cold - Evodia rutaecarpa, Cinnamomum cassia, Zingiber officinale dried, simmered Zingiber officinale, roasted Zingiber officinale, Syzygium aromaticum, Zanthoxylum bungeanum, Foeniculum vulgare, Aconitum carmichaeli.

Dispelling wind-damp pain - Clematis chinensis, Piper kadsura, Trachelospermum jasminoides, Aconitum carmichaeli, Aconitum kusnezoffii, Gentiana macrophylla, Morus alba twig, Luffa cylindrica reticulum.

(2) Those pertaining to heat: divided into heat pathogen, fire pathogen, and blood heat.

Clearing heat - Lonicera japonica, Forsythia suspensa, raw Gypsum fibrosum, floating Talcum, Anemarrhena asphodeloides, Imperata cylindrica root, Phragmites australis root (fresh Imperata cylindrica root and fresh Phragmites australis root can also be used), black Gardenia jasminoides, Scutellaria baicalensis, light Phyllostachys nigra leaf, stir-fried Phyllostachys nigra shavings (fresh Phyllostachys nigra leaf and fresh Phyllostachys nigra shavings can also be used).

Purging fire - Coptis chinensis, Phellodendron chinense, Gentiana scabra, Sophora tonkinensis, raw Glycyrrhiza uralensis.

Clearing blood heat - fresh Rehmannia root, Moutan bark, Cynanchum atratum, Lycium bark, Scrophularia, Rhinoceros horn, Isatis leaf, Isatis root.

(3) Those pertaining to dampness: divided into damp turbidity and damp-heat.

Transforming dampness - processed Atractylodes lancea, Magnolia officinalis, Acorus calamus, simmered Amomum tsao-ko, Amomum cardamomum, stir-fried Coix seed.

Clearing damp-heat - Dioscorea collettii, Sophora flavescens, Artemisia capillaris, Dictamnus dasycarpus, Stephania tetrandra.

(4) Those pertaining to phlegm: divided into heat-phlegm, wind-phlegm, cold-phlegm, fluid retention, and phlegm nodules.

Transforming heat-phlegm - baked Aristolochia, dilute bamboo juice, Fritillaria cirrhosa, Bambusa concretio silicea, roasted Mulberry bark, sweet almond, Loquat leaf (clear roasted Loquat leaf can also be used), bile Arisaema, Belamcanda chinensis, Eleocharis dulcis, Rhopilema esculentum.

Transforming wind-phlegm - stir-fried Arctium lappa, Peucedanum praeruptorum, bitter almond, Fritillaria thunbergii, bitter Platycodon grandiflorus, Sterculia lychnophora.

Transforming cold-phlegm - ginger-processed Pinellia ternata, dried tangerine peel, roasted Perilla seed, calcined Stalactite, roasted Stemonae, roasted Aster tataricus, roasted Tussilago farfara.

Expelling fluid retention - Lepidium apetalum, processed Kansui, black Pharbitis seed, Phytolacca acinosa, Gryllotalpa orientalis, Gryllus chinensis.

Resolving phlegm nodules - light Kelp, light Seaweed, Cremastra appendiculata, roasted Bombyx batryticatus, Taraxacum mongolicum.

(5) Those pertaining to qi: divided into qi stagnation and qi rebellion.

Relieving qi stagnation - broad Curcuma longa, processed Cyperus rotundus, Tribulus terrestris, Liquidambar formosana, Melia toosendan, Toosendan fruit, Citrus medica, Citrus sarcodactylis, Citrus aurantium, Rosa rugosa, green tangerine peel, simmered Aucklandia lappa, Lindera aggregata, processed Frankincense, roasted Myrrh, Santalum album.

Calming qi rebellion - Agarwood, Inula japonica, Haematitum, calcined Magnetite, Gecko tail.

(6) Those pertaining to blood: divided into blood stasis, static blood, and bleeding.

Activating blood - whole Angelica sinensis, Ligusticum chuanxiong, Carthamus tinctorius, Spatholobus suberectus, Caesalpinia sappan, Trogopterus dung, Salvia miltiorrhiza.

Breaking static blood - Lycopus lucidus, Leonurus japonicus, Sparganium stoloniferum, Curcuma zedoaria, Vaccaria segetalis, Patrinia scabiosaefolia, mashed Prunus persica seed, Eupolyphaga sinensis.

Stopping bleeding - Panax notoginseng, Rubia cordifolia, Agrimonia pilosa, Platycladus orientalis leaf, Eclipta prostrata, carbonized Sophora japonica flower, carbonized Sanguisorba officinalis, carbonized human hair, carbonized Trachycarpus fortunei, carbonized Typha angustifolia, Nelumbo nucifera node.

(7) Those pertaining to accumulations: divided into worm accumulation and food accumulation.

Killing worms - Quisqualis indica fruit, Ulmus pumila, Carpesium abrotanoides, Omphalia lapidescens, roasted Stemonae, Areca catechu,

Melia azedarach root.

Promoting digestion - Medicated leaven, carbonized Crataegus pinnatifida, charred Hordeum vulgare germ, stir-fried Raphinus sativus seed.

Classifying drugs according to their functions is mainly for the convenience of clinical practice. However, it must be emphasized that a drug has multiple effects, and neglecting other aspects will reduce its comprehensive efficacy. Therefore, for each drug, one should fully understand its nature, flavor, and efficacy, and then grasp its main indications. In this way, it can be used flexibly in practice.

The earliest classification of drugs can be found in *Shennong Bencao Jing* (Shennong's Classic of Materia Medica), which divides them into superior, middle, and inferior grades. Superior grade refers to tonic drugs that are beneficial when taken in large amounts for a long time and are considered non-toxic; middle grade includes drugs that are either toxic or non-toxic, capable of curing diseases and nourishing the body, with their effects depending on proper usage; inferior grade mostly consists of toxic drugs used to treat diseases such as cold and heat stagnation. This general classification based on efficacy is basically correct, except for some parts that need correction. Herbal books after the Han and Decoction dynasties mostly classify drugs according to their own attributes. The most detailed one is *Compendium of Materia Medica* by Li Shizhen, which divides drugs into 16 sections and 62 categories. The 16 sections are Water, Fire, Earth, Metals and Stones, Grasses, Grains, Vegetables, Fruits, Trees, Clothing and Utensils, Insects, Scales, Shellfish, Birds, Beasts, and Humans. The 62 categories are subdivisions within each section. For example, the Grass section is divided into nine categories: Mountain Grasses, Fragrant Grasses, Marsh Grasses, Poisonous Grasses, Vines, Water Grasses, Stone Grasses, Mosses, and Miscellaneous Grasses, and the same applies to other sections.

This has provided certain favorable conditions for later studies on pharmacology.

Our predecessors also compiled works to facilitate the learning of materia medica, first *Yaoxing* Fu (Ode to Medicinal Properties), then *Xinbian Yao*fu (New Compilation of Ode to Medicinal Properties) (included in *Yijia Siyao* (Four Essentials for Physicians)). A common strength of these two works is that they classify drugs according to the four qi (cold, hot, warm, cool), briefly present their main indications, thus combining qi-flavor with efficacy. We believe that one can choose either to memorize thoroughly first, and then read other herbal books such as *Bencao Congxin* (New Compilation of Materia Medica), so as to gradually improve their knowledge.

III. Channel Tropism

Each drug has a specific effect on certain *zang-fu* organs and meridians, and predecessors attributed a drug to specific *zang-fu* organs and meridians. For example, ephedra enters the lung and bladder meridians, indicating that the effect of ephedra is mainly on the lung and bladder meridians. Whenever the lung and bladder are attacked by cold pathogens, using the pungent and warm nature of ephedra to dispel them is most appropriate. Therefore, ephedra is good at treating exterior cold in Taiyang disease and can also relieve cough and asthma. This method is called "channel tropism".

Channel tropism is of great significance in practical application. As mentioned earlier, cold drugs can treat heat diseases, hot drugs can treat cold diseases; heat-clearing drugs are mostly cold in nature, and cold-dispelling drugs are mostly warm or hot in nature. This is a basic principle. However, the same heat syndrome or cold syndrome can occur in different parts of the body, either on the exterior, in the interior, in *zang* organs, or in fu organs. For instance, a certain cold drug that can clear exterior heat may not necessarily clear interior heat, and one that can clear heat in the lung may not necessarily clear heat in the stomach; similarly, a warm or hot drug that can dispel exterior cold may not necessarily dispel interior cold, and one that can dispel cold in the lung may not necessarily dispel cold in the stomach. It can be seen that drugs have their own scope of application in the human body, and channel tropism indicates this scope.

The "channel" in channel tropism refers to the meridians and collaterals. Meridians and collaterals are distributed throughout the body; when symptoms of a certain channel appear, drugs that act on that channel are used. For example, the same headache: Pain in the forehead belongs to the Yangming channel, so Pueraria is used; pain in the back of the neck belongs to the Taiyang channel, so Ephedra is used; pain on both sides belongs to the Shaoyang channel, so Bupleurum is used. This is because Pueraria is a drug for the Yangming channel, Ephedra for the Taiyang channel, and Bupleurum for the Shaoyang channel. However, meridians and collaterals are closely connected with internal organs; therefore, a certain drug can exert its specific effect on a particular channel and organ. This specific effect is also related to the drug's qi, flavor, and nature. For instance, the bladder pertains to cold water, and its channel is the Taiyang channel. Ephedra has thin, clustered stems that are hollow and grow straight upward, with a light and clear qi and flavor, so it can unblock the yang qi in the lower jiao, bring it out through the skin and hair to induce sweating, and is a key drug for Taiyang exterior cold in cold damage. Or Qianghuo can be used instead of Ephedra, also because its deep roots and straight stems can guide the yang qi of the bladder to reach the meridians, but its flavor is more pungent and intense, and it can also dispel dampness, unlike Ephedra which is light and clear. Thus, Ephedra can also diffuse the lung and promote urination, while Qianghuo can also treat wind-dampness body pain, showing similarities with differences.

In summary, channel tropism is a rule for using drugs. After understanding the properties and efficacy of drugs, and then knowing their channel tropism, drugs can be used with perfect accuracy.

Section 3 Usage

I. Compatibility (including contraindications)

Each drug has its own effect. Through the combination of drugs, their effects can be enhanced, adverse reactions reduced, and better efficacy exerted, which is the important significance of the combined application of traditional Chinese medicines. From the application of single drugs to combined application, and then to the development of prescriptions, it is undoubtedly a process of progress.

Our predecessors, through practice, recognized the reactions of drug combinations, pointing out not only the beneficial aspects but also the adverse ones. They are divided into six categories.

1. **Mutual reinforcement:** Two drugs with the same efficacy, when used in combination, can promote and strengthen each other's effects. For example, Anemarrhena combined with Phellodendron has a stronger effect of nourishing yin and reducing fire; the prepared formulas Zhibai Bawei Wan and Dabuyin Wan are examples of Anemarrhena and Phellodendron used in combination.
2. **Mutual assistance:** Two drugs with different efficacies, when combined, can reach the diseased site directly and exert better curative effects. For example, Aconite takes Poria as an assistant; in the prepared formulas Zhenwu decoction and Fuzi decoction, Poria is used

as an assistant to Aconite.

3. **Mutual inhibition:** One drug can be restrained by another, thereby reducing or eliminating its intensity, which is called mutual inhibition. For example, Pinellia is inhibited by Ginger; therefore, Ginger is used to process Pinellia to reduce its toxicity, and those poisoned by Pinellia can also be rescued with Ginger.
4. **Mutual antagonism:** When two drugs are used together, their efficacy is reduced due to mutual restraint, which is called mutual antagonism (antagonism means dislike). For example, Ginger is antagonistic to Scutellaria, because Scutellaria is cold in nature and can reduce the warm nature of Ginger.
5. **Mutual detoxication:** One drug can eliminate the toxicity of another, such as Saposhnikovia detoxifies arsenic, and Mung Bean detoxifies Croton.
6. **Mutual incompatibility:** When used together, they can cause severe side effects, such as Aconitum is incompatible with Pinellia, and Licorice is incompatible with Kansui.

Drugs that are mutually incompatible or mutually inhibitory must be used with caution. Therefore, predecessors compiled the "Song of Eighteen Incompatibilities" and "Song of Nineteen Inhibitions".

Song of Eighteen Incompatibilities: The materia medica clearly states eighteen incompatibilities; Banxia (Pinellia), Lou (Trichosanthes), Bei (Fritillaria), Lian (Adenophora), and Gong (Kuanxiong) are incompatible with Wu (Aconitum); Zao (Seaweed), Ji (Euphorbia), Sui (Kansui), Yuan (Genkwa) all conflict with Cao (Licorice); various Shen (Ginseng), Xin (Asarum), Gou (Angelica) are incompatible with Lilu (Veratrum).

The eighteen kinds of medicines mentioned in the song indicate significant incompatibility, such as Pinellia ternata, Trichosanthes kirilowii, Fritillaria, Adenophora stricta, Bletilla striata being incompatible with

Aconitum; Sargassum, Euphorbia pekinensis, Kansui, Daphne genkwa being incompatible with Glycyrrhiza uralensis; Ginseng, Adenophora stricta, Asarum sieboldii, Paeonia lactiflora being incompatible with Veratrum nigrum.

Song of Nineteen Inhibitions: Sulfur is originally the essence of fire, and it will conflict with Mirabilite at first sight; Mercury should not meet Arsenic, and Stellera chamaejasme fears Lithargyrum the most; Croton is extremely intense in nature and is particularly incompatible with Pharbitis; Clove should not meet Curcuma, and Natrii sulfas exsiccatus hardly mixes with Sparganium stoloniferum; Aconitum carmichaeli and Aconitum kusnezoffii are incompatible with Rhinoceros horn; Ginseng fears Trogopterus dung the most; Cinnamomum cassia is good at regulating cold qi, but it will be opposed if it meets Halloysitum rubrum. In general, when preparing medicines, one should check for compatibility and incompatibility, and processing methods such as roasting, stir-frying, and calcining should not be neglected.

The nineteen kinds of medicines mentioned in the song indicate significant inhibition, such as Sulfur being inhibited by Mirabilite, Mercury by Arsenic, Stellera chamaejasme by Lithargyrum, Croton by Pharbitis, Clove by Curcuma, Natrii sulfas exsiccatus by Sparganium stoloniferum, Aconitum carmichaeli and Aconitum kusnezoffii by Rhinoceros horn, Ginseng by Trogopterus dung, Cinnamomum cassia by Halloysitum rubrum.

In addition, pregnancy contraindication drugs, also known as abortifacient drugs, have long been recorded in herbal books, and by the time of *Compendium of Materia Medica*, the number had increased to 87. Some of these drugs are no longer used at all, and the ones still in use are listed below. They should be avoided as much as possible in prescriptions to prevent accidents. Plant drugs such as Euphorbia pekinensis, Croton,

Veratrum nigrum, Paeonia suffruticosa, Achyranthes bidentata, Cinnamomum cassia, Gleditsia sinensis, Coix lacryma-jobi, Dianthus superbus, Aconitum carmichaeli, Aconitum kusnezoffii, Pharbitis, Pinellia ternata, Arisaema heterophyllum, Prunus persica, Daphne genkwa, Sophora japonica, Rubia cordifolia, Carthamus tinctorius, Imperata cylindrica, Hordeum vulgare, Sparganium stoloniferum, Zingiber officinale, Magnolia officinalis, Tetrapanax papyrifer, Caesalpinia sappan, Malva verticillata, Dichroa febrifuga, Zingiber officinale; animal drugs such as Calculus bovis, Scolopendra subspinipes, Mylabris, Hirudo nipponica, Tabanus bivittatus, Cimex lectularius, Gryllotalpa orientalis, Erinaceus europaeus, Lacerta agilis, Elaphe carinata, Moschus; mineral drugs such as Realgar, Mirabilite, Haematitum, Sal ammoniac, Arsenic. Pregnancy-prohibited drugs are mainly to prevent miscarriage, but they are not all prohibited. For example, *Jiyin Gangmu*, the most popular gynecological monograph, uses drugs such as Aconitum carmichaeli, Cinnamomum cassia, Pinellia ternata, Achyranthes bidentata, Paeonia suffruticosa, Magnolia officinalis, Imperata cylindrica, Tetrapanax papyrifer, Prunus persica, Mirabilite in preventing miscarriage and treating various diseases during pregnancy. *Huangdi Neijing* also said: “What about using toxic drugs on a pregnant woman? If there is a cause, it will not cause damage, and there will be no damage. For large accumulations and aggregations, they can be attacked, but only until more than half of them are reduced.” However, some drugs that are prohibited during pregnancy should still be used cautiously and not carelessly.

Experience tells us that predecessors were very careful about the combination of drugs, because proper combination can achieve higher curative effects.

Now, a few examples are given for reference in prescriptions. Cinnamomum cassia combined with Coptis chinensis: named Jiaotai Pill, which can treat disharmony between the heart and kidney.

(1) Evodia rutaecarpa combined with Coptis chinensis: named Zuojin Pill, which can calm the liver and reduce acid.

(2) Zingiber officinale combined with Coptis chinensis: can eliminate cold and heat evil accumulation in the chest.

(3) Pinellia ternata combined with Coptis chinensis: can resolve phlegm-turbidity, damp-heat stagnation, relax the chest and stop vomiting.

(4) Magnolia officinalis combined with Coptis chinensis: can resolve damp-heat in the spleen and stomach.

(5) Cinnamomum cassia twig combined with Paeonia lactiflora: can regulate ying and wei.

(6) Angelica sinensis combined with Paeonia lactiflora: can nourish blood.

(7) Angelica sinensis combined with Ligusticum chuanxiong: named Foshou Powder, which can promote blood circulation.

(8) Typha angustifolia combined with Trogopterus dung: named Shixiao Powder, which can dispel blood stasis and relieve pain.

(9) Prunus persica combined with Carthamus tinctorius: can promote blood circulation and unblock menstruation.

(11) Bupleurum chinense combined with Scutellaria baicalensis: can clear heat in the liver and gallbladder.

(12) Bupleurum chinense combined with Paeonia lactiflora: can soothe the liver and harmonize the liver.

(13) Morus alba combined with Chrysanthemum morifolium: can clear wind-heat in the head and eyes.

(14) Alpinia officinarum combined with Cyperus rotundus: named Liangfu

Pill, which can relieve stomach pain.

(15) Corydalis yanhusuo combined with Melia toosendan: named Jinlingzi Powder, which can treat abdominal pain.

(16) Aconitum carmichaeli combined with Cinnamomum cassia: can warm the lower origin.

(17) Phellodendron chinense combined with Anemarrhena asphodeloides: can clear damp-heat in the lower jiao.

(18) Atractylodes lancea combined with Phellodendron chinense: can treat damp-heat induced flaccidity.

(19) Armeniacae Semen Amarum combined with Fritillaria: can resolve phlegm and stop cough.

(20) Pinellia ternata combined with Citri Reticulatae Pericarpium: can transform damp-phlegm.

(21) Massa Medicata Fermentata combined with Crataegus pinnatifida: can eliminate meat food stagnation.

(22) Amomum kravanh combined with Amomum villosum: can invigorate the spleen and stomach.

(23) Dichroa febrifuga combined with Amomum tsao-ko: can stop malaria.

(24) Os Draconis combined with Concha Ostreae: can astringe essence and qi.

(25) Eucommia ulmoides combined with Dipsacus asperoides: can treat soreness and pain in the waist and knees.

(26) Asparagus cochinchinensis combined with Ophiopogon japonicus: can clear and nourish the lung and kidney.

(27) Pinellia ternata combined with Sulfur: named Banliu Pill, which treats

deficiency-cold constipation.

(28) Ligustrum lucidum combined with Eclipta prostrata: named Erzhi Pill, which can tonify kidney yin.

(29) Morus alba leaf combined with Sesamum indicum: named Sangma Pill, which can treat liver yang dizziness.

(30) Dioscorea opposita combined with Dolichos lablab: can tonify the spleen and stop diarrhea.

(31) Cimicifuga foetida combined with Bupleurum chinense: can lift the sinking middle qi.

(32) Trionyx sinensis shell combined with Artemisia annua: can nourish yin and reduce steaming heat.

(33) Prunus mume combined with Glycyrrhiza uralensis: can promote fluid production and quench thirst.

(34) Atractylodes lancea combined with Magnolia officinalis: can expel damp turbidity.

(35) Fermented soybean combined with Allium fistulosum white: named Congchi Decoction, which can unblock yang and induce sweating.

(36) Gleditsia sinensis combined with Alum: named Xixian Powder, which can induce vomiting of wind-phlegm.

(37) Aucklandia lappa combined with Areca catechu: can soothe the intestines and relieve pain.

(38) Sparganium stoloniferum combined with Curcuma zedoaria: can eliminate hard masses and resolve abdominal masses.

(39) Citrus aurantium combined with Bamboo Shavings: can harmonize the stomach and stop vomiting.

(40) Paeonia suffruticosa bark combined with Gardenia jasminoides: can clear blood heat.

(41) Inula japonica combined with Haematitum: can calm belching.

(42) Syzygium aromaticum combined with Diospyros kaki calyx: can stop hiccups.

(43) Psoralea corylifolia combined with Myristica fragrans: named Ershen Pill, which can stop spleen-kidney diarrhea.

(44) Morus alba bark combined with Lycium chinense bark: can purge lung fire.

(45) Anemarrhena asphodeloides combined with Fritillaria: named Ermu Powder, which can clear lung heat.

(46) Aucklandia lappa combined with Coptis chinensis: named Xianglian Pill, which can stop dysentery with red and white stools.

(47) Alum combined with Curcuma longa: named Baijin Pill, which can treat mania.

(48) Citrus aurantium combined with Atractylodes macrocephala: named Zhizhu Pill, which can invigorate the spleen and resolve abdominal masses.

(49) Halloysitum rubrum combined with Limonitum: named Chishizhi Yuyuliang Decoction, which can astringe the large intestine.

(50) Rosa laevigata combined with Euryale ferox: named Shuilu Erxian Dan, which can stop spermatorrhea.

(51) Lycium barbarum combined with Chrysanthemum morifolium: can improve eyesight.

(52) Zingiber officinale combined with Ziziphus jujuba: can harmonize qi and blood.

There are many examples of such combinations of two medicinal flavors. By paying attention to the compositions of previous works and prepared formulas, more information can be obtained. These materials are methods of using drugs, such as combining cold and heat, combining tonification and purgation, combining upper and lower, exterior and interior, qi and blood, etc., which are very rich and flexible.

II. Dosage

The dosage of traditional Chinese medicines is determined based on the following conditions.

1. **Nature of the drugs:** Drugs with strong and intense qi and flavor are used in small doses, while those with mild properties are used in relatively large doses. Examples of the former include Aconitum, Cinnamon, Dried Ginger, etc.; examples of the latter include Chinese Yam, Poria, Hyacinth Bean, etc. Drugs with heavy texture are used in large doses, and those with light and loose texture are used in small doses. Examples of the former include Turtle Shell, Oyster, Magnetite, etc.; examples of the latter include Mulberry Leaf, Cicada Slough, Rice Paper Pith, etc.
2. **Composition of the prescription:** The dosage of the principal drug is large, and that of the auxiliary drugs is relatively small. For instance, in Baihu Decoction, Gypsum should be used in a large dose, while the dosages of Anemarrhena and Licorice are smaller. In terms of compatibility, such as in Zuojin Pill, the dosage of Evodia should be smaller than that of Coptis. Generally speaking, for the composition of the whole prescription, if there are many types of drugs, the dosage of each is relatively small; if there are few types of drugs, the dosage of each is relatively large.
3. **Condition of the disease:** For severe diseases requiring emergency treatment, the dosage is large; for mild diseases or those suitable for long-term conditioning, the dosage is small. Examples of the former

include Sini Decoction, Dachengqi Decoction, etc.; examples of the latter include Sangju Decoction, Ginseng Nutritive Decoction, etc.

4. **Constitution of the patient:** For patients with a strong constitution, the dosage can be large; for those with a delicate constitution, the dosage should be small. Generally, the dosage in the northwest region is larger than that in the southeast region, mainly due to the difference in physical strength.
5. **Age:** The dosage for adults can be large, and that for children should be small. Generally, the dosage for children is half of that for adults.

Although the dosage depends on specific circumstances, it should be pointed out that there is a certain standard for general dosage. The adjustment of dosage based on this standard is not arbitrary. One must master the standard dosage and then increase or decrease it appropriately to achieve the desired effect.

The dosage has a great impact on the efficacy of the prescription. A good prescription often loses its effect or even causes adverse reactions due to improper dosage. The appropriateness or inappropriateness mainly depends on two aspects: on the one hand, whether the dosage is appropriate according to the condition and constitution; on the other hand, whether the dosage is appropriate according to the compatibility of drugs. For severe diseases with a strong constitution, the dosage should be large; for severe diseases with a weak constitution, the dosage should be reduced appropriately. For mild diseases with a strong constitution, a large dosage is not needed; for mild diseases with a weak constitution, a large dosage is even more inappropriate. In addition, the effect of drugs and the effect after compatibility change with the dosage. For example, a small dose of Tibetan Saffron can harmonize blood, while a large dose can break blood stasis; when Cinnamon Twig and White Peony Root are used in equal amounts, they can regulate nutrient and defensive qi; if the dosage of Cinnamon Twig is increased, it tends to act on the defensive aspect; if the dosage of White Peony Root is increased, it tends to act on the nutrient aspect. This requires careful work in clinical practice.

Regarding the ancient system of weights and measures, which is different from the modern system, the ancient system is smaller than the modern one. According to recent research, approximately one *liang* (tael) in the Han Dynasty is equivalent to a little more than 4.8 *qian* (mace) in the modern market weight, and one *sheng* (liter) in the Han Dynasty is about 0.2 *he* (deciliter) in the modern system. This is provided for reference to illustrate that the dosage in ancient prescriptions cannot be used as the standard for current prescription dosag.

Essentials for TCM Clinical Practice

Preface

This book is primarily intended as a reference for clinical practice in TCM and serves as a clinical handbook, but it differs from general clinical handbooks that introduce content classified by diseases. This book starts from symptoms and conducts syndrome differentiation and treatment based on different syndromes. Syndrome differentiation and treatment are based on analyzing symptoms; through this analysis, etiology and disease location are explored, leading to the determination of the treatment method. For example, cough is a symptom; to distinguish between exogenous cough and internal injury cough, and to further determine whether exogenous cough is due to wind-cold or wind-heat, it is necessary to conduct a comprehensive analysis in combination with other symptoms. Another example: Even if diseases have been named according to etiology and *zang-fu* organs, such as cold damage and stomach pain, treatment still needs to be carried out by distinguishing them into Taiyang disease, Yangming disease, cold stomach pain, stomach qi pain, etc., based on different symptoms. At the same time, syndrome differentiation and treatment are also procedures and methods for dealing with diseases, which must be closely combined with the four diagnostic methods. The four diagnostic methods include many contents, such as changes in facial complexion, tongue coating, phlegm, blood, urine and stool, etc., which are actually various symptoms reflected by pathological changes. It can be seen from this that syndrome differentiation and treatment cannot be separated from the four diagnostic methods, and the four diagnostic methods themselves are also based on symptoms. The complex and intricate occurrence of symptoms is an important basis for syndrome differentiation and treatment. If one deviates from symptoms, or ignores the main symptoms, or is not familiar with their mutual combinations, it is impossible to correctly apply syndrome differentiation and treatment. To be proficient in the method of syndrome differentiation and treatment, it is necessary to conduct in-depth analysis from the perspective of symptoms, understand the occurrence, changes of each symptom and its connection with *zang-fu* organs, further study the common symptoms and special symptoms of the same disease, and pay attention to the relationship between the increase or decrease of symptoms and the transformation of the disease condition throughout the course of the disease, so as to achieve a clear diagnosis and correct treatment.

Symptoms are objectively existing; if we are allowed to regard symptoms as indicators, then TCM's diagnosis and treatment of diseases through syndrome differentiation and treatment have certain objective indicators. These indicators are a summary of TCM practical experience, a set of rules explored in distinguishing symptoms and syndromes, and also theories that guide clinical practice. Regarding these examples, anyone who has studied the basic theories and clinical disciplines of TCM will understand, so they will not be elaborated here. The problem lies in that a disease contains many symptoms; in clinical practice, how to analyze them and how to synthesize scattered symptoms. That is, for a certain disease syndrome, how to analyze and summarize based on different symptoms, draw clear conclusions, so as to obtain a confirmed diagnosis and correct treatment.

The above are my personal views and also my subjective thoughts. I have discussed this with three doctors: Li Yan, Zhang Tianren, and Wei Zhizhen, and they share the same feelings. After discussing the structure, we decided to compile this book jointly on the basis of previous theories and empirical knowledge, combined with some of our own experiences and insights, integrating theory with practice. The core methodology involves focusing on symptoms, classifying them according to their locations, connecting symptoms with diseases (or: syndrome patterns), and implementing the treatment principles of Theory, Method, Formula, and Medicine. Of course, this is not yet mature and can be said to be an attempt. We hope that readers will put forward valuable opinions for future revision and gradual improvement.

Qin Bowei
March 1963

Notes on the Use of the Book

The purpose of compiling this book is to help readers, after mastering the basic theories of TCM, apply the method of syndrome differentiation and treatment in clinical practice to diagnose and treat diseases. Based on internal medicine, this book appropriately incorporates gynecology, pediatrics, surgery, ophthalmology, laryngology, and other disciplines, with prescriptions and medicines as the main treatment methods, and appropriately includes some treatment methods such as acupuncture and moxibustion, tuina, etc., for general reference in clinical practice, hence the name *Essentials for Traditional Chinese Medicine Clinical Practice*.

TCM syndrome differentiation mainly relies on symptoms combined with the four diagnostic methods. Therefore, this book focuses on common symptoms, explains complex and intricate disease syndromes based on the etiology and pathogenesis of each symptom, thereby pointing out treatment methods and relating them to prescriptions and medicines. For the convenience of reference, symptoms are classified according to body parts into 20 categories, totaling 417 symptoms, including systemic symptoms, head and face symptoms, eye symptoms, ear symptoms, nose symptoms, lip and mouth symptoms, tongue symptoms, tooth symptoms, throat symptoms, neck symptoms, shoulder and back symptoms, chest, hypochondrium, armpit and breast symptoms, waist symptoms, abdominal and umbilical symptoms, limb symptoms, hand and foot symptoms, anterior genital symptoms, posterior genital symptoms, internal organ symptoms, and gynecological symptoms. For example, aversion to cold, fever, chills, tidal fever, alternating chills and fever, external heat with internal cold, external cold with internal heat, body heat with cold feet, half-body coldness, etc., are all included in systemic symptoms; local symptoms such as back coldness, head and face heat, cold limbs, heat in the palms and soles, etc., are respectively included in shoulder and back, head and face, limb, hand and foot categories. Except for women's menstruation, leukorrhea, pregnancy, and childbirth, which are separately listed under gynecological symptoms, others are not classified by discipline.

The names of symptoms are not unified across ancient and modern times, nor consistent in different regions, and it is also difficult to force integration with diseases diagnosed by Western medicine in recent years. This book temporarily focuses on popularity, with specialized terms included in the text. For example, "fengshui" (wind edema), "pishui" (skin edema), "zhengshui" (true edema), "shishui" (stone edema), "yinshui" (yin edema), "yangshui" (yang edema), etc., are all attached to the entry of "edema";又如: measles, "fengsha" (wind rash), and skin bleeding points diagnosed by Western medicine as thrombocytopenia are all included in the entry of "red rash".

Starting from clinical practice and adhering to the principle of closely integrating theory with practice, this book provides a brief discussion based on the achievements of predecessors, combined with the research results from various regions in recent years and personal experiences. For each category of symptoms, a general introduction is given first, and then for each symptom, its causes, pathology, and treatment methods are explained respectively, striving to be both comprehensive and concise. Key issues such as the similarities and differences of certain symptoms, the contraindications of treatment methods, and the modifications of established prescriptions are elaborated in detail for clarity. In addition, disease syndromes that belong to specialized fields or require surgical treatment, as well as those currently mostly handled by hospitals, are generally explained and separately indicated to be managed by specialists or other departments.

TCM formulas are quite abundant, including general formulas and main therapeutic formulas. The formulas selected in this book are based on the criteria of being commonly used and effective for specific disease syndromes, and some proven formulas and single-ingredient formulas are also included as appropriate. For the convenience of clinical reference and to compare different treatment methods for the same disease syndrome, the formulas are listed after each symptom. Meanwhile, each disease and syndrome includes several symptoms, and it is impossible to make a diagnosis and treatment based on a single symptom. Therefore, some symptoms do not have corresponding formulas; for example, "yellowing of the eyes" is noted to refer to the entry of "jaundice". As for the dosage of formulas, due to differences in ancient and modern systems of weights and measures, variations in traditional habits across regions, and especially differences in the severity of illness, physical strength, and age, it is difficult to enforce uniformity. Hence, the attached formulas do not specify dosages. For some pills, powders, ointments, pellets, etc., that are already available as proprietary medicines, and those that cannot be casually manufactured or converted into decoctions, the word "proprietary medicine" is noted after the formula. For special formulas, the dosage, treatment method, and usage are still attached to avoid affecting the therapeutic effect.

This book is mainly intended to provide materials for syndrome differentiation and treatment. Based on the author's experience, an article titled "A Brief Explanation of Syndrome Differentiation and Treatment" is attached at the end to facilitate discussion.

Section 1 Systemic Symptoms

Systemic symptoms refer to a type of symptoms that appear throughout the body, are not limited to a certain part, or can spread from a local area to the entire body. These include aversion to cold, fever, pain, itching, sweating, macular eruption, rashes, edema, emaciation, fatigue, muscle twitching and numbness, dry and withered skin, rough and discolored skin (jia cuo), as well as frostbite, burns, scalds, and snake and insect bites, etc. The causes of such symptoms are quite complex, with many similar and ambiguous syndromes, and they occupy an important position among general symptoms. Although they appear on the body surface, it is necessary to distinguish between exterior and interior, deficiency and excess, cold and heat, especially conditions such as external cold with internal heat or external heat with internal cold, which are easily obscured by false appearances. Therefore, in clinical practice, one cannot only look at the surface phenomena but must explore the main cause of the disease and treat it fundamentally. Some severe skin diseases, burns, scalds, etc., can also affect the internal organs and should be consulted by internal and surgical specialists together.

I. Aversion to Cold

Aversion to cold refers to feeling cold. Generally, there is a feeling of cold at the initial stage of exogenous syndromes, followed by fever. Some patients have fever while still feeling cold, and some have reduced aversion to cold after fever, which are generally referred to as "exterior syndromes". For all exogenous syndromes, whether cold damage or warm disease, regardless of the duration, the severity of cold and heat, the presence of a certain degree of aversion to cold indicates a certain degree of exterior syndrome. A characteristic of aversion to cold in exogenous syndromes is that the feeling of cold becomes more severe when exposed to wind; even in a warm room without cold invasion, the whole body feels cold, and some patients still do not want to remove their clothes and quilts even though they have a fever. However, due to the complexity of exogenous syndromes, aversion to cold is an early symptom, and it is difficult to confirm a diagnosis of a specific disease at the initial stage; most cases require observation for several days before a decision can be made. At the same time, it should be combined with other symptoms; for example, if accompanied by head distension and nasal congestion, it can be diagnosed as "wind damage". As stated in *Treatise on Cold Damage*, "Taiyang disease may have fever or not yet have fever, but there must be aversion to cold, body pain, nausea and vomiting, and tight pulses both yin and yang; this is called 'cold damage'." The treatment method is mainly to induce sweating and dispel pathogens, refer to the entry of "fever" in this section.

Constant fear of wind and cold, which subsides when warmed, even reluctance to open windows in summer, is mostly a yang deficiency syndrome, commonly seen in patients with long-term diarrhea due to spleen and kidney deficiency, as well as phlegm-fluid cough and asthma. Such aversion to cold due to insufficient yang qi in the body, along with other syndromes caused by yang deficiency, are collectively called deficient cold syndromes, all belonging to interior syndromes. The treatment must fundamentally tonify yang, which is completely different from the treatment of exogenous diseases.

Aversion to wind is similar to aversion to cold. Although literatures distinguish them, stating that cold damage syndromes involve aversion to cold and wind damage syndromes involve aversion to wind, generally those with aversion to cold often have aversion to wind, and those with aversion to wind often have aversion to cold, making it extremely difficult to distinguish them clinically. In short, it must be determined in combination with other symptoms, and one should not be rigidly adheret.

II. Aversion to Cold with Shivering

Shivering accompanied by aversion to cold, referred to as "chills" for short, is common in "malaria". Refer to the entry "alternating chills and fever" in this section.

During the course of cold damage and warm diseases, there may be sudden chills, extreme fatigue, and gradual calmness and improvement after sweating, which is called "zhan han" (fighting sweat). This is a phenomenon where the patient's healthy qi, although weak, rises up when there is an opportunity to recover, engaging in a struggle with pathogenic qi. If healthy qi prevails, sweating occurs and pathogenic qi is resolved. Therefore, sweating after the fight indicates survival, while failure to sweat indicates danger, which is indeed a critical juncture. If there is no sign of collapse, let it take its natural course without panic; if necessary, use modified Fumai Decoction to support primordial qi.

"Zhen han" (trembling cold) is similar to chills, both involving shivering. The difference is that chills originate from within, while zhen han is merely a trembling of the body. Zhen han is mostly caused by yang deficiency failing to protect the exterior, often accompanied by abdominal pain, diarrhea, heavy limbs, and difficulty in urination. The disease is in the Shaoyin channel, and treatment should tonify yang, using Zhenwu Decoction.

Fumai Decoction: Ginseng, Rehmannia, Cinnamon Twig, Ophiopogon, Donkey-hide Gelatin, Honey-fried Licorice, Hemp Seed, Ginger, Jujube

Zhenwu Decoction: Aconite, White Peony Root, Atractylodes, Poria, Ginger

III. Fever

Also known as "body heat", it is most common in exogenous syndromes. General differentiations are as follows: accompanied by aversion to wind, headache, nasal congestion, and cough, it is "wind damage"; accompanied by aversion to cold, headache, and pain in the nape, back, and body, it is "cold damage"; similar to wind damage but with dryness in the mouth, it is "wind-warmth"; occurring after being caught in cold rain or walking in fog and dew, with a heavy, wrapped sensation in the head, it is due to exogenous dampness. In all cases of initial exogenous fever, pathogenic qi is on the body surface, with a pulse mostly floating and rapid, and treatment should promote sweating. *The Inner Canon* states: "For pathogenic qi in the skin, induce sweating to expel it." This is the meaning. Also, due to the different natures of pathogenic qi, it is divided into pungent-cool diaphoresis and pungent-warm diaphoresis. For wind-cold, pungent-warm diaphoresis is appropriate, such as Congchi Decoction and Mahuang Decoction; for exogenous dampness, Shenshu Powder is used; for wind-warmth, pungent-cool diaphoresis is appropriate, such as Yinqiao Powder. However, exogenous fever may present with or without spontaneous sweating: Those without sweating should be induced to sweat, while those with spontaneous sweating should not be sweated again. Hence, there is also the method of using Guizhi Decoction to regulate nutrient and defensive qi for resolving the exterior. The pulse in exogenous fever is mostly floating and rapid, but it may also be accompanied by tightness, smoothness, or softness depending on the disease syndrome. If the pulse is not floating but deep, or appears thin and weak, it indicates inconsistency between pulse and syndrome, and one must not rashly induce sweating to prevent deterioration.

In the initial stage of exogenous syndromes, fever is mostly accompanied by aversion to wind or cold. If after sweating, there is no aversion to wind or cold, but fever persists or gradually increases, it means pathogenic qi has transformed into heat and transmitted to the interior. Generally, it mostly locates in the middle jiao (Yangming), presenting with thirst and desire for cold drinks, yellow and greasy tongue coating, and smooth and large pulse, which should be treated with the sweet-cold and slightly pungent method, such as Baihu Decoction.

In internal injury miscellaneous syndromes, there is also fever, but the fever patterns are different. Li Dongyuan wrote *Treatise on Differentiating Internal and External Injuries*, stating, for example, "In external injury, cold and heat occur simultaneously without interruption; in internal injury, cold and heat occur alternately and irregularly; in external injury, the back of the hands is hot while the palms are not; in internal injury, the palms are hot while the back of the hands is not," etc. Refer to the entries "fever with fixed timing" and "alternating chills and fever" in this section.

Congchi Decoction: Fermented Soybean, Fistular Onion Stalk

Mahuang Decoction: Ephedra, Cinnamon Twig, Almond, Licorice

Shenshu Powder: Atractylodes, Saposhnikovia, Licorice, Fistular Onion Stalk, Ginger

Yinqiao Powder: Schizonepeta, Fermented Soybean, Mint, Honeysuckle, Forsythia, Platycodon, Licorice, Bamboo Leaf, Arctium, Reed Rhizome

Guizhi Decoction: Cinnamon Twig, White Peony Root, Licorice, Ginger, Jujube

Baihu Decoction: Gypsum, Anemarrhena, Licorice, Rice

IV. Fever with Fixed Timing

Fever without aversion to cold, with rises and falls at fixed times like the regular tides, is called "tidal fever." This syndrome can be either deficient or excessive, both belonging to interior syndromes. The distinction is: Deficient syndromes are caused by deficiency of qi and blood, and in most cases, the heat can subside completely; excessive syndromes result from external pathogens transmitting inward, with heat not subsiding completely and rising at fixed times.

Excessive tidal fever mostly starts with external infection, presenting with steaming body heat and sweating, constipation, abdominal distension and pain that worsens with pressure, and the heat tends to increase around 4 p.m. It is thus also called "afternoon fever," belonging to excess in the Yangming stomach. In severe cases, it can cause delirium and confusion. Treatment should involve purgation using Dachengqi Decoction. This is the treatment method from *Treatise on Cold Damage*, which must be used only when the syndrome and body are excessive and the healthy qi can withstand it. Later, *Systematic Differentiation of Warm Diseases* mentioned that heat pathogens easily damage yin and that after purgation, deficiency of healthy qi may lead to reaccumulation of pathogens, thus establishing formulas like Huwei Chengqi Decoction and Zengye Chengqi Decoction, which can also be used as appropriate. Wu Youke said: "Each day the healthy qi is deficient, yin fluid is consumed day by day; one must take care to protect yin, and must not act impetuousl." This is the significance.

Deficient tidal fever, mostly due to blood deficiency and yin deficiency, often occurs in the afternoon or at night, accompanied by deficiency symptoms such as palpitations, sweating, fatigue, and a thin and rapid pulse. It is often caused by massive blood loss, severe diarrhea, or chronic illness, leading to exhaustion of fluid and hyperactivity of fire, consumption of true yin, gradual emaciation, and heat steaming from between the muscles and bones. Over time, yin becomes increasingly consumed and qi also weakens, so it is also called "bone-steaming consumption heat." Treatment should involve nourishing blood and yin, using the method of Qinggu Powder. There is also morning tidal fever with subsidence in the afternoon, or fever due to injury to middle qi from hunger, satiety, overexertion, with concurrent deficiency of nutrient blood, presenting with body heat, irritability, reluctance to speak, bodily fatigue, and a large but weak pulse, belonging to qi deficiency. Li Dongyuan proposed the sweet-warm method to reduce heat using Buzhong Yiqi Decoction; in this formula, Cimicifuga and Bupleurum have heat-reducing effects and should not be regarded merely as lifting herbs.

In summer, children's fever, either rising in the morning and subsiding in the evening or rising in the evening and subsiding in the morning, accompanied by polydipsia, frequent urination, irritability, and restless sleep, often persists and resolves naturally with the coolness of autumn. It is often seen in the southeast and central south regions, with no definite disease name, tentatively called "summer fever," which can be treated with modified Qingshu Yiqi Decoction from Wang Mengying.

Dachengqi Decoction: Rhubarb, Magnolia Bark, Aurantium, Mirabilite

Huwei Chengqi Decoction: Rhubarb, Scrophularia, Rehmannia, Moutan Bark, Anemarrhena, Ophiopogon

Zengye Chengqi Decoction: Rehmannia, Scrophularia, Ophiopogon, Rhubarb, Mirabilite

Qinggu Powder: Starwort Root, Picrorhiza, Turtle Shell, Wormwood, Gentiana, Wolfberry Bark, Anemarrhena, Licorice

Buzhong Yiqi Decoction: Astragalus, Ginseng, Atractylodes,

Angelica, Honey-fried Licorice, Cimicifuga, Bupleurum, Tangerine Peel, Ginger, Jujube

Qingshu Yiqi Decoction: Adenophora, Ophiopogon, Anemarrhena, Licorice, Bamboo Leaf, Coptis, Dendrobium, Watermelon Peel, Lotus Leaf, Rice

V. Alternating Chills and Fever

Sudden chills and sudden fever, occurring once a day or several times a day, are called "alternating chills and fever". This kind of fever can sometimes subside completely, and sometimes not. All cases that develop from the transmission of exogenous pathogens belong to Shaoyang meridian syndrome, often accompanied by symptoms such as bitter taste in the mouth, dry throat, dizziness, chest and hypochondrium fullness, and a string-like and rapid pulse. Xiaochaihu Decoction is used for harmonizing and resolving, and sweating, vomiting, or purging must not be used.

Women with irregular menstruation often have phenomena such as sudden chills and fever, head distension, and chest and hypochondrium stuffiness before menstruation, which are caused by stagnation of liver qi or liver fire. Tiaojing Decoction can be used, which is Xiaochaihu Decoction plus Siwu Decoction. There are also cases where women catch wind-cold and develop fever just before or after menstruation, or menstruation occurs during the fever period, and pathogenic heat invades the uterus taking advantage of deficiency, leading to binding of stasis and heat, which also causes alternating chills and fever. *Synopsis of the Golden Chamber* calls this "heat entering the blood chamber", and Xiaochaihu Decoction can also be used to purge heat. However, once heat has entered the blood chamber, it should be assisted with clearing the nutrient aspect and dispelling stasis; Danshen, Red Peony Root, Zelan, and Charred Gardenia can be added to the formula as appropriate, and for severe heat, Ginseng should be removed and Fresh Rehmannia added.

The main symptom of "malaria" is also recurrent chills and fever, occurring once a day, once every two days, or once every three days, but the condition is quite different from alternating chills and fever. Generally, the onset of malaria starts with a cold sensation in the back, skin goosebumps, frequent yawning, followed by shivering with clenched teeth, body soreness, then high fever like burning, headache like splitting, thirst with a preference for cold drinks, and finally sweating all over the body, with fever subsiding and the body feeling comfortable. The entire process takes about six to eight hours. Its characteristics are: chills and fever occur at a fixed time, each episode has the same symptoms; the pulse is mostly deep and string-like during chills, turns surging, large, and rapid during fever, and gradually calms down after sweating. Commonly used formulas include Qingpi Decoction and Jieyao Qibao Decoction. The medicine should be taken about two hours before the onset; if taken after the onset, it will instead aggravate the condition. Acupuncture and moxibustion also have good effects on this disease, with main acupoints such as Dazhui, Taodao, Jianshi, and Houxi, but it is also important to perform the treatment before the onset. Therefore, *The Inner Canon* states: "Do not needle when there is blazing heat, do not needle when the pulse is confused, do not needle when there is profuse sweating, because the disease is in a reverse state and cannot be treated. This applies to all cases of malaria, whether in terms of medicine, methods, or diet."

Among malaria, there are "pin malaria" with more cold than heat, "wind malaria" with heat first then cold, "warm malaria" and "dan malaria" with only heat without cold, as well as "summer-heat malaria", "damp malaria", "phlegm malaria", "food malaria", "miasma malaria" classified by cause. It can be seen that predecessors made detailed observations on malaria, but some are malaria-like conditions rather than true malaria. Among them, miasma malaria is more common in miasma-stricken areas in Lingnan. For heat miasma, during onset, there is severe heat and mild cold, flushed face and eyes, irritability, thirst with desire for cold drinks, chest stuffiness, vomiting, headache, severe limb pain, reddish urine, constipation, and even delirium. Treatment should clear heat and dispel filth, using Qingzhang Decoction. For cold miasma, during onset, there is chills and shivering, mild heat, headache, lumbago, weak legs, and even confusion and inability to speak. Treatment should aromatically transform turbidity, using Jiawei Buhuanjin Zhengqi Powder. During the period of confusion, orifice-opening emergency treatment can be used together, refer to the entry "coma" in internal organ symptoms.

Chronic malaria most readily depletes qi and blood, manifesting as a sallow complexion, emaciated muscles, and diminished capacity for labor. Even when chills and fever subside, relapse occurs after exertion, giving rise to what is called "consumptive malaria." At this stage the usual methods are contraindicated; the treatment should instead tonify and replenish qi and blood, employing the formula "He Ren Drink." In some cases, long-standing malaria leaves a mass beneath the ribs; when exertion provokes chills, and fever it is termed "malaria mother." For its treatment, consult the section on chest, rib, axilla, and breast disorders under "hard mass beneath the ribs."

When damp-heat and turbid phlegm stagnate in the middle burner, symptoms resembling malaria appear—alternating chills and fever, sweating that does not clear the heat, oppression in the chest with nausea, a dry mouth with little desire to drink, dark yellow urine, and stools that are either constipated or loose and foul-smelling. In this case use Da Yuan Drink. This formula was originally designed for pestilential pathogens lodged in the membrane source; hence it employs areca seed (bing lang), tsaoko fruit (cao guo), and magnolia bark (hou po) to drain and transform the stomach and intestines, assisted by poria (fu ling), white peony (bai shao), anemarrhena (zhi mu), fresh ginger (sheng jiang), and jujube (da zao) to clear and harmonize. Clinically, however, it is not limited to pestilential disorders; whenever alternating chills and fever are accompanied by a greasy, dirty tongue coating, the formula proves effective. One may add bupleurum (chai hu) to open the exterior or rhubarb (da huang) to attack the interior, thereby separating and dispersing the entangled pathogens of cold, heat, dampness, and turbidity.

Minor Bupleurum Decoction: Bupleurum, Scutellaria, Pinellia, Ginseng, Licorice, Fresh Ginger, Jujube

Four-Substance Decoction: Rehmannia, Angelica, White Peony, Ligusticum

Spleen-Clearing Beverage: Green Tangerine Peel, Magnolia Bark, Scutellaria, Pinellia, Bupleurum, Atractylodes, Tsaoko Fruit, Poria, Licorice

Malaria-Cutting Seven-Treasure Beverage: Dichroa Root, Tsaoko Fruit, Magnolia Bark, Green Tangerine Peel, Aged Tangerine Peel, Areca Seed, Licorice

Clear Pestilential Decoction: Sweet Wormwood, Bupleurum, Anemarrhena, Pinellia, Aged Tangerine Peel, Poria, Coptis, Immature Bitter Orange, Scutellaria, Dichroa Root, Bamboo Shavings, Yi Yuan San

Augmented "Priceless" Qi-Righting Powder: Magnolia Bark, Atractylodes, Aged Tangerine Peel, Agastache, Eupatorium, Tsaoko Fruit, Pinellia, Areca Seed, Acorus, Lotus Leaf, Licorice

He-Ren Beverage: Polygonum Multiflorum, Ginseng, Angelica,

Aged Tangerine Peel, Baked Ginger, Jujube

Da Yuan Beverage: Magnolia Bark, Tsaoko Fruit, Areca Seed, Anemarrhena, White Peony, Scutellaria, Licorice, Fresh Ginger, Jujube

VI. External Heat and Internal Cold

Mostly belonging to the syndrome of false heat and true cold, that is, the root is a cold syndrome, but there appear heat signs on the surface. For the identification of false heat syndrome, Zhang Jingyue once pointed out: "In false heat, there is heat externally but cold internally; the pulse is faint and weak, or rapid but deficient, or floating and large without root, or string-like and hollow with interruptions; the body may be burning hot but the spirit is calm; there may be delirious speech but the voice is faint; there may be wild and restless movements but they stop when restrained; there may be mosquito-bite-like false macules that are light red with patchy coating; there may be a desire for cold drinks but only a small amount is consumed; the tongue coating may be red but the patient does not want to uncover the clothes and quilts; there may be profuse urination; or the stool may not be constipated. This kind of dislike of heat is not true heat, it is clearly a cold syndrome, which is called 'extreme cold accompanied by heat transformation' or 'exuberant yin separating yang'." Such syndromes are all manifestations of severe illness, and treatment must target the root cause. If mistakenly treated as exogenous fever, it often leads to collapse due to sweating.

VII. External Cold and Internal Heat

It is the syndrome of false cold and true heat. Zhang Jingyue said: "In false cold, there is cold externally but heat internally; the pulse is rapid and increasing, or deep but forceful on palpation; there may be bodily cold but dislike of wearing clothes; or hot and dry stool; or irritability and thirst with a desire to drink; or foul-smelling intestinal residues. This kind of dislike of cold is not true cold, it is clearly a heat syndrome, which is called 'extreme heat accompanied by cold transformation' or 'exuberant yang separating yin'." Clearing heat will make the cold disappear naturally; pungent-warm diaphoresis is strictly prohibited.

VIII. Upper Heat and Lower Cold

Coldness in the shins, with a slightly red face like a flush, accompanied by fear of cold, a deep and thin pulse, or accompanied by diarrhea. It is due to deficiency and cold in the lower origin, with yang qi escaping upward, called "upward floating yang", which is one of the collapse syndromes. Urgently use Baitong Decoction to restore yang, and a small amount of pig bile or coptis can be added as a counteraction to prevent mutual rejection of cold and heat. If sweating occurs on the head after taking the medicine and the pulse suddenly becomes floating and large, the condition is difficult to treat.

IX. Body Heat with Cold Feet

Body heat with islated coldness of the feet is commonly seen in "damp-warmth" syndrome. It is mostly caused by excessive damp turbidity stagnating yang qi. Treatment should focus on clearing and transforming dampness with mild diuresis, allowing pathogenic factors to dissipate and yang qi to circulate naturally. As Ye Tianshi stated, "Unblocking yang does not rely on pungent-heat but on promoting urination." It must not be mistaken for yang deficiency.

X. Half-Body Coldness

This syndrome is relatively rare. Patients experience coldness from head to foot on either the left or right half of the body, with sweating absent on the affected side alone. When exposed to wind, the affected side first feels piercing cold, while joint movement remains unobstructed, accompanied by soreness, weakness, and a deep, thin pulse. Use Yougui Decoction with added Angelica and Asarum to warm and activate yang qi, and unblock blood vessels.

Yougui Decoction: Aconite, Cinnamon, Prepared Rehmannia, Cornus, Yam, Eucommia, Wolfberry, Honey-fried Licorice

XI. Body Pain

Generalized body pain often appears in exogenous syndromes such as cold damage and damp damage, all caused by meridian obstruction and disharmony of qi and blood. Treatment focuses on dispelling pathogens. If body pain persists after sweating (when external pathogens have been eliminated) with a deep, slow pulse, regulate nutrient and defensive qi. This syndrome requires distinguishing between the presence or absence of pathogens: Prioritize relieving the exterior for external pathogens, and harmonize qi and blood when pathogens are absent. "Body pain" refers to pain in all muscles; if only limb soreness occurs, it belongs to impediment syndrome (see "Limb Pain" under Limb Symptoms).

For traumatic injuries with body pain and purple-blue skin ecchymoses (due to qi stagnation and blood stasis), modify Fuyuan Huoxue Decoction.

Body pain resembling trauma, with purple-blue skin, blue complexion, and sore throat is called "yin toxin" in *Synopsis of the Golden Chamber*. If accompanied by crimson macules like brocade patterns, sore throat, and vomiting of pus and blood, it is "yang toxin." Treat yang toxin with Shengma Biejia Decoction; for yin toxin, remove Realgar and Sichuan Pepper from the formula. Interpretations of yin-yang toxins have long varied, but *Chaoshi Bingyuan* (Chao's Origins of Diseases) includes chapters on cold damage yin-yang toxin and seasonal qi yin-yang toxin, suggesting similarities to "macule eruption" in seasonal diseases. Macule eruptions can present two external signs, customarily divided into "yang macules" and "yin macules" (see "Red Macule Eruption" in this section).

Fuyuan Huoxue Decoction: Angelica, Peach Kernel, Safflower, Pangolin, Rhubarb, Bupleurum, Trichosanthes Root, Licorice

Shengma Biejia Decoction: Cimicifuga, Turtle Shell, Angelica, Sichuan Pepper, Realgar, Licorice

XII. Body Heaviness

Common in damp syndromes. Internal obstruction of damp turbidity impairs qi movement and prevents clear yang from rising, causing heaviness in movement and lethargy. Use Pingwei Powder to warm, transform, and harmonize the middle jiao.

In chronic or deficient conditions, inability to turn over due to extreme body heaviness—even with assistance—indicates severe physical exhaustion, with a poor prognosis.

Pingwei Powder: Atractylodes, Magnolia Bark, Tangerine Peel, Licorice

XIII. Body Itching

Wind-cold invading the skin surface, failing to disperse through mild sweating or transform into heat and enter the interior, causes generalized itching (like insects crawling) without skin abnormalities. Use Guizhi Mahuang Ge Ban Decoction (Cinnamon and Ephedra Half-and-Half Decoction).

Body itching with tiny blood spots after scratching indicates wind-heat stagnating in the minute collaterals; use Siwu Xiaofeng San (Four-Substance Wind-Dispelling Powder). If scratching produces excessive white scales, it is blood deficiency generating dryness; use Zizao Yangrong Decoction (Nourishing and Moisturizing Decoction).

In surgical skin diseases, “impetigo” starts with small papules like millet grains, which itch and ooze fluid. As the fluid spreads into patches with pain, treatment should dispel wind, overcome dampness, cool blood, and clear heat. Use Shengma Xiaodu Yin (Cimicifuga Detoxifying Decoction) with added Atractylodes lancea, Coptis chinensis, and apply Qingge San (Indigo and Clam Powder) externally. Another condition, “millet sores,” appears as red, itchy millet-sized bumps. If prolonged, they consume blood, leaving the skin dry like snake scales. Treat with Xiaofeng San (Wind-Dispelling Powder).

“Tinea sores” cause intense itching, mostly localized, resulting from damp-heat, blood dryness, or wind-toxin. There are dry and wet types: “dry tinea” is dry without fluid, scaling when scratched; “wet tinea” is moist, exuding mucus when scratched. This stubborn condition is also called “stubborn tinea.” Internal medicines rarely work, so external treatments are preferred: tinea lotion for dry tinea and Qingdai San (Indigo Powder) for wet tinea.

Those exposed to or allergic to lacquer toxin first develop facial itching and swelling, progressing to limb involvement with unbearable itchiness and pain. Scratching leads to oozing ulcers, termed “lacquer sores.” Lacquer toxin is pungent, hot, and toxic. Treat with Huaban Jiedu Decoction (Macule-Resolving Detoxifying Decoction) plus Schizonepeta tenuifolia, Cicada slough, Duckweed, and raw Glycyrrhiza uralensis. External application of Qingdai San is also advisable; bathing is not recommended.

"Wind rashes" and "prickly heat" also cause itching (see respective entries in this section).

Guizhi Mahuang Geban Decoction (Cinnamon and Ephedra Half-and-Half Decoction): Cinnamomum cassia twig, Paeonia lactiflora, Ephedra sinica, Armeniacae semen, honey-fried Glycyrrhiza uralensis, Zingiber officinale, Ziziphus jujuba

Siwu Xiaofeng San (Four-Substance Wind-Dispelling Powder): Rehmannia glutinosa, Angelica sinensis, Schizonepeta tenuifolia, Saposhnikovia divaricata, Paeonia lactiflora (red), Ligusticum chuanxiong, Dictamnus dasycarpus, Cicada slough, Mentha haplocalyx, Angelica pubescens, Bupleurum chinense, Ziziphus jujuba

Zizao Yangrong Decoction (Moisturizing and Nourishing Decoction): Rehmannia glutinosa (raw), Rehmannia glutinosa (processed), Angelica sinensis, Paeonia lactiflora, Scutellaria baicalensis, Gentiana macrophylla, Saposhnikovia divaricata, Glycyrrhiza uralensis

Shengma Xiaodu Yin (Cimicifuga Detoxifying Decoction): Cimicifuga foetida, Angelica sinensis (tail), Paeonia lactiflora (red), Lonicera japonica, Forsythia suspensa, Arctium lappa, Gardenia jasminoides, Notopterygium incisum, Angelica dahurica, Carthamus tinctorius, Saposhnikovia divaricata, Platycodon grandiflorus, Glycyrrhiza uralensis

Qingge San (Indigo and Clam Powder): 30g clam powder, 9g indigo naturalis, 30g gypsum, 1.5g calomel, 15g Phellodendron chinense (ground into powder). Mix with sesame oil to form a block; dissolve in cold water for application.

Xiaofeng San (Wind-Dispelling Powder): Schizonepeta tenuifolia, Saposhnikovia divaricata, Angelica sinensis, Rehmannia glutinosa, Sophora flavescens, Atractylodes lancea, Cicada slough, Sesamum indicum, Arctium lappa, Anemarrhena asphodeloides, Gypsum fibrosum, Glycyrrhiza uralensis, Akebia quinata

Tinea Lotion: 240g Stemona sessilifolia, 240g Cnidium monnieri, 300g Hibiscus syriacus bark, 240g sulfur, 6g white arsenic, 60g Mylabris, 36g camphor, 36g calomel, soaked in 100 liters of rice vinegar.

Qingdai San (Indigo Powder): 60g indigo naturalis, 120g gypsum, 60g talc, 120g Phellodendron chinense (ground into powder). Mix with sesame oil for application.

Huaban Jiedu Decoction (Macule-Resolving Detoxifying Decoction): Cimicifuga foetida, Gypsum fibrosum, Forsythia suspensa, Arctium lappa, Licoriceproducts, Coptis chinensis, Anemarrhena asphodeloides, Scrophularia ningpoensis, Phyllostachys nigra leaves

XIV. Spontaneous Sweating

Spontaneous sweating occurs without diaphoretic drugs or other stimuli, as seen in "wind damage" or "wind-warmth." However, the term typically refers to internal disorders, mainly due to unconsolidated defensive qi causing fluid leakage, often with post-sweating chills and fatigue. For mild cases, use Muli San (Oyster Powder); for severe cases, Buyang Decoction (Yang-Tonifying Decoction). External application of equal parts Dragon Bone, Oyster, and glutinous rice powder (ground) is also helpful.

Localized sweating, common on the head, hands, and feet, is discussed under "head sweating" (Head and Face Symptoms) and "palmar and plantar heat" (Hand and Foot Symptoms).

Muli San (Oyster Powder): Oyster, Astragalus membranaceus, Ephedra root, floating wheat

Buyang Decoction (Yang-Tonifying Decoction): Ginseng, Astragalus membranaceus, Atractylodes macrocephala, Glycyrrhiza uralensis, Schisandra chinensis

XV. Night Sweating

Also known as "sleep sweat", it refers to sweat secretly oozing out during sleep and stopping upon waking, with no feeling of cold after stopping but rather a sensation of heat and restlessness. It is mostly caused by yin deficiency disturbing heat, which prevents heart fluid from being contained. As stated in *The Inner Canon*, "Yang added to yin is called sweat." Therefore, the treatment of night sweating focuses on nourishing yin and clearing heat, different from spontaneous sweating which emphasizes replenishing qi and securing the exterior. Yiyin Decoction is used. For individuals with pronounced internal heat or a propensity for the fire of the five emotions to flare up, the combination with Danggui Liuhuang Tang (Angelica and Six-Yellow Decoction) is recommended.

Yiyin Decoction: Raw Rehmannia, Cornus, Moutan Bark, White Peony Root, Ophiopogon, Yam, Alisma, Wolfberry Bark, Lotus Seed, Rush, Schisandra

Danggui Liuhuang Decoction: Angelica, Astragalus, Raw Rehmannia, Prepared Rehmannia, Scutellaria, Coptis, Phellodendron

XVI. Profuse Sweating Unabated

Excessive sweating in general consumes primordial qi and body fluids, and since sweat is the fluid of the heart, the heart is prone to weakness, so Shengmai Powder is appropriate for treatment. In exogenous syndromes, if sweating persists after diaphoresis, heat subsides but there is instead fear of cold, difficulty in urination, and tetany of the limbs with impaired flexion and extension, it is due to unconsolidated defensive qi, called "yang exhaustion", which is in danger of collapse. It is essential to support yang with Shaoyao Gancao Fuzi Decoction or Guizhi Jia Fuzi Decoction. It must be noted that although this syndrome is named yang exhaustion, yin fluids are also exhausted, so White Peony Root is also a main ingredient.

Sweat coming out like beads that do not flow, or sweat like oil that is sticky to the touch, often accompanied by panting with a faint voice, is a dissipation of primordial qi, one of the critical signs, called "final sweat".

Shaoyao Gancao Fuzi Decoction: White Peony Root, Honey-fried Licorice, Aconite

Guizhi Jia Fuzi Decoction: Cinnamon Twig, White Peony Root, Aconite, Honey-fried Licorice, Ginger, Jujube

XVII. Hemihidrosis

Sweating on either the left or right half of the body is mostly due to qi and blood disharmony, which cannot be cured by merely stopping sweating. Modified Shiquan Dabu Decoction is used to replenish qi, nourish the nutrient aspect, assist yang, and secure the defensive aspect. After half-body sweating, the skin becomes deficient and loose, making it most susceptible to wind pathogens, leading to hemiplegia. As *The Inner Canon* states, "Sweating on one side leads to hemiplegia", so prevention should be done early.

In lower limb paralysis syndrome, sweating mostly occurs above the chest, with no sweat in the affected area. As the condition gradually improves, sweating gradually extends downward. If due to exogenous pathogens, sweating cannot be achieved all over the body, forced sweating should not be done.

Shiquan Dabu Decoction: Astragalus, Cinnamon, Codonopsis, Atractylodes, Prepared Rehmannia, White Peony Root, Angelica, Ligusticum, Poria, Licorice

XVIII. Tinea Versicolor

In summer, wiping sweat with a just sun-dried towel often leaves marks. A folk recipe: grind litharge and lead powder in equal parts, mix well, and wipe with ginger dipped in the powder. Another recipe: grind borax into a fine powder and wipe.

"Purple macule wind" and "white macule wind" also belong to the category of tinea versicolor, caused by wind-dampness invading the hair follicles and blocking the pores. Purple is due to blood stagnation, white is due to qi stagnation. Initially, there is no pain or itching, and after a long time, there is slight itching. For both, Huma Pills should be taken internally, and Litharge Powder applied externally.

Huma Pills: Sesame, Saposhnikovia, Sophora, Acorus, Clematis, White Aconite, Angelica Pubescens, Licorice

Litharge Powder: Realgar (2 *qian*), Sulfur (2 *qian*), Cnidium (2 *qian)*, Litharge (1 *qian*), Stone Yellow (1 *qian*), Calomel (5 *fen*), ground into powder, mixed with vinegar and applied to the affected area.

XIX. Erythema

When warm diseases and cold damage transform into heat, and pathogenic factors enter the nutrient phase, the body heat persists, and erythema appears on the skin, varying in shape from round to oval; or they connect with each other like clouds. They initially appear on the chest, then rapidly spread to the back, abdomen, and limbs, with the color gradually deepening. The patient is thirsty and drinks a lot, restless and unable to sleep, with a red tongue, dry and rough coating with little fluid, and in severe cases, delirium. This is a condition where pathogenic factors move from the qi phase to the nutrient phase, spreading from the inside to the outside, belonging to diseases of the muscles. In treatment, since the stomach governs the muscles and pathogenic heat is already intense, pungent and penetrating methods are inappropriate. Therefore, blood-clearing ingredients are mostly added to stomach-clearing formulas, using Huaban Decoction (Macule-Resolving Decoction). However, although macule eruption is caused by stomach heat, it is also related to fire in various meridians. When necessary, it is still necessary to assist in penetrating and draining, so modified Xiaoban Qingdai Yin (Macule-Reducing Indigo Drink) is commonly used. For those with delirium, Zixue Dan (Purple Snow Pellet) is used together to open the orifices and clear the spirit. Generally, the macules gradually subside after seven days, and the body heat decreases accordingly, though some may persist for a longer period.

Macule eruption is a severe syndrome; improper treatment can lead to death. If the eruption is incomplete or exposed to cold, causing the macules to turn dark purple due to blood stasis, consideration should be given to using herbs like Red Peony Root, Safflower, and Pangolin to disperse the stasis. A purely cold and cool approach is strictly avoided.

Huaban Decoction (Macule-Resolving Decoction): Gypsum, Anemarrhena, Scrophularia, Rhinoceros Horn, Licorice, Rice

Xiaoban Qingdai Yin (Macule-Reducing Indigo Drink): Indigo Naturalis, Coptis, Gardenia, Scrophularia, Anemarrhena, Raw Rehmannia, Rhinoceros Horn, Gypsum, Bupleurum, Ginseng, Licorice, Ginger, Jujube

Zixue Dan (Purple Snow Pellet): Talc, Gypsum, Calcite, Magnetite, Antelope Horn, Rhinoceros Horn, Costus Root, Aquilaria, Clove, Cimicifuga, Scrophularia, Licorice, Glauber's Salt, Nitre, Cinnabar, Musk

(proprietary medicine)

XX. Red Rash

In warm diseases with persistent body heat, the appearance of small red dots is called "red rash," caused by the same factors as macule eruption. However, macules are more severe, rashes are slightly milder; macules are deeper in the muscles, while rashes are shallower in the blood collaterals. Although they can appear simultaneously, they should not be confused. Generally, with proper treatment of warm diseases, macules and rashes may not occur. Both develop due to heat stagnation in the nutrient phase unable to dissipate externally. Therefore, once they appear, clearing the nutrient phase should be assisted. Pungent, warm, ascending, and dispersing methods are strictly avoided, as are cold, greasy substances that suppress and contain, to prevent complications such as vomiting of blood, nosebleeds, and delirium. Additionally, macules and rashes should gradually subside with the heat, and the body cooling down. If they suddenly disappear completely, it is mostly due to inward penetration of pathogenic factors, with a poor prognosis. For treating red rashes, Yinqiao San (Honeysuckle and Forsythia Powder) without Fermented Soybean, plus Raw Rehmannia, Moutan Bark, Folium Isatidis, and Scrophularia is appropriate. For severe heat with clouded consciousness, Qinggong Decoction (Palace-Clearing Decoction) is used in combination.

Note: Western medicine-diagnosed thrombocytopenia, mainly characterized by a tendency to bleed, particularly with skin petechiae. These petechiae closely resemble red rashes, often accompanied by low-grade fever in the afternoon. However, they are distinctly different from red rashes in warm diseases. Treatment should focus on nourishing yin and clearing blood, using herbs such as Raw Rehmannia, Turtle Shell, Donkey-Hide Gelatin, White Peony Root, Cimicifuga, and Arnebia Root.

Yinqiao San (Honeysuckle and Forsythia Powder): Forsythia, Honeysuckle, Fermented Soybean, Schizonepeta, Mint, Platycodon, Bamboo Leaf, Arctium, Licorice, Reed Rhizome

Qinggong Decoction (Palace-Clearing Decoction): Scrophularia (heart), Lotus Seed (heart), Bamboo Leaf (heart), Forsythia (heart), Ophiopogon (heart), Rhinoceros Horn

XXI. White Papules

In damp-warm diseases with unresolved alternating chills and heat, restlessness, chest tightness, nausea, and a yellow greasy tongue coating, white papules (bái pò) are most likely to appear. These are small, white blisters on the skin; due to their clear and plump appearance, they are also called "crystal papules" (jīng pò) and, when occurring with red rashes, "red-white rashes" (hóng bái zhěn). Caused by damp-heat pathogens stagnating in the muscle surface unable to disperse, they emerge with bodily fluids, and after eruption, the condition often feels slightly relieved. They first appear on the neck and chest, gradually spreading to the abdomen and back, sometimes extending to the limbs, starting sparse and becoming dense, with a characteristic sour, rotten odor. They typically erupt once or twice a day, diminishing after 3–4 days, with body heat gradually lowering, and clearing completely within 7 days, followed by peeling skin. In severe cases, they may persist for over half a month; in some cases, later papules lose their brightness, resembling louse shells, called "withered papules" (kū pò), indicating qi and yin deficiency with a poor prognosis. White papules belong to the qi phase; if heat is severe and the nutrient phase is also affected, they often appear with red rashes, making the condition more serious. White papules are a way for pathogens to exit, with each eruption reducing the severity—they cannot clear in a single episode, hence the analogy by predecessors to "peeling a cocoon" or "unfolding a banana leaf." Treatment should clear, transform, disperse, and penetrate on the basis of reducing fever, using modified Yīnyūn Tāng (Mist-like Decoction). For qi and yin deficiency, add ginseng fibrils, adenophora, or dendrobium; for concurrent red rashes, add moutan bark, red peony root, or arnebia; for recovery, use Yìyǐ Zhúyè Sǎn (Coix and Bamboo Leaf Powder).

Yīnyūn Tāng (Mist-like Decoction): Fermented soybean sprouts, agastache, eupatorium, artemisia annua, charred gardenia peel, forsythia, talc, akebia, curcuma, acorus

Yìyǐ Zhúyè Sǎn (Coix and Bamboo Leaf Powder): Coix seed, bamboo leaf, talc, amomum, forsythia, poria, akebia

XXII. Measles

This condition is regionally termed "shāzi" (rash) or "dázi" (pock), and "kāngchuāng" (bran sore) in Northern China. Most children are susceptible, with occasional adult cases, caused by congenital fetal toxin combined with seasonal pathogens; once contracted, immunity is life-long. Epidemics occur mostly in winter and spring. Initial symptoms resemble wind-cold, with mild chills and fever. Characteristics include teary eyes, cool earlobes, frequent sneezing, and uncomfortable coughing. Before eruption, the face is puffy with flushed cheeks, white spots inside the cheeks, and a red, prominent fingerprint. During eruption, the child is restless; rashes first appear behind the ears, at the hairline, and on the neck, then spread to the forehead, face, shoulders, back, chest, and abdomen—small, uniform, sand-like granules under the skin, gradually rising and palpable. After full eruption, body heat and other symptoms subside, rashes fade, and skin sheds branny scales. The entire course has three stages: fever, eruption, and resolution, each averaging two days, totaling nine days. Measles should erupt fully and completely; generally, rashes on the head, feet, and face indicate a favorable course. Full eruption is confirmed by dense red dots on the nose and palms/soles; full penetration by a rough, raised texture on the skin. Poor eruption (incomplete or sudden regression) or pale, non-red, or purplish-dark rashes indicate an unfavorable course. Treatment focuses on clearing and dispersing lung and stomach pathogens, using Fángfēng Jiědú Tāng (Saposhnikovia Detoxifying Decoction) or modified Zhúyè Liǔbàng Tāng (Bamboo Leaf and Willow Pith Decoction). After resolution, only clear residual heat in the blood. Key is preventing deterioration and sequelae: avoid pungent-hot, bitter-cold, or tonifying-astringent herbs, which may cause wheezing, nasal flaring, delirium, convulsions, abdominal distension, or diarrhea. Common sequelae include wasting with bone steaming, dry, frizzy hair, and dry skin (measly consumptive disease), or persistent cough, asthma, and blood-tinged sputum, often lingering.

Fángfēng Jiědú Tāng (Saposhnikovia Detoxifying Decoction)

Zhúyè Liǔbàng Tāng (Bamboo Leaf and Willow Pith Decoction)

The child has only a slight fever, with skin faintly flushed and a rash that appears as small spots resembling measles but lacking the characteristic features of measles. The rash spots are small, sparse, spread quickly, fully erupt within one-two days, and clear completely in three-four days. There is no desquamation after resolution. Caused by wind-heat, unrelated to congenital toxin, it is called "wind rash" (fēng shā). Modified Xiāodú Yǐn (Detoxifying Drink) is used.

Fángfēng Jiědú Tāng (Saposhnikovia Detoxifying Decoction): Saposhnikovia, Schizonepeta, Mentha, Arctium, Platycodon, Glycyrrhiza, Phyllostachys leaves, Forsythia, Gypsum, Anemarrhena, Akebia, Aurantium

Zhúyè Liǔbàng Tāng (Bamboo Leaf and Willow Pith Decoction):

Phyllostachys leaves, Salix babylonica, Pueraria, Arctium, Anemarrhena, Cicada slough, Schizonepeta, Mentha, Gypsum, Scrophularia, Ophiopogon, Glycyrrhiza, Oryza sativa

Jiāwèi Xiāodú Yǐn (Modified Detoxifying Drink): Schizonepeta, Saposhnikovia, Arctium, Cimicifuga, Glycyrrhiza, Paeonia rubra, Forsythia, Crataegus

XXIII. Urticaria

Ancient names include "pǐ zhǒng" (wheal swelling) and "yǐn zhěn" (hidden rash). The skin develops wheals, initially like broad bean slices, gradually forming patches, white without redness, similar to bedbug bites, hence the common name "fēng zhèn kuài" (wind patches). The more it is scratched, the more itchy and numerous the wheals become, covering the entire body, with intense itching even in the hair, ears, and palms/soles. They appear and disappear periodically, recurring frequently. It is mostly caused by exposure to wind after sweating, leading to wind–heat rebelling in the superficial muscles, and is also related to blood heat. Xiāo Fēng Sǎn (Wind-Dispelling Powder) is appropriate; adding fresh Polygonum multiflorum and purple-backed duckweed enhances efficacy. External washing with camphor wood decoction provides temporary relief. Excessive scratching leading to broken skin and ulceration can be treated with decoctions of Artemisia capillaris and Sophora flavescens (30g each) or silkworm excrement (90g), applied while hot.

Xiāo Fēng Sǎn (Wind-Dispelling Powder): Schizonepeta, Saposhnikovia, Cicada slough, Arctium, Atractylodes lancea, Gypsum, Anemarrhena, Rehmannia glutinosa, Cannabis sativa, Akebia, Glycyrrhiza

XXIV. Prickly Heat

In summer, when sweating, children and obese individuals often develop dense, sharp red papules on the skin, with severe itching and stinging, called "prickly heat" (fèi zǐ). They quickly turn into small pustules, dry out after a few days, and form fine scales. Due to summer heat blocking sweat pores, Liù Yī Sǎn (Six-to-One Powder) is taken internally, and prickly heat powder is applied externally.

Liù Yī Sǎn (Six-to-One Powder): Talc, Glycyrrhiza

XXV. Smallpox

Ancient name "dòu chuāng" (pock sore), in pediatrics, it is as severe as "measles" and collectively referred to as "rash and pock". The cause is the same as measles, arising from congenital fetal toxin combined with external pathogens, but it is more prevalent in spring and summer. The entire course, from fever, eruption, swelling, pustulation, scabbing to crusting, takes approximately 15 days. Onset is acute, starting with chills and high fever, with eruptions appearing after three days. Generally, the pustules have pointed tops and rounded bases, with distinct red and white colors, spreading from the face to the chest, back, and limbs, covering the entire body. They quickly swell, with white tops and red bases, then pustulate, surrounded by tight red halos, followed by gradual scabbing. The pocks change from waxy yellow to chestnut shell color, forming thick crusts that fall off. This is the normal progression of smallpox. In recent years, with vaccination, this disease has been basically eradicated.

"Chickenpox", similar to smallpox, initially presents with chills and fever, with red spots appearing on the head and face, gradually spreading to the trunk, with fewer on the limbs. They then turn into blisters with bright white tops and red halos at the base, and like smallpox, appear in pairs. However, the blisters have thin, delicate walls, with unclear, loose bases. From eruption to swelling and crusting, the course is only five-six days. Another characteristic is the irregular progression of eruptions, so red spots, blisters, and dry crusts are present simultaneously on the skin, unlike smallpox, which erupts uniformly in stages. Chickenpox generally has few complications and a good prognosis. It is mostly caused by wind-heat stagnating in the skin surface, and treatment is with modified Dà Liánqiào Yǐn (Great Forsythia Drink).

Dà Liánqiào Yǐn (Great Forsythia Drink): Forsythia, Angelica, Red Peony Root, Saposhnikovia, Arctium, Cicada Slough, Akebia, Talc, Dianthus, Schizonepeta, Bupleurum, Scutellaria, Gardenia, Gypsum, Plantain Seed, Rush

XXVI. Yellowing of the Skin

Yellowing of the entire skin is a characteristic of "jaundice" (huángdǎn), accompanied by yellowing of the eyes and dark yellow urine. It can be divided into two types: "yang jaundice" with a bright orange-yellow color, accompanied by fever, thirst, chest tightness, restlessness, abdominal fullness, constipation, and a yellow greasy tongue coating, caused by damp-heat in the stomach; "yin jaundice" with a dull, smoky yellow color, accompanied by chills, loss of appetite, loose stools, and a white greasy tongue coating, caused by cold-dampness in the spleen. The former is treated with Yinchenhao Decoction, the latter with Yinchen Wuling Powder or Yinchen Zhufu Decoction. Whether yang or yin jaundice, the main cause is related to dampness, so jaundice is often accompanied by difficult urination, and promoting diuresis is the main treatment method. Artemisia capillaris is the key herb for jaundice, actually because it can dispel stagnation and promote dampness, so it is often used in damp-heat syndromes even without jaundice.

Yellowing of the skin with normal urination, a pale and lusterless yellow color, and no yellowing of the eyes is a syndrome of spleen deficiency and blood deficiency due to nutritional deficiency, often accompanied by fatigue, dizziness, and palpitations, commonly called "fatigue jaundice" (tuōlì huáng), treated with Xiaojianzhong Decoction.

Prolonged illness with yellow, dry, loess-like skin is mostly a sign of spleen failure, which is called "fading color" in *The Inner Canon,* and is difficult to treat.

Yinchenhao Decoction: Artemisia capillaris, Gardenia, Rhubarb

Yinchen Wuling Powder: Artemisia capillaris, Atractylodes, Cinnamon Twig, Alisma, Poria, Polyporus

Yinchen Zhufu Decoction: Artemisia capillaris, Atractylodes, Aconite, Dried Ginger, Licorice

Xiaojianzhong Decoction: Cinnamon Twig, White Peony Root, Licorice, Maltose, Ginger, Jujube

XXVII. Darkening of the Skin

Dark and dull skin color is called "black jaundice" (hēidǎn); because it is caused by kidney damage from excessive sexual activity, it is also called "sexual fatigue jaundice" (nǚláo dǎn). It is a type of jaundice, mostly transformed from jaundice, so it is yellow with a blackish tint; in mild cases, only the forehead is slightly black, with yellow eyes and yellow urine. In severe cases, there are emaciation, abdominal fullness, heat in the palms and soles, loose and slightly black stools, and a deficient and string-like pulse. In the later stage, loss of appetite, nausea and vomiting, anuria, and coma occur, which are difficult to save. Xiaoshi Fanshi Powder and Heidan Decoction should be used in combination with the treatment methods for jaundice. Refer to the entry "Yellowing of the

Skin" in this section.

Note: In Addison's disease diagnosed by Western medicine, the face is significantly dark, the skin color of the arms is also dark, and the lips and gums are grayish-brown. Combined with other symptoms such as listlessness, loss of appetite, frequent urination, impotence in men, especially a craving for salty foods, and a deep and thin pulse, all belong to insufficient kidney yang with water qipathology.Prepared Rehmannia, Aconite, Psoralea, Epimedium, Angelica, Deer Horn Glue, Amomum, etc., can be used to warm and nourish the kidney and life gate.

Xiaoshi Fanshi Powder: Nitre, Alum

Heidan Decoction: Artemisia capillaris, Trichosanthes Root

XXVIII. Reddening of the Skin

Reddening of the skin, as if stained with rouge or cinnabar, is called "erysipelas" (dāndú). Due to different locations of occurrence, the causes, names, specific symptoms, and treatment methods vary slightly. When occurring all over the body, it is called "wandering erysipelas" (chìyóu dāndú); initially, there are red cloud-like patches, often wandering without a fixed location, or swollen and painful, accompanied by chills, fever, and headache. In mild cases, it subsides in seven days; in severe cases, the redness and swelling expand to the surrounding area, accompanied by chest tightness, vomiting, or delirium. Mostly caused by excessive heart fire, plus invasion by wind-heat; in children, it is related to fetal toxin. Use Huaban Jiedu Decoction. The most common local occurrence is "flowing fire" (liúhuǒ); refer to the entry "Swelling and Redness of the Lower Limbs" in Limb Symptoms.

Huaban Jiedu Decoction: Cimicifuga, Gypsum, Forsythia, Arctium, Renzhonghuang (processed human excrement), Coptis, Anemarrhena,

Scrophularia, Bamboo Leaves

XXIX. Edema

There are two types of skin edema: “water edema” and “qi edema”, with water edema being more common. In water edema, the skin is bright and thin; when pressed, it leaves a pit like a sagging pouch that does not quickly rebound. The swelling may spread from top to bottom, bottom to top, or start from the abdomen and gradually extend to the limbs and the whole body. It is mostly caused by wind pathogens and water-dampness, with pathological changes mainly involving the lung, spleen, and kidney, but also related to the triple energizer and bladder. It is generally divided into “yang water” and “yin water”. Yang water refers to edema in the upper body and exterior, tending to be heat syndromes and excess syndromes, with an acute onset; yin water refers to edema in the lower body and interior, tending to be cold syndromes and deficiency syndromes, with a slow onset. *Zhengzhi Yaojue* (Essentials of Syndrome and Treatment) states: “Generalized edema with irritability, thirst, reddish and scanty urine, and mostly constipation belongs to yang water; generalized edema without irritability and thirst, with normal or loose stools, and scanty but not reddish urine belongs to yin water.” However, the exterior-interior and deficiency-excess of edema are often complicated and intertwined, so in clinical practice, they must be distinguished according to the characteristics of symptoms. Predecessors divided it into four types: “wind water”, “skin water”, “true water”, and “stone water”. Edema first appearing on the face and eyes, with eye sockets like silkworms, throbbing neck vessels, aversion to wind, fever, cough, joint pain, and a floating pulse is wind water; edema starting from the limbs and abdomen, with a large but not full abdomen, heavy limbs, a floating pulse, and no aversion to wind is skin water; edema with shortness of breath and inability to lie flat, and a deep and slow pulse is true water; edema with obvious abdominal swelling, or radiating to hypochondriac fullness, a deep pulse, and no shortness of breath is stone water. Therefore, to distinguish edema, attention should be paid to whether the head and face are more swollen, the limbs are more swollen, the lower limbs are more swollen, or the waist and abdomen are more swollen. Secondly, in water edema, urine is scanty; attention should be paid to whether it is yellowish-red or not, and whether the stool is constipated or loose. At the same time, the degree of swelling is also crucial; for example, no lines in the palms, a flat waist and protruding navel, swelling of the scrotum and penis, and knees like buckets are all severe, with a poor prognosis. Treatment based on the cause, symptoms, and involved *zang-fu* organs includes methods such as inducing sweating, promoting diuresis, warming transformation, regulating qi, strengthening transportation, and attacking stagnation. These methods must be used in appropriate combination. Commonly used formulas include Maxing Yicao Decoction, Yuebi Jiazhu Decoction, Wupi Decoction, Daoshui Fuling Decoction, Fangji Fuling Decoction, Zhenwu Decoction, Shipi Decoction, Weiling Decoction, Fangji HuangqiDecoction, Shuzao Yinzi, Zhouche Pill, Yugong Powder, etc. For post-illness conditioning, Xiangsha Liujun Decoction and Shenling Baizhu Powder are often used. Edema patients should avoid salt, otherwise, the swelling is not easy to subside. *Dexiao Fang* (Effective Prescriptions) states: "For all edema, only salt is forbidden, even a tiny bit should not enter the mouth" and emphasizes that "if you cannot avoid salt, do not take medicine; if you really want to cure the disease, you must avoid salt."

"Qi edema" is obvious in the abdomen and limbs, with unchanged skin color, and the depression rebounds immediately when pressed; although the abdomen is large, it sounds like an empty drum when tapped, also called "skin distension". Due to the dysfunction of qi movement in the spleen, stomach, and triple energizer, it is often accompanied by chest tightness and abdominal distension after eating. Treatment should promote qi and resolve stagnation, using Kuanzhong Decoction plus Aucklandia, Cyperus, and Green Tangerine Peel. If qi does not circulate, water cannot be transformed, and water can gradually accumulate, so attention must be paid to the amount of urine and whether the abdomen is hard at any time. Once water accumulates, it should be treated as water edema.

Edema accompanied by yellowish skin, sweat staining clothes like cork tree juice, cold shins, oliguria, and a deep pulse is called "yellow sweat". It is caused by bathing with cold water when sweating, and the accumulation of spleen heat and water-dampness. Huangqi Shaogui Kujiu Decoction is used; for severe swelling, add Saposhnikovia and Stephania.

Edema during pregnancy in women is called "fetal edema" (zǐ zhǒng), which is related to fetal qi. Refer to the entry "Edema During Pregnancy" under Gynecological Symptoms.

Maxing Yicao Decoction: Ephedra, Almond, Coix Seed, Licorice

Yuebi Jiazhu Decoction: Ephedra, Gypsum, Licorice, Atractylodes, Ginger, Jujube

Wupi Decoction: Poria Peel, Ginger Peel, Tangerine Peel, Mulberry Bark, Areca Peel

Daoshui Fuling Decoction: Red Poria, Alisma, Atractylodes, Areca Peel, Aucklandia, Amomum, Areca Nut, Perilla, Ophiopogon, Mulberry Bark, Rush, Tangerine Peel, Papaya

Fangji Fuling Decoction: Stephania, Poria, Astragalus, Cinnamon Twig, Licorice

Zhenwu Decoction: Aconite, Atractylodes, White Peony Root, Poria, Ginger

Shipi Decoction: Aconite, Processed Ginger, Atractylodes, Poria, Licorice, Tsaoko, Magnolia Bark, Aucklandia, Papaya, Areca Peel, Ginger, Jujube

Weiling Decoction: Atractylodes Lancea, Atractylodes Macrocephala, Cinnamon Twig, Poria, Polyporus, Alisma, Magnolia Bark, Tangerine Peel, Licorice, Stephania

Huangqi Decoction: Stephania, Astragalus, Atractylodes, Licorice

Shuzao Yinzi: Areca Nut, Phytolacca, Poria Peel, Areca Peel, Pepper Seed, Adzuki Bean, Gentiana, Notopterygium, Alisma, Akebia, Ginger Peel

Zhouche Pill: Black Morning Glory Seed, Rhubarb, Kansui, Euphorbia, Genkwa, Green Tangerine Peel, Tangerine Peel, Aucklandia, Calomel

Yugong Powder: Black Morning Glory Seed, Fennel

Xiangsha Liujun Decoction: Ginseng, Atractylodes, Poria, Licorice, Aucklandia, Amomum

Shenling Baizhu Powder: Ginseng, Atractylodes, Poria, Yam, Hyacinth Bean, Amomum, Coix Seed, Tangerine Peel, Lotus Seed, Licorice, Platycodon

Kuanzhong Decoction: Atractylodes, Aurantium, Magnolia Bark, Tangerine Peel, Poria, Pinellia, Hawthorn, Medicated Leaven, Radish Seed, Ginger

Huangqi Shaogui Kujiu Decoction: Astragalus, White Peony Root, Cinnamon Twig, Rice Vinegar

XXX. Emaciation

Gradual emaciation is common in deficiency syndromes. Since the spleen governs the muscles, treatment should focus on nurturing qi and blood in the middle jiao in conjunction with the main symptoms. For example, the most prominent is "lung consumption" (tuberculosis), which should be treated with the method of nourishing the earth to generate metal (nurturing the spleen to benefit the lung).

Muscle emaciation, especially the complete wasting of large muscles in the limbs, is most severe. Refer to the entry "Limb Emaciation" under Limb Symptoms.

Women who are otherwise healthy but become extremely thin, as particularly noted in *Dongyi Baojian* (Treasured Mirror of Oriental Medicine), are considered to have insufficient qi and blood. Ginseng decoction is used to deliver Guling Pills.

Persistent hunger with daily emaciation should raise suspicion of "consumptive thirst" (diabetes); gradual weight loss in obese individuals, accompanied by excessive phlegm, cough, and gurgling sounds in the intestines, is mostly a fluid retention syndrome. Refer to the entries "Excessive Hunger and Voracious Appetite" under Internal Organ Symptoms and "Abdominal Rumbling" under Abdominal and Umbilical Symptoms.

Guling Pills: Astragalus, Achyranthes, Angelica, Aconite, Prepared Rehmannia, Poria, Eucommia, Atractylodes Lancea, Atractylodes Macrocephala, Cinnamon, Wolfberry

XXXI. Fatigue

Generalized fatigue and weakness in movement are mostly deficiency syndromes, suitable for replenishing both qi and blood with Bazhen Decoction. However, shortness of breath during activity indicates a predominance of qi deficiency; a sensation of heat, palpitations, and sweating during movement indicates a predominance of blood deficiency. Medications should be adjusted accordingly.

Dampness can stagnate qi, and summer heat can damage qi. In summer, internal obstruction of summer heat and dampness often causes severe fatigue without major illness, commonly called "summer lassitude" (zhù xià). For mild cases, soak Agastache and Eupatorium for drinking; for severe cases, modify Qingshu Yiqi Decoction.

Qingshu Yiqi Decoction: Ginseng, Astragalus, Licorice, Angelica, Ophiopogon, Schisandra, Pueraria, Cimicifuga, Atractylodes Lancea, Atractylodes Macrocephala, Green Tangerine Peel, Tangerine Peel, Phellodendron, Medicated Leaven, Alisma, Ginger, Jujube

XXXII. Muscle Twitching

This condition is commonly seen in patterns of blood deficiency, resulting from malnourishment of the tendons and vessels. Referred to as "tendon spasm and muscle twitching" in *Treatise on Cold Damage*, it is not treated as a primary symptom.

XXXIII. Skin Numbness

Numbness refers to loss of sensation, also called "unfeelingness," commonly seen in the collateral syndrome of wind stroke. As stated in *Synopsis of the Golden Chamber*, "When pathogenic factors are in the collaterals, the skin and muscles are unfeeling." Refer to the entry "Facial Numbness" under Head and Face Symptoms.

"Leprosy," ancient name "li wind," initially presents with skin numbness, followed by white scales and red swelling, spreading into scars, shaped like snake skin, falling off in patches, and in severe cases, breaking down with thick swelling but no pus. If the pathogenic toxin invades the interior, causing symptoms such as loss of eyebrows, collapse of the nose, eversion of the lips, and rupture of the eyelid margins, all are difficult to treat. General treatment should dispel wind, transform dampness, killparasites, supplemented by nourishing qi and blood. Initially, Wanding Pills are used for bathing to induce sweating, followed by Shenying Yangzhen Pills. For broken skin, Bisheng Powder is used first, then Wanding Pills. Others such as Agkistrodon Wine and Polygonum Multiflorum Wine can also be used as appropriate.

Wanding Pills: Atractylodes, Notopterygium, Schizonepeta, Saposhnikovia, Asarum, Ligusticum, Lindera, Angelica, Aconitum Carmichaeli, Dendrobium, Ephedra, Gastrodia, Realgar, Licorice, Polygonum Multiflorum, Scorpion (proprietary medicine)

Shenying Yangzhen Pills: Notopterygium, Papaya, Gastrodia, White Peony Root, Angelica, Cuscuta, Prepared Rehmannia, Ligusticum

Bisheng Powder: Rhubarb, Areca, White Morning Glory Seed (each one *qian*), Calomel (one *qian* two *fen*), ground into powder. For strong adults, divide into five doses; for middle-aged and long-term deficient patients, divide into seven doses.

Agkistrodon Wine: One agkistrodon, drowned in twojin of white wine, add five *qian* of ginseng.

Polygonum Multiflorum Wine: Polygonum Multiflorum (four *liang*), Angelica (body), Pangolin, Raw Rehmannia, Prepared Rehmannia, Toad (each one *liang*), Oriental Arborvitae Leaf, Pine Needle, Acanthopanax Bark, Aconitum Carmichaeli, Aconitum Kusnezoffii (each four *qian*), soaked in 20 jin of yellow rice wine.

XXXIV. Dry and Rough Skin

Dry and rough skin is mostly caused by blood deficiency generating dryness. *The Inner Canon* calls it "suoze" (dry lusterlessness), and Liu Hejian stated, "All astringency, dryness, withering, dryness, hardness, chapping, and peeling are attributed to dryness." Use Shengxue Runfu Drink, in which a small amount of peach kernel and safflower are added to moisten dryness and harmonize blood, different from dispelling stasis.

Internal obstruction of static blood, failure to generate new blood, and loss of nourishment to the skin and muscles, often appearing as dry, scaly, and rough like fish scales, is called "dry and rough skin like fish scales." It is accompanied by blurred vision, abdominal fullness, and inability to eat. Treatment should gently soothe the middle jiao and tonify deficiency, using Dahuang Zhechong Pills. However, its stasis-breaking effect is strong, and it should not be used lightly unless the syndrome is correctly identified.

Shengxue Runfu Drink: Raw Rehmannia, Prepared Rehmannia, Asparagus, Ophiopogon, Angelica, Astragalus, Scutellaria, Peach Kernel, Safflower, Trichosanthes, Schisandra

Dahuang Zhechong Pills: Rhubarb, Scutellaria, Licorice, Peach Kernel, Almond, White Peony Root, Rehmannia, Dry Lacquer, Horsefly, Leech, Grub (proprietary medicine)

XXXV. Infantile Five Delays

Infantile five delays refer to "delayed standing," "delayed walking," "delayed hair growth," "delayed tooth eruption," and "delayed speech." During the normal developmental period, it manifests as weak limbs, unconsolidated muscles and bones, weakness in the four limbs, unsteady standing, difficulty in walking, delayed tooth eruption, sparse and withered yellow hair, inability to speak even at two or three years old, and dull expression. This syndrome is caused by congenital insufficiency or postnatal malnutrition, which hinders the growth and development of infants. Treatment should tonify the five *zang* organs and nurture qi and blood. For delayed standing, delayed walking, and delayed tooth eruption, the focus is on tonifying the kidney, using Bushen Dihuang Pills; for delayed hair growth, the focus is on nourishing blood, using Huma Dan; for delayed speech, the focus is on nourishing the heart, using Changpu Pills.

Bushen Dihuang Pills: Prepared Rehmannia, Cornus, Yam, Deer Antler, Achyranthes, Alisma, Moutan Bark, Poria

Huma Dan: Sesame, Rehmannia, Polygonum Multiflorum, Angelica, White Peony Root, Oyster

Changpu Pills: Ginseng, Acorus, Ophiopogon, Polygala, Ligusticum, Angelica, Frankincense, Cinnabar

XXXVI. Infantile Five Flaccidities

It refers to "soft head", "soft neck", "soft limbs", "soft muscles" and "soft mouth". It manifests as a weak and tilted head and neck that cannot be lifted, a soft mouth and loose lips with weak chewing ability, soft hands that hang down and cannot grasp, soft feet that cannot stand, soft and flabby muscles, loose skin and emaciated flesh, and at the same time, dull intelligence. This syndrome is caused by weakness of the spleen and kidney qi, which fails to nourish the bones and flesh. Fuyuan Powder with added antler glue is used.

Fuyuan Powder: Ginseng, Atractylodes, Poria, Fushen, Astragalus, Prepared Rehmannia, Yam, Honey-fried Licorice, Angelica, White Peony Root, Ligusticum, Acorus, Ginger, Jujube

XXXVII. Infantile Five Stiffnesses

It refers to "stiff head", "gasping", "hard palms and soles", "tight mouth" and "hard flesh". Due to stagnation of wind-cold, yang qi fails to circulate, resulting in insufficient nourishment of the head and neck, muscles, hands and feet, etc., manifesting as stiff head and neck, inability to look down, difficulty in turning, blue face and cold breath, chest and diaphragm congestion, big belly with visible blue veins, tense muscles, and stiff limbs. It mostly occurs in children aged one or two years old. The treatment should dispel wind and cold, and regulate qi and blood at the same time, using Wuyao Shunqi Powder. All infantile five delays and five weaknesses are caused by congenital and postnatal deficiencies. Although five stiffnesses are caused by external pathogens, they are also due to insufficient qi and blood nourishment, so treatment must pay attention to nurturing, otherwise they often become chronic diseases.

Wuyao Shunqi Powder: Ephedra, Angelica Dahurica, Ligusticum, Platycodon, Aurantium, Bombyx Batryticatus, Lindera, Processed Ginger, Licorice, Tangerine Peel, Fistular Onion Stalk

XXXVIII. Frostbite

Working in the wild in winter, being attacked by severe cold, causes local qi and blood stagnation. At the beginning, the skin is pale and insensitive, after relief, it turns purple-red, slightly swollen and itchy, gradually forming hard lumps, the skin is chapped, the itching and pain are unbearable, and sometimes it is also numb. It mostly occurs on the hands, feet and ears, called "chilblains", also known as "frostbite". In severe cases, the surrounding area of the wound is purple, swollen and painful, or bleeding and purulent, and some muscles are black, causing tissue death and shape damage, bone detachment and tendon connection, transforming into "gangrene". For mild cases, before ulceration, use Hongling Wine or ginger to rub frequently, and for those already ulcerated, treat according to ulcers. Those with weak qi and blood can take Renshen Yangrong Decoction and yellow rice wine internally.

Hongling Wine: Angelica and Cinnamon each two *liang*, Safflower, Zanthoxylum and Dried Ginger each 1 *liang*, Camphor and Asarum each five *qian,* soaked in two jin of alcohol, dip cotton in it to rub the affected area.

Renshen Yangrong Decoction: Ginseng, Angelica, White Peony Root, Prepared Rehmannia, Atractylodes, Astragalus, Cinnamon, Licorice, Schisandra, Poria, Polygala, Tangerine Peel

XXXIX. Scalds and Burns

Scalded by boiling water or burned by intense fire, mild ones are shallow in the skin surface, only the skin is flushed and painful, or blisters gradually form, and if the epidermis is removed, the exposed red flesh gradually dries and heals. Severe ones are deep in muscles or bones, and blisters form immediately after injury. If the epidermis is removed to expose grayish white or dark red flesh, it indicates that the muscles have been injured. More severe scalds cause the skin to collapse and the flesh to rot, burns cause the skin to scorch and the flesh to curl, then exude sebum and pus, with severe pain. In particular, the fire toxin can damage the internal organs, causing restlessness, asthma, and coma. Therefore, two aspects must be paid attention to: on the one hand, the size and depth of the wound, on the other hand, whether there are internal symptoms. In terms of treatment, mild cases can be cured with external treatment, and severe cases must be treated with medicine. General external treatment methods are divided into: ① washing the wound surface with Coptis water or phellodendron water or water decoction of honeysuckle and licorice for irrigation; ② Treatment of blisters: larger ones are pricked with a needle to release the toxic fluid, smaller ones need not be pricked; ③ Wound surface treatment: apply cooling ointment, etc. internally, the main treatment is to clear fire, detoxify and nourish yin, using modified Huanglian Jiedu Decoction. If there are residual scar wheals, Heibu Gao can be applied.

Qingliang Gao (Cooling Ointment): one *sheng* of air-slaked lime, clarified with four bowls of water, mix one part of the clear water with one part of sesame oil, dip a chicken feather in it and apply to the affected area.

Huanglian Jiedu Decoction (Coptis Detoxifying Decoction): Coptis, Scutellaria, Phellodendron, Gardenia

Heibu Gao (Black Cloth Paste): two *liang* and eight *qian* of gallnut, one centipede, ground into powder, mixed with six *qian* of honey and half a jin of black vinegar.

XL. Bites

Common ones are bites by poisonous insects, snakes, and dogs. Mild cases cause swelling, pain, and decay; severe cases are life-threatening. For poisonous insect bites such as centipede bites, the injured area is slightly swollen, with excruciating pain, or numbness all over the body. Use saliva from a rooster's mouth to apply, or mix licorice and realgar powder with vegetable oil for application, or mash fresh mulberry leaves for external application. Scorpion stings cause itching, pain, and swelling, and in severe cases, the pain radiates to the whole body. Mash a large snail for application, or mix chalcanthite with rice vinegar for application. For bee stings, if the stinger is embedded in the flesh, it must be picked out, and then apply saliva immediately. For caterpillar stings in trees, the hairs scatter into the skin, causing initial itching followed by pain, as if burned by fire. Mash fermented soybeans and soybean oil for application. Bites by other insects, although swollen, are not painful or only slightly itchy, and generally subside on their own.

For snake bites, it is necessary to distinguish between poisonous snake bites and non-venomous snake bites. Non-venomous snake bites leave tooth marks mostly in six rows, i.e., four rows on one side and two rows on the other; poisonous snake bites leave four rows. There is obvious edema near the wound of a snake bite, initially burning pain, then numbness, mostly on the hands and feet, with swelling gradually spreading upward. Generally, swelling occurs on the day of the bite, becomes more severe on the second day, remains the same on the third day, starts to subside on the fourth day, and completely disappears in about seven days. On the night after the snake bite, the eyelids droop, vision is blurred, unable to see people across, breathing is difficult, vomiting occurs, the pulse is thin and rapid, and body heat rises with the swelling, but the heat subsides when the swelling subsides, and the heat subsides faster than the swelling. It should be noted that poisonous snake bites can cause death within a few hours or more than ten hours. Immediately take five Jidesheng Snake Bite Tablets orally, and dissolve the tablets in warm water to apply around the wound about half an inch away from it; do not apply the medicine to the wound to allow the venom to be discharged.

Dog bites should be divided into domestic dog bites and mad dog bites. Mad dogs have abnormal postures, with their tongues sticking out and salivating, heads lowered and ears drooping, red eyes and tails dragging, running around aimlessly. Domestic dog bites only leave local tooth marks, and in severe cases, decay, but there is no danger to life. Mad dog bites, initially the same as domestic dog bites, have no special symptoms, but later, symptoms such as listlessness, fear, insomnia, irritability, thirst, painful and difficult urination appear. Over time, they become sensitive to colors and light, afraid of fire, startled by the sound of forging, and twitch with slight stimulation. If there is difficulty in urination and defecation, restlessness, abdominal distension, foaming at the mouth, madness and barking at people, with a voice like a dog, and white eyes, it is a critical condition. Take Fuwei Powder initially, then Yuzhen Powder, and often eat almonds to prevent the toxin from attacking the heart.

Sheyao Pian (Snake Bite Tablets): Omitted (proprietary medicine)

Fuwei San (Crisis-Assisting Powder): Mylabris, one for each day since the dog bite, one *liang* of talc stir-fried with glutinous rice, one *qian* of realgar, two *fen* of musk, ground into powder, one *qian* per dose, taken with yellow rice wine or rice soup.

Yuzhen San (Jade Truth Powder): one *liang* each of arisaema, saposhnikovia, angelica dahurica, gastrodia, notopterygium, and white aconite, ground into powder, three *qian* per dose, taken with a cup of hot wine.

XLI. Traumatic Injuries

Generally speaking, traumatic injuries include injuries from knives, guns, falls, beatings, abrasions, sports, martial arts practice, etc., with various external injury manifestations such as skin lesion, pain, injured tendons, broken bones, dislocation, bleeding, and purple-blue skin, as well as internal injury symptoms such as vomiting blood and internal stabbing pain during breathing. The scope is quite extensive and should be handled by emergency treatment and surgical treatment in traumatology. In terms of internal medicines, the main focuses are stopping bleeding, dissipating blood stasis, promoting qi circulation, relieving pain, relaxing tendons, and strengthening bones. Prescriptions such as Qili Powder, Shenhuang

Powder, Zijin Powder, Fuyuan Huoxue Decoction, Zhuangjin Yangxue Decoction, and Zhenggu Dan can be used appropriately.

Qili Powder: Frankincense, Myrrh, Angelica, Catechu, Safflower, Dragon's Blood, Cinnabar, Musk, Borneol (proprietary medicine)

Shenhuang Powder: Panax Notoginseng, Rhubarb, Magnolia Bark, Aurantium, Peach Kernel, Angelica Tail, Red Peony Root, Safflower, Pangolin, Turmeric, Corydalis, Cinnamon, Bupleurum, Licorice, Green Tangerine Peel

Zijin Powder: Redbud Bark, Drynaria, Pollen Typhae, Moutan Bark, Angelica Tail, Safflower, Ligusticum, Dipsacus, Ground Beetle, Peach Kernel, Frankincense, Myrrh, taken with hot yellow rice wine.

Fuyuan Huoxue Decoction: Angelica, Peach Kernel, Safflower, Rhubarb, Pangolin, Trichosanthes Root, Bupleurum, Licorice

Zhuangjin Yangxue Decoction: Angelica, Prepared Rehmannia, White Peony Root, Moutan Bark, Safflower, Ligusticum, Dipsacus, Eucommia, Achyranthes

Zhenggu Dan: Angelica Tail, Rhubarb, Myrrh, Frankincense, Acanthopanax Bark, Green Tangerine Peel, Ligusticum, Cyperus, Pyrite, Borax

Section 2 Head and Face Symptoms

The head is located at the highest part of the human body. The clear yang qi of the *zang-fu* organs ascends to the head, the three yang meridians of the hands and feet all converge at the head, and the governor vessel, which dominates the yang of the whole body, also reaches the top of the head, so it is called the convergence of all yang. Because of its high position and belonging to yang, among internal and external causes, wind pathogens and fire qi are most likely to cause head diseases. It is said that fire tends to flame upward, and only wind can reach the top of the head. On the other hand, due to weakness of internal organs, failure of clear qi to ascend, or invasion of wind-cold, leading to stagnation of yang qi, deficiency and cold syndromes can also appear. In addition, the brain is the sea of marrow; its excess or deficiency can affect the energy of the whole body, and the complexion can also reflect pathological changes of internal organs. This section includes symptoms such as headache, head distension, dizziness, brain tinnitus, brain distension, facial swelling, abnormal facial complexion, as well as symptoms of the fontanel, eyebrows and hair, and appropriately includes some surgical diseases. Clinically, it is necessary to distinguish internal and external causes, cold, heat, deficiency and excess, and conduct treatment in combination with *zang-fu* organs and meridians.

I. Headache

Headache can occur in both exogenous diseases and internal miscellaneous illnesses, and is one of the common symptoms, sometimes even serving as the main symptom. Due to the numerous causes and varying degrees of pain, diagnosis and treatment are quite complex. Among exogenous factors, those caused by wind-cold, wind-heat, and external dampness from fog and dew are the most common. Their differentiations are as follows: "wind-cold headache" initially feels like coldness and head distension, gradually turning into pain, spreading to the back of the head with a stiff sensation, and the distending pain worsens when exposed to wind, accompanied by general joint discomfort and mental fatigue. Treatment should dispel wind and cold, using Chuanxiong Chatiao Powder. "Wind-heat headache" also has a distending sensation when it hurts, worsening when exposed to wind, accompanied by dry mouth, red eyes, and flushing of the face. It is appropriate to dispel wind and dissipate heat, using modified Sangju Decoction. This formula originally treats the initial stage of wind-warm diseases, so it is suitable for mild cases of wind-heat headache. If the distending pain is severe, accompanied by internal heat symptoms such as scanty and reddish urine, constipation, and sores on the lips and nose, Huanglian Shangqing Pills, which are bitter-cold to reduce fire, should be used, focusing on treating the interior. "Dampness pathogen headache" is characterized by a dizzy, distended, and heavy pain, as if wrapped in cloth, with aching and tired limbs and a white greasy tongue coating. Although this headache is mainly caused by dampness, it is also related to wind-cold. It is appropriate to dispel the exterior and overcome dampness, using Qianghuo Shengshi Decoction, aiming to expel wind-dampness through sweating. Exogenous headache, caused by external pathogens, has a basic treatment similar to that of the initial stage of exogenous diseases. However, if headache is the main symptom, pain-relieving and head-clearing ingredients should be added to the treatment principle of pungent dispersion and light elevation. Generally, Jingjie, Fangfeng, Bohe, and Juhua are used as basic medicines. For those with a tendency to cold, add Qianghuo and Congbai; for those with a tendency to heat, add Sangye and Jiaoshanzhi; for those with a tendency to dampness, add Cangzhu and Shengjiang. As for Baizhi, Gaoben, Xixin, etc., although they have analgesic effects and are generally used as essential medicines for headache, due to their pungent-warm, fragrant-dry, and volatile nature, improper use can easily cause dizziness. They can be omitted when not necessary, and even when used, the dosage should not be large. Acupuncture treatment must be based on the location of the pain; refer to the entry "Migraine" in this section.

If exogenous headache persists for a long time, or if there is a pre-existing phlegm-fire, and then wind-cold invades due to taking coolness in the wind, the pathogen enters the brain from Fengfu, resulting in "head wind pain". It comes and goes, triggered by a touch, often worsening on the day before a windy day and relieving on the windy day itself. In addition, anger, overwork, and emotional depression can also trigger it. When it occurs, the pain is generally severe, radiating to the tips of the eyebrows, often with a pulling sensation, making it impossible to open the eyes or lift the head, and the scalp is numb. It is appropriate to take Xiaofeng Powder mixed with tea internally and use Tou Ding Powder for nasal insufflation. There is also the syndrome of "Leitoufeng" (thunder head wind), which has the same name but is actually different; refer to the entry "Brain Tinnitus" in this section.

The causes of internal headache are commonly blood deficiency, qi deficiency, liver fire, phlegm turbidity, and cold reversal. "Blood deficiency headache" is accompanied by dizziness when it hurts, attacking from the tips of the eyebrows upward, along with a pale complexion, a feeling of heat in the palms, and a thin and weak pulse. It is mostly caused by post-hemorrhage, post-severe illness, and post-childbirth, etc. Buyang Yangying Decoction is appropriate. Insufficient blood can easily lead to deficiency yang disturbing upward, with headache focusing on both sides, more obvious dizziness, orbital pain, heavy and sore eyelids, photophobia, preference for quietness and dislike of noise, nausea and vomiting, and restless sleep. In severe cases, there is a feeling of heavy pressure on the top of the head, accompanied by numbness, called "liver yang headache". Since this syndrome is basically due to blood deficiency, treatment should focus on nourishing blood for the root cause and suppressing yang for the symptom, using modified Xunlong Decoction. "Liver fire headache" is characterized by pain with head distension; "cold reversal headache" is characterized by pain with cold in the brain. The characteristic of "liver-fire headache" is a distending pain in the head; "cold-reversal headache" manifests as a cold sensation in the brain; qi-deficiency and phlegm-turbidity headaches present as a heavy, dizzy pain with a hollow feeling. For treatment, consult the sections on "head distension," "head heaviness," and "cold brain" in this section. Headache that is extremely severe and unbearable, spreading to the entire nape, with the hands and feet turning blue up to the elbows and knees, is called "true headache." Predecessors believed that the brain, as the sea of marrow, is where genuine qi gathers; once invaded by pathogens, death occurs within twelve hours. Emergency moxibustion at Baihui acupoint combined with large doses of ginseng and aconite may save one in ten cases. However, if accompanied by backward bending of the occipital vertebrae, rescue is ultimately impossible.

Chuanxiong Chatiao Powder: Ligusticum, Mint, Schizonepeta, Saposhnikovia, Angelica Dahurica, Notopterygium, Asarum, Licorice

Sangju Yin: Mulberry Leaf, Chrysanthemum, Mint, Platycodon, Forsythia, Almond, Licorice, Reed Rhizome

Huanglian Shangqing Wan: Coptis, Scutellaria, Phellodendron, Gardenia, Chrysanthemum, Mint, Pueraria, Platycodon, Forsythia, Trichosanthes Root, Scrophularia, Rhubarb, Turmeric, Angelica, Ligusticum (proprietary medicine)

Qianghuo Shengshi Decoction: Notopterygium, Angelica Pubescens,

Saposhnikovia, Ligusticum, Vitex, Ligusticum, Licorice

Xiaofeng Powder: Notopterygium, Schizonepeta, Saposhnikovia, Agastache, Magnolia Bark, Bombyx Batryticatus, Cicada Slough, Ginseng, Poria, Tangerine Peel, Licorice

Touding Powder: 2 stems of Asarum, 7 melon pedicel, 3 cloves, 0.5 *fen* each of Borneol and Musk, 7 glutinous rice grains. First grind the medicines, then add borneol and musk and grind evenly; use a bean-sized amount for nasal insufflation.

Bugan Yangying Decoction: Raw Rehmannia, Angelica, White Peony Root, Ligusticum, Chrysanthemum, Tangerine Peel, Licorice

Xunlong Decoction: Raw Rehmannia, Angelica, White Peony Root, Antelope Horn, Pearl Shell, Dragon's Tooth, Chrysanthemum, Mint, Taxillus, Uncaria, Angelica Pubescens, Aquilaria

II. Migraine

Generally refers to pain on the left or right side. In a broader sense, many headaches localized to one part fall under migraine. Hence, there are differential treatments based on the three yang meridians: Pain at the back of the head is "Taiyang headache," treated with Notopterygium and Ephedra as guides, with acupuncture at Hou Ding, Fengchi, Dazhu, and Kunlun acupoints; pain at the forehead is "Yangming headache," treated with Pueraria and Cimicifuga as guides, with acupuncture at Shangxing, Yintang, Touwei, Yangbai, and Cuanzhu acupoints; pain at both sides is "Shaoyang headache," treated with Bupleurum and Scutellaria as guides, with acupuncture at Taiyang, Touwei, Shuaigu, Lieque, Zhongzhu, and Xiaxi acupoints. Refer to the entry "Headache" in this section.

III. Pain at Both Temples

Belongs to the Shaoyang meridian; refer to the entry "Migraine" in this section. A folk remedy: apply thin slices of ginger to both temple acupoints to relieve pain.

IV. Vertex Pain

Pain at the vertex, precisely at Baihui acupoint, is caused by hyperactivity of ministerial fire disturbing upward along the Governor Vessel. Pungent-dispersing methods are inappropriate; use Sancai Decoction with oyster and turtle shell, and acupuncture at Baihui, Tongtian, Kunlun, Zhiyin, and Taichong acupoints.

Sancai Decoction: Asparagus, Prepared Rehmannia, Ginseng

V. Pain at the Supraorbital Ridges

Often accompanies Yangming or Shaoyang headache. If occurring alone, it is mostly due to external binding of wind-heat, with inability to open the eyes during pain; use Xuanqi Decoction.

Xuanqi Decoction: Saposhnikovia, Notopterygium, Scutellaria, Licorice

VI. Head Distension

Mostly caused by anger leading to upward reversal of liver fire, with head distension and pain, muddledness and heat sensation, prominent head veins, bitter taste and dry mouth, and in severe cases, sudden deafness in both ears, with a string-taut pulse; use Longdan Xiegan Decoction.

Head distension due to external dampness, feeling as if wrapped in cloth: refer to the entry "Headache" in this section.

Damp-heat obstruction after drunkenness also causes cloudy head distension; use Gehua Jiecheng Decoction.

Longdan Xiegan Decoction: Gentiana, Raw Rehmannia, Angelica, Scutellaria, Gardenia, Akebia, Plantain, Bupleurum, Licorice

Gehua Jiecheng Decoction: Pueraria Flower, Amomum, Cardamom, Aucklandia, Green Tangerine Peel, Tangerine Peel, Ginseng, Atractylodes, Dried Ginger, Poria, Polyporus, Alisma, Medicated Leaven

VII. Heavy Head Sensation

After a long illness or excessive fatigue, deficiency of middle qi and failure of clear yang to raise cause a heavy, dull headache with an empty sensation, which is classified as "qi deficiency headache." Buzhong Yiqi Decoction is used.

Obstruction of the middle jiao by phlegm-dampness and turbidity also causes a heavy, distending headache, often accompanied by chest and diaphragm fullness, nausea, vomiting, phlegm, and a thick, white or sticky tongue coating. Banxia Tianma Baizhu Decoction is used. Although this type of heavy headache also involves failure of clear yang to rise, it differs from qi deficiency headache: The latter arises from insufficient middle qi preventing clear yang from ascending, while the former results from phlegm-dampness blocking and suppressing clear yang. Thus, the former requires lifting and tonifying, while the latter focuses on strengthening the middle jiao, resolving phlegm, and draining dampness.

Buzhong Yiqi Decoction: Astragalus, Codonopsis, Atractylodes, Angelica, Cimicifuga, Bupleurum, Tangerine Peel, Licorice, Ginger, Jujube

Banxia Tianma Baizhu Decoction: Pinellia, Tangerine Peel, Poria, Dried Ginger, Alisma, Gastrodia, Codonopsis, Astragalus, Atractylodes

Lancea, Atractylodes Macrocephala, Medicated Leaven, Malt, Phellodendron

VIII. Dizziness

A spinning sensation as if objects are whirling and one is about to fall; in severe cases, the eyes cannot be opened, as opening them brings a feeling of the world turning upside down, with nausea and a desire to vomit. It is often caused by deficiency of liver and kidney yin, with deficient yang transforming into wind and disturbing upward, also called liver wind or internal wind. Pungent-dispersing methods must not be misused; Heche Dazao Wan is appropriate. Additionally, yin-nourishing and wind-calming substances such as turtle shell, donkey-hide gelatin, hawksbill shell, black sesame, and antelope horn can be added as appropriate, and regular consumption of dried mussels (also called "tribute dried") is helpful. Generally speaking, dizziness is more often due to deficiency than excess; patients with middle deficiency are more prone to nausea and vomiting, for which Aurantium, Bamboo Shavings, and Tangerine Peel can be used to harmonize the stomach, without needing to descend rebellious qi. Furthermore, obese individuals with frequent dizziness must be cautious of sudden collapse, which may lead to "wind stroke."

A severe blow to the head from a fall from a height often causes unconsciousness, described in *Golden Mirror of Medicine* as "severe injury involving the brain marrow." Emergency treatment by traumatologists is required, but most cases leave residual dizziness, heavy distension, photophobia, and a preference for quiet and aversion to noise, similar to internal wind, which is difficult to completely cure.

Dizziness and vomiting when traveling by boat or vehicle, called "motion sickness" or "seasickness," can be prevented or treated with

Rendan (a proprietary medicine).

Heche Dazao Wan: Placenta, Prepared Rehmannia, Asparagus, Ophiopogon, Turtle Shell, Codonopsis, Eucommia, Achyranthes, Phellodendron, Poria

IX. Head Shaking

Sudden, involuntary shaking of the head, mostly caused by wind-fire agitation; use Xiaochaihu Decoction without Ginseng, adding Saposhnikovia. Chronic head shaking, often due to internal wind, is difficult to treat.

Xiaochaihu Decoction: Bupleurum, Scutellaria, Ginseng, Pinellia, Licorice, Ginger, Jujube

X. Head and Eyes Tilting Upward

Head leaning backward and eyes rolling upward are commonly seen in infantile "tiandiao" (heavenly hook) syndrome. Tiandiao is one of the syndromes of acute convulsions, characterized by prominent upward tilting of the head and eyes, rolling eyes, tearing without tears, high fever, and hand-foot convulsions. When pathogenic heat and phlegm–saliva congest the chest and diaphragm so that qi cannot be freed, first give Suhexiang Wan, then follow with Gouteng Yin.

Suhexiang Wan: Styrax, Benzoin, Rhinoceros Horn, Borneol, Cyperus, Aucklandia, Frankincense, Atractylodes, Aquilaria, Clove, Musk, Cinnabar (proprietary medicine)

Gouteng Yin: Uncaria, Rhinoceros Horn, Gastrodia, Scorpion, Aucklandia, Licorice, Ginger

XI. Brain Tinnitus

A sound like insects chirping inside the head, usually accompanied by tinnitus and dizziness, arises from deficiency of the brain marrow. The brain is the sea of marrow, and marrow is produced from bones, which pertain to the kidney. Tonifying kidney yin is appropriate, using Zuogui Yin.

The syndrome of "leitoufeng" (thunder head wind) involves a thunder-like rumbling in the brain, with swollen lumps on the scalp and face, chills, and high fever, mostly caused by wind, dampness, and heat pathogens stagnating in the three yang meridians. Clearing, diffusing, ascending, and dispersing are appropriate, using Qingzhen Decoction.

Zuogui Yin: Prepared Rehmannia, Cornus, Turtle Shell, Wolfberry, Ophiopogon, Yam, Eucommia, Honey-fried Licorice

Qingzhen Decoction: Cimicifuga, Atractylodes Lancea, Lotus Leaf

XII. Cold Sensation in the Brain

When wind-evil enters the brain upward through Fengfu (GV-16), the patient feels a cold sensation at the occipital gate, accompanied by headache and chills along the nape and back; this is called "brain-wind," and is treated with Shen-sheng Powder. It is appropriate to dispel wind and dissipate cold, using Chuanxiong Chatiao Powder with added Asarum and Xanthium. Refer to the entry "Headache" in this section.

Wind pathogens invading the brain through Fengfu acupoint cause headache with a cold sensation at Naohu, and chills in the nape and back, known as "naofeng" (brain wind). Shengshen Powder is used.

"Cold inversion headache" is caused by upward inversion of cold qi in the liver meridian, also called "jueyin headache". During the pain, there is a cold feeling inside the brain, and the patient often wants to sleep covered with quilts even in mild wind. The face looks gloomy and melancholy, slightly cyanotic, with vomiting of clear saliva and sticky froth, cold limbs, and a deep string-like or deep tight pulse. Treatment should warm the liver and harmonize the stomach, using Danggui Sini Decoction or Wuzhuyu Decoction with added Angelica and Cinnamon.

Headache radiating from the vertex to the forehead, with marked aversion to cold; the patient feels as though wind were blowing straight into the brain gate. The pain is localized mainly to the vertex and forehead, is not severe, and is relieved by warmth; the pulse is weak and thready. Due to deficient cold in the Governor Vessel and decline of the Yangming meridian, warm and nourishing treatment is applied with antler glue, prepared Rehmannia, processed aconite slices, Angelica dahurica, Ligusticum, Cimicifuga, and baked ginger.

Shengshen Powder: Pueraria, Ephedra, Asarum, Agastache

Danggui Sini Decoction: Angelica, Cinnamon Twig, White Peony Root, Asarum, Akebia, Licorice, Jujube

Wuzhuyu Decoction: Evodia, Ginseng, Ginger, Jujube

XIII. Head Sweating

Sweating only on the head is common in Yangming heat syndrome and damp-heat syndrome. Because heat is stagnated internally and cannot disperse, it rises along the meridians. The sweating stops when internal heat subsides. Lung heat also often causes head sweating, which can be cleared with mulberry leaves and mulberry bark.

Excessive head sweating in conditions such as post-illness and asthma in the elderly are all deficiency syndromes.

It is not a pathological sign when children usually have head sweating during sleep without other symptoms, commonly known as "steamer head".

XIV. Facial Edema

It is one of the symptoms of edema, commonly seen in "wind edema". As stated in *The Inner Canon*, "Facial edema is called wind, and edema of the ankles is called water". Refer to the entry "Edema" in systemic symptoms.

XV. Red and Swollen Head and Face

The head and face are as swollen and red as a bucket, with the eyes narrowed into slits, and in severe cases, sore throat and deafness, caused by infection with warm-toxic seasonal pathogens, known as "datouwen" (severe head pestilence) or "xiamawen" (toad pestilence). Treatment should clear heat and detoxify, using Puji Xiaodu Yin.

"Mianyoufeng" (wandering wind on the face) initially also has red and swollen face and eyes, but with itching like insects crawling, dry skin, occasional white scales, bleeding when scratched, and unbearable pain, treated with Xiaofeng Powder.

In case of wild vegetable poisoning, with chills and fever, red and swollen face, dry mouth, nausea, and constipation, Puji Xiaodu Yin can also be used with modifications.

Puji Xiaodu Yin: Coptis, Scutellaria, Scrophularia, Isatis root, Bombyx batryticatus, Platycodon, Licorice, Arctium, Bupleurum, Cimicifuga, Puffball, Tangerine Peel, Forsythia, Mint

Xiaofeng Powder: Schizonepeta, Saposhnikovia, Angelica, Raw Rehmannia, Sophora flavescens, Atractylodes, Cicada slough, Sesame, Arctium, Anemarrhena, Gypsum, Licorice, Akebia

XVI. Flushing and Heat Sensation of the Head and Face

Episodic heat sensation in the head and face, with flushed cheeks and ears, or accompanied by sweating, commonly known as "shanghuo" (internal heat), is one of the yin deficiency syndromes. If there are no other symptoms, Liuwei Dihuang Wan can be taken regularly.

Liuwei Dihuang Wan: Rehmannia, Cornus, Moutan bark, Yam, Poria, Alisma

XVII. Malar Flush

The cheeks belong to the kidney. Reddened cheeks are all caused by deficient fire floating upward due to kidney yin deficiency, commonly seen in consumptive diseases, especially "feilao" (lung consumption). The malar flush in lung consumption is also caused by the failure of the metal (lung) to generate water (kidney), with yin deficiency and yang floating upward, not the primary disease of the lung. Therefore, treatment often involves both the lung and the kidney, using Baxian Changshou Wan.

Baxian Changshou Wan: Ophiopogon, Schisandra, Raw Rehmannia, Cornus, Yam, Moutan bark, Poria, Alisma

XVIII. Facial Numbness

It is the zhongluo syndrome in "stroke" (apoplexy). It is characterized by sudden loss of sensation on half of the face, deviation of the mouth and eyes – if the disease is on the left, the deviation is to the right; if on the right, the deviation is to the left. It is mostly caused by wind pathogens attacking the collaterals when sweating in the wind, treated with Qianzheng Powder taken internally, combined with external fumigation.

Qianzheng Powder: White Aconite, Bombyx Batryticatus, Scorpion

External Fumigation Method: Decoct Chuanxiong, Fangfeng, Juhua, and Bohe; cover the head with a cloth to fumigate, two to three times a day.

XIX. Non-Closure of Skull Sutures

In children, the separation of skull sutures and the failure of the anterior fontanel to close are called "jielu" (split skull). Due to congenital insufficiency and insufficient brain marrow, it is often accompanied by visible blue veins on the head, a pale complexion, and dull expressions. In severe cases, the skull enlarges, the neck bones are thin and weak and cannot support the head, and there is also downward displacement of the eyeballs, abnormal exposure of the white of the eyes, and dull eyesight. Treatment should combine internal administration and external application: take Fuyuan Powder internally and apply Fengsuo Powder externally.

Fuyuan Powder: Ginseng, Atractylodes, Poria, Fushen, Astragalus, Prepared Rehmannia, Yam, Honey-fried Licorice, Angelica, White Peony Root, Chuanxiong, Acorus, Ginger, Jujube

Fengsuo Powder: Equal parts of Platycladus Seed, Fangfeng, and Arisaema, ground into powder; use 1 *qian* each time, mix well with pig bile, apply to the fontanel, change once a day, and keep it moist with water from time to time to prevent drying.

XX. Sunken Fontanel

A significant sinking of the fontanel in children, even like a pit, accompanied by a sallow complexion, alusterlessface, cold limbs, and a pale and stagnant fingerprint, is called "xixian" (fontanel sinking). It is due to congenital deficiency; use Guzhen Decoction. In infants under six months old, a slight sinking of the head is not considered pathological.

Guzhen Decoction: Ginseng, Atractylodes, Poria, Honey-fried Licorice, Coptis, Aconite, Cinnamon, Yam

XXI. Bulging Fontanel

A bulging of the fontanel in children like a mound is called "xitian" (fontanel filling). Some cases are due to upward blazing of fire qi, with a soft and floating feel when pressed, accompanied by a red face and lips, and a purple fingerprint; take Huadu Dan internally and apply indigo naturalis mixed with cold water externally. Others are due to cold qi stagnation, with a harder feel when pressed and no heat, and cold fingers and toes; use Lizhong Decoction.

Huadu Dan: Rhinoceros Horn, Coptis, Platycodon, Scrophularia, Mint, Indigo Naturalis, Licorice, Rhubarb

Lizhong Decoction: Ginseng, Atractylodes, Processed Ginger, Licorice

XXII. Pale Complexion

A pale complexion lacking luster, with pale lips and nails, is one of the symptoms of blood deficiency. A sudden pale complexion is mostly a sign of cold exposure or pain. A paper-white complexion indicates the impending exhaustion of heart qi.

XXIII. Sallow Complexion

A yellow and haggard complexion is one of the symptoms of spleen deficiency, commonly seen in conditions such as chronic diarrhea and poor appetite.

XXIV. Dull and Stagnant Complexion

A complexion as if covered with dust, dull and lusterless, is a characteristic of "damp-warm" disease and also seen in blood stasis syndrome.

XXV. Hair Loss

Hair is the surplus of blood; general hair loss is due to blood deficiency. Hair loss after severe illnesses such as cold damage is also caused by qi and blood deficiency, which can be treated with Erxian Pills or Guben Wine for nourishment.

The syndrome of "youfeng" (oily wind), commonly known as "ghost shaving head", is characterized by dry hair and patchy hair loss, caused by blood deficiency with wind invasion, excessive wind generating dryness, and inability to nourish the skin. Take Shenying Yangzhen Dan internally, and applymao jiang (rhizome of Drynaria) externally, or apply Sichuan Aconite powder mixed with vinegar externally.

Erxian Pills: Platycladus Leaves, Angelica Body

Guben Wine: Two *liang* each of Raw Rehmannia, Prepared Rehmannia, Asparagus, Ophiopogon, and Poria; one *liang* of Ginseng; soaked in yellow rice wine.

Shenying Yangzhen Dan: Notopterygium, Gastrodia, White Peony Root, Angelica, Cuscuta, Papaya, Prepared Rehmannia, Chuanxiong

XXVI. White Hair

Except for senile white hair, white hair caused by diseases is mainly due to insufficient kidney yin and liver blood. Use Shouwu Yanshou Dan, or take raw Polygonum multiflorum powder regularly.

Shouwu Yanshou Dan: Polygonum multiflorum, Siegesbeckia, Cuscuta, Eucommia, Achyranthes, Ligustrum lucidum, Mulberry Leaves,

Honeysuckle, Raw Rehmannia, Mulberry Fruit, Rosa laevigata, Eclipta, Black Sesame

XXVII. Yellow Hair

Yellow and dry hair, lacking luster, is mostly due to spleen and stomach deficiency and insufficient qi and blood. It is common in children with "malnutrition" and can be treated with Shiquan Dabu Decoction or Wumei Pills.

Shiquan Dabu Decoction: Ginseng, Atractylodes, Poria, Licorice, Angelica, Prepared Rehmannia, White Peony Root, Chuanxiong, Astragalus, Cinnamon

Wumei Pills: Mume, Aconite, Dry Ginger, Cinnamon, Asarum, Coptis, Scutellaria, Ginseng, Angelica, Habitat

Hair that is withered, yellow, and lusterless is mostly due to blazing fire and blood dryness. Use Caohuan Dan internally and Juhua Powder for external washing.

Caohuan Dan: Raw Rehmannia, Wolfberry Bark, Acorus, Achyranthes, Polygala, Cuscuta

Juhua Powder: Chrysanthemum, Vitex, Arborvitae Leaf, Ligusticum, Angelica Dahurica, Asarum, Mulberry Bark, Eclipta

XXVIII. Eyebrow Loss

Eyebrow loss is one of the symptoms of "leprosy," caused by pathogenic toxin attacking the lung. Refer to the entry "Skin Numbness" in Systemic Symptoms.

XXIX. Scalp Itching

Dry and itchy scalp with white scales falling off when scratched is due to wind-heat. Use Xiaofeng Powder.

Xiaofeng Powder: Schizonepeta, Licorice, Bombyx Batryticatus, Saposhnikovia, Ligusticum, Agastache, Cicada Slough, Ginseng, Poria, Notopterygium, Tangerine Peel, Magnolia Bark

XXX. Scalp Lumps

Scalp lump is one of the symptoms of "thunder head wind." Refer to the entry "Brain Tinnitus" in this section.

XXXI. Pungent Sensation between the Eyebrows

A pungent sensation between the eyebrows, called "xin'e" in *The Inner Canon*, is one of the symptoms of sinusitis (deep nasal disorder). Refer to the entry "Nasal Discharge of Turbid Mucus" in Nasal Symptoms.

XXXII. Acne

Small lumps on the face, shaped like millet grains, red, swollen, and painful, which exude white powdery fluid when squeezed, are called "acne." They are caused by heat in the lung meridian and blood. Occasional ones may not require treatment; for frequent ones, take Pipa Qingfei Yin.

Pipa Qingfei Yin: Ginseng, Loquat Juice, Licorice, Coptis, Phellodendron, Mulberry Bark

XXXIII. Freckles

Freckles appear on the face as pale-yellow, countless tiny spots. They are formed when heat becomes depressed in the minute collaterals and wind evil externally constricts them. Use Shizhen Zhengrong Powder externally.

Shizhen Zhengrong Powder: One *liang* each of Pig Tooth Soap, Duckweed, White Plum Pulp, and Cherry Branch, 3 *qian* of Hawk Dung White; bake and grind into powder. Apply a little mixed with water to the face morning and evening, and wash off with warm water after some time.

XXXIV. Moles

Moles on the face, small as millet or large as beans, slightly raised above the skin, may appear from childhood or middle age. They are caused by stagnation of blood in the small collaterals and are not painful. For treatment, try applying Shuijing Gao (Crystal Paste).

Shuijing Gao: Dissolve lime in water, take 5 *qian* of the powder, soak the lime powder in alkaline water to a depth of two fingers, scatter 50 glutinous rice grains on the lime. Add water as it decreases, soak for a day and night, take out the rice and mash into a paste. Prick the mole, apply a little paste, and the mole will fall off after scabbing.

XXXV. Parotid Swelling

Swelling, redness, and heat in the fleshy part of the cheeks (not on the bone), either left or right, with alternating chills and fever, is called "mumps" or "cheek-containing sore." Caused by wind-heat in the Yangming meridian, clear and resolve with Chaihu Gegen Decoction. For cases with thirst and constipation, use Sisheng Qingliang Yin, and apply Jinhuang Powder externally to help reduce swelling; avoid incision.

"Fayi" (submandibular abscess) is similar to mumps, initially with pain and tension at the angle of the mandible, difficulty opening the mouth, swelling gradually spreading to the front and back of the ears, and chills and fever. However, the initial swelling is like a nodule, growing to the size of a peach or plum. Often caused by poor sweating in cold damage or warm diseases, with pathogens stagnating in the collaterals of the Shaoyang and Yangming meridians, it is also called "sweat toxin," differing from primary mumps. Initially, use Jingfang Baidu Powder; avoid excessive cold medicines, which may trap the toxin internally and cause swelling of the throat. Treat as an ulcer after rupture.

Chaihu Gegen Decoction: Bupleurum, Pueraria, Gypsum, Trichosanthes Root, Scutellaria, Licorice, Arctium, Forsythia, Platycodon, Cimicifuga

Sisheng Qingliang Yin: Saposhnikovia, Gardenia, Forsythia, Licorice, Angelica, Red Peony Root, Notopterygium, Rhubarb, Rush

Jinhuang Powder: Arisaema, Tangerine Peel, Atractylodes, Phellodendron, Turmeric, Licorice, Angelica Dahurica, Trichosanthes Root, Magnolia Bark, Rhubarb (proprietary medicine)

Jingfang Baidu Powder: Schizonepeta, Saposhnikovia, Bupleurum, Peucedanum, Notopterygium, Aurantium, Platycodon, Poria, Ligusticum, Licorice, Ginseng, Ginger

XXXVI. Hot Furuncles

Mostly occur on the head and face, and are more common in summer and in children, which mainly caused by exposure to summer heat that cannot be released, blocking between the skin and muscles, so they are also called "summer furuncles". Initially, the local skin is flushed, and the next day there is swelling and pain, but without a root, with a limited range, and a pus head appears, which heals after spontaneous rupture and pus discharge. At the beginning, Qianchui Gao, commonly known as red plaster, can be applied externally, and honeysuckle dew or Liushen Pills can be taken internally to clear heat and detoxify. Although furuncles are minor illnesses, they appear one after another, with as few as several or as many as dozens, often making children unable to sleep peacefully, irritable and crying, and emaciated. In summer, 0.2 to 0.3 *fen* of Xihuang Powder can be taken internally for prevention.

Qianchui Gao: Rosin, Castor Seeds, Verdigris, Almonds, Catechu, Frankincense, Myrrh, Dragon's Blood, Calomel, Pearl (proprietary medicine)

Liushen Pills: Omitted (proprietary medicine)

XXXVII. Favus of the Scalp

Initially, white scabs form on the head, with unbearable itching. Over time, they spread into patches, with the hair becoming dry and falling off, also known as "bald sore", which mostly caused by damp-heat generating parasites. The treatment method is to wash with onion soup and apply Runji Gao. A proven recipe: wash live shrimps, mash them and apply to the affected area, wrap with cloth. After application, there will be severe itching, which must be endured. Wash off after one day, apply again the next day, and it can take effect after two or three times.

Runji Gao: Five *qian* of Angelica, one *liang* of Arnebia, decoct with four *liang* of sesame oil until withered, filter to get the oil, decoct the oil again, add five *qian* of yellow wax to melt, and when cold, dip ginger in it to wipe the affected area.

Section 3 Eye Symptoms

The eyes are one of the five sense organs and are closely connected with the *zang-fu* organs. Therefore, *The Inner Canon* states: "The essence of the five *zang* and six fu organs all flows upward to the eyes and becomes their essence." In ophthalmic diagnosis, the eye is customarily divided into five wheels: The black eyeball is the wind wheel belonging to the liver, the canthi are the blood wheel belonging to the heart, the eye sockets are the flesh wheel belonging to the spleen, the white of the eye is the qi wheel belonging to the lung, and the pupil is the water wheel belonging to the kidney. It is also divided into eight regions: The pupil is the water region belonging to the bladder, the black eyeball is the wind region belonging to the gallbladder, the white of the eye is the heaven region belonging to the large intestine, the eye sockets are the earth region belonging to the stomach, the upper inner canthus is the fire region belonging to the small intestine, the lower inner canthus is the thunder region belonging to the life gate, the upper outer canthus is the mountain region belonging to the pericardium, and the lower outer canthus is the marsh region belonging to the triple energizer. It can be seen that although eye diseases are local disorders, they are mostly caused by internal organ lesions. Based on these different parts, the root cause of the disease can be detected. Therefore, in addition to external treatments such as eye drops, ointments, fumigation and washing, and technical operations using instruments and manipulations, internal medicines are generally used focusing on overall treatment. From the perspective of internal medicine, the eyes are the orifices of the liver, so eye symptoms focus on the liver, and are also treated in relation to the meridians related to the eyes - the foot taiyang, yangming, and shaoyang meridians. This section mainly deals with internal medicine, and also includes some ophthalmic disorders, including symptoms such as dizziness, eye pain, eye swelling, red eyes, yellow eyes, tearing, photophobia, dryness, nebula, star-like opacity, dilated pupils, and inverted eyelashes. In special cases, treatment should be sought from an ophthalmologist.

I. Dizziness

Xuan (dazzling) refers to blurred and confused vision, such as suddenly seeing everything black after standing up from a squat, or seeing black spots or floating threads, commonly known as "dizziness in the eyes". Habitually, xuan (dazzling) and yun (dizzy) are mentioned together, and they often appear simultaneously clinically. However, xuan means dimness, and yun means a spinning sensation; there is a difference between the two. Mild cases of this symptom are related to the liver, as Shen Jin'ao put it, "When qi and blood decline, the liver lobes become thin, and bile decreases"; severe cases are related to the kidney, as Zhu Danxi stated, "The causes of eye diseases are nothing more than deficiency and excess; deficiency leads to blurred vision, resulting from the depletion of true water in the kidney meridian". Due to insufficient yin and blood, the rebellious yang transforms into wind and disturbs upward, hence *The Inner Canon* says, "All wind-induced tremors and dizziness are related to the liver". And because liver yang disturbs upward, it often affects the stomach's qi harmony and descent, easily causing nausea and vomiting. In treatment, combine with the main symptoms and add ingredients such as wolfberry, chrysanthemum, tribulus terrestris, oyster, and gastrodia. For severe vomiting, appropriately add aurantium and bamboo shavings. The elderly can often take Zhujing Pills.

Zhujing Pills: Prepared Rehmannia, Cuscuta, Plantain Seed

II. Diminished Vision

Diminished vision is mostly caused by deficiency of liver and kidney yin, and insufficient essence and blood, generally without signs of pupil deformation or discoloration. Except for natural decline in the elderly, severe cases can gradually develop into "qingmang" (green blindness) leading to blindness. In the early stage of qingmang, there are no opacity, and the appearance is the same as normal, but vision continuously decreases. It is advisable to take Xiongui Mingmu Pills and Shihu Yeguang Pills. Avoid impatience and anger, and often close the eyes to rest.

Diminished vision leading to "hyperopia" or "myopia" was discussed by predecessors mostly from the perspective of excess or deficiency of water and fire. They believed that inability to see far is due to qi deficiency and blood excess, treated with Dingzhi Pills; inability to see near is due to blood deficiency and qi excess, treated with Dizhi Pills.

Xiongui Mingmu Pills: Rehmannia, Angelica, Ligusticum, Asparagus, Wolfberry, White Peony Root, Chrysanthemum, Achyranthes, Licorice

Shihu Yeguang Pills: Dendrobium, Ginseng, Asparagus, Ophiopogon, Prepared Rehmannia, Raw Rehmannia, Cistanche, Cuscuta, Poria, Chrysanthemum, Yam, Celosia, Wolfberry, Antelope Horn, Cassia Seed, Almond, Schisandra, Tribulus Terrestris, Ligusticum, Licorice, Coptis, Saposhnikovia, Aurantium, Rhinoceros Horn, Achyranthes (proprietary medicine)

Dingzhi Pills: Acorus, Polygala, Fushen, Ginseng

Dizhi Pills: Prepared Rehmannia, Asparagus, Aurantium, Chrysanthemum

III. Dull Eyesight

Patients feel weak when looking at things, and their eyes get sore and tired after looking for a while, all of which are signs of yin deficiency. If the eyes are sunken and lack luster, seen in deficiency syndromes and chronic diseases, the prognosis is poor.

IV. Red Eyes

Red eyes with photophobia, excessive tearing and discharge, gritty sensation and difficulty in opening, or starting in one eye and spreading to both, or both eyes being red at the same time, commonly known as "red eyes" or "fire eyes". Mostly caused by internal heat, it is an acute infectious eye disease. Take Qufeng Sanshuo Yin internally, wash with chrysanthemum soaked in water externally, or beat egg white with coptis water until frothy, take the foam to drop into the canthi, which can also be used for prevention. In severe cases, due to latent heat in the lung and subsequent invasion of wind pathogens, it breaks out suddenly with severe onset, accompanied by headache, nasal congestion, chills and fever, use Jiu Diao Powder. If there is swollen eyelids, swollen white of the eyes, sunken cornea, severe eye pain, and restlessness, take Xiefei Yin. Generally, in ophthalmic medicines, saposhnikovia and chrysanthemum are often used to dispel wind, red peony root and moutan bark to harmonize blood, coptis and scutellaria to clear heat, and rhubarb to purge severe heat.

Qufeng Sanshuo Yin: Forsythia, Arctium, Notopterygium, Mint, Rhubarb, Red Peony Root, Saposhnikovia, Angelica Tail, Licorice, Ligusticum, Gardenia

Jiu Diao Powder: Angelica Tail, Ephedra, Atractylodes, Red Peony Root, Chrysanthemum, Licorice, Notopterygium, Rhubarb, Leonurus, Mantis Egg Case, ground into powder, taken with warm yellow rice wine.

Xiefei Yin: Gypsum, Red Peony Root, Scutellaria, Mulberry Bark, Aurantium, Akebia, Forsythia, Schizonepeta, Saposhnikovia, Gardenia, Angelica Dahurica, Notopterygium, Licorice

V. Yellow Eyes

Yellow eye is one of the symptoms of “jaundice”. Refer to the entry “Yellow Skin” in Systemic Symptoms.

VI. Eyes Rolling Upward

The black part of the eye rolling upward, resulting in more white and less black, is called “pupil elevation” or “eyeballs looking upward”, which indicates exhaustion of essence in the Taiyang Meridian. It often appears in “convulsion disease” and infantile “convulsions”, “umbilical wind” and other syndromes, all of which are dangerous.

VII. Staring Eyes

The eyes do not move. Due to excessive pathogenic qi and failure of *zang-fu* essence to ascend and nourish the eyes, it is mostly difficult to treat. It may also appear together with upward rolling, called “eyes rolling backward and staring”, which is incurable.

VIII. Diplopia

Diplopia often sees one object as two. If due to liver and kidney deficiency, use Dizhi Pills; if due to pathogenic invasion of the eye connective tissues, use Qufeng Yizi Powder.

Dizhi Pills: Prepared Rehmannia, Asparagus, Aurantium, Chrysanthemum

Qufeng Yizi Powder: Ligusticum, Schizonepeta, Sichuan Aconite, Notopterygium, Mint, Saposhnikovia

IX. Protruding Eyeballs

Accumulation of wind-toxin, phlegm and heat in the *zang-fu* organs, surging upward to the eyes, causing protruding, itching and painful eyeballs, called “eye swelling”, treated with Xiegan Powder. If only a bean-sized protrusion appears on the black part of the eye with a thin membrane around it and unbearable pain, it is due to accumulated heat in the liver meridian surging upward, causing the spiritual paste inside the eye to burst out of the black eye from the break, called “crab eye”. Over time, it becomes flaccid without pain, vision is blurred, and the pupil is damaged, which can lead to blindness. Initially, use Lingyang Powder, then Zhenshe Jueming Pills. Eye swelling and crab eye caused by trauma must be treated according to trauma first aid.

Xiegan Powder: Rhubarb, Licorice, Prunus japonica Seed, Schizonepeta

Lingyang Jiao Powder: Chrysanthemum, Saposhnikovia, Ligusticum, Notopterygium, Plantain, Sichuan Aconite, Asarum, Pinellia 曲, Antelope Horn, Mint

Zhenshe Jueming Pills: Abalone Shell, Cuscuta, Schisandra, Asarum, Yam, Raw Rehmannia, Anemarrhena

X. Corneal Opacity

White opacity in the cornea, flake-like like floating clouds, called “cloudy opacity”, is one of the “external obstacles”. Generally, those that are white and tender and do not cover the pupil are mild and easy to treat. Those with thick white or yellow opacity but still able to distinguish light and dark can also be treated. If the entire opacity covers the eye and light and dark cannot be distinguished, it is difficult to treat; or if the opacity is thick and yellowish-brown with blood vessels around it, even if it does not affect the entire cornea, it is also difficult to treat. Corneal opacity is mostly caused by wind-heat and liver fire, redness, swelling and pain.

Commonly used formulas include Shijueming Powder and Lianqiao Powder.

Shijueming Powder: Abalone Shell, Cassia Seed, Notopterygium, Gardenia, Equisetum, Celosia, Red Peony Root, Rhubarb, Schizonepeta

Lianqiao Powder: Forsythia, Scutellaria, Notopterygium, Chrysanthemum, Cassia Seed, Tribulus terrestris, Buddleja officinalis, Gentiana, Licorice

XI. Corneal Star-like Opacity

Round spots of varying sizes on the cornea are called "star opacity". Because star opacity develops into cloudy opacity, and cloudy opacity initially has white spots, they are actually indistinguishable. So initially, only one or two sparse spots that do not expand are mild; several connected or clustered or scattered spots that quickly form rice-like depressions are most likely to damage the cornea and become cloudy opacity leading to blindness. For treatment, refer to the entry "Corneal Opacity" in this section.

XII. Pterygium

Yellowish-red fleshy growth at the inner canthus, like fat or tough ointment, slightly pungent and astringent, gradually thickening over time, spreading across the cornea and covering the pupil, causing blindness. Pterygium is mostly caused by eating pungent and hot foods, accumulated heat in the spleen and lung, or excessive wind-heat in the heart and lung meridians, and stagnation of meridians and collaterals. Treatment should be surgical removal, and take Zhizi Shengqi Powder internally.

Zhizi Shengqi POwder: Tribulus terrestris, Cicada slough, Eriocaulon, Equisetum, Scutellaria, Cassia Seed, Chrysanthemum,

Gardenia, Ligusticum, Schizonepeta, Notopterygium, Buddleja officinalis, Saposhnikovia, Vitex

XIII. Milium-like Granules on Eyelids

Sharp-tipped milium-like granules growing between the upper and lower eyelids, slightly itchy and swollen, followed by redness, pain, and pus formation, which dissipate on their own after rupture, called "needle eye". Milium-like granules on eyelids are mostly caused by excessive consumption of spicy foods, with heat toxin in the stomach meridian attacking upward. Initially, use hot compress; when pus forms, prick with a needle and take Qingpi Powder internally.

"Eye erysipelas" occurs on the upper and lower eyelids, with burning redness, swelling, and pain, more severe than needle eye, often accompanied by chills, fever, headache, thirst, etc. The cause is roughly similar, only differing in severity.

Qingpi Powder: Scutellaria, Mint, Cimicifuga, Gypsum, Red Peony Root, Gardenia, Agastache, Aurantium, Tangerine Peel, Licorice, Saposhnikovia

XIV. Inverted Eyelashes

The disease name is "inverted and curled eyelashes", abbreviated as "inverted eyelashes", a secondary condition. For example, untreated "trachoma" initially causes itching of the eyelids, frequent rubbing, leading to gradual contraction of the upper and lower eyelid skin, curling of eyelashes, which stab the eyeball internally, causing astringent pain, tearing, difficulty in opening the eyes, and inability to look straight, only sideways. Over time, it can cause cloudy opacity and blindness; surgical treatment is generally used.

XV. Eye Discharge

Eye discharge is mostly caused by internal heat in the lung. Abundant and hard discharge is excessive heat; abundant but non-hardened discharge is deficient heat. It not only appears in eye diseases but also often accompanies internal wind-heat syndrome and infantile measles, etc.

XVI. Eye Bleeding

Stagnant fire in the lung causes blood to overflow outside the collaterals, appearing on the surface of the white of the eye. It may be a spot or a patch, bright red in color, gradually turning purplish dark. Generally, it subsides on its own in about ten days, with no pain, swelling, photophobia, tearing, or other lesions. Treatment should clear the lung and disperse blood, using Zhijin Jian.

Zhijin Jian: Scrophularia, Mulberry Bark, Aurantium, Coptis, Almond, Inula, Saposhnikovia, Scutellaria, Chrysanthemum, Lepidium

XVII. Photophobia

Photophobia is commonly seen in patterns of excess heat and yin-deficiency internal heat—for example, in Yangming-stage illness the patient shuns both people and fire, while in liver-yang headache the sufferer prefers to stay in dark places. Photophobia appearing in wind-fire red eyes is called "photophobia", treated along with the main symptoms. However, yang deficiency syndrome also often involves sleeping with eyes closed, which is due to mental fatigue, different from photophobia.

XVIII. Tearing

Excessive tearing, or more when exposed to wind. Due to external invasion of wind-heat and stagnation of liver fire and external wind, often accompanied by redness, swelling, burning pain, photophobia, etc., called "hot tears". It is appropriate to clear the liver and dispel wind, using Sangju Qufeng Decoction, which can be taken internally or used for fumigation and washing.

Liver and kidney deficiency, or prolonged sad crying, with constant tearing, worse in wind, no redness or pain in the eyes, called "cold tears". Treatment should tonify and nourish, using Juhua Wan, and moxibustion can also be applied to Yingxiang, Ganshu, Jingming, Linqi acupoints, etc.

Tears are one of the five bodily fluids. Prolonged tearing in deficiency syndrome can cause blurred vision and difficulty in distinguishing objects, leading to blindness. *The Inner Canon* states: "Fluids are used to irrigate essence and moisten the orifices. Therefore, when the upper fluid passage opens, tears flow; if tears flow incessantly, the fluids are exhausted; when exhausted, essence is not irrigated; when essence is not irrigated, the eyes cannot see, which is called deprivation of essence."

Sangju Qufeng Decoction: Mulberry Leaf, Chrysanthemum, Honeysuckle, Saposhnikovia, Angelica, Red Peony Root, Coptis

Juhua Wan: Chrysanthemum, Wolfberry, Morinda, Cistanche

XIX. Dry Eyes

After overworking the mind, insomnia, or reading for a long time, the eyes feel dry, the eyelids are heavy, and it improves slightly after resting with eyes closed. Mostly due to blood deficiency and yin deficiency, it is appropriate to nourish the liver and kidney along with the main symptoms. Commonly used medicines include raw Rehmannia, Dendrobium, Chrysanthemum, Wolfberry, etc.

XX. Itchy and Painful Eyes

Initially, there is slight itching, gradually followed by astringent pain, excessive discharge and tearing, photophobia, difficulty in opening the eyes, blurred vision, and the inner eyelids are covered with red fine granules, called "pepper sore", commonly known as "trachoma". The condition lasts for a long time and is highly contagious, which can cause eye opacity and endanger eyesight. Treatment should clear and resolve dampness and fire in the spleen meridian, using Chufeng Qingpi Yin. To prevent progression, local eye drops and ophthalmic surgery should be applied.

Chufeng Qingpi Yin: Saposhnikovia, Schizonepeta, Forsythia, Anemarrhena, Tangerine Peel, Scutellaria, Coptis, Scrophularia, Raw Rehmannia, Platycodon, Rhubarb, Sodium Sulfate

XXI. Orbital Pain

Sore pain in the orbit, heavy eyelids with photophobia, commonly seen in liver yang headache; refer to the entry "Headache" in Head and Face Symptoms.

XXII. Heavy Eyelids

Heavy eyelids mostly refer to ptosis of the upper eyelid, generally caused by qi and blood deficiency and listlessness. If there is frequent dizziness accompanied by a numb feeling in the eyelids, it is pathogenic wind attacking collaterals due to deficiency; Use Huangqi Pills.

Huangqi Pills: Astragalus, Tribulus terrestris, Angelica pubescens, Bupleurum, Raw Rehmannia, Licorice, Gardenia, Sophora flavescens, Atractylodes, Agkistrodon, Lycium bark, Chrysanthemum, Saposhnikovia,

Cornus, Fushen, Gentiana macrophylla, Asparagus, Aurantium, Areca

XXIII. Eyelid Twitching

Twitching of the eyelids spread to the eyebrows, commonly known as "eyebrow twitching". Mostly caused by liver-spleen disharmony after illness or occasional attack by wind pathogens, it is not treated as a main symptom. However, if the twitching is too frequent day and night accompanied by blurred vision, it is necessary to prevent it from developing into "internal obstruction"; use Danggui Huoxue Decoction.

Danggui Huoxue Decoction: Angelica, Ligusticum, Prepared Rehmannia, Astragalus, Atractylodes, Saposhnikovia, Notopterygium, Mint, Licorice, White Peony Root

XXIV. Swollen Eyelids

It is one of the symptoms of "edema". *The Inner Canon* states: "Slight swelling of the eye sockets, like the shape of a silkworm just waking up, is called water." Refer to the entry "Edema" in Systemic Symptoms.

First, there is redness of the eyes, followed by swollen eyelids like peaches or plums and pain in the eyeballs, called "clam closure". Due to excessive heat in the lung and spleen attacking upward, the more the heat is stagnated, the more severe the swelling; the more severe the swelling, the more excessive the spleen. It is appropriate to clear fire, dispel wind and detoxify; use Sanshu Xiaodu Yin.

Swelling and puffy upper eyelids like balls, which flatten slightly when wiped but swell again after a while, belong to spleen deficiency with dampness and fire. Initially, there is no abnormality in the eyes; over time, slight red threads appear, and the eyelids are slightly red. It is appropriate to mainly tonify the spleen with a little assistance in dispelling dampness and clearing fire; use Shenxiao Huangqi Decoction with added Alisma and Phellodendron.

Sanshu Xiaodu Yin: Arctium, Notopterygium, Coptis, Scutellaria, Mint, Saposhnikovia, Forsythia

Shenxiao Huangqi Decoction: Astragalus, Ginseng, White Peony Root, Vitex, Licorice, Tangerine Peel

XXV. Dilated Pupils

Dilated pupils found in chronic diseases, deficiency syndromes or excessive sweating are all signs of depletion of primordial qi, indicating a severe condition. In ophthalmology, changes in color and shape of the pupil, depletion of eye spirit, blurred vision, etc., are classified into the scope of "internal obstruction", which is divided into five evolutionary processes: "blue wind", "black wind", "dark wind", "green wind" and "yellow wind". Among them, green wind internal obstruction is more common, with turbid and unclear pupil color showing light greenish white, and dilated pupils as its main feature, with the dilation width almost equal to that of the cornea. In terms of causes, it can be due to wind-heat attacking upward, anger injuring the liver, or yin deficiency with fire excess and disharmony between the heart and kidney. Generally, after an acute attack, there is often a relatively long static period before recurrence; each attack leads to a sharp decrease in vision. When the pupil turns golden yellow, i.e., the yellow wind stage, it is the end stage of the disease, which is difficult to cure.

XXVI. Night Blindness

Night blindness refers to inability to see objects at dusk, with normal vision restored at dawn, also known as "sparrow's eye". It is divided into two types: "high wind sparrow's eye internal obstruction" and "liver deficiency sparrow's eye internal obstruction". The former is due to insufficient primordial yang, and the latter is due to liver deficiency and blood deficiency. The difference between the two is that the former can only see objects above, but cannot see clearly on both sides; the latter can only see objects directly below, and is often accompanied by itching and astringency. In sparrow's eye syndrome, there is no opacity in the pupil. Liver deficiency is more common in children, with a good prognosis, treated with Yanggan Pills; yang deficiency is more common in adults, and if it persists for a long time without healing, it can easily develop into "green blindness", treated with Juhua Pills.

Yanggan Pills: Yeming Sha (Bat Feces), Angelica, Equisetum, Cicada Slough, Sheep Liver

Juhua Pills: Chrysanthemum, Morinda, Cistanche, Wolfberry

XXVII. Sudden Blindness

Sudden loss of vision in eyes that were previously healthy, without external damage to the eye contour or internal damage to the pupil, all belong to sudden blindness. The main difference between this syndrome and "green blindness" lies in the course of the disease: Green blindness leads to blindness slowly, while this syndrome causes blindness rapidly. Precisely because of its acute onset, early diagnosis and treatment must be sought; delay will lead to stagnation of qi, making it difficult to cure. Generally, if accompanied by emotional tension, it is due to anger injuring the liver, treated with Shengtieluo Yin; if accompanied by mental fatigue, it is due to anger damaging primordial yin and yang, treated with Chaihu Shenzhu Decoction. If it occurs after massive blood loss, gynecological metrorrhagia, or childbirth, emergency treatment to secure and rescue from collapse is needed, using large doses of ginseng decoction.

Shengtieluo Yin: Iron Filings, Gypsum, Dragon's Tooth, Poria, Saposhnikovia, Scrophularia, Gentiana Macrophylla, Bamboo Sap

Chaihu Shenzhu Decoction: Ginseng, Atractylodes, Prepared Rehmannia, White Peony Root, Licorice, Ligusticum, Angelica Body, Green Tangerine Peel, Bupleurum

XXVIII. Foreign Body in the Eye

When dust, spider webs, etc., blow into the eye, there is an immediate gritty sensation, tearing, and difficulty in opening the eye. The eyelid can be everted and rinsed with light salt water; if rinsing fails, gently remove the foreign body with cotton dipped in light salt water. Iron filings, etc., that fly into the eye often cause severe eye pain, and in serious cases, damage to the eyeball and cornea, requiring treatment by an ophthalmologist.

Section 4 Ear Symptoms

The ear is the orifice of the kidney, and the hand and foot Shaoyang meridians all converge in the ear. Therefore, ear diseases are most closely related to the kidney, gallbladder, and triple energizer. *Feng's Brocade Bag* states: "There are seven causes of ear diseases: excessive heat, yin deficiency, phlegm, fire, qi obstruction, liver wind, and diseases arising from fetal origin. There are five symptoms: tinnitus, pain, swelling, deafness, and ear discharge." Generally, new diseases are mostly excessive, related to the meridians; chronic diseases are mostly deficient, related to the *zang* organs. However, individual syndromes are related to the heart and lung, so the overall condition should be considered, and one should not be rigidly confined.

I. Tinnitus

Tinnitus, which may sound like cicadas chirping, water rushing, or bells and drums beating, is a subjective symptom. It is divided into excessive and deficient types. The excessive type is due to upward adverse flow of liver and gallbladder fire, as stated in *The Inner Canon*: "The solitary roaring of the lesser yang is the reversal of the Shaoyang." It is often accompanied by headache, head distension, irritability, and a wiry and slippery pulse, treated with Chaihu Qinggan Powder; for those with dry stools, add Aloe to descend fire. The deficient type is due to kidney deficiency with upward flaming of yin fire, or excessive use of the brain, as stated in *The Inner Canon*: "Insufficiency of the sea of marrow leads to dizziness and tinnitus." It is often accompanied by dizziness, palpitations, and lumbar soreness, with a thready and weak pulse. The brain is the sea of marrow, and marrow belongs to the kidney, so treatment focuses on nourishment, using Bushen Pills, and magnetite can be added for sedation. A folk remedy is to often eat black sesame and walnut meat mashed together, which also has a laxative effect for those with constipation.

Patients with "palpitations" (zhengchong) experience a rumbling sound in the ears, which corresponds to the heartbeat and becomes clearer at night, disturbing sleep. This is mostly related to the heart. *The Inner Canon* states: "The southern [direction corresponds to the] red color, which connects to the heart in humans and opens into the ears." It is advisable to add Acorus and Polygala to blood-nourishing and mind-calming formulas to unblock heart qi.

Chaihu Qinggan Powder: Bupleurum, Raw Rehmannia, Red Peony Root, Arctium, Angelica, Forsythia, Ligusticum, Scutellaria, Gardenia, Trichosanthes Root, Saposhnikovia, Licorice

Bushen Wan: Prepared Rehmannia, Cuscuta, Angelica, Cistanche, Cornus, Phellodendron, Anemarrhena, Psoralea

II. Deafness

Deafness mostly develops from tinnitus; except for sudden deafness due to qiobstruction, which occurs without tinnitus, all other cases start with tinnitus and gradually lose hearing. Therefore, although predecessors classified it into "wind deafness," "damp deafness," "deficiency deafness," "overwork deafness," "reversal deafness," "sudden deafness," etc., clinically, treatment is often based on that of tinnitus. Refer to the entry "Tinnitus" in this section.

Deafness is closely related to lung qi, especially wind deafness and sudden deafness caused by external wind pathogens. It is necessary to regulate qi and relieve stagnation using modified Guixiang Powder, and it should not be mistakenly treated as a kidney, liver, or gallbladder disorder.

Deafness refers to a complete blockage of sound, with no hearing at all. There is also a condition where hearing is not completely lost but sounds are unclear, called "hard of hearing," which is mostly due to deficiency of the lower origin and insufficient essence, common in the elderly. It is advisable to regularly take Heche Dazao Wan.

Loss of hearing accompanied by inability to speak is called "deaf-mutism." It can be congenital or a sequela, and is difficult to treat. Recently, acupuncture has shown some effectiveness; generally, treatment starts with deafness, mainly selecting Yifeng and Tinghui acupoints. When deafness improves, Yamen and Lianquan acupoints are added to treat mutism. However, if there is no improvement after 20 acupuncture sessions, it is difficult to cure.

Guixiang Powder: Ephedra, Cinnamon Twig, Ligusticum, Angelica

Dahurica, Angelica, Asarum, Acorus, Aucklandia, Arisaema, Akebia, Licorice, Tribulus terrestris

Heche Dazao Wan: Placenta, Codonopsis, Prepared Rehmannia, Asparagus, Ophiopogon, Turtle Shell, Phellodendron, Poria, Eucommia, Achyranthes

III. Itchy Ears

Moisture and itching in the ears due to damp-heat in the liver meridian are treated with Qinggan Decoction. There is also a condition where ear itching stops temporarily after scratching until bleeding but recurs later, which is due to kidney deficiency with wind-heat, treated with Xuanshen Beimu Decoction.

Qinggan Decoction: Artemisia annua, Chrysanthemum leaves, Mint, Forsythia, Kudingcha, Lotus leaf

Xuanshen Beimu Decoction: Scrophularia, Saposhnikovia, Fritillaria, Trichosanthes Root, Phellodendron, Poria, Angelica Dahurica, Vitex, Gastrodia, Pinellia, Licorice, Ginger

IV. Ear Pain

Mild cases are mostly due to wind-heat congestion or blockage by condensed fluid and earwax, causing distending pain, treated with Zhizi Qinggan Decoction. Severe pain is often seen in conditions like “er ting” (ear boils), etc. Refer to the entry “Ear Discharge” in this section.

Zhizi Qinggan Decoction: Gardenia, Acorus, Bupleurum, Angelica, Scutellaria, Coptis, Moutan Bark, Licorice, Arctium

V. Ear Discharge

It is called "purulent ear." In surgery, yellow pus is termed "ting ear," and white pus is "chan ear." Generally caused by external wind-damp-heat or induced by water entering the ear during bathing, it starts with swelling, followed by pain, then purulent discharge, accompanied by chills and fever, and a wiry, slippery, and rapid pulse. It is advisable to take Yigan Xiaodu Powder internally; for severe pain, add antelope horn. For external use, pound Jinsi Heye (creeping Jenny) to extract juice, add a little borneol, and instill into the ear. If pus does not drain smoothly and redness and swelling around the ear root occur, apply Yulu Powder mixed with sesame oil.

Cases induced by deficiency fire or post-illness initially also present with swelling, pain, chills, and fever, with a thready and rapid pulse, often discharging black, foul-smelling, greenish-white thin pus. Especially in children after measles, the pus often persists, and even ulceration with pus behind the ear may occur, eroding bones, making healing extremely difficult. Internally, take Zhibai Bawei Wan with a small amount of cinnamon to guide fire back to its origin; for external use, blow Chui'er Powder into the ear.

For all cases of purulent ear, it is essential to wipe away the pus with cotton to prevent ear blockage leading to deafness or other complications. Severe cases should be treated by a surgeon.

Yigan Xiaodu Powder: Gardenia, Bupleurum, Scutellaria, Forsythia, Saposhnikovia, Schizonepeta, Licorice, Red Peony Root, Angelica Tail, Rush, Honeysuckle

Yulu Powder: Hibiscus leaf, ground into powder

Zhibai Bawei Wan: Phellodendron, Anemarrhena, Raw Rehmannia, Cornus, Moutan Bark, Yam, Alisma

Chui'er Powder: one *qian* each of Cuttlefish Bone, Dried Alum, Dragon Bone, Red Stonecrop, Rouge, Litharge, Chalcanthite, Indigo Naturalis, Borax, Coptis; two *fen* of Borneol; one *fen* of Musk, ground into fine powder

VI. Growth of Flesh in the Ear

Small fleshy growths in the ear, shaped like cherries or goat's milk nipples, are called "ear hemorrhoids"; those with a large head and small stalk like mushrooms are "ear fungi"; those long and thin like jujube stones protruding outside the ear, causing pain when touched, are "ear projections". These three are named differently based on their shapes, all formed by stagnation of liver meridian fire, kidney meridian ministerial fire, and stomach meridian accumulated fire. Take Zhizi Qinggan Decoction internally and apply Naosha Powder externally. A folk remedy can also be used: three *qian* of dried alum, two *qian* of dark plum, a little borneol, ground into powder, and sprinkled on the affected area; another folk remedy: nine parts of Brucea javanica seed oil and one part of glycerin, mixed as ear drops, instilled once or twice a day.

Zhizi Qinggan Decoction: Gardenia, Ligusticum, Angelica, Bupleurum, White Peony Root, Moutan Bark, Licorice, Gypsum, Arctium, Scutellaria, Coptis

Naosha Powder: one *qian* of Sal Ammoniac, three *qian* each of Calomel and Realgar, five li of Borneol, ground into powder, mixed with water and applied to the affected area.

VII. Insects Entering the Ear

For ants, lice, and other insects crawling into the ear, folk external remedies are mostly used, such as instilling sesame oil, or juice of Chinese chives, green onions, ginger, etc.

Section 5 Nasal Symptoms

The nose is the orifice of the lung and is responsible for breathing. Also, since the Yangming meridian connects at the chin and runs along the sides of the nose, nasal diseases are mainly related to the lung and stomach meridians. External causes are mostly invasion by wind-cold or wind-heat pathogens, and internal causes are mostly upward fumigated and steamedby accumulated damp-heat and fire, which are relatively common. Clinically, the color of the nose is also used as part of inspection: For example, a slightly black nose indicates water retention, a yellow nose indicates cold in the chest, and a white nose indicates blood loss, which must be carefully observed.

I. Nasal Congestion

Nasal congestion and obstruction are often a precursor symptom of a cold, or due to nasal polyps, resulting in loss of smell. Refer to the entries "Clear Nasal Discharge" and "Nasal Polyps" in this section.

II. Clear Nasal Discharge

Invasion by wind-cold or wind-heat pathogens in a cold, with clear nasal discharge, often accompanied by nasal congestion and sneezing, is called "biqiu" (allergic rhinitis). If there are chills and fever, focus on treating chills and fever; if there is cough, focus on treating cough. In both cases, appropriately add aromatic orifices-opening medicines such as magnolia flower and cocklebur fruit to the prescription. If nasal congestion and discharge persist alone for a long time, hindering inhalation, Changpu Powder can be inserted into the nose. It can also turn into greenish-yellow turbid discharge, developing into "naoyou" (rhinorrhea).

Elderly people often have excessive nasal discharge, which is due to insufficient primordial qi. *The Inner Canon* states: “At the age of sixty, yang declines, qi is greatly weakened, the nine orifices are dysfunctional, there is deficiency below and excess above, and both nasal discharge and tears occur.”

Changpu Powder: Equal parts of Acorus and Saponaria, ground into powder, wrapped in cotton and stuffed into the nose.

III. Turbid Nasal Discharge

Constant discharge of greenish-yellow turbid nasal mucus with a fishy smell is called “biyuan” (sinusitis), commonly known as “naolou” (brain leakage). Caused by internal heat from the gallbladder meridian moving upward and external wind-cold stagnation, take Qishou Huoxiang Wan with Xangerzi Decoction, or Xinyi Jingjie Powder. If this syndrome persists for a long time, it can lead to deficiency, so qi tonification should be considered, and one should not rely solely on pungent-dispersing methods. In addition, the daoyin (guidance) method: rub the tip of the middle finger in the palm until extremely hot, then iron and rub the Yingxiang acupoints.

Xangerzi Decoction: Cocklebur Fruit, Magnolia Flower, Angelica Dahurica, Mint

Qishou Huoxiang Wan: Agastache, Pig Bile

Xinyi Jingjie Powder: Magnolia Flower, Schizonepeta, Scutellaria, Arisaema, Pinellia, Medicated Leaven, Angelica Dahurica, Atractylodes

IV. Epistaxis

Bleeding from the nose is called “bixue” (nosebleed), which is mostly seen in heat syndromes. In exogenous syndromes such as wind-warm syndrome, add Moutan Bark, Imperata Rhizome, and Imperata Flower to the pungent-cool resolving formula. For those with inherent heat in the lung forcing blood to overflow upward, use Jisu Powder. For cases caused by excessive drinking or consumption of spicy foods, with heat in Yangming, use Yunü Jian with added Reed Rhizome and Imperata Rhizome. For those with hyperactive liver fire, often accompanied by irritability and head distension, use Qingnü Decoction. There are also cases of upward flaming of deficiency fire due to yin deficiency, with nosebleeds occurring even with slight exertion or easily during face washing, which persists for a long time; use Yunü Jian without Gypsum, adding Scrophularia, Donkey-Hide Gelatin, Asparagus, and Lotus Node, etc.

In epistaxis, if bleeding is uncontrollable and causes severe dizziness, it is called "bihong" (severe nosebleed); it is appropriate to use Xijiao Dihuang Decoction to cool blood and stop bleeding. First-aid methods: take 2 *qian* of Baicaoshuang (plant soot) mixed with glutinous rice soup, or take fresh Lotus Rhizome Juice, Fresh Rehmannia Juice, and Cirsium Juice mixed with honey. For external treatment, apply a wet towel or ice pack to the forehead, or tightly tie the middle joint of the middle finger with a string—tie the right hand for left nosebleed, the left hand for right nosebleed, and both hands for bleeding from both nostrils.

In cold damage syndrome, when sweating is supposed to occur but does not, excessive heat forces blood to cause epistaxis, and often the heat is relieved with the nosebleed, which is called "red sweat". However, there are cases where the heat is not relieved after epistaxis or bleeding is uncontrollable, which should not be taken lightly.

Jisu Powder: Mint, Astragalus, Raw Rehmannia, Donkey-Hide Gelatin, Imperata Rhizome, Ophiopogon, Cattail Pollen, Fritillaria,

Mulberry Bark, Licorice, Platycodon

Yunü Jian: Raw Rehmannia, Gypsum, Ophiopogon, Anemarrhena, Achyranthes

Qingnü Decoction: Raw Rehmannia, Red Peony Root, Angelica, Cyperus, Scutellaria, Gardenia, Arborvitae Leaf, Coptis, Red Poria, Platycodon, Licorice, Lotus Node

Xijiao Dihuang Decoction: Rhinoceros Horn, Raw Rehmannia, White Peony Root, Moutan Bark

V. Dry Nose

Dryness inside the nose is one of the symptoms of yin deficiency with internal heat or stagnant heat in the lung and stomach.

"Nasosinusitis" also initially feels dry, followed by the growth of millet-like grains with pain, and in severe cases, redness and slight swelling outside the nose, caused by excessive heat in the lung meridian attacking upward; use Huangqin Decoction, and for severe dryness, apply Huanglian Gao.

Huangqin Decoction: Scutellaria, Licorice, Ophiopogon, Mulberry Bark, Red Peony Root, Platycodon, Mint, Schizonepeta, Gardenia

Huanglian Gao: Coptis, Phellodendron, Turmeric, Angelica, Raw Rehmannia, Sesame Oil, Yellow Wax (proprietary medicine)

VI. Itchy Nose

Itchy nose is mostly seen in colds, causing sneezing.

In children, itching inside the nose, frequent picking with hands, excessive crying, emaciation, or accompanied by fever and sores around the lips, is "biggan" (nasal malnutrition). Due to improper diet and stagnation in the upper jiao, take Wufu Huadu Dan internally. If itching only occurs on both sides under the nose, with redness and greasy discharge, caused by wind-heat invading the lung, it is also called "nasal boils"; take Zexie Powder internally and apply Qingdai Powder externally.

Wufu Huadu Dan: Raw Rehmannia, Prepared Rehmannia, Asparagus, Ophiopogon, Scrophularia, Licorice, Feng Hua Xiao (weathered saltpeter), Indigo Naturalis

Zexie Powder: Alisma, Curcuma, Gardenia, Licorice

Qingdai Powder: Two *liang* each of Indigo Naturalis and Phellodendron, four *liang* each of Gypsum and Talc, ground into powder, mixed with sesame oil for application.

VII. Nose Pain

Pain inside the nose is mostly due to internal stagnation of wind pathogens. If there is swollen obstruction with distending pain extending to the forehead, it is "nasal furuncle" caused by fire toxin in the lung meridian. In severe cases, with swelling of the cheeks and lips, urgently take Chansu Wan, then grind Chansu Wan into powder and put it into the nose; for hard swelling outside the nose, apply Ligong Dingzi.

Chansu Wan: Toad Venom, Calomel, Verdigris, Dried Alum, Chalcanthite, Calcite, Frankincense, Myrrh, Musk, Cinnabar, Realgar, Snail (proprietary medicine)

Ligong Dingzi: Dragon's Blood, Cinnabar, Chalcanthite, Beijing Ink, Toad Venom, Musk (proprietary medicine)

VIII. Nasal Swelling

Diffuse swelling of the nose, caused by excessive fire in the lung meridian. For mild cases, blow saponaria powder into the nose; sneezing repeatedly will lead to recovery. For severe cases with unbearable pain, use Jieyu Decoction. If the swelling has a root, beware of external conditions such as "nasal abscess".

Jieyu Decoction: Platycodon, Asparagus, Ophiopogon, Scutellaria, Licorice, Trichosanthes Root, Aster, Perilla, Stemona

IX. Nasal Flaring

Flaring of the nostrils with shortness of breath, commonly seen in children when "measles" erupts and suddenly subsides, which is a severe syndrome of lung qi obstruction. Refer to the entry "Measles" in systemic symptoms.

In children, invasion by wind-cold or heat pathogens stagnating in the lung, with chills, fever, cough, and shortness of breath, and in severe cases, nasal flaring, accompanied by absence of nasal discharge and tears, and pale complexion. Since the lung opens into the nose, pathogenic stagnation in the lung leads to obstruction of clear qi, a condition called "lung wind". Treatment should prioritize opening the lung; descending and astringing should not be used, with ephedra as the main herb. For wind-cold cases, use Huagai Powder; for heat pathogen cases, use Maxing Shigan Decoction.

Huagai Powder: Ephedra, Almond, Tangerine Peel, Mulberry Bark, Licorice, Red Poria

Maxing Shigan Decoction: Ephedra, Almond, Gypsum, Licorice

X. Red Nose

Redness, even purplish, of the tip and sides of the nose, is common in drinkers. Caused by stomach fire fumigating the lung and stagnation of blood stasis, it is called "alcohol nose", which is lingering and difficult to cure. Take Liangxue Siwu Decoction internally and apply Diandao Powder externally. A proven recipe: equal parts of gardenia seed and campsis flower, ground into powder, 2 *qian* each dose, taken with green tea, avoiding spicy foods.

Redness of the nose during illness is mostly due to warm pathogens entering the spleen meridian. *The Inner Canon* states: "In spleen heat disease, the nose is the first to turn red."

Liangxue Siwu Decoction: Angelica, Red Peony Root, Raw Rehmannia, Ligusticum, Red Poria, Tangerine Peel, Safflower, Licorice, Ginger

Diandao Powder: Equal parts of Rhubarb and Sulfur, ground into powder, mixed with cold water for application.

XI. Cyanotic Nose

Cyanotic nose is one of the severe symptoms of yin-cold syndrome, indicating exhaustion of yang qi in the middle jiao. *Synopsis of the Golden Chamber* states: "If the tip of the nose is blue, with abdominal pain and severe cold, it is fatal."

XII. Cold Nose

Cold nose is common in spleen yang deficiency syndrome, with a yellow or white complexion, appropriate to use large doses of ginseng, atractylodes, dried ginger, etc., for warm tonification. If the nose is cold or the breath from the nose is cold during a severe illness, it is a fatal syndrome.

XIII. Nasal Smoke-like Discoloration

The nostrils are black as if coated with smoke, one of the symptoms of extreme heat in yang toxin syndrome. It is appropriate to add coptis, raw rehmannia, etc., to the main prescription to purge fire, clear the nutrient level, and detoxify.

XIV. Collapse of the Nasal Bridge

Collapse of the nasal bridge is rotting and depression of the nose, more common in "yangmei jiedu" (syphilitic gummata). Yangmei jiedu is one of the syndromes of "syphilis", where the toxin attacks outward, causing swelling anywhere, rotting after ulceration, and mostly damaging the appearance. If it occurs in joints, it damages tendons and bones, often resulting in stiffness after healing; if it occurs on the top of the head, it causes headache and eye swelling, gradually leading to collapse of the top of the skull; if it occurs in the mouth and nose, it often results in a collapsed nose and a split lip; if it occurs in the throat and eyes, it can even cause throat damage, blindness, and hoarseness; if it occurs in the hands, feet, and limbs, it eventually leads to contracture and stiffness. Therefore, yangmei jiedu can appear in various parts of the body, but a collapsed nose is the most prominent. After liberation, active prevention and treatment were carried out, and the system of prostitution in the old society was eliminated, eradicating the main route of syphilis transmission, so such diseases are now extremely rare.

"Leprosy" virus also causes collapse of the nasal bridge. Refer to the entry "Skin Numbness" in systemic symptoms.

XV. Nasal Polyps

Fleshy growths in the nose like pomegranate seeds, gradually growing larger and hanging down, purple in color and slightly hard, blocking the nostrils and making breathing difficult, are called "nasal hemorrhoids", which is mostly caused by stagnation of wind-damp-heat pathogens in the lung meridian. Take Xinyi Qingfei Yin internally, apply Naosha Powder externally, or use Guading Powder wrapped in cotton into a bean-sized ball and stuffed into the nostrils.

Xinyi Qingfei Yin: Magnolia Flower, Gypsum, Anemarrhena, Gardenia, Scutellaria, Loquat Leaf, Cimicifuga, Lily, Ophiopogon, Licorice

Naosha Powder: One *qian* of Sal Ammoniac, three *fen* each of Calomel and Realgar, five li of Borneol, ground into powder, mixed with water and applied to the affected area.

Guading Powder: Equal parts of Melon Pedicel and Asarum, ground into powder.

Section 6 Lip Symptoms

The lips belong to the spleen, and the spleen and stomach are internally-externally related, so most lip symptoms are caused by steaming of spleen dampness and stomach heat, with a very small part caused by external pathogens and infantile fetal toxins. Generally, excess syndromes are more than deficiency syndromes, heat syndromes more than cold syndromes, and interior syndromes more than exterior syndromes. Also, since the body fluids in the mouth are connected to the five *zang* organs, an excess of zang qi will be reflected in the mouth with different tastes, serving as a basis for diagnosis.

I. Bland Taste in the Mouth

Bland taste in the mouth embodies a bland, tasteless mouth with no pleasure in eating. It can be seen in exogenous wind-cold, where dispelling pathogens is the main treatment; it can also be seen in post-illness stomach deficiency, treated with Liujunzi Decoction for regulation. Generally, a bland taste in the mouth during illness is mostly due to damp turbidity in the stomach, which is bland and greasy, with a greasy tongue coating, and even nausea and vomiting. It is not treated as a main symptom; instead, agastache, amomum, tangerine peel, etc., are added to the main prescription to aromatically transform and harmonize the middle jiao.

Liujunzi Decoction: Ginseng, Atractylodes, Pinellia, Tangerine Peel, Poria, Licorice

II. Bitter Taste in the Mouth

Bitter taste in the mouth is common in gallbladder heat or liver heat syndromes, so *The Inner Canon* calls it "gallbladder heat". It states: "This person often plans but cannot decide, so the gallbladder is deficient and qi overflows upward, causing a bitter taste in the mouth." It also says: "When liver qi is hot, the gallbladder leaks and the mouth is bitter, and the fascia dries up." Treatment should be modified Longdan Xiegan Decoction. However, bitter and dry mouth are common in febrile diseases and are not treated as main symptoms; when heat is cleared, the bitter taste will disappear.

Longdan Xiegan Decoction: Gentiana, Scutellaria, Akebia, Plantain Seed, Angelica, Raw Rehmannia, Bupleurum, Licorice

III. Sweet Taste in the Mouth

A constant sweet taste in the mouth, even when drinking plain water, is due to damp-heat accumulated in the spleen, called "spleen heat" in *The Inner Canon*, and it is said that "treat it with lan". Lan cao (orchid grass) is eupatorium, which is used for its aromatic clearing and transforming properties; modified Xiehuang Powder can also be used.

Xiehuang Powder: Agastache, Gardenia, Gypsum, Licorice, Saposhnikovia

IV. Salty Taste in the Mouth

It is due to upward flow of kidney fluid. For deficiency fire, use Zishen Wan to guide fire downward; for deficient cold, use Fugui Bawei Wan with added schisandra.

Zishen Wan: Phellodendron, Anemarrhena, Cinnamon

Fugui Bawei Wan: Aconite, Cinnamon, Prepared Rehmannia, Cornus, Yam, Poria, Moutan Bark, Alisma

V. Sour Taste in the Mouth

Liver heat attacking the spleen, use Zuojin Wan with added medicated leaven.

Zuojin Wan: Coptis, Evodia

VI. Pungent Taste in the Mouth

A pungent taste in the mouth, accompanied by a numb and spicy feeling on the tongue, or a fishy smell, is all due to lung heat, treated with modified Xiebai Powder.

Modified Xiebai Powder: Mulberry Bark, Platycodon, Wolfberry Bark, Licorice, Scutellaria, Ophiopogon, Schisandra, Anemarrhena

VII. Greasy Taste in the Mouth

An unpleasant greasy taste in the mouth, often accompanied by a thick and greasy tongue coating, indicates extremely severe damp turbidity and dysfunction of the spleen and stomach, treated with Pingwei Powder with added agastache.

Pingwei Powder: Atractylodes, Magnolia Bark, Tangerine Peel, Licorice

VIII. Foul Breath

Foul smell from the mouth is mostly due to excessive stomach fire, often appearing in warm febrile diseases, "oral ulcers", "gingival bleeding", etc., treated with modified Ganlu Yin. If the smell is like rotten food, it is due to indigestion and should not be treated as a pure heat syndrome.

Persistent foul breath in the mouth can be managed by frequently gargling with decocted Agastache. For bad breath after eating chives or garlic, take two *qian* of Forsythia powder with green tea, or chew several black thorny dates to reduce the odor.

Modified Ganlu Yin: Rehmannia, Asparagus, Scutellaria, Loquat Leaf, Capillary Wormwood, Aurantium, Dendrobium, Rhinoceros Horn, Licorice

IX. Thirst

Thirst is a common symptom and of great significance in diagnosis. Whether one is thirsty is reflected in whether one drinks water or not. Those who are thirsty and desire to drink are mostly suffering from interior or heat syndromes. For example, in exogenous diseases with fever, there is no thirst at the onset, and even if there is thirst, little water is drunk, indicating the disease is in the exterior. If the fever persists, and there is intense thirst with a preference for cold drinks, it means the pathogen has transformed into heat and entered the interior. Generally, thirst is not treated as a primary symptom; for mild cases, appropriately add Reed Rhizome or Snakegourd Peel to the prescription. For severe cases, it is necessary to distinguish between excessive fire and fluid damage: For excessive fire, use bitter-cold herbs such as Coptis and Scutellaria to purge heat, and the thirst will subside once the heat is relieved; for fluid damage, use Dendrobium, Polygonatum, Trichosanthes Root, etc., to clear heat and generate fluids. If heat lingers and injures yin, causing unrelenting thirst, the Lianmei Decoction method can be used, which employs sour and bitter flavors to drain heat and sweet and sour flavors to transform yin. There are also cases of excessive heat in the intestines and stomach, accompanied by constipation, thirst, dry throat, and a yellow and dry tongue coating, where purgative methods should be used to clear heat and preserve fluids, known as "urgent purgation to preserve yin" or "taking fuel from under the cauldron".

Generally, thirst is mostly due to heat in the qi level. If there is thirst with restlessness, a crimson tongue, or red prickles on the tip of the tongue, it indicates stagnant heat in the nutrient level, and Qingzao Decoction is appropriate. However, when heat pathogens have just entered the nutrient level, there is often no thirst. As Wu Jutong stated, "A crimson and dry tongue should typically be accompanied by thirst; if there is no thirst, the heat is in the nutrient level." This is because pathogenic heat enters the nutrient level and steams the nutrient qi upward, making the condition more severe than heat in the qi level.

Thirst as the main symptom is seen in the upper consumption syndrome of "xiaoke" (diabetes). The characteristic of upper consumption is frequent thirst and frequent drinking, with the consumed water being quickly eliminated. Generally, due to heat in the lung injuring fluids, use Tianhuafen Powder; if there is excessive heart fire consuming the lung's qi and yin, use Huangqi Zhuye Decoction and Shengjin Yin. If lung cold fails to transform water, with one part intake and two parts urination, it is difficult to treat. If there is intense thirst with a desire to drink, but the person does not want to drink, drinks little, or prefers hot drinks, it is due to internal obstruction by damp turbidity and fluid retention, preventing fluids from ascending, known as false thirst. Clearing heat and generating fluids is inappropriate; instead, aromatic and warm-transforming methods should be used. Once water-dampness is resolved, the thirst will naturally subside. Additionally, water-damp syndromes should not involve thirst; if thirst occurs after taking medicine, it is a sign that the water-dampness has been resolved and should not be treated as a thirst syndrome. Therefore, in thirst syndromes, it is necessary to distinguish between the desire to drink or not, the amount consumed, preference for cold or warm drinks, and whether the heat is in the qi or nutrient level, combined with other symptoms. One should not assume it is a heat syndrome upon seeing dryness and thirst.

Lianmei Decoction: Coptis, Dark Plum, Ophiopogon, Raw Rehmannia, Donkey-Hide Gelatin

Qingzao Decoction: Ophiopogon, Anemarrhena, Renzhonghuang (Human Feces Processed), Raw Rehmannia, Scrophularia

Tianhuafen Powder: Trichosanthes Root, Raw Rehmannia, Ophiopogon, Pueraria, Schisandra, Licorice, Japonica Rice

Huangqi Zhuye Decoction: Ginseng, Astragalus, Angelica, White Peony Root, Raw Rehmannia, Ophiopogon, Ligusticum, Scutellaria, Licorice, Gypsum, Bamboo Leaves

Shengjin Yin: Asparagus, Ophiopogon, Raw Rehmannia, Prepared Rehmannia, Angelica, Schisandra, Licorice, Trichosanthes Root, Snakegourd Seed, Hemp Seed

X. Excessive Clear Fluid in the Mouth

Excessive clear fluid in the mouth is common in stomach cold and acid regurgitation syndromes, treated by taking two *fen* of Clove powder with boiled water.

XI. Drooling from the Corners of the Mouth

One of the symptoms of "zhongfeng" (stroke), caused by stiff tongue and deviated mouth failing to contain saliva. Refer to the entry "Deviated Mouth" in this section.

Drooling in children is divided into cold and heat types, both caused by the spleen's inability to contain fluids. For spleen cold, use Atractylodes, Green Tangerine Peel, Roasted Ginger, Pinellia, Aucklandia, Clove; for spleen heat, use Atractylodes, Talc, Hyacinth Bean, Poria, Dendrobium, Coptis, Pueraria, etc.

XII. Deviated Mouth

Deviated mouth is also called "mouth deviation", commonly seen in "stroke" syndrome, presenting together with eye deviation, known as "facial deviation". *The Inner Canon* states: "When the channels of the Foot Yangming and Hand Taiyang are tense, the mouth and eyes become deviated, and the canthi are tense, making it impossible to look straight." First, it is appropriate to moisten dryness and dispel wind with Da Qinjiao Decoction, followed by nourishing blood. Combined with acupuncture, select Jiache and Dicang points, taking the opposite side for the affected side, and also needling Hegu and Taichong, etc.

Da Qinjiao Decoction: Gentiana Macrophylla, Ligusticum, Notopterygium, Angelica Pubescens, Raw Rehmannia, White Peony Root, Angelica Body, Asarum, Atractylodes, Poria, Angelica Dahurica, Gypsum, Scutellaria, Saposhnikovia, Licorice, Ginger

XIII. Lockjaw

The Yangming channel ascends to wrap around the lips; invasion by wind-cold causes spasm and lockjaw, but it mainly manifests as tightly closed jaws. Therefore, local treatments are generally adopted: grind Dark Plum, Borneol, Raw Arisaema into powder to rub the teeth; or grind Veratrum, Curcuma into powder to blow into the nose to induce sneezing; or decoct Saponaria, Frankincense, Astragalus, Saposhnikovia for fumigation and washing; or needle Renzhong and Jiache points.

XIV. Oral Erosion

Local erosion in the mouth, white in color, shaped like moss, called "koumi" (oral erosion). Wiping it off with green cloth dipped in water or mint water reveals a red, painful area. Mostly due to yang excess and yin deficiency, and internal stagnation of damp-heat in the spleen channel, which overs time transforms into pure heat, with heat steaming the stomach orifice, as *The Inner Canon* states: "Obstructed intestines and difficulty in defecation lead to oral erosion above." In severe cases, it spreads throughout the mouth, extending to the throat, making eating and drinking impossible. For mild cases, use Daochi Powder; for severe cases, use Shaoyin Ganjie Decoction; for external use, blow Jiangbo Powder onto the affected area and rinse with warm water. This syndrome can also involve stomach heat with spleen deficiency and dampness, accompanied by bad breath and diarrhea, treated with Jiawei Lianli Decoction. When it appears after warm febrile diseases, it is mostly due to yin deficiency with blazing fire; if accompanied by confusion and convulsions, it is even more dangerous.

Newborn babies with white scales all over the mouth and tongue, resembling coagulated milk films, are called "e's mouth sore", commonly known as "snow mouth". It is due to latent heat in the fetus, accumulating in the heart and spleen. Severe cases are accompanied by fever, restlessness, and incessant crying. Or the white scales may extend to the throat, causing phlegm rales in the throat, blue face and purple lips, leading to death. Early internal administration of Qingre Xiepi Powder, external use of Coptis and Licorice decoction to wipe the mouth, followed by application of Bingpeng Powder, can lead to recovery in three to four days.

Daochi Powder: Akebia, Raw Rehmannia, Bamboo Leaves, Licorice

Shaoyin Ganjie Decoction: Platycodon, Licorice, Ligusticum, Scutellaria, Tangerine Peel, Scrophularia, Bupleurum, Notopterygium, Cimicifuga

Jiangbo Powder: Equal parts of Dried Ginger and Phellodendron, ground into powder

Jiawei Lianli Decoction: Atractylodes, Ginseng, Poria, Coptis, Dried Ginger, Licorice

Qingre Xiepi Powder: Gardenia, Gypsum, Coptis, Raw Rehmannia, Scutellaria, Red Poria, Rush

Bingpeng Powder: Five *fen* of Borneol, five *qian* each of Borax and Sodium Sulfate, six *fen* of Cinnabar, ground into fine powder.

XV. Oral Ulcers

Small white ulcerated blisters on the cheeks, lips, or tongue edges, with redness and pain, sometimes accompanied by slight fever, also called "oral malnutrition" or "broken mouth". Due to accumulated heat in the heart and spleen channels steaming upward, it is necessary to distinguish between excess and deficiency. Excess fire presents with bright red color, numerous ulcer spots, and in severe cases, swollen cheeks and tongue, red urine, and constipation, suitable for internal administration of Liangge Powder and external application of Fuyan Powder. Deficiency fire presents with pale red color, white spots without other heat symptoms, internal administration of Siwu Decoction with added Phellodendron, Anemarrhena, Moutan Bark, and a small amount of Cinnamon for counter-treatment, external application of Liuhua Powder.

Liangge Powder: Scutellaria, Mint, Gardenia, Forsythia, Gypsum, Licorice, Sodium Sulfate, Rhubarb

Fuyan Powder: Equal parts of Scutellaria, Coptis, Gardenia, Dried Ginger, Phellodendron, Asarum, ground into fine powder

Siwu Decoction: Raw Rehmannia, White Peony Root, Ligusticum, Angelica

Liuhua Powder: One *liang* of Phellodendron, three *qian* of Indigo

Naturalis, one *qian* of Cinnamon, two *fen* of Borneol, ground into fine powder

XVI. Crimson Lips

Crimson red around the lips is one of the symptoms of internal heat. Mostly caused by accumulated heat in the heart and spleen, it is also seen in the late stage of pulmonary tuberculosis.

XVII. Pale White Lips

Pale white lip is one of the symptoms of blood deficiency, also seen in syndromes such as spleen deficiency with salivation and vomiting.

XVIII. Cyanotic Lips

Bluish lips indicate deep cold in the interior, stagnation of blood vessels, and failure of nourishment to reach the exterior, so they are often accompanied by dark blue nails. There are also cases of cyanosis due to heat stagnation, which must be accompanied by deep purple in the cyanosis.

In pregnant women, a blue tongue indicates fetal death in the womb, and blue lips indicate the death of the mother.

XIX. White Spots on Lips

The presence of small white spots inside the lips when examined is a characteristic of intestinal parasitosis.

XX. Dry and Chapped Lips

Dry and chapped lip is mostly caused by dry weather or spleen heat, and in severe cases, chapped and bleeding. Grind peach kernels into a paste, mix with lard for external application, and take Qingliang Yin internally.

Qingliang Yin: Scutellaria, Coptis, Mint, Scrophularia, Angelica, Red Peony Root, Licorice, Honey

XXI. Lip Tremor

Lip tremor is involuntary tremor of the lips. If caused by blood deficiency and wind-dryness, use Siwu Xiaofeng Yin. If it appears in deficiency syndromes, it is mostly due to spleen deficiency with failure to contain, and treatment should focus on tonifying the middle jiao.

Siwu Xiaofeng Yin: Raw Rehmannia, Angelica Body, Red Peony Root, Schizonepeta, Mint, Ligusticum, Cicada Slough, Bupleurum, Scutellaria, Licorice

XXII. Contraction of Lips and Mouth

Called "lip inversion", it is a sign of spleen failure. *The Inner Canon* states: "In cases of lip inversion, the flesh dies first."

Narrow lips and mouth, inability to open and close, and inability to eat or drink, called "tight lips". Mostly caused by wind-phlegm invading the collaterals, use equal parts of Galla Chinensis and Terminalia Chebula, ground into powder, mixed with sesame oil for external application, or apply Huangbai Powder externally.

Contraction of the lips and mouth in infants, inability to suckle, called "pursed mouth", is a severe symptom of "umbilical wind". Caused by infection from external pathogens and water-dampness due to improper umbilical cord cutting at birth, it has the same etiology as "tetanus" in adults. It generally occurs four to seven days after birth, commonly known as "four-six wind" and "seven-day wind". Before the onset, the infant cries incessantly, suckles weakly, sneezes from time to time, and soon develops mouth pursing, inability to cry, neck stiffness, limb convulsions and other critical signs. Examination revealing umbilical swelling and abdominal distension confirms the diagnosis. If the area around the umbilicus is blue-black, the face is blue, the lips are purple, and the nails are black, death is likely. Take Cuofeng Powder internally; for constipation, add Heibai Powder. Externally, blow Qifeng Suokou Fang into the nose, or use the lampwick moxibustion method from *Youke Tiejing*: take lampwick the size of rice grains, dip in sesame oil and burn to moxibustion the fontanelle, between the eyebrows, philtrum, Chengjiang, and both Shaoshang points, one moxibustion each; six moxibustions around the umbilicus; if the umbilical cord has not fallen off, one moxibustion at the cord opening; if it has fallen off, one moxibustion at the fallen site, totaling thirteen moxibustions.

Huangbai Powder: Two *qian* each of Galla Chinensis and Litharge, two *fen* of Licorice, ground into powder; additionally, two *qian* of Phellodendron, mix the powder with water, apply, dry over fire, then cool the Phellodendron thoroughly, make into thin slices and apply to the lips.

Cuofeng Powder: Centipede, Uncaria, Scorpion Tail, Musk, Bombyx Batryticatus

Heibai Powder: Black Semen Pharbitidis, White Semen Pharbitidis, Rhubarb, Areca, Tangerine Peel, Licorice, Sodium Sulfate

Qifeng Suokou Fang: One centipede, five scorpion tails, seven Bombyx Batryticatus, five *fen* of Dianthus Superbus, ground into fine powder, use one *fen* each time, blow into the nose. If there is a reaction with crying, decoct three *fen* of Mint, mix with two *fen* of the powder for administration.

XXIII. Swollen, Itchy and Painful Lips

Itching, redness, and swelling of the lips, which over time crack and ooze fluid, with a burning pain, is called "lip wind". Initially appearing as a bean-sized lump, gradually growing as large as a silkworm cocoon, hard and painful, hindering eating and drinking, it is called "cocoon lip". Purple in color with a head, frequently feeling numb and painful, and even accompanied by alternating chills and fever, it is named "lip abscess". Additionally, at the corners of the upper and lower lips, initially shaped like millet grains, purple and hard, severely swollen with numbness, itching, and pain, along with alternating chills and fever, they are called "reverse lip boil" and "lockjaw boil", which can cause the lips to turn outward and the mouth to be unable to open, all requiring prompt surgical treatment.

Generally, swollen and red lips are due to accumulated heat in the stomach; use Yiyiren Decoction.

Yiyiren Decoction: Coix Seed, Stephania, Adzuki Bean, Licorice

Section 7 Tongue Symptoms

The heart is the *zang* organ of fire and opens into the tongue; generally, tongue syndromes are mostly attributed to excessive heart fire. Moreover, since the primary meridian of the heart is connected to the root of the tongue, the liver meridian is connected to the base of the tongue, the spleen meridian is connected to the sides of the tongue, and the kidney's fluid flows out from under the tongue, pathological changes caused by external pathogenic factors and emotional excitement can also affect the tongue through the meridians. Just as *De Xiao Fang* states: "Attack by the four qi (climatic factors) causes the tongue to curl and inability to speak;

stagnation of the seven emotions causes the tongue to swell and inability to speak; heart heat causes the tongue to break and form sores; liver congestion causes profuse bleeding; spleen obstruction causes white coating like snow—these are the diseases of the tongue." Examining the tongue is also an important part of inspection, distinguishing the vitality or decline, hardness or softness, trembling or atrophy, swelling or shrinking, dryness or moisture, maturity or immaturity, thickness or thinness, looseness or greasiness of the tongue proper and tongue coating, which also includes tongue symptoms, and are included here as appropriate.

I. Swollen Tongue

Swollen tongue filling the mouth with pain, due to stagnation of the seven emotions, excessive heart fire and blood congestion, is called "purple tongue swelling". A swollen and enlarged tongue, hard as armor, with alternating chills and fever, is called "wooden tongue". Both can block the throat and cause death; it is advisable to pierce to let out blood and take modified Liangge Powder internally. For swelling protruding outside the mouth, soak it in a strong decoction of holly leaves.

Modified Liangge Powder: Schizonepeta, Gardenia, Arctium, Mint, Scutellaria, Forsythia, Gypsum, Licorice

II. Fat Tongue

A puffy tongue proper, pale and tender, is a syndrome of deficiency-cold and severe water-dampness; treatment should focus on warming and transforming the lower jiao.

III. Long Tongue

The tongue extending out of the mouth and not retracting is called "protruding tongue", caused by intense internal fire; apply five *fen* of borneol to the tongue.

In cold damage syndrome, a protruding tongue mostly indicates death.

A child's protruding tongue is called "tongue thrusting", mostly due to accumulated heat in the heart and spleen. Usesedimentof human urine and borneol, or grind borneol, borax, and realgar into powder and apply to the tongue; additionally, decoct coptis alone for oral administration.

IV. Short Tongue

A short, curled, and atrophied tongue that cannot be extended is called "atrophied tongue", also known as "curled tongue". It is mostly seen in extreme deficiency of qi or cold pathogenic stagnation in the chest and abdomen; if it appears in chronic illness along with scrotal contraction, it is a sign of exhaustion of Jueyin meridian qi, which is incurable.

V. Deviated Tongue

A tongue that protrudes crookedly, either to the left or right, is one of the symptoms of "stroke", often seen together with facial paralysis; refer to the entry "facial deviation" in lip symptoms.

VI. Trembling Tongue

A tongue that trembles uncontrollably when protruded is one of the symptoms of deficiency syndrome and "apoplectic-like syndrome".

VII. Stiff Tongue

Mostly due to wind-phlegm obstructing the base of the tongue, manifested as inability to move and slurred speech, it is one of the symptoms of "stroke". Use Ditan Decoction in the early stage; for long-standing cases, use Zishou Jieyu Decoction.

Ditan Decoction: Pinellia, Arisaema cum Bile, Tangerine Peel, Ginseng, Acorus, Poria, Bamboo Shavings, Aurantium, Licorice, Ginger

Zishou Jieyu Decoction: Notopterygium, Saposhnikovia, Aconite, Antelope Horn, Jujube Seed, Gastrodia, Cinnamon, Licorice, Bamboo Sap, Ginger Juice

VIII. Numb Tongue

A tingling, numb, or prickling sensation on the tongue is called "tongue numbness" (shebi). It arises from emotional disturbances, worry, anger, and the stagnation of qi, phlegm, and fire. Use five *fen* each of schizonepeta and realgar, ground into powder, and take with a decoction of akebia; alternatively, dust saponaria powder onto the tongue.

IX. Tongue Pain

A stabbing pain in the tongue during eating, apart from tongue ulcers, is generally caused by a peeled, cracked tongue coating or red prickles on the tongue tip, belonging to yin deficiency or internal heat syndromes.

X. Tongue Wagging

Children frequently protrude and move their tongues up, down, left, and right, as if a snake is flicking its tongue. This is mostly due to heat accumulated in the heart and stomach, accompanied by liver wind. Internally, use Qingwei Powder; externally, apply a little bezoar to the tongue.

Qingwei Powder: Cimicifuga, Raw Rehmannia, Angelica, Coptis, Moutan Bark

XI. Self-Biting Tongue

Biting one's own tongue is one of the symptoms of "internal wind". *The Inner Canon* states: "When a person bites their own tongue, it is due to reversed qi ascending, with all vessel qi arriving. When shaoyin qi arrives, they bite the tongue; when shaoyang qi arrives, they bite the cheeks; when yangming qi arrives, they bite the lips." Treat with modified Shengshen Fuyuan Decoction.

Shengshen Fuyuan Decoction: Coptis, Phellodendron, Raw Rehmannia, Aurantium, Asarum, Ligusticum, Vitex, Notopterygium, Bupleurum, Ligusticum Sinense, Licorice, Pinellia, Angelica, Saposhnikovia, Ginseng, Prunus japonica Seed, Dried Ginger, Aconite, White Sunflower, Astragalus, Cardamom, Tangerine Peel

XII. Fissured Tongue

There are cracks on the tongue—some have one or two, others have crisscrossing cracks, and some are as deep as grooves. Generally, cracks with a coating indicate internal heat; those without a coating indicate yin deficiency.

Individual cases of congenital fissures are not considered pathological.

XIII. Peeled Tongue

A patch of the tongue coating peeled off like a coin, several patches peeled off, or the entire tongue with scattered peeling like a map, all indicate yin deficiency and insufficient fluids, commonly known as "fluid depletion". Even if heat signs are not obvious, avoid using drying and aromatic herbs with caution.

XIV. Dry Tongue

A shiny, dry tongue is a severe yin deficiency syndrome, common in the late stage of warm diseases, requiring nourishing blood and increasing fluids. A greasy yet dry coating indicates consumption of stomach fluids, more common in the middle and late stages of damp-warm diseases, with a thick, greasy, rough coating that feels like sandpaper when touched. Treatment should first generate fluids; wait until fluids return and the tongue becomes moist before resolving dampness. To nourish blood and increase fluids, use raw rehmannia, ophiopogon, donkey-hide gelatin, and white peony root; to generate fluids, use dendrobium, trichosanthes root, reed rhizome, imperata rhizome, etc.

XV. Greasy Tongue

A tongue coating thicker than normal is called "greasy tongue", mostly due to damp turbidity in the stomach. It can be slightly thick or extremely thick, allowing observation of the severity of damp turbidity. Generally, a white greasy coating indicates cold-dampness, and a yellow greasy coating indicates damp-heat, but it is necessary to distinguish between dryness/moisture and the depth of yellow. In particular, a greasy, gray-black, and dry coating indicates extreme fire mimicking water; a slippery and moist one indicates water overcoming fire, with significant differences in treatment.

The tongues of nursing infants are often white, greasy, and slippery; the tongues of healthy people immediately after drinking milk or soy milk are also white and greasy, but the greasiness is relatively superficial, making it easy to distinguish.

XVI. Shiny Tongue

A shiny, coating-free tongue is characteristic of yin deficiency syndrome. A tongue shiny like a skinned pig's kidney indicates severe damage to liver and kidney yin, which is difficult to treat.

XVII. Pale Tongue

A pale tongue proper indicates blood deficiency—the more deficient the blood, the paler the color, and even a pale white color without any redness indicates severe qi and blood deficiency.

XVIII. Crimson Tongue

A crimson tongue proper indicates heat in the blood phase. A crimson tip alone indicates warm pathogens initially entering the nutrient phase or yin deficiency with blazing fire, mostly involving the upper jiao.

XIX. Bluish-Purple Tongue

Bluish-purple spots or patches on the tip or edges of the tongue are common in yin-cold syndromes and blood stasis syndromes. A purely blue tongue like that of a water buffalo is incurable.

A bluish tongue in pregnant women indicates fetal death in the womb.

XX. Serrated Tongue Edges

Uneven, sawtooth-like edges of the tongue indicate stagnation of liver qi and blood.

XXI. Red Spots on the Tongue Tip

Red spots or red prickles on the tip of the tongue, or extending to the edges of both sides of the tongue, all indicate heat in the blood phase or excessive fire in the heart and liver. If they are red and purple-dark, it is blood stasis.

XXII. Bleeding on the Tongue

Bleeding on the tongue is called “she nǜ” (tongue bleeding). Initially, small pinhole-like openings appear on the tongue, with blood oozing from the openings. It is due to upward blazing of heart fire and reckless movement of hot blood. Purple-colored openings indicate excessive heat, and black ones indicate potential putrefaction. It is advisable to take Shengma Decoction and apply Bisheng Powder externally. A folk recipe: pound Cirsium japonicum and Cirsium setosum, mix with a little yellow rice wine for internal administration; or first rinse the mouth with decocted Typha angustifolia, then dust with stir-fried and ground Sophora japonica.

Shengma Decoction: Cimicifuga, Cirsium setosum, Rubia cordifolia, Artemisia argyi, Calcite, Rehmannia glutinosa, yellow juice

Bisheng Powder: One *qian* each of Indigo naturalis and stir-fried Typha angustifolia, ground into powder

XXIII. Blood Blisters on the Tongue

Purple blood blisters the size of mung beans appear on the tongue, often breaking and bleeding on their own, then subsiding, and appearing elsewhere after subsiding. Mostly caused by stagnant heat in the heart and spleen. Initially, hold three-four Chan Su Wan in the mouth to dissolve and swallow; after breaking, apply Zi Xue Powder, also swallowing slowly. If fire toxin is intense, with hardness, pain, and accompanied by chills and fever, it is called “she ding” (tongue boil), also treated with the previous method, and internally take Huanglian Jiedu Decoction.

Chan Su Wan: Toad venom, Calomel, Verdigris, Dried alum, Chalcanthite, Calcite, Frankincense, Myrrh, Musk, Cinnabar, Realgar,

Snail (proprietary medicine)

Zi Xue Powder: Rhinoceros horn, Antelope horn, Gypsum, Calcite, Cimicifuga, Scrophularia ningpoensis, Licorice, Agarwood, Aucklandia lappa, Sodium nitrate, Cinnabar, Borneol, Gold leaf (proprietary medicine)

Huanglian Jiedu Decoction: Coptis chinensis, Phellodendron amurense, Scutellaria baicalensis, Gardenia jasminoides

XXIV. White Blisters on the Tongue

White blisters of varying sizes on the tongue are called "she shang zhu" (pearls on the tongue), belonging to accumulated heat in the heart and spleen, treated with Powder Huang Decoction plus Gypsum, Paris polyphylla, and Viola yedoensis. Those under the tongue are called "she xia zhu" (pearls under the tongue), belonging to deficiency of the spleen and kidney, treated with Zhibai Bawei Wan plus Scrophularia ningpoensis and Akebia quinata.

San Huang Decoction: Coptis chinensis, Scutellaria baicalensis, Rheum palmatum

Zhibai Bawei Wan: Rehmannia glutinosa, Cornus officinalis, Dioscorea opposita, Anemarrhena asphodeloides, Phellodendron amurense, Paeonia suffruticosa, Poria cocos, Alisma orientale

XXV. Sore Poison on the Tongue

Initially appearing like a bean on the tongue, gradually growing like a fungus, with a large head and a small stalk, painful, red, and rotten without skin, mild in the morning and severe in the evening, it is called "she yan" (tongue cancer), also known as "she jun" (tongue fungus). It often swells and protrudes like a cockscomb, with shortening of the tongue base, unbearable pain when touched, and a foul-smelling saliva. This syndrome is mostly formed by stagnant fire in the heart and spleen; due to difficulty in moving the tongue, insufficient food intake leads to emptiness of the stomach and gradual decline. Initially, use Daochi Powder plus Coptis chinensis; for excessive heat, use Qingliang Ganlu Yin; for external use, apply Bei Ting Dan.

Daochi Powder: Rehmannia glutinosa, Phyllostachys nigra, Akebia quinata, Licorice

Qingliang Ganlu Yin: Rhinoceros horn, Dendrobium nobile, Stellaria dichotoma, Artemisia capillaris, Ophiopogon japonicus, Citrus aurantium, Rehmannia glutinosa, Scutellaria baicalensis, Anemarrhena asphodeloides, Licorice, Eriobotrya japonica

Bei Ting Dan: Sal ammoniac, Human urine sediment, Orostachys fimbriata, Moss on tiles, Chicken feces, Musk, Borneol (proprietary medicine)

XXVI. Mass Under the Tongue

A swollen mass under the tongue, shaped like a small tongue, hindering eating and speaking, is called "chong she" (double tongue), which is caused by excessive heat in the heart and spleen, surging upward along the meridians, causing blood vessels to swell. Take a decoction of Coptis chinensis alone internally, and apply Qingdai Powder externally.

A swollen mass under the tongue like a gourd, smooth and soft like cotton, formed by accumulation of fire and phlegm, is called "tan bao" (phlegm bag). It needs to be pricked with a needle to release viscous fluid, then apply Bingpeng Powder, and take Jiawei Erchen Decoction internally.

Qingdai Powder: Three *qian* each of Coptis chinensis and

Phellodendron amurense, six *fen* each of Indigo naturalis, Sodium nitrate, and Cinnabar, three *fen* each of Realgar, Bezoar, and Borax, one *fen* of Borneol, ground into powder

Bingpeng Powder: Five *fen* of Borneol, five *qian* each of Borax and Sodium sulfate, six *fen* of Cinnabar, ground into fine powder

Jiawei Erchen Decoction: Tangerine Peel, Pinellia, Poria, Scutellaria, Coptis, Mint, Licorice, Ginger

Section 8 Tooth Symptoms

Teeth are the surplus of bones and belong to the kidney. The Foot Yangming Meridian runs through the upper gums, and the Hand Yangming Meridian runs through the lower gums, so tooth symptoms are mostly treated from these three meridians. The causes of tooth symptoms vary, with kidney yin deficiency, upward flaming of deficiency fire, wind-fire, and damp-heat being more common. This section includes symptoms of teeth, gums, and jaw joints, many of which fall within the scope of surgery and require surgical treatment, but most can still be treated internally with decoctions.

I. Toothache

Toothache is closely related to gum swelling. If there is simple toothache: those that hurt when inhaling cold air are cold pain, treated with Wenfeng Powder; those that hurt when exposed to heat or eating spicy food are heat pain, treated with Qingwei Powder; those that hurt regardless of cold or hot stimuli are cold-heat pain, treated with Danggui Longdan Powder.

Pain from tooth decay is called “tooth worm” and “tooth moth”, treated with Dingtong Powder by holding and swallowing, or externally with Yixiao Powder.

Wenfeng Powder: One *qian* each of Angelica, Ligusticum, Asarum, Angelica Dahurica, Piper Longum, Ligusticum Sinense, and Honeycomb, decocted in water, used as a mouthwash and then spat out.

Qingwei Powder: Cimicifuga, Moutan Bark, Angelica, Raw Rehmannia, Coptis

Danggui Longdan Powder: One *qian* each of Ephedra, Cimicifuga, Gentiana, Coptis, and Cardamom; five *fen* each of Raw Rehmannia, Angelica, Angelica Dahurica, and Sheep Tibia Ash, ground into powder, applied to the painful area.

Dingtong Powder: Angelica, Raw Rehmannia, Asarum, Dried Ginger, Angelica Dahurica, Forsythia, Sophora Flavescens, Sichuan Pepper, Coptis, Platycodon, Dark Plum, Licorice

Yixiao Powder: Sichuan Pepper, ground into powder; one croton seed, mashed, mixed with rice to make pills, wrapped in cotton and placed in the decayed hole.

II. Loose Teeth

Loose teeth in the elderly without swelling are mostly due to insufficient kidney qi, a precursor to tooth loss. Take Huanshao Dan regularly; for loose teeth with pain, apply Laoya POwder.

Huanshao Dan: Prepared Rehmannia, Wolfberry, Yam, Achyranthes, Polygala, Cornus, Morinda, Poria, Schisandra, Acorus, Cistanche, Broussonetia, Eucommia, Fennel, Jujube

Laoya Powder: One *liang* and five *qian* of Gentiana, one *liang* each of Notopterygium and Wolfberry Bark, four *fen* of Cimicifuga, ground into fine powder.

III. Scorched Black Teeth

Scorched black tooth is one of the symptoms of excessive heat damaging yin in warm febrile diseases, with a poor prognosis. *The Classic of Difficult Issues* states: "A patient with swollen lips and black teeth will die, as the spleen and kidney are exhausted."

IV. Weak and Sensitive Teeth

Excessive consumption of sour foods leading to weak and sensitive teeth is called "chi cuo" (tooth hypersensitivity); chewing walnut meat thoroughly can relieve it.

V. Teeth Gritting

Teeth gritting during illness is called "xie chi" (teeth grinding), also known as "jia chi", mostly seen in heat syndromes. Grinding sounds from teeth in sleep in both adults and children are also due to excessive stomach fire; soak reed rhizome in water for drinking.

VI. Swollen and Painful Gums

Swollen and painful gums mostly belong to "ya yong" (tooth abscess). Initially, a hard, swollen area appears on the gums, gradually becoming highly swollen, red, and painful, often involving swelling of the cheeks, with loose teeth and inability to chew, but the jaw can still open and close, accompanied by chills and fever, and thirst. Pus forms in about three to four days, and it gradually subsides after being lanced. All are caused by stomach fire; clear it with Zhuye Shigao Decoction. For initial cases with chills and fever, appropriately add Schizonepeta, Saposhnikovia, and Charred Gardenia. Apply Bingpeng Powder whether it has ulcerated or not. This condition is relatively common and heals quickly; there is no need to extract the tooth because of the pain. If the ulcer does not heal for a long time, it can develop into "ya lou" (tooth fistula) with constant pus discharge. Check for sequestered bone; if present, wait for the bone spicule to protrude and remove it for healing.

Zhuye Shigao Decoction: Bamboo Leaves, Gypsum, Platycodon, Mint, Akebia, Licorice, Ginger

Bingpeng Powder: Five *fen* of Borneol, five *qian* each of Borax and Sodium Sulfate, six *fen* of Cinnabar, ground into fine powder.

VII. Gum Decay

This syndrome is most prominent in "ya gan" (gingival necrosis), divided into "zouma ya gan" (galloping gingival necrosis) and "fengre ya gan" (wind-heat gingival necrosis). "Zouma ya gan" describes the rapid decay, as swift as a galloping horse. This syndrome is mostly caused by intense internal heat after sha (measles-like) toxin, cold damage, malaria, or dysentery, and is a severe acute disease. Initially, it starts with decay at the gum margin, grayish-white in color, which then turns black and rotten, oozing purple blood, with a particularly foul odor. In cases of severe toxic fire, the cheeks and lips become red and swollen, and the black decay spreads; within a few days, a cyan-brown color appears on the nose, around the nostrils, or around the cheeks and lips, indicating deep internal ulceration. In more severe cases, the lips decay, teeth fall out, the cheeks and palate are perforated, and the nasal bridge collapses, allowing the throat to be seen through the hole beside the nose. The decayed area is mostly itchy with little pain, accompanied by chills and fever, inability to eat, diarrhea, shortness of breath, and clouded consciousness, often leading to death due to excessive pathogen and deficient vital qi. If the black decay is easily removed, revealing red flesh and fresh blood, and the fever gradually subsides, there is a possibility of cure even with tooth loss and cheek perforation. Initially, use Luhui Xiaogan Yin to clear the fire toxin; for those with spleen-stomach weakness, concurrently take Renshen Fuling Zhou; for external use, apply Renzhongbai Powder or Luhui Powder.

"Fengre ya gan" is caused by the struggle between accumulated heat in the stomach meridian and externally contracted wind pathogens. The onset is rapid; after two to three days of chills and fever, gum decay, bleeding, and bad breath occur. The difference from "zouma ya gan" is severe pain without cheek decay, and it generally gradually heals within half a month. Only a few cases persist for a long time, leading to exposed gums and occasional pus discharge. Initially, use Qingwei Decoction; for prolonged cases, add Ershen Decoction; externally, apply Wutonglei Powder or Renzhongbai Powder to the affected area.

Luhui Xiaogan Yin: Aloe, Picrorhiza, Gypsum, Antelope Horn, Gardenia, Arctium, Starwort Root, Platycodon, Rhubarb, Scrophularia, Mint, Licorice, Bamboo Leaves

Renshen Fuling Zhou: One *qian* of Ginseng, six *qian* of Poria (ground into powder), cooked with one teacup of japonica rice to make a thin porridge.

Renzhongbai Powder: Human Urine Sediment, Catechu, Phellodendron, Mint, Indigo Naturalis, Borneol (proprietary medicine)

Luhui Powder: One *qian* of Aloe, five *qian* of Phellodendron, five *fen* of White Arsenic, ground into fine powder.

Qingwei Powder: Gypsum, Coptis, Scutellaria, Raw Rehmannia, Moutan Bark, Cimicifuga

Ershen Decoction: Ginseng, Scrophularia

Wutonglei Powder: One *qian* and five *fen* each of Manna, Asarum, Ligusticum, Angelica Dahurica, one *qian* of Raw Rehmannia, two *qian* of Calcite, two *fen* of Green Salt, ground into fine powder.

VIII. Gum Atrophy

In the elderly, gradual decline of kidney qi leading to gum shrinkage and elongated teeth is not considered a pathological sign but makes teeth prone to loosening and falling out. *Yixue Rumen* states: "Exposed and loose gums indicate deficient kidney origin." If gums first swell and gradually decay and shrink, leading to exposed tooth roots, it is called "yaxuan" (exposed gums). For those who prefer cold drinks and dislike heat, with bad breath and oozing gums, use Qingwei Decoction. For those who prefer hot drinks and dislike cold, with severe pain upon exposure to wind, use Duhuo Powder. For foul-smelling gums and loose teeth due to kidney deficiency with deficient fire in the stomach, use Sanyin Anshen Wan.

Qingwei Decoction: Gypsum, Coptis, Scutellaria, Raw Rehmannia, Moutan Bark, Cimicifuga

Duhuo Powder: Notopterygium, Angelica Pubescens, Saposhnikovia, Schizonepeta, Mint, Ligusticum, Raw Rehmannia, Asarum

Sanyin Anshen Wan: Psoralea, Trigonella, Fennel, Toosendan Fruit, Dipsacus, Yam, Almond, Poria, Peach Kernel

IX. Gum Granulation

Granulation growing between the gums, varying in size, is called "chi yong" (gum overgrowth). Take one cup of raw rehmannia juice, heat several pieces of saponaria on fire, quench them in the juice, repeat heating and quenching until the juice is exhausted, dry in the sun, grind into powder and apply, or grind mirabilite into fine powder and apply.

X. Gum Bleeding

Bleeding mostly oozing from between the teeth is called "chi nǜ" (gum bleeding), divided into excess heat in the stomach meridian and upward flaming of deficient fire in the kidney meridian. The former has relatively more blood, foul breath, but no gum decay; use modified Yunü Jian, or decoct three *qian* of wine-processed rhubarb and five *qian* of aurantium, add a little boy's urine for adjustment and administration. The latter drips out, with slight tooth pain, and even loosening or falling out of teeth; use Liuwei Dihuang Decoction with a small amount of cinnamon to guide fire downward. For external treatment, rinse the mouth with salt water and apply Xiaoji Powder.

Modified Yunü Jian: Raw Rehmannia, Gypsum, Anemarrhena, Ophiopogon, Achyranthes, Moutan Bark

Liuwei Dihuang Decoction: Rehmannia, Cornus, Yam, Moutan Bark, Alisma, Poria

Xiaoji Powder: Five 5 *qian* each of Small Thistle, Plant Soot, Stir-fried Cattail Pollen, Cyperus, ground into fine powder.

XI. Swollen and Painful Jaw Joints

Swelling and pain between the cheek and the gum at the back of the molar teeth, with inability to open or close the jaw, difficulty in taking food and water, accompanied by chills and fever, is mostly "ya yao yong" (molar abscess). Due to steaming of damp-fire in the Yangming meridian, take Shengma Shigao Decoction internally and blow Bingpeng Powder externally. It usually resolves easily or heals after pus discharge; if the ulcer does not close, leading to sequestered bone, it can develop into "gucao feng" (osteomyelitis of the jaw).

"Gucao feng" occurs in the area in front of the ear extending to the cheek, persisting for a long time, often with jaw bone defect, becoming a stubborn disease, which is mostly caused by rich and greasy food accumulated in the intestines and stomach, and wind-fire stagnation in the collaterals of Shaoyang and Yangming meridians. It develops rapidly, with initial swelling and pain of the jaw joint, redness, swelling, heat and pain of the cheek, chills and high fever; after three to five days, pus discharges at the back of the molar teeth, and the external swelling gradually subsides, but the swelling and hardness of the cheekbone remain. After more than ten days, the cheek ulcerates, discharging foul-smelling pus, with loose teeth; if it persists for a long time, sequestered bone forms internally, and even the teeth and gums fall off together. Initial treatment: take Shengma Shigao Decoction internally, blow Bingpeng Powder, and apply Chonghe Gao externally. For stiff and immobile jaw, moxibustion the cheekbone point with 27 cones of ginger-partitioned moxibustion, or needle Hegu point. For sequestered bone, blow Tuiche Powder into the sore. This syndrome can also be caused by wind-cold, phlegm-dampness invading deficiency, leading to qi and blood stagnation, with a slower onset: initial vague soreness, or a small nodule first, gradually becoming diffusely swollen and hard, white in color without heat, and not ulcerating for a long time. After ulceration, the hard swelling in the cheek does not subside, and the wound does not close. *Waike Quansheng Ji* states: "Gucao feng with numbness, no swelling, and pain radiating to the cheekbone." Initial treatment: use Shengyang Sanhuo Decoction; for severe phlegm-dampness, add Pinellia and Tangerine Peel; for long-standing cases, use Yanghe Decoction; after ulceration, use Zhonghe Decoction, and apply Yanghe Jie'ning Gao externally mixed with Guisha Powder.

Shengma Shigao Decoction: Cimicifuga, Gypsum, Saposhnikovia, Schizonepeta, Angelica Tail, Red Peony Root, Forsythia, Platycodon, Licorice, Mint, Scutellaria, Rush

Bingpeng Powder: five *fen* of Borneol, five *qian* each of Borax and Sodium Sulfate, six *fen* of Cinnabar, ground into fine powder.

Chonghe Gao: five *liang* of Redbud Bark, three *liang* of Angelica Pubescens, two *liang* of Red Peony Root, one *liang* of Angelica Dahurica, one *liang* and five *qian* of Acorus, ground into powder, mixed with green onion soup and yellow wine for application.

Tuiche Powder: one roasted Dung Beetle, five *fen* of Dried Ginger, ground into fine powder.

Shengyang Sanhuo Decoction: Ligusticum, Vitex, White Peony Root, Saposhnikovia, Notopterygium, Angelica Pubescens, Licorice, Ginseng, Bupleurum, Cyperus, Pueraria, Cimicifuga, Bombyx Batryticatus, Ginger, Jujube

Yanghe Decoction: Ephedra, Prepared Rehmannia, White Mustard Seed, Roasted Ginger, Licorice, Cinnamon, Deer Horn Glue

Zhonghe Decoction: Angelica Dahurica, Platycodon, Ginseng, Astragalus, Agastache, Cinnamon, Licorice, Atractylodes, Ligusticum, Angelica, White Peony Root, Ophiopogon, Ginger, Jujube

Yanghe Jie'ning Gao: Burdock Root, Leaf, Stem, Garden Balsam Stem, Ligusticum, Aconite, Cassia Twig, Rhubarb, Angelica, Cinnamon, Sichuan Aconite, Kusnezoff Monkshood, Earthworm, Bombyx Batryticatus, Red Peony Root, Angelica Dahurica, Ampelopsis, Bletilla, Frankincense, Myrrh, Dipsacus, Saposhnikovia, Schizonepeta, Trogopterus Dung, Aucklandia, Citrus medica, Tangerine Peel, Styrax, Musk, Minium, Rapeseed Oil (boiled into paste and spread for use, proprietary medicine)

Guisha Powder: Five *qian* each of Ephedra and Asarum, one *liang* each of Cinnamon and Clove, eight *qian* each of Raw Pinellia and Raw Arisaema, three *qian* of Saponaria, six *fen* of Musk, four *fen* of Borneol, ground into fine powder.

XII. Failure of Teeth to Erupt

In children, failure of teeth to erupt at the appropriate developmental stage is one of the "five delays". Refer to the entry "Five Delays in Children" in systemic symptoms.

Section 9 Throat Symptoms

The larynx is responsible for breathing and belongs to the lung; the pharynx is the esophagus and belongs to the stomach. The pharynx and larynx are adjacent in location but different in function. Also, due to the connection with internal organs such as the liver and kidney and the passage of meridians, throat disorders can also be caused. This syndrome generally has an acute onset; external causes are mostly wind-heat, and internal causes are mainly phlegm-fire and yin deficiency with yang hyperactivity. In syndrome differentiation, attention is generally paid to whether there is a sudden mass, the location and shape of the mass, whether the surface is smooth or uneven, the color is dark red or light red, whether the mass is eroded, whether there are small white, grayish-white, or yellowish-white dots and patches, whether there is difficulty in opening and closing the jaw, and whether there is diffuse swelling in the front, back, and sides of the neck. Among these, the local redness and swelling, pain, and degree of erosion are more important for diagnosis. TCM has always had specialized departments for throat diseases; when necessary, they should be treated by specialists. In addition, *The Inner Canon* states: "The epiglottis is the door of the voice; the lips are the fan of the voice; the tongue is the mechanism of the voice; the uvula is the gate of the voice." Therefore, symptoms such as loss of voice and hoarseness are also included in this section.

I. Sore and Swollen Throat

Generally speaking, a sore throat is accompanied by redness, swelling, and pain, with a rapid onset. Among them, sudden swelling and pain on one or both sides of the throat, difficulty in swallowing, accompanied by general fatigue, chills, and fever, with more severe swelling and pain within a few hours, which can spread to the entire throat, and swelling and drooping of the uvula, accompanied by excessive phlegm, constipation, and a surging rapid or slippery rapid pulse. All are caused by accumulated heat in the lung and stomach, invasion by wind pathogens, leading to fire stirring up phlegm, mostly "houfeng" (throat wind). Take Qingyan Lige Decoction internally, blow Jinsuoshi externally, and prick Shaoshang and Shangyang points to bleed to discharge heat toxin. This syndrome is heat-related, mostly occurring in young and middle-aged adults, and can lead to death due to internal invasion of toxin and difficulty in breathing within two to three days. If it does not subside immediately, white spots can appear in the swollen area, initially scattered, then merging into patches, eroding like soybeans or broad beans, and even spreading to the uvula, called "lanhoufeng" (erosive throat wind); Wubao Dan can be added to the topical powder. If accompanied by trismus and inability to speak, it is called "suohoufeng" (lockjaw throat wind); first blow Tongguan Powder into the nose to induce sneezing, or needle Jiache point to relax the jaw, then treat as throat wind. There is also "chanhoufeng" (wrapping throat wind), with symptoms similar to throat wind and the same treatment, except that there is simultaneous diffuse swelling in the front and back of the neck, red in color and pitting when pressed, like a snake wrapping around, and in severe cases, swelling extending to the chest; apply Yulu Powder mixed with honeysuckle dew.

Initially, one or both sides of the throat feel dry and burning, slightly red, slightly swollen, slightly painful, or small red spots like prickly heat appear on the mucosa, hindering swallowing, or accompanied by chills and fever. Later, the redness and swelling gradually worsen, or become red with a purplish tint, the pain intensifies, there is a sensation of blockage in the throat, with profuse thick phlegm, and there may be lumps in the neck that are tender to touch. Caused by exogenous wind pathogens stirring up accumulated heat in the lung and stomach, which rises to steam the throat, it is called "wind-heat throat obstruction". Blow Bingshe Powder externally, take Qingyan Shuanghe Yin internally; if there are interior symptoms such as constipation, appropriately add rhubarb for mild purgation. Cases due to yin deficiency where water fails to control fire, with deficiency fire flaring upward, are called "deficiency-fire throat obstruction", characterized by mild throat pain, slight redness and swelling, a sensation of obstruction when swallowing, pain being mild in the morning, worse in the afternoon, and even more severe at night, often accompanied by dry mouth and tongue, heat in the palms and soles, and a thready rapid pulse; take Zhibai Bawei Wan internally. If there is mild throat pain without redness or swelling, cold hands and feet, and a weak pulse, it also belongs to deficiency-fire throat obstruction, due to yang deficiency with rootless fire disturbing upward; it is appropriate to use Fugui Bawei Wan to guide fire back to its origin.

"Throat abscess" occurs beside the uvula, often on one side, initially presenting with bright red, raised swelling and pain, difficulty in eating, increased sticky phlegm, and alternating chills and fever. In severe cases, the pain radiates to the ear, the uvula swells and tilts, there are hard swollen lumps in the neck, and the jaw is stiff; at this time, the body temperature is higher, the throat feels blocked, and even liquids are difficult to swallow. Pus can form within five to seven days; when the pus matures, the swelling becomes localized, and signs such as a raised center with a hollow underneath, reduced pain, and lessened chills and fever may appear. Treatment: first prick the Shaoshang point to let blood out, gargle with Gargle Formula, and blow Bingpeng Powder; take Qingyan Lige Decoction and Liushen Wan internally; when the pus has matured, use a knife or throat spear to puncture and drain the pus; after ulceration, modify Qingyan Shuanghe Yin and blow Zhuhuang Powder.

Qingyan Lige Decoction: Forsythia, Gardenia, Scutellaria, Mint, Saposhnikovia, Schizonepeta, Sodium Sulfate, Platycodon, Honeysuckle, Scrophularia, Rhubarb, Licorice, Coptis

Jinsuoshi: One *liang* and five *qian* of Nitre, two *qian* each of Bombyx Batryticatus and Realgar, five *qian* of Borax, four *fen* of Borneol, ground into fine powder.

Wubao Dan: Five *qian* each of calcined gypsum and Borax, one *qian* of Yao Huang (yellow orpiment), five *fen* of Chalcanthite, four *fen* of Borneol, ground into fine powder.

Tongguan Powder: One *liang* of Saponaria, five *qian* of Ligusticum, ground into fine powder.

Yulu Powder: XIAORONG Ye...

Bing She Powder: Take one *qian* each of Phellodendron bark, Coptis, and Mirabilite; five *qian* of deer-antler frost; five *fen* each of bile-processed copperas and licorice; two *qian* and five *fen* of borax; four *fen* of Borneol; and one *fen* of musk. Grind together into an extremely fine powder.

Qing-yan Shuang-he Drink: Platycodon root, Lonicera flower, Angelica, red peony, raw Rehmannia, Scrophularia, Poria in red, Schizonepeta, Moutan bark, Fritillaria, licorice, Pueraria, and Peucedanum.

Zhi-bai Ba-wei Pills (Anemarrhena & Phellodendron Eight-Ingredient Formula): Anemarrhena, Phellodendron bark, prepared Rehmannia, Cornus, Chinese yam, Moutan bark, Alisma, and Poria.

Fu-gui Ba-wei Pills (Aconite & Cinnamon Eight-Ingredient Formula): Prepared Rehmannia, Cornus, Chinese yam, Moutan bark, Alisma, Poria, prepared Aconite lateral root, and cinnamon bark.

Mouth-Rinse Formula: One *qian* each of Saposhnikovia, licorice, Lonicera flower, peppermint, Schizonepeta, salted plum, chestnut calyx, and shell. Decoct in water and use as a gargle.

Bing Peng Powder: Four *fen* of Borneol, five *qian* each of borax and Mirabilite, and six *fen* of cinnabar. Grind into an extremely fine powder.

Liu-shen Pills (a prepared proprietary medicine—details omitted).

Zhu Huang Powder: Five *qian* each of calcined gypsum and borax, two *qian* of realgar (lumbus), three *qian* of Ren Zhong Bai (processed human calculus), and four *fen* of Borneol. Grind together into an extremely fine powder.

.II Throat mass

Prominent lumps on both sides of the pharynx, shaped like nipples or silkworm moth, are called “ru’e” (tonsillitis) or “hou’e” (throat moth). When occurring on one side, it is “dan ru’e” (single tonsillitis); when occurring on both sides, it is “shuang ru’e” (double tonsillitis), which is mostly caused by accumulated heat in the lung and stomach, further congealed by wind pathogens. Initially, there is redness, swelling, and pain, hindering swallowing, accompanied by chills and fever; in more severe cases, the pain radiates to the ears, with cervical lymph node swelling and difficulty in turning the neck. Treatment involves externally applying Bingpeng Powder, internally taking Shufeng Qingre Decoction, and placing a small amount of Tiehou Yigong Powder under an ordinary plaster to stick on the neck corresponding to the sore throat—on the side where the pain is, or on both sides if both are painful. Remove after half a day when blisters appear, and prick them with a needle to release fluid. If this condition does not subside within four-five to six-seven days, with small white spots or yellowish-white pus-like membranes appearing on the lumps, this is a sign of erosion, commonly called "lan ru'e" (erosive tonsillitis). Continue using the previous formula but remove wind-dispelling herbs, increase the dosage of Scrophularia, shift from pungent-cool clearing to nourishing yin and clearing, and switch to Jinbuhuan to blow on the throat for removing decay.

Hard lumps protruding like nipples on either side of the pharynx, neither red nor painful, with slight swelling and pain when fatigued, difficulty in eating, and few systemic symptoms. The swelling and pain can subside on their own after rest, but the hard lumps cannot disappear. Called "shi'e" (stone moth), it is easily confused with tonsillitis. Its characteristic is the absence of subjective symptoms when not attacking.Regularly eating less spicy food and avoiding excessive fatigue can reduce or prevent episodes; even whenattacking, it is not as severe as tonsillitis and does not erode. During episodes, Bingpeng Powder can be applied externally, and Qingyan Lige Decoction can be taken internally with modifications.

Both tonsillitis and stone moth are difficult to fully resolve, and they tend to recur. Consider specialized treatments such as incision and cauterization, but these must be performed when the swelling and pain have subsided.

Bingpeng Powder: four *fen* of Borneol, five *qian* each of Borax and Sodium Sulfate, six *fen* of Cinnabar, ground into fine powder.

Shufeng Qingre Decoction: Schizonepeta, Saposhnikovia, Arctium, Licorice, Honeysuckle, Forsythia, Mulberry Bark, Red Peony Root, Platycodon, Angelica Tail, Trichosanthes Root, Scrophularia, Ligusticum, Angelica Dahurica

Tiehou Yigong Powder: Four *qian* of Mylabris, six *fen* each of Frankincense, Myrrh, Scorpion, Scrophularia, Dragon's Blood, three *fen* each of Musk and Borneol, ground into fine powder.

Jinbuhuan Powder: Five *qian* each of Watermelon Frost and Borax, six *fen* of Cinnabar, five *fen* each of Bombyx Batryticatus and Borneol, one *qian* of Human Urine Sediment, three *fen* each of Indigo Naturalis, Calculus Bovis, and Pearl Powder, ground into fine powder.

Qingyan Lige Decoction: Forsythia, Gardenia, Scutellaria, Mint, Schizonepeta, Saposhnikovia, Sodium Sulfate, Platycodon, Honeysuckle, Scrophularia, Rhubarb, Coptis, Licorice

III. White Erosion of the Throat

General sore and swollen throat conditions such as "throat wind" and "tonsillitis" may all present with white erosion, with the prominent and severe one being "diphtheria". Initially, there is slight fever or no fever, mental fatigue, redness and swelling in the throat, with pain or slight pain. Subsequently, white spots appear on both sides of the pharynx, which may also emerge after two to three days. The white spots can turn into strip-like or block-like membranes, grayish-white or slightly yellowish in color. The white membranes gradually expand, spreading to the inside and outside of the throat or the uvula, etc. The surface of the white membranes is smooth, with distinct edges, and they are not easy to peel off. If forced to peel off, bleeding will occur, exposing a layer of red and swollen fleshy surface, but it will be covered by newly formed white membranes in a very short time. In severe cases, the body temperature rises, the complexion is pale, the spirit is dull, there is a foul odor in the mouth, the white membranes expand rapidly, accompanied by hoarseness, phlegm and asthma, choking during eating, and other associated symptoms. If the white membranes extend to the trachea, they often block breathing and cause suffocation. The difference from the white erosion in "throat wind" etc. is that in throat wind and the like, there is mostly a yellowish-white pus-like substance covering the lumps, with scattered white spots that do not form tough flakes, which are easy to wipe off and do not bleed easily. Previous generations believed that the cause of this syndrome is related to seasonal epidemic toxins, so it is also called "epidemic throat". Those inclined to wind-heat often have accompanying chills, fever, headache, and a floating and rapid pulse. Treatment first involves relieving the exterior, clearing heat and detoxifying, using Sangge Decoction and taking Chuoyao Powder. After the exterior symptoms are relieved, continue with Yangyin Qingfei Decoction plus earth achyranthes. Those inclined to yin deficiency have no exterior symptoms initially, with a rapid and weak pulse, and should immediately nourish yin, clear heat and detoxify, using Yangyin Qingfei Decoction plus earth achyranthes, and taking Chuoyao Powder concurrently. In all cases, Qingliang Powder is blown into the throat. If generalized rashes appear after taking the medicine, it is a sign that pathogenic factors are exiting the body; do not mistake them for ordinary rashes, avoid nourishing yin, and thus cause delay.

"Throat gan" is also a condition where erosion occurs on the epidermis of the throat, mostly growing outside the throat pass near both sides of the uvula, and rarely found at the bottom of the throat. It is caused by the struggle between external wind and internal heat attacking the throat upward. Initially, there is flushing and pain, or blisters, followed by erosion, with scattered white spots, varying in number, up to more than ten, and inconsistent in size. There must be a red halo around the white spots, which is its characteristic. Generally, there are accompanying systemic symptoms such as chills and fever, with more pediatric patients, and some complicated with "mouth gan". Internally, take modified Puji Xiaodu Yin, and externally blow Xilei Powder.

"Lanhousha" (erosive throat with rashes), also known as "housha" or "lanhou dansha", initially presents with chills, fever, headache, vomiting, redness, swelling and pain in the throat, with erosion appearing after three to four days. Meanwhile, scarlet rashes emerge on the neck, gradually spreading to the chest, back, abdomen or limbs, and can cover the entire body within a day, except for the pale, spot-free area around the lips. This syndrome, caused by epidemic toxins steaming the lung and stomach, with blazing fire from the Jueyin and Shaoyin meridians upward excessively, is extremely severe. Treatment can be divided into three stages: In the initial stage, with chills, fever, restlessness, nausea, vomiting, sore, swollen and eroded throat, and a thin, greasy yellow or white tongue coating like accumulated powder, indicating epidemic pathogens stagnated in the qi level, pungent-cool exterior-releasing methods should be used to expel pathogens outward, using modified Jingfang Baidu Powder; for cases with severe interior heat such as foul breath and constipation, use Qingyan Lige Decoction. In the middle stage, with high fever, thirst, restlessness, sore, swollen and eroded throat, crimson tongue with a yellow coating in the center, dense scarlet rashes, and clouded consciousness, indicating epidemic pathogens transforming into fire and entering the nutrient level from the qi level, clearing the nutrient level, detoxifying, and assisting with dispersion and penetration are appropriate, using modified Heigao Decoction or modified Xichi Decoction. In the late stage, when rashes have subsided, heat is mild, and throat pain is relieved, nourishing fluids and yin is advisable, using Qingyan Yangying Decoction. For external treatment, blow Yuyaoshi Powder for sore and swollen throat, and Xilei Powder for erosion; meanwhile, pricking Shaoshang or Weizhong points to bleed can alleviate the condition.

Sangge Decoction: Mulberry Leaf, Pueraria, Mint, Bulbus Fritillaria Cirrhosae, Licorice, Akebia, Bamboo Leaf, Honeysuckle, Snakegourd Peel

Chuoyao Powder: Three *qian* each of Bulbus Fritillaria Cirrhosae, Earth Achyranthes, Phellodendron, one *qian* of Licorice, five *fen* each of Watermelon Frost, Human Urine Sediment, ten bamboo bees, ground into fine powder, add one *qian* of Bezoar and five *fen* of Borneol; take one *fen* each time, mixed with one tablespoon of boiled water, sipped slowly.

Yangyin Qingfei Decoction: Raw Rehmannia, Scrophularia, Rhubarb, Ophiopogon, Bulbus Fritillaria Cirrhosae, Moutan Bark, White Peony Root, Licorice, Mint

Qingliang Powder: Three *qian* of Borax, two *qian* of Human Feces Processed, one *qian* of Coptis, six *fen* of Mint, four *fen* of Indigo Naturalis, five *fen* of Borneol, ground into fine powder.

Modified Puji Xiaodu Yin: Forsythia, Mint, Puffball, Arctium, Schizonepeta, Bombyx Batryticatus, Scrophularia, Honeysuckle, Isatis Root, Platycodon, Human Feces Processed

Xilei Powder: Ivory Shavings, Pearl, Indigo Naturalis, Borneol, Uroctea, Calculus Bovis, Human Nail (proprietary medicine)

Modified Jingfang Baidu Powder: Schizonepeta, Arctium, Honeysuckle, Forsythia, Mint, Bamboo Leaf, Platycodon, Fermented Soybean, Puffball, Cicada Slough, Bombyx Batryticatus, Belamcanda

Qingyan Lige Decoction: Forsythia, Gardenia, Scutellaria, Mint, Saposhnikovia, Schizonepeta, Sodium Sulfate, Platycodon, Honeysuckle, Scrophularia, Rhubarb, Licorice, Coptis

Modified Heigao Decoction: Fresh Rehmannia, Fermented Soybean, Mint, Forsythia, Bombyx Batryticatus, Gypsum, Red Peony Root, Cicada Slough, Dendrobium, Licorice, Bulbus Fritillaria Thunbergii, Duckweed, Bamboo Leaf

Modified Xichi Decoction: Rhinoceros Horn, Dendrobium, Gardenia, Moutan Bark, Rehmannia, Mint, Coptis, Red Peony Root, Scrophularia, Gypsum, Licorice, Forsythia, Bamboo Leaf, Reed Rhizome, Imperata Rhizome, Golden Juice

Qingyan Yangying Decoction: Rehmannia, American Ginseng, Scrophularia, Asparagus, Ophiopogon, Trichosanthes Root, White Peony Root, Poria with Hostwood, Platycodon, Licorice, Anemarrhena

Yuyaoshi Powder: Five *qian* each of Watermelon Frost and Borax, six *fen* of Cinnabar, five *fen* each of Bombyx Batryticatus and Borneol, ground into fine powder.

IV. Itchy Throat

Itching in the throat with coughing is one of the symptoms of exogenous cough; refer to the entry “Cough” in visceral symptoms.

Dryness in the throat, with more itching than pain, pale red and slightly swollen, gradually developing red nodules in the throat, numerous ones resembling bayberry thorns, is called “throat lichen”. When stomach fire smolders and scorches the lung, use Guangbi Shunian Decoction and blow Qingliang POwder externally. If left untreated for a long time, it can develop moldy erosion, with successive layers of necrotic tissue, and small holes like ant bites around, mostly leading to death. Hence, it is commonly known as "heavenly white ants".

Guangbi Shunian Decoction: Raw Rehmannia, Bulbus Fritillaria Thunbergii, Scrophularia, Licorice, Arctium, Trichosanthes Root, Belamcanda, Forsythia, Bombyx Batryticatus, Bamboo Leaf

Qingliang Powder: Three *qian* of Borax, two *qian* of Human Feces Processed, one *qian* of Coptis, six *fen* of Mint, four *fen* of Indigo Naturalis, five *fen* of Borneol, ground into fine powder.

V. Dry Throat

Generally, dry mouth is due to heat in the lung and stomach damaging fluids, occurring during the day. Dry throat is mostly due to insufficient kidney yin, feeling dry after lying down, thus often being one of the yin deficiency symptoms. *The Inner Canon* states: "Dry throat, heat in the mouth like glue, select Foot Shaoyin."

VI. Hoarseness

Hoarse voice unable to form sounds is called "yin" (loss of voice), even completely unable to make sounds, commonly known as "aphonia". Sudden onset is mostly due to external pathogens attacking the lung; those developing from chronic illnesses are mostly due to damage to the lung's qi and yin, all related to the lung meridian. Previous generations compared it to "metal that is solid does not ring, and metal that is broken also does not ring". For wind-cold, use San'ao Decoction; for cold wrapping fire, use Maxing Shigan Decoction; for lung deficiency, use Qingyin Decoction; for lung deficiency with heat, use Yangjin Decoction.

Aphonia in pregnant women is related to fetal qi, called “zi yin” (gestational aphonia); refer to the entry “Hoarseness during Pregnancy” in gynecological symptoms.

San’ao Decoction: Ephedra, Almond, Licorice

Maxing Shigan Decoction: Ephedra, Almond, Gypsum, Licorice

Qingyin Decoction: Ginseng, Poria, Angelica, Raw Rehmannia, Asparagus and Ophiopogon, Dark Plum, Terminalia, Donkey-Hide Gelatin, Human Milk, Cow’s Milk, Pear Juice, Honey

Yangjin Decoction: Raw Rehmannia, Mulberry Bark, Almond, Donkey-Hide Gelatin, Anemarrhena, Adenophora, Ophiopogon, Honey

VII. Choking

Often caused by eating leading to reversed qi and coughing fits, except for occasional occurrences, it is more common in “yin fei” (aphonia and flaccidity) syndrome. Due to the epiglottis being unable to close the laryngeal cavity, food mistakenly enters the trachea, which is a severe symptom. Most sufferers have stiff tongue and slurred speech; use Acorus and Polygala to dredge heart qi, which cannot be treated by clearing the lung and smoothing qi.

VIII. Throat Sounding like Sawing

Qi obstructed by phlegm, with noisy breathing and throat sounds like sawing, is one of the symptoms of phlegm asthma; refer to the entry “Shortness of Breath” in visceral symptoms.

IX. Throat Sounding like Waterfowl

A characteristic of asthma, with a sharp waterfowl-like sound in the throat during asthma attacks; refer to the entry "Shortness of Breath" in visceral symptoms.

X. Throat Obstruction

Throat not red or swollen, no pain, food can be swallowed smoothly, but feeling as if there is roasted meat or a plum pit stuck in the throat, unable to spit out or swallow down, called "plum pit qi". Due to stagnation of the seven emotions and phlegm stagnation blocking the throat, it can be alleviated when in a good mood. Treat with Jiawei Siqi Decoction.

Jiawei Siqi Decoction: Poria, Magnolia Officinalis, Perilla Stem, Pinellia, Tangerine Peel, Green Tangerine Peel, Aurantium, Amomum, Arisaema, Medicated Leaven, Cardamom, Areca, Ginger

XI. Swollen and Painful Uvula

The uvula, also called the "small tongue" or "suspended yong", general swelling and pain of the uvula is called "suspended yong ptosis". Caused by eating spicy hot food or contracting wind-heat, blow Bingshe Powder externally; a folk remedy is to dip the tip of a chopstick in vinegar and then a little fine salt, apply to it, which can cure mild cases.

A blood blister at the tip of the lower end of the uvula, purple like a cherry, painful and hindering eating, called "suspended flag abscess". In addition to blowing Bingshe Powder, take Jiawei Ganjie Decoction internally; if necessary, pierce the blood blister to release purple blood.

Bingshe Powder: One *qian* each of Phellodendron, Coptis, and Sodium Sulfate, five *qian* of deer antler frost, five *fen* each of Chalcanthite and Licorice, two *qian* and five *fen* of Borax, four *fen* of Borneol, one *fen* of Musk, ground into fine powder.

Jiawei Ganjie Decoction: Raw Rehmannia, Scrophularia, Platycodon, Aurantium, Arctium, Saposhnikovia, Honeysuckle, Forsythia, Moutan Bark, stir-fried pangolin scales), Dandelion, Licorice

XII. Bone Stuck in Throat

Bones stuck in the throat, mostly fish bones. Folk remedies include slowly swallowing rice vinegar, or decocting Clematis Chinensis for slow drinking. *Sanyin Fang* contains Yuxie Wuyou Powder, but it can only treat pain from thin and soft fish bones. For hard and thick bones that can cause redness and swelling at the injured site, surgical removal should be performed.

Yuxie Wuyou Powder: Three *qian* each of Calcite and Borax, five *qian* each of Scrophularia, Cyrtomium Rhizome, Talc, Amomum, Sophora Tonkinensis, Coptis, Licorice, Aloe, and Schizonepeta, ground into powder; take one *qian* each time with water.

Section 10 Neck and Nape Symptoms

The front is the neck, the back is the nape. The Ren Meridian runs along the front, the Du Meridian runs along the back, and the three Yang Meridians of the hands and feet run along both sides. Due to the small area, there are not many clinical symptoms, and most appear simultaneously with other symptoms. However, when presenting as the main symptom, some can be extremely severe and stubborn, especially common in surgery. This section includes stiff nape, flaccid nape, pain, qi toxin, scrofula, goiter, locked-throat abscess, nape carbuncle opposite the mouthabscess, etc.

I. Stiff Nape

Stiffness of the back of the nape, inability to bend forward or turn left and right, gradually involving stiffness of the back, with opisthotonos, which is the main symptom of "convulsive disease". Convulsive disease is caused by consumption of body fluids and blood, leading to insufficient nourishment of the tendons and vessels, often appearing after blood loss, excessive sweating, or high fever damaging yin, with a thready, string-like, rapid pulse, and a shiny, dry, crimson tongue. It is advisable to nourish yin and calm wind, using Dadingfeng Zhu. Those caused by external pathogens are accompanied by chills, fever, headache, etc.; those with sweating are "soft convulsion", treated with Gualou Guizhi Decoction; those without sweating are "rigid convulsion", treated with Gegen Decoction. This syndrome must focus on preserving body fluids, so trichosanthes root and pueraria become the main medicines; for those with heat transformation and constipation, cooling and purging should be used to preserve yin. A few are caused by external dampness obstructing the meridians, as stated in *The Inner Canon*: "All convulsions and stiff nape are related to dampness". Accompanied by head distension and heaviness, soreness and pain in the neck tendons, use Qianghuo Shengshi Decoction.

Knife wounds infected with wind pathogens at the injured site can also easily cause stiffness of the nape and back, with frequent limb convulsions, called "golden wound convulsion" in *Chaoshi Bingyuan* (Chao's Etiology of Diseases), commonly known as "tetanus". Initially accompanied by chills and fever, with the risus sardonicus, it is advisable to dispel pathogens and detoxify, using Yuzhen Powder. In severe cases with internal invasion of pathogenic toxins, accompanied by increased nausea and vomiting, the injured site is not very red and swollen, with white scabs forming on the wound and discharge of dirty black water, use Wuhu Zhuifeng Powder. When convulsions stop and the condition improves, focus on nourishing blood and regulating.

If a child has persistent fever with stiff nape, "infantile convulsion" must be prevented; refer to the entry "Coma" in visceral symptoms.

Stiffness and immobility of the nape caused by improper head position during sleep or cold exposure, with soreness and distension when turning, called "stiff neck". It is advisable to perform massage on Fengchi, Fengfu, Jianjing points, etc., or needle Dazhu, Jinggu, Jianwaishu, Houxi points, etc.

Dadingfeng Zhu: White Peony Root, Donkey-Hide Gelatin, Turtle Shell, Rehmannia, Ophiopogon, Hemp Seed, Schisandra, Oyster, Turtle Shell, Licorice, Egg Yolk

Gualou Guizhi Decoction: Trichosanthes Root, Cinnamon Twig, White Peony Root, Licorice, Ginger, Jujube

Gegen Decoction: Pueraria, Ephedra, Cinnamon Twig, White Peony Root, Licorice, Ginger, Jujube

Qianghuo Shengshi Decoction: Notopterygium, Angelica Pubescens, Saposhnikovia, Ligusticum Sinense, Ligusticum, Vitex, Licorice

Yuzhen Powder: Saposhnikovia, Arisaema, Angelica Dahurica, Gastrodia, Notopterygium, White Aconite, Cicada Slough

Wuhu Zhuifeng POwder: Cicada Slough, Arisaema, Gastrodia, Scorpion, Bombyx Batryticatus

II. Flaccid Nape

Softness of the nape in children after a severe illness is due to severe deficiency of qi and blood. Since the back of the nape is traversed by the Du Meridian, tonics should be supplemented with yang-supporting ingredients, using Banlong Wan. If caused by congenital insufficiency, it is one of the "five flaccidities"; refer to the entry "Five Flaccidities in Children" in systemic symptoms.

Flaccid nape in chronic illnesses is mostly due to yang exhaustion and disorder of the Du Meridian, called "collapse of the heavenly pillar bone", which is difficult to treat. *The Inner Canon* states: "The head is the residence of clarity; when the head tilts and the gaze is deep, clarity is lost." The "head tilt" mentioned here refers to nape flaccidity.

Banlong Wan: Deer Antler Glue, Deer Antler Cream, Poria, Platycladi Seed, Cuscuta, Psoralea, Prepared Rehmannia

III. Thick Neck

A thick neck without redness, swelling, or pain, accompanied by chills, fever, and dizziness, is called "qi toxin", treated with Jiawei Huoxiang Powder. There are also cases marked enlargement deviated to the anterior neck, presenting with increased appetite, restlessness, palpitations, restless sleep, difficulty breathing, irritability, melancholy, and other manifestations of liver fire and liver qi stagnation; treat with Dayu Decoction method plus Prunella, Indigo Naturalis, Moutan Bark, and Sargassum.

Jiawei Huoxiang Powder: Agastache, Platycodon, Licorice, Green Tangerine Peel, Tangerine Peel, Bupleurum, Perilla, Atractylodes, Angelica Dahurica, Poria, Magnolia Officinalis, Ligusticum, Cyperus, Prunella

Dayu Decoction: Cimicifuga, Bupleurum, Ligusticum, Cyperus, Mulberry Bark, Tangerine Leaf, Tribulus Terrestris

IV. Throbbing Neck Vessels

The arteries of the Foot Yangming Meridian on both sides of the

Adam's apple are called "renying". In syndromes such as "edema", "asthma", and "palpitation", their pulsation is often obvious, serving as one of the diagnostic signs.

V. Cervical Lateral Nodules

Nodules found under the skin and above the fascia on the lateral side of the neck, either on the left, right, or both sides, with a few as one-two or more than four-five, are generally called "phlegm nodules" or "scrofula". There are various names in literature such as "phlegm scrofula", "stringed scrofula", "overlapping scrofula", and "mache and axillary goiter". Generally speaking, this syndrome can be divided into acute and chronic types: The acute type is caused by exogenous wind-heat with phlegm stagnating in the collaterals of Shaoyang and Yangming meridians. The nodules are pigeon egg-sized, with a diffused base, white in color, hard and swollen, accompanied by chills, fever, and stiff neck pain. It is advisable to dispel wind, clear heat, and resolve phlegm, using Niubang Jieji Decoction, and externally apply Jinhuang Powder mixed with tea juice. If fever persists after four-five days, swelling and pain worsen, and the top of the nodule gradually turns light red, suppuration and ulceration should be prevented. However, after ulceration, the pus drains and pathogens subside, making it easy to heal, which can be managed as ordinary ulcers. The chronic type is mostly caused by worry, anxiety, depression, and anger, emotional distress, with liver qi carrying phlegm-fire stagnating in the Liver and Gallbladder meridians. Initially, the nodules are bean-sized, one or three-five in number, gradually spreading, with unchanged skin color, hard on palpation, movable when pushed, no chills or fever, and no pain. Over time, there is slight pain, and the nodules become immovable. Treatment should soothe the liver, nourish blood, relieve depression, and resolve phlegm, using Xiaoyao Powder plus Pinellia and Tangerine Peel; for those with excessive liver fire, use Chaihu Qinggan Powder, and take Neixiao Luoli Wan, Xiaojin Dan, and Yunai Wan concurrently. Among them, Xiaojin Dan can prevent spreading, and Yunai Wan can promote pus and tissue growth for ulcerated cases, so they are more commonly used. This syndrome is not easy to ulcerate; when approaching ulceration, the skin first turns cyanotic. After ulceration, the pus is thin, mixed with cheese-like substances, and it is difficult to drain and heal in a short time. With proper management, it takes about two-three months; some patients have long-term unhealed wounds or recurrent ulceration leading to fistulas, or recurrence due to physical deficiency after healing. Recently, external application of Stellera chamaejasme powder has been effective in removing necrosis and promoting granulation.

Chronic scrofula is a stubborn disorder that not only occurs in the neck but can also extend to the submandibular area, supraclavicular fossa, chest, and armpits. It persists for a long time and can present with tidal fever, night sweats, emaciation, and mental fatigue, gradually developing into consumptive disease. Therefore, regardless of whether it is ulcerated or not, those with qi and blood deficiency should first strengthen the healthy qi and then treat the symptoms, using Xiangbei Yangrong Decoction. If the hardness does not subside or remains unulcerated, ulceration-inducing methods can be used: take a thin needle, heat it red-hot, pinch the nodule with fingers, and pierce the top four-five *fen* deep. For larger nodules, multiple holes can be needled. Phlegm or blood will flow out from the nodule; after it is exhausted, cover with Taiyi Gao. The next day, pus will form in the needle holes; insert Baijiang Dan strips to corrode, and still cover with Taiyi Gao to make the nodule fall off. However, the ulceration-inducing method is inevitably painful, and the medicinal strips used are highly irritating, so strict control is necessary—avoid deep and large punctures, and it is contraindicated for the elderly and weak. In addition, moxibustion can be used in combination. Zhu Danxi once said: " Locate one point at the bony cleft where the tip of the shoulder (acromial extremity) and the tip of the elbow (olecranon) meet, moxibustion seven cones; for left-sided disease, moxibustion the left side; for right-sided disease, moxibustion the right side; for bilateral disease, moxibustion both sides, which is often effective. Gu Shicheng also believed that selecting acupoints such as Jianjing, Feishu, Danzhong, Fengchi, Bailao, and Quchi, moxibustion three cones each, combined with internal treatment, yields quicker results."

Niubang Jieji Decoction: Arctium, Mint, Schizonepeta, Forsythia, Gardenia, Moutan Bark, Dendrobium, Scrophularia, Prunella

Jinhuang Powder: Arisaema, Tangerine Peel, Atractylodes Lancea, Phellodendron, Turmeric, Licorice, Angelica Dahurica, Trichosanthes Root, Magnolia Officinalis, Rhubarb (proprietary medicine)

Xiaoyao Powder: Angelica, White Peony Root, Bupleurum, Atractylodes Macrocephala, Poria, Licorice, Mint, Ginger

Chaihu Qinggan Powder: Raw Rehmannia, Angelica, White Peony Root, Ligusticum, Bupleurum, Scutellaria, Gardenia, Trichosanthes Root, Saposhnikovia, Arctium, Forsythia, Licorice

Neixiao Luoli Wan: Prunella, Scrophularia, Seaweed, Fritillaria, Green Salt, Mint, Trichosanthes Root, Clam Powder, Ampelopsis, Forsythia, Processed Rhubarb, Licorice, Raw Rehmannia, Platycodon, Aurantium, Angelica, Nitre (proprietary medicine)

Xiaojin Dan: White Frankincense, Aconitum Kusnezoffii, Trogopterus Dung, Earthworm, Momordica Cochinchinensis, Frankincense, Myrrh, Angelica, Musk, Ink Carbon (proprietary medicine)

Yunai Wan: Take an appropriate amount of fragrant stem taro, slice and dry in the sun, grind into fine powder, and make pills with soaked and desalted old jellyfish and decoction of water chestnut.

Xiangbei Yangrong Decoction: Cyperus, Fritillaria, Ginseng, Poria, Tangerine Peel, Prepared Rehmannia, Ligusticum, Angelica, White Peony Root, Atractylodes Macrocephala, Platycodon, Licorice, Ginger, Jujube

Taiyi Gao: Scrophularia, Angelica Dahurica, Angelica, Cinnamon, Red Peony Root, Rhubarb, Raw Rehmannia, Eupolyphaga Sinensis, Ferula, Calomel, Willow Twigs, Pagoda Tree Twigs, Human Hair, Dongdan (red lead), Frankincense, Myrrh, Sesame Oil (proprietary medicine)

Tumors growing in the neck are mostly caused by stagnation of qi and blood, hence the name. They gradually grow larger and, resembling tassels, are also called "yingliu" (goiter and tumor). The shapes of the tumors vary: some shrink and grow alternately, soft but not hard, with normal skin color; some are as soft as cotton or as hard as steamed buns, neither tight nor loose, shaped like an inverted bowl; some are hard with a purple color, covered with coiled blue veins like earthworms; some are purplish red with visible veins, a mix of hardness and softness, occasional pulling pain, and uncontrollable bleeding when broken; some are purplish black, hard as stone, immovable when pushed, and tightly adhering to the bone; others have a pale red color, soft but not hard. Generally speaking, the causes of goiter and tumor are mostly internal injury from the seven emotions, worry, anger, and stagnation of phlegm-dampness and blood stasis. Those with a soft texture that discharge pus or powdery pus after ulceration, with gradually subsiding swelling, are easy to cure; those that are hard, ulcerate and bleed, with increasing swelling and unrelenting pain, are difficult to treat. Internal medicines can be divided into three categories: resolving phlegm and softening hardness with Haizao Yuhu Decoction; regulating qi and breaking stagnation with Tongqi Sanjian Wan;

clearing the liver and relieving depression with Qinggan Luhui Wan. For external treatment, apply Taiyi Gao mixed with Hongling Dan.

The therapeutic effect on goiter and tumor is not very significant. Except for those with pale red skin that is soft but not hard, which can be surgically incised, others should not be easily pierced with knives or needles. In some areas, those caused by mountain mists and dampness have unchanged skin color, no pain or itching. *Shenshi Zunsheng Shu* (Mr. Shen's Book of Respecting Life) once formulated Yingnang Wan for its treatment.

Haizao Yuhu Decoction: Sargassum, Tangerine Peel, Fritillaria, Forsythia, Kelp, Pinellia, Green Tangerine Peel, Angelica Pubescens, Ligusticum, Angelica, Licorice, Sea Tangle

Tongqi Sanjian Wan: Ginseng, Platycodon, Ligusticum, Angelica, Trichosanthes Root, Scutellaria, Aurantium, Tangerine Peel, Pinellia, Poria, Arisaema with Bile, Fritillaria, Sargassum, Cyperus, Acorus, Licorice

Qinggan Luhui Wan: Angelica, Raw Rehmannia, White Peony Root, Ligusticum, Coptis, Green Tangerine Peel, Clam Powder, Saponaria, Licorice, Kelp, Aloe

Taiyi Gao: Scrophularia, Angelica Dahurica, Angelica, Cinnamon, Red Peony Root, Rhubarb, Raw Rehmannia, Eupolyphaga Sinensis, Ferula, Calomel, Willow Twigs, Pagoda Tree Twigs, Human Hair, Dongdan (Red Lead), Frankincense, Myrrh, Sesame Oil (proprietary medicine)

Hongling Dan: Six *qian* each of Realgar, Frankincense, Myrrh, and Nitre; one *liang* of calcined Borax; three *qian* each of Chlorite Schist and Borneol; two *liang* of Cinnabar; one *qian* of Musk, ground into fine powder.

Yingnang Wan: Realgar, Green Wood Aromatic, Areca, Kelp, Clam, Ampelopsis, Pinellia Ferment, Cinnamon, White Mustard Seed

VII. Sore Poison on the Neck

Sore poison on the neck is most severe when occurring at the front and back midlines. Those growing outside the Adam's apple are called "suohou yong" (locked-throat abscess), referred to as "meng ju" (fierce abscess) in *The Inner Canon*, indicating the dangerous nature of the condition. Initially, there is redness and swelling around the throat, high fever, and thirst, with a violent onset, even blocking the throat and making it difficult to swallow fluids. If the base is loose and suppuration occurs easily, it is a favorable condition; if it is hard and difficult to suppurate, it is severe; if pus forms but does not burst externally but penetrates inward, it is also a critical condition. This syndrome is mostly caused by upward congestion of wind-fire and phlegm-heat in the lung and stomach. Initially, use Niubang Jieji Decoction; for those with a tendency to suppuration, add pangolin scales and saponaria thorns to promote pus drainage. For external use, apply Yulu Powder mixed with honeysuckle dew, leaving a small hole in the center and keeping it moist to facilitate the penetration of medicinal effects; do not apply plaster. After ulceration, it can be managed like ordinary abscesses.

Those occurring at the midline of the back of the nape are called "duikou ju" (counterpart abscess). They are mostly caused by excessive consumption of rich and greasy foods, internal abundance of fire toxin and damp-heat, combined with external contraction of wind pathogens, leading to qi and blood stasis blocking the meridians. Initially, there is a millet-sized sore head on the hard lump, with itching and pain; the lump expands, the sore heads multiply, appearing red, hot, and increasingly painful. Pus forms inside the sore, and the sore heads start to decay, shaped like a beehive. It is necessary to wait for the pus to drain smoothly, the necrotic tissue to gradually fall off, and new tissue to start growing. This syndrome is accompanied by chills, fever, headache, and loss of appetite from the onset; these symptoms worsen as the condition progresses, and in severe cases, due to internal invasion of pathogenic toxins, it may be accompanied by delirium and convulsions. The area of decay varies in size, with the largest extending up to the occipital bone, down to the Dazhui acupoint, and sideways to the back of the ears. Weak individuals find it difficult to heal and generate new tissue. Therefore, the speed of the course and the prognosis (favorable or unfavorable) must be diagnosed based on the patient's qi and blood status and the severity of the pathogenic toxins. Generally, for excess syndrome in the initial stage, it is advisable to clear heat, dispel wind, promote blood circulation, and resolve stasis, using Xianfang Huoming Yin. For those with difficulty in pus drainage, use Tougong Powder. For those with deficiency of both qi and blood, use Tuoli Xiaodu Powder to strengthen healthy qi and expel toxins, with external application of Chonghe Gao. During the pus-draining stage, add Jiuyi Dan; during the healing stage, use Shengji Yuhong Gao mixed with Shengji Powder.

All those occurring on both sides of the neck are generally called "neck abscess". The treatment method is roughly the same as that for locked-throat abscess, except that locked-throat abscess is caused by accumulated heat in the lung and stomach, while this is caused by stagnant fire in the triple energizer attacking upward, leading to qi and blood stagnation.

Niubang Jieji Decoction: Arctium, Mint, Schizonepeta, Forsythia, Gardenia, Moutan Bark, Dendrobium, Scrophularia, Prunella

Yulu Powder: Hibiscus leaf, ground into powder.

Xianfang Huoming Yin: Angelica Tail, Red Peony Root, Saposhnikovia, Honeysuckle, Trichosanthes Root, Tangerine Peel, Angelica Dahurica, Pangolin Scales, Saponaria, Thorns, Fritillaria, Licorice, Frankincense, Myrrh

Tougong Powder: Angelica, Astragalus, Pangolin Scales, Ligusticum, Saponaria Thorns

Tuoli Xiaodu Powder: Ginseng, Astragalus, Angelica, Ligusticum, White Peony Root, Atractylodes, Honeysuckle, Poria, Angelica Dahurica, Platycodon, Saponaria Thorns, Licorice

Chonghe Gao: Redbud, Angelica Pubescens, Red Peony Root, Angelica Dahurica, Acorus (proprietary medicine)

Jiuyi Dan: Nine *qian* of calcined gypsum, one *qian* of elevator powder, ground into fine powder.

Shengji Yuhong Gao: Angelica, Angelica Dahurica, White Wax, Calomel, Licorice, Lithospermum, Dragon's Blood, Sesame Oil (proprietary medicine)

Shengji Powder: One *liang* each of Calcite, Talc, Cuttlefish Bone, Dragon's Bone; five *qian* each of Starch, Litharge, Alum Ash, Dried Cochineal, ground into fine powder.

Section 11 Shoulder and Back Symptoms

The shoulder is the meeting point of the three Yang meridians of the hands and feet, and also the domain of the lung. Diseases of the shoulder are mostly caused by direct invasion of external pathogens or lung disorders affecting the meridians. On the back, the Du Meridian runs through the spine in the middle, and the Foot Taiyang Meridian runs in four lines on the left and right alongside the spine. Therefore, back disorders caused by external pathogens mostly belong to the Taiyang Meridian; internal injury syndromes are mainly related to the Du Meridian, often accompanied by spinal deformation. In addition, the back is the residence of the chest, and the chest is where the lung is located; chest and lung diseases can also affect the back. Furthermore, the shoulders and back often suffer sprains and strains due to heavy lifting; this section also includes some traumatic symptoms.

I. Shoulder Pain

Shoulder pain focused on the back is often accompanied by back pain, caused by the Foot Taiyang Meridian being affected by wind-dampness, treated with Qianghuo Shengshi Decoction. Pain focused on the front, often radiating to the arm, is caused by the lung being affected by wind-heat, treated with Qianghuo Powder. Acupuncture and moxibustion at Jianjing, Jianyu, and other points are also advisable.

Excessive weight-bearing or forceful lifting of heavy objects can easily cause sprains and pain in the muscles around the shoulder. Initially, this manifests as restricted forward and backward movement of the arm at the painful area, with inability to lift it upward. In severe cases, the pain radiates to the neck, and over time, it becomes soreness and weakness, which should be treated by traumatic surgery.

Qianghuo Shengshi Decoction: Notopterygium, Angelica Pubescens, Ligusticum, Ligusticum Sinense, Saposhnikovia, Vitex, Licorice

Qianghuo Powder: Notopterygium, Saposhnikovia, Asarum, Ligusticum, Chrysanthemum, Scutellaria, Gypsum, Vitex, Peucedanum, Aurantium, Aloe, Licorice, Ginger

II. Shoulder Lifting

It is one of the symptoms of asthma. When lung qi rebels upward, breathing becomes difficult, with the mouth open and eyes protruding, and at the same time, the shoulders rise and fall, which is called "shoulder breathing". *Synopsis of the Golden Chamber* states: "Upper qi, facial edema, shoulder breathing, with a floating and large pulse, incurable." But generally, it appears in severe cases, especially during severe "asthma" attacks.

III. Drooping Shoulders

Both shoulders droop, unable to lift with strength, due to qi deficiency failing to raise, also called "shoulder collapse". *The Inner Canon* states: "The back is the residence of the chest; a curved back and collapsed shoulders mean the residence is decaying."

IV. Back Pain

Stiff back pain, involving discomfort in the back of the neck and shoulder blades, accompanied by chills, is caused by wind-cold attacking the Foot Taiyang Meridian, leading to sluggish meridians, generally treated with Jianghuang Powder. For treating back pain, Notopterygium and Saposhnikovia must be used to guide the medicine to the meridian. Also, since the lung governs the skin and hair, and the back is the residence of the chest, during treatment, methods to diffuse the lung can be combined to make it easier to dispel external pathogens. Use Sanhe Decoction, which is a compound of Xiangsu Powder, Erchen Decoction, and Wuyao Shunqi Powder.

Back soreness after sleeping, which gradually eases after getting up and moving, is due to qi and blood stagnation and disharmony of the collaterals. Use Shujin Decoction, combined with massage therapy.

Back pain from injury due to bending over and lifting weights, often accompanied by stiff neck, numb fingers, and inability to move the arm. Traumatic treatment should be applied.

Jianghuang Powder: Turmeric, Notopterygium, Atractylodes, Licorice

Sanhe Decoction: Ephedra, Perilla, Platycodon, Atractylodes Lancea, Tangerine Peel, Lindera, Ligusticum, Bombyx Batryticatus, Angelica Dahurica, Aurantium, Licorice, Dried Ginger, Poria, Pinellia, Cyperus

Shujin Decoction: Angelica, White Peony Root, Atractylodes, Licorice, Notopterygium, Turmeric, Pittosporum

V. Back Pain Radiating to the Heart

Back pain involving chest pain, called "chest impediment". It is one of the stomach pain syndromes, so *The Inner Canon* states: "The back and heart are interconnected in pain; treat Tiantu, the tenth vertebra, and Shangji. Shangji refers to the stomach duct." Refer to the entry "Chest Pain" in chest, hypochondrium, abdomen, and breast symptoms.

VI. Back Cold

People with yang deficiency often feel back cold, treated with Shengyu Decoction plus Cinnamon Twig. *Gujin Yijian* has the method of external application with Yuhan Gao.

Severe "phlegm-fluid retention" disease is often accompanied by a cold sensation in the center of the back, which is a phenomenon of spleen and kidney yang deficiency; refer to the entry "Cough" in visceral symptoms.

Shengyu Decoction: Astragalus, Ginseng, Raw Rehmannia,

Prepared Rehmannia, Angelica, Ligusticum

Yuhan Gao: Mash half a piece of ginger to get juice, add three *liang* of gelatin, one *qian* and five *fen* each of Frankincense and Myrrh, decoct and stir into a paste, then add a little Sichuan pepper powder and mix well, spread on leather paper and apply to the affected area, remove after five to seven days. It doesn't matter if small sores appear.

VII. Spinal Pain

Spinal pain mostly starts in the waist, involving the back, unable to straighten up; even if straightening up occasionally feels more comfortable, it cannot be maintained for long. In severe cases, there is a cold sensation in the middle line of the spine, and the waist is also cold, often as if wind-cold is invading, with a weak pulse, or accompanied by frequent and clear urination, and weak lower limbs. For kidney yang deficiency, it is advisable to warm and tonify the lower origin, using Yougui Wan plus Deer Antler Glue and Cibotium, or Wenshen Powder, and moxibustion at Shenshu point.

Spinal pain accompanied by a waist that feels as if it is breaking, a neck that feels as if it is being pulled, and headache radiating upward is due to obstructed qi movement in the Taiyang Meridian, treated with Qianghuo Shengshi Decoction.

Yougui Wan: Aconite, Cinnamon, Cornus, Yam, Prepared Rehmannia, Wolfberry, Roasted Licorice, Eucommia

Wenshen Powder: Prepared Rehmannia, Achyranthes, Morinda, Cistanche, Ophiopogon, Roasted Licorice, Schisandra, Poria with Hostwood, Dried Ginger, Eucommia

Qianghuo Shengshi Decoction: Notopterygium, Angelica Pubescens, Ligusticum, Ligusticum Sinense, Saposhnikovia, Vitex, Licorice

VIII. Protruding Spine

Partial protrusion of the vertebrae, which feel raised when pressed, mostly belongs to disorders of the Du Meridian. Due to severe yang deficiency and insufficient marrow failing to connect the bones, it leads to a hunched back, widened chest, and abnormal gait, called "hunchback" or "great hunchback", commonly known as "curved back". *The Inner Canon* states: "Yang qi, when refined, nourishes the spirit; when gentle, it nourishes the tendons. When opening and closing are impaired, cold qi invades, giving rise to great hunchback." This refers to this syndrome. It can also be caused by damp-heat: When large tendons are affected by heat, they contract and shorten; when small tendons are affected by dampness, they stretch and lengthen, gradually leading to a curved back and protruding joints. However, clinical cases are mostly deficient; in children, it is often due to congenital insufficiency. Treatment should use substances with rich nutritional properties to tonify the kidney and life gate, such as Banlong Wan or Guilu Erxian Jiao taken regularly.

Newborn infants whose backs are exposed to wind-cold invading the spinal bones, resulting in a curved back, called "turtle back", often becomes a chronic condition, treated with Songrui Dan. *Dongyi Baojian* (Korean Medical Treasures) points out: "If infants sit too early, it can also lead to hunchback with a high back like a turtle." Care should be taken.

Banlong Wan: Deer Antler Glue, Deer Antler Cream, Cuscuta, Platycladi Seed, Prepared Rehmannia

Guilu Erxian Jiao: Deer Antler, Turtle Shell, Ginseng, Wolfberry (proprietary medicine)

Songrui Dan: Pine Pollen, Aurantium, Saposhnikovia, Angelica Pubescens, Ephedra, Rhubarb, Peucedanum, Cinnamon

IX. Back Retraction

Backward bending and retraction of the back with inflexible meridians is called "opisthotonos". It often develops gradually from a stiff nape, mostly seen in "convulsive diseases" and "tetanus", etc. Refer to the entry "Stiff Nape" in neck symptoms.

X. Coccygeal Pain

The coccyx is at the lower end of the spine, traversed by the Du Meridian and Foot Shaoyin Meridian. Pain often radiates to the waist, making it difficult to straighten the back, with a preference for warmth and fondness for manual massage. Generally caused by kidney deficiency, so treatment focuses on tonifying the kidney, but blood stasis, qi stagnation, and invasion by cold-dampness can also cause pain. *Shenshi Zunsheng Shu* (Mr. Shen's Book of Respecting Life) records modified Bushen Decoction: for wind, add processed Aconitum Kusnezoffii and Gastrodia; for cold, add Cinnamon Twig and Aconite; for dampness, add Atractylodes Lancea, Atractylodes Macrocephala, and Peach Kernel; for heat, remove Psoralea and add Notopterygium and Black Soybean; for phlegm, reduce Anemarrhena and Phellodendron, add Arisaema, Pinellia, and Poria; for qi stagnation, reduce Anemarrhena and Phellodendron, add Cardamom, Sandalwood, Lindera, and Green Tangerine Peel; for blood stasis, remove Anemarrhena and Phellodendron, replace Angelica with Angelica Tail, add Cinnamon, Bupleurum, and Peach Kernel, with Trogopterus Dung for severe cases; for falls or sprains, remove Anemarrhena and Phellodendron, add Notopterygium, Angelica Pubescens, Frankincense, Myrrh, and Peach Kernel, or add Cinnamon and Red Peony Root. For external treatment, moxibustion at Baliao and other points, or apply Baozhen Gao.

Bushen Decoction: Psoralea, Fennel, Corydalis, Achyranthes,

Angelica, Eucommia, Anemarrhena, Phellodendron, Ginger

Baozhen Gao: Angelica, Astragalus, Ligusticum, Raw Rehmannia, Cinnamon, Sichuan Aconite, Kusnezoff Monkshood, Kaempferia, Fermented Soybean, Rhubarb, Angelica Dahurica, Atractylodes Lancea, Safflower, Cimicifuga, Evodia, Ephedra, Asarum, Galangal, Moutan Bark, Red Peony Root, Polygonum Multiflorum, Saposhnikovia, Notopterygium, Angelica Pubescens, Castor Bean, Guangdan (red lead), Ginger, Green Onion, Sesame Oil (proprietary medicine)

XI. Back Sore Poison

Back sore poison, with "fabei" (back abscess) as a major condition, is divided into upper, middle, and lower back abscesses, all belonging to the Du Meridian area, caused by stagnation of fire toxin. The upper back abscess grows below the heavenly pillar bone, affecting the lung, also called "fei hou fa" (abscess behind the lung); the middle back abscess grows in the center of the back, affecting the liver, also called "dui xin fa" (abscess facing the heart); the lower back abscess grows in the middle of the waist, affecting the kidney, also called "dui qi fa" (abscess facing the navel). Initially, all are millet-sized, with burning pain, numbness, and itching, general stiffness, alternating chills and fever, and sudden severe swelling after several days. It is advisable to perform moxibustion with garlic as a partition; if moxibustion is ineffective, moxibustion should be applied directly on the affected area until pain is felt, which indicates effectiveness. After moxibustion, pierce a hole at the top of the sore with a needle, then use a medicinal cylinder to draw out pus and blood, allowing toxic qi to drain outward without internal invasion. For those with exterior symptoms such as fever, chills, and absence of sweating, use Jingfang Baidu Powder to induce sweating; for those with both exterior and interior symptoms such as fever, aversion to heat, and dry stool, use Neishu

Huanglian Decoction to purge; for those with both exterior and interior symptoms, use Shenshou Weisheng Decoction to resolve both. When pus is about to form, supporting therapy is necessary; the rest is the same as the treatment for general swollen sores and ulcers. Regardless of age, this condition is favorable if it is highly swollen, red, lively, and painful; it is unfavorable if it is diffusely swollen, collapsed, scorched, withered, purple, or black. Heat toxin is easy to treat, yin deficiency is difficult to treat, and those with deficiency in both body and qi are even more challenging, requiring specialist treatment.

Jingfang Baidu Powder: Schizonepeta, Saposhnikovia, Notopterygium, Angelica Pubescens, Peucedanum, Bupleurum, Platycodon, Ligusticum, Aurantium, Poria, Ginseng, Licorice

Neishu Huanglian Decoction: Coptis, Scutellaria, Gardenia, Forsythia, Mint, Licorice, Platycodon, Rhubarb, Angelica, White Peony Root, Aucklandia, Areca

Shenshou Weisheng Decoction: Saponaria Thorn, Saposhnikovia, Notopterygium, Angelica Dahurica, Pangolin, Forsythia, Angelica Tail, Frankincense, Agarwood, Honeysuckle, Abalone Shell, Trichosanthes Root, Licorice, Safflower, Rhubarb

Section 12 Chest, Hypochondrium, Axilla, and Breast Symptoms

The area above the diaphragm is the chest, where the heart and lung reside. The heart and lung are two yang organs, gathering clear yang, also known as the clear and open region. Yu Jiayan once said: "The yang qi in the chest is like the sun shining in the sky; if the earthly qi rises, it will cause obstruction." Therefore, the yang qi in the chest is too weak to stir, which can allow cold turbidity to attack upward; similarly, upward counterflow of cold turbidity can also prevent yang qi from spreading, resulting in stuffiness, pain, and other symptoms. In terms of the functions of the heart and lung, restlessness of the heart spirit and failure of the lung to depurate can lead to symptoms such as heat, irritability, and fullness. The hypochondria are the regions of the liver and spleen; the Foot Jueyin and Shaoyang meridians also traverse the hypochondria and axillae. Therefore, symptoms of the hypochondria and axillae, whether distending pain, palpable masses, or external sores, are treated from the liver and spleen, with particular emphasis on the liver and gallbladder. It must be noted that the liver is located on the right, but its qi circulates on the left; Hua Boren once said: "The liver, as an organ, its treatment is on the left, and its storage is in front of the right hypochondrium and right kidney." Thus, left hypochondriac disorders are also treated from the liver. As for breast disorders, they mostly occur in women; since the nipple belongs to the liver and the breast belongs to the stomach, treatment generally focuses on the liver and stomach meridians.

I. Chest Pain

The chest is a yang position; insufficient yang qi or invasion by cold pathogens can block qi movement, hence it is called "chest impediment" in *Synopsis of the Golden Chamber*. The cold pathogens mentioned here include accumulated cold in the middle jiao, consumption of raw and cold foods, and phlegm-dampness, which are closely related to the stomach. Therefore, in addition to upper jiao symptoms such as panting, coughing and spitting, qi congestion, and shortness of breath, there also appear middle jiao symptoms such as pain radiating to the back, epigastric fullness, belching, and nausea. *Synopsis of the Golden Chamber* mainly uses Gualou Xiebai Baijiu Decoction to acridly warm and unblock yang, and also uses ingredients like cinnamon twig, pinellia, immature bitter orange, ginger, and poria, modifying according to symptoms, with this purpose in mind. Since chest impediment is caused by yang deficiency and cold obstruction, unblocking yang and dispersing cold will stop the pain; there are also cases of lingering cold-dampness with incessant pain, alleviated when yang prevails and exacerbated when yin prevails, called "chest impediment with alternating severity", for which Yiyi Fuzi Powder should be used. There are also cases of long-term recurrence, mostly due to qi stagnation leading to blood stasis, characterized by stabbing pain with fixed location, suitable for Gualou Xiebai Baijiu Decoction plus curcuma, immature bitter orange, angelica tail, peach kernel, etc., to promote qi and activate blood.

Chest pain on the left side, sudden onset like stabbing, accompanied by qi stagnation and congestion, or radiating to the left shoulder and arm, each episode lasting extremely briefly, most likely to occur after exposure to cold, labor, and mental stimulation, with a thready rapid pulse or irregular intermittent pulse, belonging to the category of heart pain. "True heart pain" is caused by sudden cold exposure, severe unrelenting pain, inability to speak, blue complexion, cold breath, hands and feet turning blue up to the joints, mostly fatal; emergency treatment with cinnamon, asarum, aconite, dried ginger, etc., may save a life. This condition is due to insufficient heart qi affecting the circulation of nutrient and defensive qi, with a mild and transient course, pain radiating to the shoulder and arm. Based on the "arm reversal" syndrome of the Hand Shaoyin and Taiyin meridians in *The Inner Canon*, ginseng, salvia, rehmannia, cinnamon twig, notoginseng, saffron, frankincense, etc., should be used to regulate heart qi and harmonize blood vessels.

Chest pain with a constant desire to press or pound the area for relief, craving hot water before the pain starts, and feeling more comfortable after drinking, called "liver stagnation", treated with Xuanfuhua

Decoction plus safflower and curcuma.

Chest pain radiating to umbilical abdominal pain with hardness, unbearable to touch, tidal fever in the afternoon, constipation, called "bound chest", treated with Daxianxiong Decoction; mild cases with only epigastric pain and shortness of breath, treated with Xiaoxianxiong Decoction. There is also "blood-bound chest" syndrome with chest and abdominal pain radiating to the waist, hypochondria, back, and spine, stabbing pain unbearable, even convulsions, mostly caused by menstrual onset during exogenous diseases like typhoid, leading to internal stagnation, or residual blood at the end of menstruation, treated with Yanhusuo Powder.

When a cough lingers and causes a pulling pain in the chest, it indicates blood stasis obstructing the collaterals; add an appropriate amount of peach kernel and safflower to the prescription. Chest pain from falls or impacts, painful breathing or coughing up blood, treated with Qili Powder taken with yellow wine.

Gualou Xiebai Baijiu Decoction: Trichosanthes, Chinese Chive, White Wine

Yiyi Fuzi Powder: Coix Seed, Aconite

Xuanfuhua Decoction: Inula, New Cinnabar, Scallion

Daxianxiong Decoction: Rhubarb, Glauber's Salt, Kansui

Xiaoxianxiong Decoction: Coptis, Pinellia, Trichosanthes

Yanhusuo Powder: Corydalis, Angelica, Cattail Pollen, Red Peony Root, Cinnamon, Turmeric, Frankincense, Myrrh, Aucklandia, Roasted Licorice, Ginger

Qili Powder: Frankincense, Myrrh, Angelica, Catechu, Safflower, Dragon's Blood, Cinnabar, Musk, Borneol (proprietary medicine)

II. Chest Distension

Feeling of blockage in the chest with difficulty in breathing is called "chest stuffiness" (xiong pi), commonly known as "chest oppression". The difference between chest stuffiness and chest pain is that chest stuffiness is a feeling of fullness without pain, while chest pain involves both fullness and pain; it also differs from distension, where distension involves internal swelling with an external visible shape, whereas chest stuffiness is an internal sense of fullness and oppression without an externally urgent swollen appearance. Li Dongyuan once said: "The Taiyin damp earth governs obstruction, which is earth ascending to the heart region causing stuffiness." Therefore, it is commonly seen in patterns of damp obstruction and qi stagnation, often treated with aromatic qi-moving herbs such as Agastache stem, finger citron, Turmeric, and Aurantium. For cases caused by liver-stomach qi stagnation, Turmeric, Aurantium, as well as Green Tangerine Peel, Tangerine Peel, and Cyperus are also commonly used. In cases of wind-induced cough with phlegm, accompanied by chest and diaphragm stuffiness, ancient physicians used Platycodon and Aurantium together, leveraging their ascending and descending properties to regulate qi movement.

In cases of insufficient heart qi and middle qi deficiency, patients often experience chest and diaphragm stuffiness due to difficulty in breathing; treatment should target the main symptoms, and general qi-regulating methods should not be used.

The "epigastric stuffiness" pattern in *Treatise on Febrile Diseases* refers to exterior pathogens transmitting inward, involving stuffiness in the middle epigastrium; refer to the entry "Abdominal Fullness" in abdominal symptoms.

III. Chest Heat and Irritability

A sensation of heat and restlessness in the chest is mostly an internal heat pattern. In exogenous diseases, the presence of heart vexation and restlessness indicates that external pathogens have transmitted inward but remain shallow; use Zhizi Chi Decoction to induce vomiting (Zhizi Chi Decoction uses raw Gardenia for its bitter properties to induce upward drainage and dispersion, and Fermented Soybean to resolve turbidity, dispel stagnation, and release the exterior, functioning as an emetic; if Gardenia is stir-fried black, it no longer induces vomiting but transforms into a method to release the exterior and clear heat). After fever subsides, chest heat and irritability, or accompanied by nausea, vomiting, and cough with counterflow, indicate residual heat lingering internally; use Zhuye Shigao Decoction.

In miscellaneous diseases, chest heat and irritability are mostly due to excessive heart fire; use Daochi Powder. For blood deficiency with fire flaring leading to insomnia and difficulty sleeping, use Huanglian Ejiao Decoction or Tianwang Buxin Dan. However, inability to fall asleep due to insomnia can also easily cause heat and irritability, accompanied by dry mouth and sweating; treatment should target the various causes of insomnia rather than focusing on heat and irritability.

Chest heat and irritability accompanied by heat in the palms and soles is called "five-center heat" (wuxin fanre); it may also occur together with tidal fever, both belonging to patterns of yin deficiency with internal heat, treated with modified Shengliao Liuwei Wan.

Restlessness during pregnancy is called "fetal restlessness" (zi fan); refer to the entry "Restlessness during Pregnancy" in gynecological symptoms.

Zhizi Chi Decoction: Gardenia, Fermented Soybean

Zhuye Shigao Decoction: Bamboo Leaf, Gypsum, Pinellia, Ophiopogon, Ginseng, Roasted Licorice, Japonica Rice

Daochi Powder: Raw Rehmannia, Akebia, Bamboo Leaf, Licorice

Huanglian Ejiao Decoction: Coptis, Donkey-Hide Gelatin, Scutellaria, White Peony Root, Egg Yolk

Tianwang Buxin Dan: Raw Rehmannia, Scrophularia, Ginseng, Salvia, Poria, Platycodon, Polygala, Jujube Seed, Platycladi Seed, Asparagus, Ophiopogon, Angelica, Schisandra

Shengliao Liuwei Wan: Raw Rehmannia, Cornus, Moutan Bark, Yam, Poria, Alisma

IV. Chest Sweating

Sweating only in the chest with no sweating elsewhere is called "heart sweat" (xin han), commonly seen in patterns of heart qi weakness. *Zhengzhi Zhunsheng* (Standards of Syndrome and Treatment) includes Shengui Zhuxin Fang, or use Shengmai Powder with Floating Wheat and Roasted Licorice.

Shengui Zhuxin Fang: one *liang* each of Ginseng and Angelica, placed inside a pig's heart, cooked, remove the herbs, and eat the heart.

Shengmai Powder: Ginseng, Ophiopogon, Schisandra

V. Protruding Sternum

Abnormal outward protrusion of the chest in children, resulting in a deformed chest, is called "pigeon chest" (jixiong). It is mostly caused by insufficient prenatal and postnatal qi, with wind pathogens, phlegm, and heat obstructing lung qi. Clinical symptoms include emaciation, cough, and rapid breathing. Treatment should first eliminate phlegm with Kuanqi

Yin; for severe heat, use Baihe Dan, followed by gradual nurturing and regulation.

Kuanqi Yin: Almond, Mulberry Bark, Tangerine Peel, Perilla Seed, Aurantium, Loquat Leaf, Ophiopogon, Licorice, Lepidium

Baihe Dan: Lily, Almond, Asparagus, Mulberry Bark, Akebia, Rhubarb, Glauber's Salt

VI. Chest Pain Radiating to the Back

Chest pain involving back pain is one of the symptoms of "chest impediment". Refer to the entry "Chest Pain" in this section.

VIII. Hypochondriac Pain

The hypochondria are the domain of the liver; anger-induced qi counterflow and melancholy-induced qi stagnation can both cause distension and pain. Thus, clinically, it is mostly attributed to liver qi disorders. The pain may be on one side, with intervals, and over time becomes a constant dull ache, worsening with fatigue, and can affect the chest, back, and lower abdomen, with a thready, string-like or string-like, slippery pulse. Treatment should soothe the liver and regulate qi, using Chaihu Shugan Powder; for qi stagnation transforming into fire, accompanied by dry mouth and a hot sensation at the pain site, use Qinggan Decoction plus Scutellaria; for liver blood deficiency, accompanied by blurred vision, tinnitus, and timidity with palpitations, use Siwu Decoction plus Bupleurum and Green Tangerine Peel. For acupuncture treatment, select points such as Ganshu, Danshu, Riyue, Qimen, Zhangmen, Zhigou, and Yanglingquan. For liver qi hypochondriac pain, initially involving qi, and over time entering the collaterals, add Salvia and Safflower to harmonize blood. If invading the stomach and overwhelming the spleen, presenting with abdominal distension, poor appetite, belching, flatulence, and irregular bowel movements, add Magnolia Officinalis, Amomum, and Areca Peel. For liver-spleen deficiency, use Xiaoyao Powder for nourishment. In severe deficiency, with persistent pinpoint pain under the hypochondrium, called “dry hypochondriac pain” in *Yixue Rumen* (Introduction to Medicine), use Ba Wu Decoction plus Aucklandia, Green Tangerine Peel, and Cinnamon; for heat, remove Cinnamon and add Gardenia and Coptis.

Hypochondriac pain like stabbing, fixed in location, worsening with pressure, with a string-like, choppy or deep, choppy pulse, mostly due to falls, fights, or injuries causing blood stasis in the hypochondrium, with bluish-purple marks on the skin over the pain site. It is advisable to focus on dispelling stasis, using Fuyuan Huoxue Decoction, in which Bupleurum acts as a channel-guiding herb, not for soothing the liver. Alternatively, use Jiawei Sanqi Powder; Sanqi (Notoginseng) is a key herb for traumatic injuries and can also be taken alone as powder.

Hypochondriac pain occurring during the progression of exogenous diseases, accompanied by alternating chills and fever, bitter taste in the mouth, dry throat, and dizziness, is a Shaoyang syndrome of typhoid, treated with Xiaochaihu Decoction. General colds can also be accompanied by dull chest and hypochondriac pain; other possible causes should be considered and changes monitored.

Phlegm-fluid retention with hypochondriac pain radiate to the supraclavicular fossa, worsening with cough, belonging to “lingering fluid retention”, treated with Tingli Dazao Xiefei Decoction with appropriate addition of Aurantium, Cyperus, Green Tangerine Peel, and Tangerine Peel.

Note: Recently prevalent “hepatitis” generally also presents with hypochondriac pain as the main complaint. Treatment mostly focuses on harmonizing and soothing the liver, using White Peony Root, Salvia, Bupleurum, Green Tangerine Peel, Turmeric, Aurantium, and Toosendan Fruit; for internal heat sensation, add Cirsium and Cephalanoplos; for distension, add Cyperus; for severe dampness, add Atractylodes Lancea; for nausea and decreased appetite, add Medicated Leaven; for fatigue or emaciation, add Astragalus or Donkey-Hide Gelatin. Generally speaking, treatment of this condition cannot avoid regulating qi, but must also attend to liver yin, and while treating the liver, attention must be paid to the spleen and stomach. Precisely for this reason, improper diet harms the stomach, excessive overwork harms the spleen, and unresolved worry harms the liver; attention should be paid to diet and rest, and in particular, avoiding melancholy and pessimism.

When there is dull pain and slight swelling at the Qimen acupoint, followed by distension and pain in the right hypochondrium, restlessness when lying on the side, and difficulty in urination and defecation, "liver abscess" must be guarded against. It is mostly caused by anger and stagnation leading to qi counterflow. Initially, Fuyuan Tongqi Powder is used, followed by Chaihu Qinggan Decoction. It is difficult to treat after pus formation.

Chaihu Shugan Powder: Bupleurum, White Peony Root, Cyperus, Ligusticum, Aurantium, Tangerine Peel, Licorice

Qinggan Decoction: White Peony Root, Angelica, Ligusticum, Moutan Bark, Gardenia, Bupleurum

Siwu Decoction: Raw Rehmannia, Angelica, White Peony Root, Ligusticum

Xiaoyao Powder: Angelica, White Peony Root, Bupleurum, Atractylodes, Poria, Licorice, Mint, Ginger

Ba Wu Decoction: Ginseng, Atractylodes, Poria, Licorice, Prepared

Rehmannia, White Peony Root, Ligusticum, Angelica

Fuyuan Huoxue Decoction: Angelica, Safflower, Peach Kernel, Rhubarb, Pangolin Scales, Trichosanthes Root, Bupleurum, Licorice

Jiawei Sanqi Powder: Notoginseng, Cyperus, Frankincense, Myrrh, Licorice

Xiaochaihu Decoction: Bupleurum, Scutellaria, Ginseng, Pinellia, Licorice, Ginger, Jujube

Tingli Dazao Xiefei Decoction: Lepidium, Jujube

Fuyuan Tongqi Powder: Green Tangerine Peel, Tangerine Peel, Snakegourd Seed, Pangolin Scales, Honeysuckle, Forsythia, Licorice

Chaihu Qinggan Decoction: Bupleurum, Raw Rehmannia, Angelica, Red Peony Root, Ligusticum, Saposhnikovia, Forsythia, Arctium, Scutellaria, Gardenia, Trichosanthes Root, Licorice

IX. Hypochondriac Distension

Distension and discomfort in the hypochondria, belonging to liver qi stagnation, can lead to pain over time, and often affect the chest and epigastrium, causing stuffiness. In women, breast distension is felt; use Zhiqiao Powder with addition of Green Tangerine Peel, Tangerine Leaf, Turmeric, etc.

Zhiqiao Powder: Aurantium, Licorice

X. Hard Mass under the Hypochondrium

It is one of the accumulations of the five *zang* organs. The one in the left hypochondrium is called “feiqi” (fatty qi), as large as an inverted cup. If not cured for a long time, it can cause vomiting and retching, or pain radiating to the lower abdomen, cold feet, and spasms; use Daqiqi

Decoction and take Feiqi Wan concurrently. The one in the right hypochondrium is called "piqi" (stagnant qi), causing stuffiness and discomfort, affecting the chest and back with pain. Over time, it leads to abdominal fullness, vomiting, and nausea, accompanied by jaundice; Daqiqi Decoction is suitable, with concurrent use of Piqi Wan. Both Feiqi Wan and Piqi Wan contain croton cream, which is drastic; the dosage must be carefully considered and controlled.

Prolonged malaria can lead to the formation of a mass in the left hypochondrium, palpable and solid, with epigastric and abdominal discomfort, poor appetite, fatigue, emaciation, sallow complexion, and a soft, thready pulse. Slight exertion can trigger recurrence of chills and fever, called "zhengmu" (malarial mass). Treatment should soften hardness, resolve stagnation, dispel stasis, and eliminate phlegm, using Biejia Jian Wan. This pill is relatively drastic; since this condition is often accompanied by qi and blood deficiency, it should be used in combination with qi and blood-nourishing formulas. During episodes of chills and fever, it should be used together with anti-malarial formulas; refer to the entry "Alternating Chills and Fever" in systemic symptoms.

Daqiqi Decoction: Sparganium, Zedoary, Green Tangerine Peel, Tangerine Peel, Agastache, Platycodon, Cinnamon, Alpinia Oxyphylla, Cyperus, Licorice

Feiqi Wan: Bupleurum, Coptis, Magnolia Officinalis, Sichuan Pepper, Zedoary, Kelp, Ginseng, Saponaria, Poria, Sichuan Aconite, Dried Ginger, Croton Cream

Piqi Wan: Magnolia Officinalis, Coptis, Evodia, Scutellaria, Atractylodes, Artemisia Capillaris, Amomum, Dried Ginger, Poria, Ginseng, Alisma, Sichuan Aconite, Sichuan Pepper, Cinnamon, Croton Cream

Biejia Jian Wan: Turtle Shell, Scutellaria, Bupleurum, Dried Ginger, White Peony Root, Cinnamon Twig, Rhubarb, Black Fan, Mousewife, Lepidium, Pyrrosia, Magnolia Officinalis, Moutan Bark, Dianthus, Chinese Trumpet Flower, Pinellia, Ginseng, Donkey-Hide Gelatin, Eupolyphaga, Wasp Nest, Sodium Nitrate, Dung Beetle, Peach Kernel (proprietary medicine)

XI. Axillary Nodules

Nodules in the axilla as large as eggs with unchanged skin color, mostly caused by stagnation of liver qi and phlegm turbidity, commonly known as "phlegm nodules", which are actually a type of scrofula. Therefore, they often appear simultaneously with cervical nodules; treat with Xiaoke Wan. Refer to the entry "Cervical Nodules" in neck symptoms.

Xiaoke Wan: Tangerine Peel, Red Poria, Rhubarb, Forsythia, Scutellaria, Gardenia, Pinellia Ferment, Scrophularia, Oyster, Trichosanthes Root, Platycodon, Snakegourd Seed, Bombyx Batryticatus, Licorice

XII. Axillary Moisture

Axillary moisture like sweating is called "louye" (axillary leakage). Apply Liuwu Powder, which also treats moisture in the inguinal area.

Liuwu Powder: Two *liang* each of dried wolfberry root, dried rose root, and licorice; one *liang* each of lead powder, pokeweed root, and talc. Grind into powder and apply with vinegar.

XIII. Axillary Odor

Foul smell emanating from the armpits like a wild fox, commonly known as "fox odor". Apply Mituoseng Powder with a little dried alum.

Zhu Danxi once had a treatment for this condition: Keep a large field snail in water, wait for the operculum to open, use a needle to pick one piece of croton meat and place it inside the snail, place it upside down in a cup, and it will naturally turn into liquid; take it to apply on the armpits.

Mituoseng Powder: Two *qian* each of realgar, sulfur, and cnidium; one *qian* each of litharge and stone yellow; five *fen* of calomel. Grind into fine powder.

XIV. Breast Distension

Breast distension is common in liver qi syndromes. "Dysmenorrhea" caused by liver qi stagnation often presents with breast distension, even dull pain, especially before menstruation. For treatment, refer to the entries "Hypochondriac Distension" in this section and "Dysmenorrhea" in gynecological symptoms.

XV. Breast Nodules

Breast nodules vary in size, mostly with smooth surfaces, not attached to the skin, movable when pressed, with unchanged skin color, no fever, and no pain or slight pain. They have names such as "rulì" (breast nodules), "rupǐ" (breast lump), and "rǔláo" (breast consumption, also called "rǔtán" (breast phlegm)), all caused by disharmony between the liver and spleen, and stagnation of qi and phlegm. Among them, rulì mostly occurs in adolescent girls, rupǐ is more common in middle-aged and elderly women, and rǔláo is not limited by age, often growing slightly above the breast. Since the breast belongs to the stomach and the nipple belongs to the liver, treatment focuses on soothing the liver, harmonizing the stomach, regulating qi, and relieving stagnation, using Qinggan Jieyu Decoction and Lianqiao Yinzi with modifications.

In men, kidney deficiency, liver dryness, and stagnation of worry, anger, and fire can also cause nodules in the breast, which may develop dull pain over time. Use single-flavor green tangerine peel or tangerine leaves decocted for oral administration.

Qinggan Jieyu Decoction: Angelica, White Peony Root, Prepared Rehmannia, Bupleurum, Ginseng, Atractylodes, Fritillaria, Pinellia, Poria, Ligusticum, Moutan Bark, Tangerine Peel, Red Poria, Licorice, Gardenia, Ginger

Lianqiao Yinzi: Forsythia, Ligusticum, Snakegourd, Tangerine Leaf, Green Tangerine Peel, Peach Kernel, Licorice, Saponaria Thorn

XVI. Nipple Fissure

Fissures on the nipple or nipple neck are mostly caused by infants biting during breastfeeding when teething, or by infants forcefully sucking on retracted nipples, or by excessive milk overflow infiltrating and causing erosion. However, it is also related to accumulation of liver fire and damp-heat. Patients experience knife-like pain, bleeding when rubbed, or discharge of greasy fluid, or formation of yellow scabs. It tends to recur after healing, and due to pain, milk is often not fully drained, leading to secondary breast abscess. External application of Sanshi Powder is advisable; if necessary, take Longdan Xiegan Decoction internally.

Sanshi Powder: Equal parts of calamine, calcined gypsum, and red halloysite, ground into fine powder, mixed with sesame oil for application.

Longdan Xiegan Decoction: Gentiana, Scutellaria, Gardenia, Alisma, Akebia, Plantago Seed, Angelica, Raw Rehmannia, Bupleurum, Licorice

XVII. Breast Sore Poison

During lactation, breast lumps, swelling and pain, poor milk flow, chills, fever, and headache, which is mostly caused by infants blowing air while suckling, obstruction of milk collaterals, or excessive milk with infants eating less, leading to milk stasis, called "external blowing breast abscess". Internally, use Gualou Niubang Decoction plus dandelion, or add Akebia to promote lactation; for redness and swelling, apply Yulu Powder externally. After two to three days, subsidence of fever and reduction of pain indicate resolution. If fever persists, the lump enlarges, and redness and pain intensify, suppuration is imminent; add Angelica, Red Peony Root, and Pangolin to the prescription. After about ten days, the center of the hard lump gradually softens, and when pressed, it feels fluctuant, indicating mature pus, which should be incised and drained. The incision must be radial to avoid excessive damage to milk collaterals. Use Jiuyi Dan to draw out pus, with medicated thread drainage, managed as ordinary ulcers. During the sixth or seventh month of pregnancy, when fetal qi is exuberant and stomach heat is congested, abscess can also form, called "internal blowing breast abscess". Initially, the skin color is unchanged, gradually turning red and ulcerating; use Juye Powder internally, with attention to protecting the fetus. This condition is harder to resolve than external blowing breast abscess, with slower pus formation; after ulceration, it often heals only after childbirth.

Breast lumps that are hard, wood-like and painful, with unchanged or slightly red and hot skin, and mild chills and fever, called "breast abscess". Caused by stagnation of liver qi and stomach heat, unrelated to lactation or pregnancy, leaning towards yin syndromes, with slower pus formation than breast abscess—breast abscess matures in 14 days, while this takes about a month to suppurate. Initially, Gualou Niubang Decoction is also used; if chills and fever subside but swelling remains, continue with Fuyuan Tongqi Powder plus Angelica, Red Peony Root, and Safflower, with external application of Chonghe Gao mixed with Hongling Dan.

After ulceration, treat as ordinary ulcers.

Initially, a breast lump the size of a longan or walnut, uneven, hard, with skin and nucleus connected, immovable when pushed, painless, itchy, red, or hot. Breast lump gradually grows, only causing pain after years, with unrelenting pain. At this stage, the swelling is like a pile of millet or an inverted bowl, with a purple top and visible blood streaks, rotting before ulcerating. After ulceration, the root swelling becomes harder, with foul-smelling watery discharge, irregular ulcer edges, deep central depression, even severed blood vessels, or death from uncontrollable bleeding due to rage, which is mostly caused by excessive melancholy and worry, reversed liver and spleen qi blocking meridians, called "breast rock", the most intractable among breast external ulcers. Another type of breast rock occurs in the areola, initially resembling eczema, with surface erosion and bleeding, later nipple retraction, hard surrounding tissue, and purplish-brown skin. Another type has a breast lump with central elasticity, with nipple bleeding before ulceration. "Breast rock" is generally difficult to treat, avoiding surgery, moxibustion, acupuncture, and corrosive drugs. Commonly used internal prescriptions: initially use Shenxiao Gualou Powder, then Qinggan Jieyu Decoction, and when the ulcer forms, use Xiangbei Yangrong Decoction.

Gualou Niubang Decoction: Snakegourd Seed, Arctium, Trichosanthes Root, Scutellaria, Tangerine Peel, Gardenia, Forsythia, Saponaria Thorn, Honeysuckle, Licorice, Green Tangerine Peel, Bupleurum

Yulu Powder: Hibiscus leaf, ground into powder.

Jiuyi Dan: Nine *qian* of calcined gypsum, 1 *qian* of elevator powder, ground into fine powder.

Juye Powder: Tangerine Leaf, Bupleurum, Green Tangerine Peel,

Tangerine Peel, Ligusticum, Gardenia, Gypsum, Scutellaria, Forsythia, Licorice

Fuyuan Tongqi Powder: Green Tangerine Peel, Tangerine Peel, Snakegourd Seed, Pangolin Scales, Honeysuckle, Forsythia, Licorice

Chonghe Gao: Redbud Bark, Angelica Pubescens, Red Peony Root, Angelica Dahurica, Acorus (proprietary medicine)

Hongling Dan: Realgar, Frankincense, Borax, Chlorite Schist, Myrrh, Borneol, Nitre, Cinnabar, Musk (proprietary medicine)

Shenxiao Gualou Decoction: Trichosanthes, Angelica, Licorice, Frankincense, Myrrh

Qinggan Jieyu Decoction: Prepared Rehmannia, Angelica, White Peony Root, Atractylodes, Poria, Fritillaria, Gardenia, Ginseng, Pinellia, Bupleurum, Moutan Bark, Tangerine Peel, Ligusticum, Cyperus, Licorice, Ginger

Xiangbei Yangrong Decoction: Cyperus, Fritillaria, Ginseng, Poria, Tangerine Peel, Prepared Rehmannia, Ligusticum, Angelica, White Peony Root, Atractylodes, Platycodon, Licorice, Ginger, Jujube

Section 13 Waist Symptoms

The waist is the residence of the kidney. All meridians of the body, both descending from above and ascending from below, pass through the waist, especially the Dai Meridian, which encircles the waist like a belt. Therefore, although waist symptoms are not complex, their pathogenesis is relatively extensive. Generally speaking, for waist symptoms, the kidney is the main internal organ involved; in terms of meridians, it is closely related to the Foot Shaoyin, Taiyang, and Dai Meridians. Disorders involving the zang organs are mostly deficient, while those involving the meridians are mostly due to cold-dampness and sprains. Due to insufficient kidney essence, external pathogens can take advantage of the deficiency to invade; external pathogen invasion can also affect kidney qi. Clinically, these two cannot be completely separated, and particular importance should be attached to kidney function.

I. Low Back Pain

The waist is the external manifestation of the kidney. Low back pain caused by excessive sexual activity, spermatorrhea, involuntary emission, women's uterine bleeding and leukorrhea, as well as weakened essence in the elderly, all fall into the category of kidney deficiency low back pain. This kind of low back pain develops gradually; initially, there is only a feeling of soreness and weakness, with dull, lingering pain that is not severe. It is often accompanied by soreness and weakness of the spine, legs, and feet, inability to stand or walk for long, slight relief when sitting or lying down, and worsening with exertion, with a thready weak or deficient pulse. Since the kidney is the organ of water and fire, treatment must distinguish between yin deficiency and yang deficiency. For yin deficiency low back pain, accompanied by internal heat, heart vexation, dizziness, and tinnitus, nourishing yin and tonifying the kidney is appropriate, using Duzhong Wan. For yang deficiency low back pain, accompanied by fatigue, shortness of breath, fear of cold, and frequent urination, supporting yang and tonifying the kidney is appropriate, using Weishen Wan. If low back pain persists for a long time and occurs from time to time, it is often due to both kidney yin and yang deficiency; replenishing essence is appropriate, using Wubi Shanyao Wan. Ancient formulas for treating kidney deficiency low back pain also include Qing'e Wan, Busui Dan, Zhuangben Wan, and Yangshen Wan, etc. These formulas are carefully formulated; in addition to the main purpose of tonifying the kidney, they address the main and secondary symptoms. Clinically, Prepared Rehmannia, Cornus, Cistanche, Wolfberry, Psoralea, Eucommia, Fennel, and achyranthes are generally used as basic medicines; for cold bias, add Aconite and Morinda; for heat bias, add Turtle Shell and stir-fried Phellodendron. In addition, pig kidneys and sheep kidneys can also be appropriately used. A folk remedy uses a pair of pig kidneys, washed without chopping, added with one *liang* of Eucommia and two slices of ginger, boiled until very tender, and the soup and pig kidneys are eaten together, which is effective.

Low back pain caused by wind-cold invading the meridians is characterized by stiffness of the lower back, difficulty in turning, a cold sensation in the waist, relief with warmth, and a deep tight pulse, treated with Jiangfu Decoction plus Cinnamon and Eucommia. Shen Jin'ao once said: Single-flavor Eucommia, stir-fried with ginger juice and ground into powder, one *qian* taken with wine, specifically treats kidney qi low back pain and also cold-wind pain; alternatively, wine-fried Achyranthes can be used. Sitting or lying on damp ground, or exposure to dew, with a cold sensation in the waist as if sitting in water, heavy body, and the waist feeling as if carrying a heavy object, with a deep slow pulse, is cold-damp low back pain, called "kidney fixation" in *Synopsis of the Golden Chamber*, treated with Ganjiang Lingzhu Decoction. All low back pain caused by wind-cold-damp pathogens occurs in the lower back or involves both sides; if pain is also present in the Huantiao (GB30) and radiates to the thigh and knee, it should be treated as "painful obstruction"; refer to the entry "Lower Limb Pain" in limb symptoms.

Low back pain caused by strenuous lifting, sprains, or contusions is generally referred to as sprain-induced low back pain, characterized by sudden pain that restricts movement, unbearable pain during breathing or coughing, and a preference for lying prone. It is all due to qi and blood stagnation; initially, Ruxiang Chentong Powder is used, and for retained blood stasis, Tiaorong Huoluo Decoction is used. This condition is most likely to occur in manual laborers; use Shujin Powder with added Achyranthes, Peach Kernel, Frankincense, and Myrrh, grind into powder in equal parts, take 2 *qian* with warm stewed yellow wine, and undergo traction, lifting, and massage reduction by traumatologists to avoid prolonged duration.

Duzhong Wan: Eucommia, Turtle Shell, Phellodendron, Anemarrhena, Wolfberry, Galla Chinensis, Angelica, White Peony Root, Astragalus, Psoralea, Pig Spinal Cord

Weishen Wan: Cistanche, Psoralea, Cuscuta, Astragalus Complanatus, Eucommia, Achyranthes, Cinnamon, Fenugreek, Dioscorea Collettii, Pig Kidney

Wubi Shanyao Wan: Yam, Prepared Rehmannia, Cornus, Cistanche, Deer Antler Glue, Morinda, Psoralea, Cuscuta, Eucommia, Dipsacus, Achyranthes, Drynaria, Papaya, Dioscorea Collettii, Cinnamon, Poria, Alisma, Green Salt

Qing'e Wan: Eucommia, Psoralea, Walnut Meat

Busui Dan: Deer Antler, Eucommia, Psoralea, Myrrh, Walnut Meat

Zhuangben Wan: Eucommia, Psoralea, Cistanche, Morinda, Fennel, Pig Kidney

Yangshen Wan: Deer Antler, Fennel, Cuscuta, Sheep Kidney

Jiangfu Decoction: Aconite, Roasted Ginger

Ganjiang Lingzhu Decoction: Dried Ginger, Atractylodes, Poria, Licorice

Ruxiang Chentong Powder: Frankincense, Myrrh, Angelica, Red

Peony Root, Saposhnikovia, Dragon's Blood, Cinnamon, Angelica Dahurica, Turtle Shell, Achyranthes, Gastrodia, Notopterygium, Areca, Tiger Bone, Pyrite, Typhonium, Xanthium, Drynaria, Acanthopanax

Tiaorong Huoluo Decoction: Rhubarb, Achyranthes, Red Peony Root, Angelica, Almond, Notopterygium, Raw Rehmannia, Safflower, Ligusticum, Platycodon

Shujin Powder: Corydalis, Cinnamon, Angelica

II. Waist Soreness

Soreness in the waist that fails to support the body after illness or exertion is mostly a sign of insufficient kidney yin. It is also often accompanied by soreness in general low back pain; for treatment, refer to the entry "Low Back Pain" in this section.

It is common in menstrual and leukorrheal diseases in gynecology, especially in "white leukorrhea" due to insecure Dai Meridian, where waist soreness is more obvious; refer to the entries "Low Back Pain During Menstruation" and "Red and White Leukorrhea" in gynecological symptoms.

III. Heavy Sensation in the Waist

Low back pain with a heavy sensation, described in *Synopsis of the Golden Chamber* as "like carrying five thousand coins", belongs to the "kidney fixation" syndrome; refer to the entry "Low Back Pain" in this section.

IV. Cold Sensation in the Waist

A cold sensation in the waist, as if cold wind is blowing into it, is one of the symptoms of yang deficiency and also a sign of wind-cold low back pain. Treatment should warm and tonify the kidney's source; externally apply Wang Haicang Daibu Gao on the waist eyes.

Daibu Gao: Equal parts of Aconite, Cnidium, Evodia, Cinnamon, Iris Seed, Aucklandia, ground into powder, mixed with 1 spoon of wheat flour and ginger juice to make a paste, spread on paper and applied, left on overnight, its effect can replace 100 moxibustion cones.

V. Waist Feeling Bound Like a Rope

A tight, rope-like sensation around the waist is mostly a disorder of the Dai Meridian; dispersing stagnation with acrid herbs and relieving urgency with sweet herbs is appropriate, using Tiaogan Powder.

In lower limb paraplegia, waist stiffness and loss of sensation are common, gradually spreading upward with the progression of the disease, accompanied by tightness in the chest, without pain; treatment focuses on warming the kidney. Refer to the entry "Lower Limb Paralysis" in limb symptoms.

Tiaogan Powder: Cinnamon, Angelica, Ligusticum, Achyranthes, Asarum, Acorus, Jujube Seed, Roasted Licorice, Pinellia, Ginger, Jujube

VI. Waist Sore Poison

Those occurring in the fleshy depressions on both sides of the lumbar vertebrae are called "Shenshu fa" (abscess at Shenshu), and those between the waist and hip are called "Zhongshi ju" (central stone abscess). Internal and external treatments are the same as for ordinary carbuncles and abscesses. Prominent among them is "Chan yao huo dan" (waist-encircling fiery erysipelas), commonly known as "she chuan chuang" (snake-like clustered sores), which appear as bead-like clusters around the waist, with dry and wet types. The dry type is red, patchy like clouds, with wind rash-like papules, itchy and feverish, belonging to wind-fire of the heart and liver meridians, treated with Longdan Xiegan Decoction; the wet type is yellowish-white, with blisters of varying sizes that rupture and ooze fluid, more painful than the dry type, belonging to damp-heat of the spleen and lung meridians, treated with Chushi Weiling Decoction. If this condition is not treated promptly, it spreads all over the waist, and the toxin invades the navel, causing abdominal distension, stuffiness, and vomiting.

Longdan Xiegan Decoction: Gentiana, Raw Rehmannia, Forsythia, Plantago, Alisma, Akebia, Scutellaria, Coptis, Angelica, Gardenia, Rhubarb, Licorice

Chushi Weiling Decoction: Atractylodes Lancea, Atractylodes Macrocephala, Magnolia Officinalis, Tangerine Peel, Polyporus, Alisma, Red Poria, Talc, Saposhnikovia, Gardenia, Akebia, Cinnamon, Licorice, Rush

Section 14 Abdominal and Umbilical Symptoms

The abdomen belongs to yin; the three yin organs—liver, spleen, and kidney—are all located in the abdomen. Its divisions are: the upper abdomen, i.e., Zhongwan, belongs to Taiyin; the umbilical abdomen belongs to Shaoyin; the left and right lower abdomen belong to Jueyin; the area below the umbilicus, the lower abdomen, belongs to the extraordinary channels Chong and Ren. The stomach is attributed to Zhongwan, and the intestines to the umbilical abdomen. Clinically, diagnosis and treatment are mostly based on the location combined with etiology and symptoms. Etiologically, there are cold, heat, deficiency, excess, qi stagnation, stasis obstruction, worm accumulation, etc., with rather complex syndromes. This section focuses on pain and distension, and also includes external symptoms such as visible abdominal veins and cold or hot abdominal skin. The umbilicus is at the center of the abdomen, also the center of the body; below it is the dantian, the source of vital energy. It is most susceptible to cold, causing abdominal pain, diarrhea, etc., especially in infants, improper care after umbilical cord separation can lead to severe umbilical wind. This section includes local disorders such as umbilical swelling, umbilical protrusion, umbilical dampness, umbilical bleeding, and pus discharge.

I. Epigastric Pain

Pain in the upper abdomen is generally called "epigastric pain", abbreviated as "stomach pain". There are many causes, including cold pain, heat pain, deficiency pain, qi pain, stasis pain, food retention pain, worm pain, etc. Among them, stomach cold pain, directly triggered by eating raw and cold foods or inhaling cold air due to inherent stomach cold, is the most common. This syndrome mostly has a sudden onset, with a preference for pressure and hot drinks, accompanied by vomiting of clear water and sticky saliva, fear of cold, cold hands and feet, a deep slow or deep string-like pulse, and a white greasy tongue coating. Stomach cold leads to qi stagnation and damp obstruction, the so-called "pain due to obstruction"; treatment should warm the middle and dispel cold, supplemented by regulating qi and resolving dampness, using Houpu Wenzhong Decoction and *Liang*fu Wan. If pain occurs whenever exposed to cold, 2-3 *fen* of cinnamon powder taken with boiling water can relieve it. Those with greasy food retention, commonly known as "cold-food obstruction", have more severe pain and should be treated with Baohe Wan for digestion and transportation.

"Stomach qi pain" is also a common syndrome, mostly caused by indigestion and stomach qi obstruction, with distending pain in the epigastrium, stuffiness in the chest, slight relief after belching, accompanied by abdominal distension and difficulty in defecation, with a string-like slippery pulse. Due to failure of the stomach to descend and qi dysfunction, promoting qi and dispersing stagnation is appropriate, using Xiangsha Zhizhu Wan; for severe cases, combined with Chenxiang Jiangqi Powder.

Many cases are caused by liver qi, accompanied by symptoms such as hypochondriac fullness and distending pain, depression, and sighing. This is the so-called "liver wood attacking the stomach", hence also referred to as "liver-stomach qi pain". It often occurs after mental stimulation or in those with a history of emotional frustration. Treatment involves using Chaihu Shugan Powder or Tiaoqi Decoction. Stomach pain caused by liver qi that persists for a long time can often transform into fire, presenting with bitter taste in the mouth, dry mouth, acid regurgitation, heartburn, irritability, and a wiry and rapid pulse. In such cases, acrid-dispersing and bitter-descending methods are appropriate, using Huagan Jian, or combined with Zuojin Wan. If the condition lingers and damages yin, with a red tongue and scanty fluid, Yiguan Jian is used to nourish yin with a minor adjunct to drain the liver. The use of acrid-drying qi-regulating herbs is strictly avoided, as excessive dispersal will exacerbate the pain.

Stomach pain caused by middle qi deficiency is characterized by pain that mostly occurs on an empty stomach, relieved by food intake or warm compresses, accompanied by fear of cold and preference for warmth, a pale tongue with a thin white coating, and a deep, thready, weak pulse or a deficient wiry pulse. The pain fluctuates in severity, persisting for years without resolution, and in severe cases, can lead to hematemesis and melena. This condition involves not only the stomach but also has a close relationship with the spleen, as the stomach governs reception, the spleen governs transportation; the stomach tends to descend while the spleen tends to ascend; the stomach prefers coolness while the spleen prefers warmth; the stomach should be unobstructed while the spleen should be conserved. Though their functions differ, they complement each other. Deficient stomach pain, in terms of pathogenesis, tends toward spleen cold deficiency, and Huangqi Jianzhong Decoction should be used to warm and nourish middle qi. In cases of bleeding, fresh ginger is replaced with roasted ginger, and donkey-hide gelatin is added. It should be noted that this condition often recurs due to exposure to cold, anger, and other factors. Additionally, symptoms such as food retention may appear due to the diminished transforming and transporting function, requiring appropriate management based on distinguishing the root and branch causes, and should not be treated as simple cold pain, qi pain, or food retention pain. Acupuncture treatment mainly uses Zhongwan, Neiguan, and Zusanli points; points such as Pishu, Weishu, Shangjuxu, and Xiajuxu can also be used. Generally, excess pain is suitable for acupuncture, while deficiency pain requires moxibustion after acupuncture.

Stasis pain, characterized by stabbing pain with a fixed location, or the presence of masses or black stool, a choppy pulse that is forceful on heavy pressure, should be treated by harmonizing blood and relieving pain using Shounian Powder. Aggressive purging is not advisable unless necessary.

Heat pain, where pressure is not desired, is mostly accompanied by a yellow greasy tongue coating, a rapid and large pulse, and symptoms such as thirst, reddish urine, and constipation, indicating excess in the intestines and stomach. Treatment should clear heat with adjunctive qi regulation, using Qingzhong Yin plus Toosendan and Immature Bitter Orange.

In the syndrome of "stomach abscess", pain also occurs in the middle epigastrium, and over time, it may rupture, expectorating large amounts of pus and blood. In the initial stage, Shaoyao Decoction is used; when the abscess forms, Tuoli Powder is used; after rupture, Paiyong Powder is used. This syndrome is difficult to diagnose in the early stage. Generally, it starts with epigastric pain, initially presenting with a gray-black, dirty and greasy tongue coating, dull pain that is not severe, a sweet taste in the mouth with foul breath, and a large Renying pulse beside the Adam's apple. When the abscess has formed, there are chills and fever like malaria, a surging and rapid pulse, or rough and dry skin may be seen.

Worm pain is not limited to the middle epigastrium; refer to the entry "Umbilical and Abdominal Pain" in this section.

In miscellaneous diseases, conditions such as "bind chest" and "chest impediment" are related to stomach pain; refer to the entry "Chest Pain" in the symptoms of the chest, hypochondria, axillae, and breasts.

Houpu Wenzhong Decoction: Magnolia Officinalis, Amomum Cardamomum, Tangerine Peel, Aucklandia, Dried Ginger, Poria, Licorice

Liangfu Wan: Galangal, Cyperus

Baohe Wan: Medicated Leaven, Hawthorn, Malt, Radish Seed, Pinellia, Tangerine Peel, Poria, Forsythia

Xiangsha Zhizhu Wan: Aucklandia, Amomum, Immature Bitter Orange, Atractylodes Macrocephala

Chenxiang Jiangqi Powder: Agarwood, Cyperus, Amomum, Licorice

Chaihu Shugan Powder: Bupleurum, White Peony Root, Ligusticum, Cyperus, Tangerine Peel, Immature Bitter Orange, Licorice

Tiaoqi Decoction: Cyperus, Green Tangerine Peel, Tangerine Peel, Agastache, Aucklandia, Lindera, Amomum, Licorice

Huagan Jian: White Peony Root, Moutan Bark, Gardenia, Green

Tangerine Peel, Tangerine Peel, Fritillaria, Alisma

Zuojin Wan: Coptis, Evodia

Yiguan Jian: Raw Rehmannia, Angelica, Wolfberry, Adenophora, Ophiopogon, Toosendan

Huangqi Jianzhong Decoction: Astragalus, Cinnamon Twig, White Peony Root, Roasted Licorice, Ginger, Jujube

Shounian Powder: Corydalis, Trogopterus Dung, Cardamom, Myrrh

Qingzhong Yin: Coptis, Gardenia, Tangerine Peel, Poria, Pinellia, Licorice, Cardamom

Shaoyao Decoction: Red Peony Root, Rhinoceros Horn, Gypsum, Scrophularia, Cimicifuga, Licorice, Sodium Sulfate, Akebia, Ophiopogon, Platycodon

Tuoli Powder: Angelica, Red Peony Root, Rhubarb, Scutellaria, Sodium Sulfate, Saponaria Thorn, Trichosanthes Root, Forsythia, Honeysuckle, Oyster

Paiyong Powder: Codonopsis, Astragalus, Angelica Dahurica, Schisandra

II. Lower Abdominal Pain

Abdominal pain localized in the lower abdomen, either on the left, right, or both sides, often accompanied by a sense of distension. It mostly pertains to symptoms of the Liver Meridian, treated with Jinlingzi Powder, and can be supplemented with Bupleurum and Green Tangerine Peel for dispersing; for cold manifestations, add Cinnamon and Lindera for warming. Acupuncture can also be applied at points such as Guanyuan, Guilai, Xingjian, and Sanyinjiao.

Lower abdominal pain predominantly on the right side, worsening with pressure, often with a desire to curl up the legs while lying down, accompanied by chills, fever, nausea, and difficulty in defecation, indicates "intestinal abscess". *Synopsis of the Golden Chamber* states: "In intestinal abscess, there is swelling and stuffiness in the lower abdomen, which is painful to touch, resembling strangury, but with normal urination; there is frequent fever, spontaneous sweating, and recurrence of chills. If the pulse is slow and tight, pus has not yet formed, and purgation is permissible, which will result in blood... treated with Dahuang Mudanpi Decoction." This condition arises from stagnation of damp-heat and blood stasis in the intestines; in the initial stage, clearing heat, resolving dampness, and dispelling stasis is appropriate. For milder cases, Qingchang Yin can be used. Zhang Jingyue's single formula for intestinal abscess: first, use one *liang* of Sargentodoxa cuneata, decocted in two bowls of good wine to one bowl, taken in the morning; in the afternoon, use one *liang* of Viola yedoensis, decocted as before. If pain gradually subsides after administration, it is effective. However, once pus has formed, purgation is strictly prohibited to prevent intestinal rupture and other complications, hence the warning in *Synopsis of the Golden Chamber*: "If pus has formed, purgation is not permissible." Intestinal abscess may also have intermittent episodes with mild pain and no fever or only slight fever, belonging to the chronic type, treated with Huoxue Sanyu Decoction to harmonize and disperse. For post-illness debility with persistent purulent bloody discharge, Mudanpi Powder is used to tonify deficiency and resolve toxicity. Acupuncture for this condition mainly uses the Appendix Point, combined with Zusanli, Neiting, Gongsun, Tianshu, Fujie, Dachangshu, Neiguan, Qihai, etc.

Lower abdominal pain with a palpable elongated mass upon pressure is called "xuan pi". Refer to the entry "Hard Mass in the Abdomen" in this section.

Jinlingzi Powder: Sichuan Toosendan, Corydalis

Dahuang Mudanpi Decoction: Rhubarb, Moutan Bark, Peach Kernel, Sodium Sulfate, Winter Melon Seed

Qingchang Yin: Angelica, Honeysuckle, Sanguisorba, Ophiopogon, Scrophularia, Licorice, Coix Seed, Scutellaria

Huoxue Sanyu Decoction: Angelica Tail, Ligusticum, Red Peony Root, Sappan Wood, Moutan Bark, Aurantium, Snakegourd Seed, Peach Kernel, Areca, Rhubarb

Mudanpi Powder: Ginseng, Astragalus, Moutan Bark, White Peony Root, Poria, Coix Seed, Peach Kernel, Bailong (Bletilla?), Angelica, Ligusticum, Licorice, Cinnamon, Aucklandia

III. Umbilical and Abdominal Pain

The umbilical and abdominal region pertains to Shaoyin; pain radiates around the umbilicus, with a preference for pressure, accompanied by borborygmus, poor appetite, loose stools, and a white greasy tongue coating, mostly belonging to cold syndromes, involving the spleen and large and small intestines. Sudden pain caused by cold exposure or consumption of raw and cold foods is persistent; chronic pain due to spleen-kidney yang deficiency fluctuates in severity, lingering continuously. The former is treated with Tiantai Wuyao Powder minus Croton, with additional Cinnamon and Dried Ginger for severe cold; the latter with Lizhong Decoction, with additional Aconite for severe yang deficiency.

Umbilical and abdominal pain due to qi stagnation is often accompanied by distension, related to gastrointestinal indigestion, treated with Wumo Yin. If regulating qi is ineffective, with stabbing pain or fixed pain at the umbilicus and a deep choppy pulse, treatment should target blood stagnation, using Shounian Powder.

Heat syndrome of abdominal pain is less common, generally seen in exogenous cold diseases and warm diseases when pathogenic factors transmit to the middle jiao, mainly due to constipation, mostly treated with purgative methods.

Food retention can also cause abdominal pain, initially in the upper abdomen, accompanied by distension and stuffiness, belching with a rotten odor, then spreading to the umbilical abdomen, with irregular bowel movements; treatment should promote digestion and eliminate stagnation.

Intense abdominal colic, with a desire to vomit but unable to vomit, a desire to defecate but unable to defecate, restlessness and confusion, in severe cases, a pale and ashen complexion, cold limbs, sweating on the head, and a deep hidden pulse, called "dry cholera". It is caused by summer heat and dampness blocking the middle jiao, leading to stagnation and obstruction of qi movement. First, prick and bleed at Shixuan, Quze, and Weizhong points, induce vomiting with salt water boiled and taken hot, then use Houpu Decoction; if vomiting and diarrhea occur, the condition will stabilize.

Intermittent pain, severe and unbearable when it occurs, with normal eating when pain stops, is "worm accumulation pain", mostly seen in children. Worm accumulation is caused by unclean diet; patients usually have a good appetite but are thin, or crave raw rice, soil, etc., with a sallow complexion, bluish discoloration around the eyes and nose, bright red lips, or small sores like millet grains inside the lips, teeth grinding during sleep, nasal itching with a tendency to pick the nose, in severe cases, abdominal distension with hardness, a thready string-like pulse or irregularly large and rapid pulse. Treatment includes direct insecticidal methods, using Huachong Wan or Jixiao Wan; and worm-calming methods, using Wumei Wan. If the spleen and stomach are weak, focus on digestion and transportation, using Fei'er Wan. Generally, "worm pain" refers to roundworm infection, and abdominal pain caused by roundworms is particularly obvious. In addition, there is pinworm disease, characterized by anal itching; refer to the entry "Anal Itching" in posterior yin symptoms.

Abdominal pain around the umbilicus, with a lumpy, uneven sensation when pressed, called "cold hernia". It is mostly caused by cold in the small intestine. *Synopsis of the Golden Chamber* states: "In cold hernia, there is cold in the abdomen, qi rushing upward causing the skin to rise with visible 'heads and feet', pain moving up and down, unbearable to touch, treated with Dajianzhong Decoction." In severe cases, accompanied by vomiting, profuse sweating, and cold limbs, use Chiwan for treatment.

Abdominal pain with each episode followed by diarrhea, with unsatisfactory defecation, is "dysentery"; refer to the entry "Mucus in Stool" in visceral symptoms.

Tiantai Wuyao Powder: Lindera, Galangal, Fennel, Aucklandia, Green Tangerine Peel, Areca, Sichuan Toosendan, Croton

Lizhong Decoction: Codonopsis, Atractylodes, Roasted Ginger, Roasted Licorice

Wumo Yin: Agarwood, Lindera, Areca, Immature Bitter Orange, Aucklandia

Shounian Powder: Corydalis, Trogopterus Dung, Cardamom, Myrrh

Houpu Decoction: Magnolia Officinalis, Immature Bitter Orange, Galangal, Sodium Sulfate, Rhubarb, Areca

Huachong Wan: Carpesium, Chinaberry Root, Areca, Wuyi (Dutch Elm Fruit), Dried Alum, Quisqualis

Jixiao Wan: Carpesium, Wuyi, Areca, Aconite, Dried Ginger, Prepared Rhubarb, Terminalia, Aucklandia

Wumei Wan: Dark Plum, Asarum, Cinnamon Twig, Ginseng, Aconite, Coptis, Phellodendron, Dried Ginger, Sichuan Pepper, Angelica

Fei'er Wan: Atractylodes, Poria, Hyacinth Bean, Green Tangerine Peel, Tangerine Peel, Magnolia Officinalis, Chicken Gizzard Lining, Grain Worm, Amomum, Picrorhiza, Hawthorn, Medicated Leaven, Areca, Dried Toad Skin

Dajianzhong Decoction: Dried Ginger, Sichuan Pepper, Ginseng

Chiwan: Aconitum, Asarum, Pinellia, Poria

IV. Lower Abdominal Pain

Lower abdominal pain localized below the umbilicus, with spasmodic contraction, hardness, and fullness when painful, and normal urination. In severe cases, accompanied by mania, it is "blood amassment" syndrome, treated with Taoren Chengqi Decoction.

Heat binding in the bladder, with difficult urination, also presents with intermittent severe lower abdominal pain, treated with Wuling Powder.

Lower abdominal pain is common in gynecological menstrual diseases; refer to the entry "Dysmenorrhea" in gynecological symptoms.

Taoren Chengqi Decoction: Peach Kernel, Rhubarb, Xuanmingfen (Sodium Sulfate), Cinnamon Twig, Licorice

Wuling Powder: Atractylodes, Poria, Polyporus, Alisma, Cinnamon Twig

V. Abdominal Fullness

Abdominal fullness refers to a subjective feeling of stuffiness without an externally urgent swollen appearance, mostly caused by poor digestion of the spleen and stomach, damp obstruction, and qi stagnation. It is often accompanied by loss of appetite, postprandial fullness, nausea, belching, irregular bowel movements, heavy limbs, and a thick greasy tongue coating. Paiqi Yin is used to regulate qi and resolve turbidity.

It is difficult to distinguish between abdominal fullness and chest and diaphragm stuffiness. Some affect the abdomen from chest and diaphragm stuffiness, and some affect the chest and diaphragm from abdominal distension. Therefore, it is generally also called stuffy fullness (piman). "Pi" means blocked and unopened, and "man" means stuffy and uncomfortable. What is said in *Baoming Ji* ("The spleen fails to circulate qi to the lung and stomach") includes both the chest and abdomen. *Treatise on Febrile Diseases* has the syndrome of "epigastric stuffiness (xinxia pi)", referring to stuffiness in the middle epigastrium caused by exterior pathogens entering the interior. It requires bitter-cold to purge, acrid-sweet to disperse, using Banxia Xiexin Decoction, or adding ginger to make Shengjiang Xiexin Decoction, or removing ginseng and increasing licorice to make Gancao Xiexin Decoction, which is the method of acrid-opening and bitter-descending. For internal injury miscellaneous syndromes, regulating qi and resolving turbidity is the main approach, as stated in *The Inner Canon*: "For middle fullness, purge internally". If it is simply caused by middle deficiency leading to fullness, the method of "treating stagnation with tonification" is appropriate, using Yigong Powder, or ginseng powder with a small amount of chicken gizzard lining powder.

Paiqi Yin: Agastache, Aucklandia, Lindera, Magnolia Officinalis, Aurantium, Cyperus, Tangerine Peel, Alisma

Banxia Xiexin Decoction: Pinellia, Coptis, Scutellaria, Ginseng, Licorice, Dried Ginger, Jujube

Yigong Powder: Ginseng, Atractylodes, Poria, Licorice, Tangerine Peel

VI. Abdominal Distension

Abdominal distension is common in general diseases, mostly belonging to damp-heat and qi stagnation, tending to be excess syndrome, sometimes alleviating, sometimes worsening, more severe after eating, and slightly relieved after passing flatus. Therefore, Xu Huixi said: "For distension syndrome, even if there is healthy qideficiency, it is ultimately due to pathogenic excess; ancient people used tonifying methods cautiously. Moreover, distension must involve damp-heat; if there is a tangible substance in the distension, gentle purgation is appropriate." Generally, if the distension is in the intestines and stomach and worsens after eating, dredging the fu organs is appropriate; if the urine and bowel movements are normal, the distension is in the zang organs, and strengthening the spleen is appropriate, using Kuanzhong Decoction, Zhongman Fenxiao Wan, Jiawei Zhizhu Wan, etc., with modifications.

The most severe syndrome of abdominal distension is "tympanites (pengzhang)", also known as "simple abdominal distension (danfu zhang)" and "spider-like tympanites (zhizhu gu)". Furthermore, due to different causes, there are "qi tympanites (qigu)", "blood tympanites (xue gu)", "food tympanites (shi gu)", "worm tympanites (chong gu)","water tympanites (shui gu)", etc. But most fall into three types: qi, water, and blood. These three often interact as cause and effect, so the zang organs mainly involved are the liver and spleen, and the condition progresses from excess to deficiency, resulting in a combination of deficiency and excess. Initially, it is often due to liver qi stagnation and stagnation of spleen-stomach damp-heat, presenting with abdominal distension, sallow complexion, hot palms, afternoon fatigue, worsening bloating after meals, greasy tongue coating, and a string-like slippery pulse. Subsequently, stasis and water accumulation occur, with the abdomen growing larger daily, gradual emaciation, scanty urine, and the pulse turning deep, thready, string-like, and rapid, showing root deficiency with branch excess. Finally, the abdomen becomes greatly distended with visible veins, the complexion turns sallow or dark, difficulty in urination and defecation, dry mouth with drinking leading to more bloating, swollen feet, jaundice, gum oozing, crimson or prickly tongue, greasy yellow dry tongue coating, and a thready rapid or floating large weak pulse, manifesting as qi stagnation and blood stasis, dampness with heat stagnation, worsening branch excess, and severe depletion of true yin. At this stage, the prognosis is poor, with most dying from hematemesis, bloody stool, or coma. Treatment must distinguish the degree of deficiency and excess, appropriately using methods such as soothing the liver, strengthening the spleen, resolving accumulation, expelling water, clearing heat, dispelling stasis, nourishing blood, and nourishing yin. Formulas such as Jiawei Xiaoyao Powder, Zhongman Fenxiao Wan, Jijin Powder, Yugong Powder, Danggui Huoxue Decoction, Zhuling Decoction, and Dabuyin Wan can be selected. Treatment of this disease must consider consequences and not rush; excessive dispersal is inappropriate initially, and aggressive water-expelling and acrid-hot warming methods should be used cautiously for ascites to prevent qi deficiency and yin damage, which would make it more intractable. *Gezhi Yulun* states: "This disease arises over three to five years or more than ten years; it has deep roots and is severe. Seeking quick results brings disaster. Only those who understand the royal way can treat this disease." It also says: "Physicians who fail to recognize the disease arises from deficiency, rush for results to show off their skills and seek reward, and patients suffering from severe distension, eager to take diuretics for temporary relief, only gain a day or half a day of relief, but the swelling worsens, and the pathogen becomes more severe."

"Schistosomiasis" is prevalent in the Yangtze River basin, causing the greatest harm to the health of laboring people. Initially, symptoms are not obvious, with occasional abdominal pain and diarrhea, and a dull complexion. In adolescents, it can retard development. In severe stages, it presents with abdominal distension, visible veins, general emaciation, and scanty urine. Treatment should consider the prosperity and decline of pathogens and healthy qi, managed according to tympanites.

Infantile "ganji" (infantile malnutrition) is also mainly characterized by abdominal distension, mostly caused by improper intake of rich, sweet foods and milk, with accumulated heat consuming qi and blood, hence commonly known as "ganpeng shiji" (malnutrition with distension and food stagnation). Ancient physicians classified it into gan syndromes of the five *zang* organs; clinically, "spleen gan" is the most common, and gan syndromes of the other four zang organs mostly result from the further progression of spleen gan. Spleen gan is also called "fei gan" (fatty malnutrition) or "shi gan" (food malnutrition), with symptoms including a large hard abdomen, abdominal pain with passing roundworms, sallow and emaciated complexion, large head with thin neck, sparse hair in tufts, difficulty in taking milk and food, dry mouth and polydipsia, craving for soil, occasional tidal fever, listlessness and drowsiness, foul sticky stools, and rice-water-like urine. "Liver gan" is also called "jin gan" (tendon malnutrition) or "feng gan" (wind malnutrition), with symptoms such as upright hair, excessive eye discharge, head shaking and eye rubbing, large abdomen with visible blue veins, extreme emaciation, and 青苔-like green stools. "Heart gan" is also called "jing gan" (convulsion malnutrition), with symptoms including restlessness and palpitations, red cheeks and lips, oral and tongue ulcers, five-center heat, teeth grinding and tongue protrusion, and preference for lying prone during sleep. "Lung gan" is also called "qi gan" (qi malnutrition) or "gan sheng" (malnutrition with snoring), with symptoms such as dry skin, withered and scorched hair, pale complexion, cough and asthma, and nasal ulcers. "Kidney gan" is also called "gu gan" (bone malnutrition) or "ji gan" (acute malnutrition), with symptoms including gum bleeding, foul breath, feet as cold as ice, abdominal pain and diarrhea, and incessant crying. During the entire development of gan syndrome, ancient physicians also named it according to certain prominent accompanying symptoms, such as "gan re" (malnutrition with heat), "gan xie" (malnutrition with diarrhea), "gan li" (malnutrition with dysentery), "gan zhang" (malnutrition with distension), and "gan lao" (malnutrition with consumption). More specific names include "dingxi" characterized by a large abdomen, thin neck, sallow and emaciated appearance; and "bulu" characterized by polydipsia, retching, vomiting, and worms. In fact, they all fall within the scope of the five *zang* organs. For treating spleen gan, it is advisable to first eliminate the accumulation, using Xiaogan Lipi Decoction; for those with accumulated heat and diarrhea, use Qingre Hezhong Decoction; for swelling, use Yuyuan Yunqi Powder. For liver gan, use Luhui Fei'er Wan; for heart gan, use Xiexin Daochi Decoction; for lung gan, use Shengdi Qingfei Yin; for kidney gan, use Jinchan Wan. For the aftercare of gan syndrome, regulating the spleen and stomach and paying attention to diet are essential.

Kuanzhong Decoction: Magnolia Officinalis, Tangerine Peel, Atractylodes, Poria, Pinellia, Immature Bitter Orange, Hawthorn, Medicated Leaven, Radish Seed, Ginger

Zhongman Fenxiao Wan: Magnolia Officinalis, Immature Bitter Orange, Coptis, Scutellaria, Anemarrhena, Pinellia, Tangerine Peel, Poria, Alisma, Polyporus, Amomum, Dried Ginger, Turmeric, Ginseng,

Atractylodes, Licorice

Jiawei Zhizhu Wan: Immature Bitter Orange, Atractylodes, Tangerine Peel, Pinellia, Poria, Perilla, Platycodon, Licorice, Cinnamon Twig, Trogopterus Dung, Areca

Jiawei Xiaoyao Powder: Angelica, White Peony Root, Bupleurum, Atractylodes, Poria, Licorice, Mint, Moutan Bark, Gardenia, Ginger

Jijin Powder: Chicken Gizzard Lining, Agarwood, Amomum, Citron

Yugong Powder: Black Cowherb Seed, Fennel

Danggui Huoxue Decoction: Angelica Tail, Red Peony Root, Raw Rehmannia, Peach Kernel, Safflower, Cyperus, Ligusticum, Moutan Bark, Corydalis, Green Tangerine Peel, Zedoary, Sparganium

Zhuling Decoction: Donkey-Hide Gelatin, Polyporus, Talc, Poria, Alisma

Dabuyin Wan: Prepared Rehmannia, Turtle Shell, Phellodendron, Anemarrhena, Pig Spinal Cord

Xiaogan Lipi Decoction: Dutch Elm Fruit, Areca, Quisqualis, Coptis, Picrorhiza, Sparganium, Zedoary, Green Tangerine Peel, Tangerine Peel, Licorice, Malt, Medicated Leaven, Aloe

Qingre Hezhong Decoction: Coptis, Magnolia Officinalis, Atractylodes, Alisma, Poria, Licorice, Quisqualis, Medicated Leaven, Malt, Rush

Yuyuan Yunqi Powder: Mulberry Bark, Platycodon, Red Poria, Licorice, Agastache, Tangerine Peel, Akebia, Rush, Ginger Peel

Luhui Fei'er Wan: Aloe, Picrorhiza, Coptis, Starwort Root, Hyacinth Bean, Yam, Grain Worm, Hawthorn, Toad, Nutmeg, Areca, Quisqualis, Medicated Leaven, Malt, Carpesium, Dutch Elm Fruit,

Cinnabar, Musk

Xiexin Daochi Decoction: Akebia, Raw Rehmannia, Coptis, Licorice, Rush

Shengdi Qingfei Yin: Mulberry Bark, Raw Rehmannia, Asparagus, Peucedanum, Platycodon, Perilla Leaf, Saposhnikovia, Scutellaria, Licorice, Angelica, Forsythia, Red Poria

Jinchan Wan: Dried Toad, Picrorhiza, Coptis, Carpesium, Nutmeg, Polyporus, Aloe, Dutch Elm Fruit, Chinaberry Root Bark

VII. Abdominal Rumbling

Also called "borborygmus", it is mostly seen in syndromes of intestinal cold-damp distension and diarrhea, with Aucklandia and Lindera as the main herbs.

In fluid-retention disease, when fluid flows into the intestines with a gurgling sound, it is called "lingering fluid retention", treated with Gansui Banxia Decoction.

Gansui Banxia Decoction: Gansui, Pinellia, Peony, Licorice

VIII. Hard Mass in the Abdomen

A palpable hard mass in the abdomen is mostly of the "zhengjia" (abdominal masses) category. There are many causes, mainly due to gradual accumulation of qi and blood stagnation, hence also called "jiju" (accumulation and aggregation), with divisions such as seven zheng, eight jia, five accumulations, and six aggregations. Generally, blood accumulation that is hard and immovable is called zheng, belonging to zang diseases; qi aggregation that is mobile is called jia, belonging to fu diseases. However, clinically, they cannot be absolutely distinguished: some first have qi aggregation that becomes accumulation over time, and some hard masses can become mobile after treatment. Generally, initially, the mass is not hard, with or without pain, and daily life and diet are normal; then it gradually enlarges, with fixed pain, occasional cold sensation, fatigue, loss of appetite; finally, it becomes hard and full with pain, emaciation, and sallow complexion. Therefore, Cheng Zhongling believed that the treatment of accumulation should follow the early, middle, and late stages, saying: "When pathogenic qi first invades and the accumulation is not yet hard, it is appropriate to directly dispel it and then harmonize. If the accumulation lasts for a long time, with excessive pathogen and deficient healthy qi, the method is middle treatment, needing to combine tonification and purgation. If the mass is half eliminated, then use late treatment, stopping the attacking herbs, only harmonizing the middle and nourishing the stomach, dredging the meridians, so that nutrient and defensive qi circulate and the mass resolves on its own." He also said: "For deficient people with accumulation, first tonify their deficiency, regulate their spleen, increase their diet, then use herbs to attack the accumulation; this is good treatment, the method of tonifying first then attacking." This is the major method for treating accumulation, with commonly used formulas such as Wuji Powder for dispersing accumulation, Muxiang Shunqi Powder for promoting qi, Xuezheng Wan for attacking stasis, Jianpi Zisheng Wan for regulating the middle, etc.; external treatment uses Awei Gao for application.

To the left and right of the navel in the lower abdomen there are painful masses: when large they feel like an arm or a cucumber, when small like a finger, and all are as taut as a bowstring. They often extend upward and pull beneath the hypochondria; this is called "xuán pǐ" (a tugging, fixed accumulation). Caused by liver qi stagnation, pain worsens with cold, treated with Muxiang Shunqi Powder plus Corydalis and Fennel.

Hard masses in women's lower abdomen, due to cold attacking the Chong and Ren Meridians and blood stasis, called "shanjia". Use Danggui Wan. There is also "shijia" syndrome, caused by injury to the uterus and blood stasis, becoming hard as stone over time, blocking the uterine orifice, with abdominal enlargement like pregnancy and absent menstruation, treated with Shiying Powder. "Changtan" syndrome, caused by cold qi invading the large intestine and forming jia, growing polyp over time, initially like a chicken egg, later like pregnancy, hard when pressed, mobile when pushed, with menstruation still occurring, more or less, treated with Daqiqi Decoction.

Wuji Powder: Angelica, Ligusticum, White Peony Root, Atractylodes Lancea, Magnolia Officinalis, Poria, Aurantium, Pinellia, Dried Ginger, Cinnamon, Angelica Dahurica, Ephedra, Tangerine Peel, Platycodon, Licorice, Scallion, Ginger

Muxiang Shunqi Powder: Aucklandia, Green Tangerine Peel, Tangerine Peel, Aurantium, Magnolia Officinalis, Lindera, Cyperus, Atractylodes Lancea, Amomum, Cinnamon, Licorice

Xuezheng Wan: Trogopterus Dung, Rhubarb, Peach Kernel, Raw Rehmannia, Achyranthes, Cinnamon, Corydalis, Angelica, Red Peony Root, Sparganium, Zedoary, Frankincense, Myrrh, Amber, Ligusticum, Licorice

Jianpi Zisheng Wan: Atractylodes, Ginseng, Poria, Coix Seed, Hawthorn, Tangerine Peel, Coptis, Cardamom, Platycodon, Agastache, Hyacinth Bean, Lotus Seed, Licorice, Medicated Leaven

Awei Gao: Asafoetida, Cinnamon, Notopterygium, Angelica Pubescens, Scrophularia, Raw Rehmannia, Red Peony Root, Pangolin Scales, Male Rat Feces, Rhubarb, Angelica Dahurica, Gastrodia, Safflower, Momordica Cochinchinensis, Yellow Lead Oxide, Sodium Sulfate,

Frankincense, Myrrh, Styrax, Musk (proprietary medicine)

Danggui Wan: Angelica, Red Peony Root, Ligusticum, Prepared Rehmannia, Sparganium, Zedoary, Medicated Leaven, Plant Soot

Shiying Powder: Fluorite, Angelica, Verbena, Safflower, Dark Plum, Zedoary, Sappan Wood, Myrrh, Amber, Licorice

Daqiqi Decoction: Sparganium, Zedoary, Green Tangerine Peel, Tangerine Peel, Platycodon, Agastache, Alpinia Oxyphylla, Cyperus, Cinnamon, Licorice, Ginger, Jujube

IX. Inguinal Masses

Masses in the inguinal region, elongated like clams, hard and painful, all caused by "syphilis". Those on the left are called "yukou" (fish mouth), on the right "biandu" (fecal toxin); some occur near the pubic hairline of the lower abdomen, with the left called "hengxuan" (transverse mass) and the right "yinju" (yin abscess). Most of these rupture after one to two months, and the ulcer is difficult to heal. After liberation, syphilis has been basically eradicated, and this syndrome is rarely seen.

Physical weakness, overwork, or forced walking with foot problems can also cause inguinal masses and pain; mild cases heal with rest, while severe cases require harmonizing nutrition and resolving hardness, using Shugan Kuijian Decoction with modifications.

Shugan Kuijian Decoction: Angelica, White Peony Root, Cyperus, Bombyx Batryticatus, Bupleurum, Prunella Vulgaris, Ligusticum, Pangolin Scales, Safflower, Turmeric, Abalone Shell, Licorice, Tangerine Peel

X. Abdominal Skin Heat

Abdomknal skin heat is one of the diagnostic indicators. *The Inner*

Canon states: "Heat in the skin above the umbilicus, heat in the intestines leads to yellowish 糜-like discharge". In febrile diseases with pathogens in the stomach and intestines, the abdominal skin is mostly very hot, burning to the touch.

XI. Abdominal Skin Cold

Abdominal skin cold is one of the diagnostic indicators. *The Inner Canon* states: "Cold in the skin below the umbilicus; cold in the stomach leads to abdominal distension, cold in the intestines leads to borborygmus and undigested diarrhea". Mostly seen in spleen-kidney yang deficiency syndromes, with not only cold abdominal skin but also intolerance to cold exposure; it also frequently appears in gynecological Chong-Ren deficiency-cold syndromes.

XII. Visible Abdominal Veins

Visible abdominal vein is one of the symptoms of "tympanites" and infantile "ganji"; refer to the entry "Abdominal Distension" in this section.

XIII. Umbilical Protrusion

Common in infants due to excessive crying or loose binding after umbilical cord separation; no treatment is needed if there is no redness, swelling, or other pathological signs.

Umbilical protrusion in cases of swelling is one of the critical signs. *Waitai Miyao* points out: "Black lips injure the liver, flat supraclavicular fossa injures the heart, umbilical protrusion injures the spleen, flat swollen feet injure the kidney, flat back injures the lung". *Dexiao Fang* also says: "Protruding umbilicus, abdominal urgency after diarrhea, prolonged illness with emaciation, restlessness with panting, called spleen-kidney failure, incurable".

XIV. Umbilical Swelling

Infantile umbilical swelling like a chestnut, painful and soft, can be gradually resolved by applying bamboo juice several times a day. If there is redness, swelling, pain, or even erosion with pus discharge, it is "umbilical sore". Umbilical swelling is mostly caused by bath water entering the umbilicus after cord separation, diaper infiltration, or premature shedding of the umbilical scab due to friction from clothing. Wash with Saposhnikovia decoction, dry, then apply Hufen Powder; for those with chills and fever, take Xijiao Xiaodu Yin internally.

Hufen Powder: 2.5 *qian* of Coptis, one *qian* each of lead powder and calcined Dragon Bone, ground into fine powder.

Xijiao Xiaodu Yin: Arctium, Licorice, Rhinoceros Horn, Schizonepeta, Saposhnikovia, Honeysuckle

XV. Umbilical Dampness

After an infant's umbilical cord falls off, if the umbilicus remains damp with slight redness and swelling, apply pine pollen powder. For cases that do not heal for a long time, sprinkle Shenqi Powder in the umbilicus.

Shenqi Powder: Two *qian* each of dried alum and calcined dragon bone, five li of musk, ground into fine powder.

XVI. Fluid Discharge from the Umbilicus

For fluid discharge from the umbilicus, use dragon bone soaked in vinegar, roasted until dry, ground into fine powder and applied externally. If foul-smelling fluid is discharged, it is called "umbilical fistula sore", mostly caused by excessive sexual activity or frequent anger. It is advisable to take Buzhong Yiqi Decoction internally, use moxibustion externally, and after moxibustion, apply Shengji Powder, sealed with plaster or gauze.

Buzhong Yiqi Decoction: Astragalus, Codonopsis, Angelica, Atractylodes, Licorice, Bupleurum, Cimicifuga, Tangerine Peel, Ginger, Jujube

Shengji Powder: Catechu, Frankincense, Myrrh, Borneol, Musk, Dragon's Blood, Notoginseng (proprietary medicine)

XVII. Bleeding from the Umbilicus

Bleeding from the umbilicus is mostly caused by kidney fire flaming upward, using Liuwei Dihuang Decoction with added Drynaria.

Liuwei Dihuang Decoction: Raw Rehmannia, Cornus, Yam, Moutan Bark, Poria, Alisma

XVIII. Pus Discharge from the Umbilicus

Li Dongyuan said, "Intestinal abscess, as a disease, causes sores around the umbilicus, or pus discharge from the umbilicus", which is an extremely dangerous condition of internal abscess suppurating and rupturing.

XIX. Bluish-Black Discoloration around the Umbilicus

It is one of the critical symptoms of "umbilical wind"; refer to the entry "Coma" in visceral symptoms.

XX. Throbbing below the Umbilicus

Throbbing below the umbilicus is called "throbbing below the umbilicus". It is due to pre-existing accumulation of water qi in the lower jiao. Excessive sweating injures heart yang, and water qi takes the opportunity to rebel. Treatment should assist yang and promote water circulation, using Fuling Guizhi Gancao Dazao Decoction. The "ben tun" (running piglet) syndrome is also water qi surging upward, first manifesting as throbbing below the umbilicus. Wang Haicang said: "Throbbing below the umbilicus is movement of kidney qi; use Lizhong Decoction minus Atractylodes plus Cinnamon. The kidney dislikes dryness, so Atractylodes is removed; to prevent the development of ben tun, Cinnamon is added; if there is palpitation, add one *liang* of Poria."

The Chong Meridian, being the sea of blood, can also cause throbbing below the umbilicus with qi rebelling upward, rushing from the lower abdomen straight to the chest and throat, causing stuffiness as if dying. *Nan Jing* (The Classic of Difficult Issues) states: "Diseases of the Chong Meridian are rebellious qi and internal urgency." Use two-three *fen* of agarwood ground and taken for temporary relief, and internally take Fuling Wuweizi Decoction.

Fuling Guizhi Gancao Dazao Decoction: Poria, Cinnamon Twig, Licorice, Jujube

Fuling Wuweizi Decoction: Poria, Schisandra, Cinnamon, Licorice

Section 15 Limb Symptoms

The upper limbs are traversed by the six hand meridians, and the lower limbs by the six foot meridians. Generally, pain and movement disorders of the limbs, muscles, and joints are mostly caused by invasion of wind, cold, and dampness pathogens into the meridians. Symptoms such as heaviness, fatigue, reluctance to move, muscle atrophy, and swelling are related to internal organs, as the spleen governs the limbs. *Nei Jing* (The Inner Canon) points out: "If there is pathogen in the lung and heart, their qi flows to the two elbows; if the liver is affected by pathogen, its qi flows to the two armpits; if the spleen is affected by pathogen, its qi flows to the two thighs; if the kidney is affected by pathogen, its qi flows to the two popliteal fossae." This explains the relationship between internal organs and limb joints. As for other miscellaneous diseases such as stroke, which also present with limb symptoms like hemiplegia and lower limb paralysis, they should not be regarded as simple meridian disorders.

I. Limb Pain

Pain in the upper or lower limbs mostly belongs to the category of "bi disease" (impediment disease). It arises due to prior deficiency of nutrient and defensive qi, loose interstices, invasion by wind-cold with dampness, stagnation in the meridians, and failure of qi and blood to circulate smoothly. Hence, *The Inner Canon* points out that "the three qi of wind, cold, and dampness converge to form bi", and distinguishes that "when wind predominates, it is 'moving bi'; when cold predominates, it is 'painful bi'; when dampness predominates, it is 'fixed bi'". That is, bi disease is often caused by a combination of wind, cold, and dampness pathogens, though with varying degrees of predominance. In diagnosis, one must differentiate: Severe and fixed pain indicates a predominance of cold; painful, heavy, and numb sensations indicate a predominance of dampness; and wandering pain indicates a predominance of wind. Since the three pathogens of wind, cold, and dampness combine and are of a yin nature, symptoms tend to worsen or recur in cold seasons and humid climates, as stated in *The Inner Canon*: "It becomes acute upon exposure to cold, and relieved upon exposure to heat". In treatment, besides differentiating the predominance of the three pathogens, due to the stagnation of qi and blood in the meridians, it is necessary to simultaneously harmonize nutrition, activate blood, and unblock yang qi, rather than relying solely on acrid-dispersing and meridian-unblocking methods. Moreover, bi disease mostly affects one arm or one leg, so *Synopsis of the Golden Chamber* states: "Only inability to move the arm is bi". When using medicines, a distinction should be made between upper and lower limbs, and the same applies to acupuncture.

Pain localized in the upper limbs and arms, often caused by exposure to cold, generally tends to affect the areas along the three yang meridians of the hand on the outer side. The shoulder blades are particularly susceptible to cold; when pain occurs, it often radiates from the shoulder down to the elbow, with inability to lift or bend backward. In the initial stage, dispelling and activating collaterals is used, with Fangfeng Decoction; for persistent cases, focusing on harmonizing blood is appropriate, using Shujin Decoction. For treating upper limb pain, cinnamon twig excels in dispelling wind and harmonizing blood, gentiana macrophylla dispels wind-dampness, notopterygium disperses wind-cold, turmeric regulates qi in the blood, and clematis expels cold and moves qi, with a strong affinity for meridians, thus often used as channel-guiding herbs. Acupuncture points include Jianjing, Jianyu, Quchi, Waiguan, Houxi, Hegu, and Shousanli.

Pain localized in the lower limbs, thighs, and shins, as these are traversed by the six foot meridians, particularly closely related to the three yin meridians of the foot. The cause is often sitting or lying in cold, damp places, thus predominantly involving cold-dampness. The pain mainly affects the hip and knee joints, sometimes radiating to the lower back, accompanied by cold intolerance, preference for warmth, and a heavy sensation. Treatment is based on Sanbi Decoction; for severe cold, combine with Qianjin Wutou Decoction; for severe dampness, combine with Yiyiren Decoction. Generally, for lower limb pain, cinnamon, pubescent angelica, Sichuan aconite, wild aconite, papaya, dipsacus, and achyranthes are commonly used; herbs for both upper and lower limbs include kadsura pepper stem, trachelospermum stem, loofah sponge, and Xiaohuoluo Dan. An empirical formula uses 1 *liang* of ailanthus fruit soaked in one *jin* of white wine, with a small amount taken each time for temporary pain relief. Acupuncture points include Huaniao, Fengshi, Zusanli, Liangqiu, Xiyan, Xuanzhong, and Kunlun.

"Ljie feng" (seasonal joint wind) also involves limb pain, with migrating pain in the joints like tiger bites, hence also called "baihu ljie" (white tiger seasonal joints), essentially a type of moving bi. However, the joints may appear red and swollen, sometimes accompanied by chills and fever, a floating slippery rapid pulse, or skin rashes, finger contracture, and inability to flex or extend due to pain. It is mostly caused by drinking alcohol in windy conditions or bathing with sweat, treated with Guizhi Shaoyao Zhimu Decoction and Baidu Powder with modifications.

Painful obstruction that persists for a long time is also called "gout". Li Dongyuan believed it is mostly due to blood deficiency, mainly using Angelica and Ligusticum, supplemented by Peach Kernel, Safflower, Cinnamon, and Clematis. Zhu Danxi thought it initially arises from blood heat, mainly using Angelica, Ligusticum, Raw Rehmannia, White Peony Root, and Scutellaria, with added Notopterygium, Cinnamon Twig, and Clematis for upper body symptoms, and added Achyranthes, Stephania, and Phellodendron for lower body symptoms. Zhang Shiwan attributed it to damp-heat with phlegm and stasis blocking the collaterals, causing persistent severe pain, requiring Aconite to expel phlegm-damp, strengthen qi and promote movement; for constipation, Rhubarb can be used to eliminatedryness-heat. Prolonged painful obstruction often transforms into heat, secretly consuming qi and blood, which should be managed based on syndrome differentiation.

Pain in the limb joints is gradually accompanied by swelling and thickening, movement disorders, and muscle atrophy. It occurs mostly in mountainous and hilly areas. In children and young people, it can affect bone growth and cause deformities, called "kashin-beck disease", commonly known as "willow stick disease" and "abacus bead disease". In the early stage, it is treated as obstruction syndrome, dispelling wind and cold, activating blood and relieving pain, combined with acupuncture and cupping.

Fangfeng Decoction: Saposhnikovia, Notopterygium, Cinnamon Twig, Gentiana Macrophylla, Pueraria, Angelica, Almond, Scutellaria, Red Poria, Licorice, Ginger

Shujin Decoction: Turmeric, Angelica, Red Peony Root, Atractylodes, Pittosporum, Notopterygium, Licorice

Sanbi Decoction: Ginseng, Astragalus, Angelica, Prepared Rehmannia, Ligusticum, White Peony Root, Cinnamon, Asarum, Pubescent Angelica, Saposhnikovia, Gentiana Macrophylla, Eucommia, Dipsacus, Achyranthes, Poria, Licorice, Ginger, Jujube

Qianjin Wutou Decoction: Aconitum, Aconite, Cinnamon, Sichuan Pepper, Asarum, Pubescent Angelica, Saposhnikovia, Dried Ginger, Gentiana Macrophylla, Angelica, White Peony Root, Poria, Licorice, Jujube

Yiyiren Decoction: Coix Seed, Atractylodes Lancea, Ephedra, Cinnamon Twig, Angelica, White Peony Root, Licorice, Ginger

Xiaohuoluo Dan: Sichuan Aconite, Wild Aconite, Earthworm, Arisaema, Frankincense, Myrrh

Guizhi Shaoyao Zhimu Decoction: Cinnamon Twig, Peony, Anemarrhena, Ephedra, Saposhnikovia, Atractylodes, Aconite, Licorice, Ginger

Baidu Powder: Notopterygium, Pubescent Angelica, Bupleurum, Ligusticum, Platycodon, Aurantium, Peucedanum, Poria, Licorice

II. Limb Weakness

Limb weakness or only lower limb weakness with inability to move, generally without pain, numbness, or other sensations, belongs to "flaccidity syndrome". It is often caused by lung heat scorching, damaging body fluids, or deficiency of heart and spleen, liver and kidney yin deficiency, failing to nourish the meridians, resulting in flaccidity and weakness. In severe cases, the hands cannot grasp objects, the feet cannot support the body, joints such as elbows, wrists, knees, and ankles feel dislocated, muscles become emaciated, leading to untreatable conditions. However, it is more common in the lower limbs, hence also called "flaccid legs". In terms of syndrome differentiation, those belonging to lung heat mostly occur during or after febrile diseases, accompanied by upset and thirst, cough with dry throat, short, red, and painful urination, a thready rapid pulse, treated with Mendong Qingfei Yin combined with Yiwei Decoction. Those belonging to heart and spleen are mostly caused by emotional factors such as irritability and proneness to sadness, accompanied by palpitations and fears, insomnia and dizziness, heat in the hands and feet, poor appetite, a weak pulse, treated with Wuwei Decoction. Those belonging to liver and kidney are mostly caused by excessive sexual activity or long-term spermatorrhea, accompanied by dizziness, tinnitus, and soreness of the waist and spine. There are also cases of yin deficiency with internal heat or gradual development to both yin and yang deficiency, treated with Huqian Wan and Lujiaojiao Wan. In addition, internal accumulation of damp-heat can also cause flaccidity, with symptoms such as heavy body and chest tightness, red and astringent urination, hot sensation in both feet, relief with coolness, and a yellow greasy tongue coating. But damp-heat can also damage yin, resulting in a red tip of the tongue or peeling in the middle of the tongue coating, treated with Jiawei Ermiao Powder. *The Inner Canon* states: “To treat flaccidity, solely select Yangming”, mainly referring to tonifying the acquired foundation to generate body fluids, essence, and blood, nourishing meridians, muscles, and bones. In short, it is necessary to appropriately handle according to specific conditions.

General post-illness limb weakness and inability to move are mostly due to qi and blood weakness, different from flaccidity syndrome, and are not treated as the main symptom.

Mendong Qingfei Yin: Ophiopogon, Ginseng, Astragalus, Angelica, Schisandra, White Peony Root, Aster, Licorice

Yiwei Decoction: Adenophora, Ophiopogon, Raw Rehmannia, Polygonatum, Rock Sugar

Wuwei Decoction: Ginseng, Atractylodes, Poria, Ophiopogon, Angelica, Phellodendron, Anemarrhena, Aucklandia, Licorice, Coix Seed, Ginger, Jujube

Huqian Wan: Turtle Shell, Prepared Rehmannia, White Peony Root, Tiger Bone, Cynomorium, Phellodendron, Anemarrhena, Tangerine Peel

Lujiaojiao Wan: Deer Antler Glue, Deer Antler Frost, Prepared Rehmannia, Ginseng, Angelica, Cuscuta, Eucommia, Tiger Bone, Turtle Shell, Atractylodes, Poria, Achyranthes

Jiawei Ermiao Wan: Phellodendron, Atractylodes Lancea, Angelica, Achyranthes, Turtle Shell, Stephania, Dioscorea Collettii

III. Limb Numbness

Limb numbness, without awareness of pain or itching, mostly belongs to qi deficiency with wind-phlegm entering the collaterals, hindering the circulation of nutrient and defensive qi. *The Inner Canon* states: "Deficiency of nutrient qi leads to numbness, deficiency of defensive qi leads to inability to move, deficiency of both nutrient and defensive qi leads to both numbness and inability to move". Li Dongyuan and Zhu Danxi both attributed it to qi deficiency with impaired circulation and internal obstruction of damp-phlegm. Treatment should focus on tonifying and moving qi, supplemented by resolving wind-phlegm and turbid dampness, and harmonizing the meridians, using Shenxiao Huangqi Decoction and Zhimi Fuling Wan. Generally, for this syndrome, Codonopsis and Astragalus are used to tonify qi, Angelica and White Peony Root to harmonize blood, Aurantium to promote qi, Pinellia to resolve phlegm, Notopterygium and Saposhnikovia to dispel wind, Clematis and Bombyx Batryticatus to unblock collaterals. Mulberry twig is used for the arms, Achyranthes for the legs, with ginger as a guide.

Numbness in one area, worsening in cold and damp conditions, due to phlegm-stasis obstruction, treated with white mustard seed powder mixed with ginger and green onion juice for external application.

Shenxiao Huangqi Decoction: Astragalus, Ginseng, Tangerine Peel, White Peony Root, Licorice, Vitex

Zhimi Fuling Wan: Pinellia, Poria, Aurantium, Effloresced Sodium Sulfate, Ginger Juice

IV. Limb Spasm

Spasm and contracture of the limbs, inability to extend, a disorder of the tendons and meridians, called "jin luan" (tendon spasm). It is mostly caused by excessive blood loss, internal heat damaging yin, excessive sweating consuming fluids, or blood being depleted along with pus in ulcers, leading to dryness of the blood and failure to nourish the tendons.

Use Yangxue Dihuang Wan minus Tianxiong (Aconitum), Qicao (Grub), Ganqi (Dried Lacquer), appropriately adding Shouwu (Polygonum Multiflorum), Baishao (White Peony Root), Lingyangjiao (Antelope Horn), etc. *Nei Jing* once said: "If damp-heat is not dispelled, the large tendons become soft and short, the small tendons become flaccid and long; soft and short leads to contracture, flaccid and long leads to flaccidity." The damp-heat mentioned here mainly refers to heat damaging the blood, which fails to nourish the tendons; thus, Yiyiren (Coix Seed), Rendongteng (Honeysuckle Vine), etc., should be added to blood-nourishing formulas, and exclusive use of clearing and resolving methods is inappropriate. Invasion of cold pathogens into the meridians, as cold is characterized by contraction, causes spasm, treated with Qianjin Yiyiren Decoction to warm.

Contracture is mostly related to the liver. Since the liver governs the tendons, dryness of the fascial membranes leads to contraction. However, the heart, which governs blood and vessels, is also involved. Those with heart weakness often first feel palpitations, shortness of breath, chest tightness and obstruction, followed by spasm of both arms, which gradually relax only when heart qi gradually flows smoothly. Therefore, Ejiao (Donkey-Hide Gelatin), Danggui (Angelica), Guizhi (Cinnamon Twig) are also commonly used.

For spastic pain due to sprain, promoting blood circulation and relaxing tendons is appropriate, using Huohua Powder.

Yangxue Dihuang Wan: Shudi (Prepared Rehmannia), Shanzhu (Cornus), Baizhu (Atractylodes), Gouji (Cibotium), Manjingzi (Vitex), Difuzi (Kochia), Tianxiong (Aconitum), Qicao (Grub), Ganqi (Dried Lacquer), Cheqianzi (Plantago), Bixie (Dioscorea Collettii), Shanyao (Yam), Zexie (Alisma), Niuxi (Achyranthes)

Qianjin Yiyiren Decoction: Bailian (Ampelopsis), Yiyiren (Coix Seed), Baishao (White Peony Root), Rougui (Cinnamon), Zaoren (Jujube Seed), Ganjiang (Dried Ginger), Niuxi (Achyranthes), Gancao (Licorice), Fuzi (Aconite) in wine

Huohua Powder: Sumu (Sappan Wood), Honghua (Safflower), Moyao (Myrrh), Ziran tong (Pyrite), Ruxiang (Frankincense), Xuejie (Dragon's Blood), Mubiezi (Momordica), Dingxiang (Clove)

V. Limb Twitching

Contraction and spasm of the limbs' meridians with uncontrollable tension and relaxation were termed "yǐn yū" in ancient texts and are colloquially called "convulsions" or "spasms."It is common in febrile diseases with yin injury, postpartum women, and children with persistent fever. Mostly arising from consumption of yin and blood, reckless movement of wind and fire, it is one of the severe symptoms. *Yuanbing Shi* states: "When heat prevails and wind struggles, combining in the meridians, wind is characterized by movement and restlessness; wind and fire interacting thus give rise to confusion and twitching." It advocates the use of wind-dispelling and heat-purging formulas. This syndrome pertains to the liver and heart meridians, generally accompanied by loss of consciousness, so Zixue Dan and Angong Niuhuang Wan are mainly used for emergency treatment; once consciousness is restored, the twitching will subside.

In children, limb twitching after vomiting and diarrhea is mostly a deficiency syndrome of spleen yang collapse, accompanied by cold limbs and a thready weak pulse as the true manifestation, while feverishness and a floating large pulse are false manifestations, called "manjing" (slow convulsion). If the twitching appears weak, with eyes rolling upward and backward arching, and sweating like pearls, it is difficult to treat;

emergency treatment should consolidate the root, using Guzhen Decoction. Additionally, moxibustion is applied to Dazhui, Pishu, Tianshu, Guanyuan, Zusanli, etc.

Zixue Dan: Huashi (Talc), Shigao (Gypsum), Hanshuishi (Calcite), Cishi (Magnetite), Lingyangjiao (Antelope Horn), Muxiang (Aucklandia), Xijiao (Rhinoceros Horn), Chenxiang (Agarwood), Dingxiang (Clove), Shengma (Cimicifuga), Xuanshen (Scrophularia), Gancao (Licorice), Punxiao (Sodium Sulfate), Xiaoshi (Niter), Zhusha (Cinnabar), Shexiang (Musk) (proprietary medicine)

Angong Niuhuang Wan: Niuhuang (Bezoar), Yujin (Turmeric), Xijiao (Rhinoceros Horn), Huanglian (Coptis), Zhusha (Cinnabar), Bingpian (Borneol), Shexiang (Musk), Zhenzhu (Pearl), Shanzhi (Gardenia), Xionghuang (Realgar), Huangqin (Scutellaria), Jinbo (Gold Leaf) (proprietary medicine)

Guzhen Decoction: Renshen (Ginseng), Baizhu (Atractylodes), Fuling (Poria), Zhigancao (Roasted Licorice), Fuzi (Aconite), Rougui (Cinnamon), Shanyao (Yam), Huanglian (Coptis)

VI. Cold Limbs

Coldness in the hands and feet is called "qing"; if the cold extends beyond the wrists and ankles, it is called "jue"; if it reaches beyond the elbows and knees, it is called "ni". Thus, mild cases are termed "jueleng" (cold limbs), and severe cases "jueni" (severe cold limbs). Generally, cold limbs are mostly cold syndromes, called "hanjue" (cold reversal) or "gangjue" (rigid reversal), accompanied by coldness in the body, blue complexion, curled-up posture, diarrhea, and a faint slow pulse, treated with Sini Decoction. Meanwhile, cold limbs seen in severe stages of typhoid, diarrhea, and all deficient conditions are signs of yang deficiency and impending collapse, treated with Fuzi Lizhong Decoction and Shenfu Decoction to support yang.

Internal heat stagnation with cold limbs is called "rejue" (heat reversal) or "yangjue" (yang reversal), accompanied by fever, red complexion, restlessness, constipation, scanty reddish urine, and a slippery rapid pulse. There are also cases where limbs alternate between cold and warm, recurring repeatedly, called "deep heat with deep reversal". In all cases, the deeper the heat is, the deeper the reversal is; the milder the heat, the milder the reversal. It must not be mistaken for yin cold, and should be treated with Sini Powder and Huoyu Decoction.

Patients with blood deficiency often have cold hands and feet, even difficulty warming the lower limbs after sleeping, which must be comprehensively differentiated.

In painful syndromes such as epigastric pain and abdominal pain, when the pain is severe, the hands and feet often become cold, but warm up as the pain eases, without the need for yang restoration.

Sini Decoction: Aconite, Dried Ginger, Licorice

Fuzi Lizhong Decoction: Aconite, Ginseng, Atractylodes, Roasted Ginger, Licorice

Shenfu Decoction: Ginseng, Aconite

Sini Powder: White Peony Root, Bupleurum, Immature Bitter Orange, Licorice

Huoyu Decoction: Notopterygium, Cimicifuga, White Peony Root, Saposhnikovia, Pueraria, Starwort Root, Licorice, Scallion White

VII. Limb Emaciation

Local muscle emaciation in the limbs is common in "flaccidity syndrome" and "crane-knee wind", etc.; refer to the entries "Limb Weakness" and "Knee Swelling" in this section.

In severe or prolonged illnesses, significant emaciation of the arm and shin muscles, anciently called "loss of fleshy parts", is one of the incurable symptoms.

VIII. Red Streaks Spreading on Limbs

Sores on the fingers or toes, with toxin spreading through the meridians, appear as a red streak on the inner side of the forearm or lower leg, spreading upward. In the upper limbs, it often stops at the elbow or armpit; in the lower limbs, at the popliteal fossa or groin. Mild cases have thin red streaks without systemic symptoms; severe cases have thicker streaks accompanied by chills and fever, most commonly seen in "ding 疮" (boils) and "liuhuo" (flowing fire). In treatment, besides addressing the boils and flowing fire, a needle can be used to prick the red streak at intervals along its path, pinching the skin around the needle holes to slightly induce bleeding.

IX. Hemiplegia

Inability to move the upper and lower limbs on one side, called "hemiplegia" or "hemiparalysis", is one of the symptoms of "stroke". Most cases occur after a sudden collapse and loss of consciousness, with paralysis of one side of the limbs, becoming a sequela after regaining consciousness. Some develop gradually, starting with numbness in the hands and feet. Stroke is caused by wind, fire, phlegm, qi, etc., thus categorized into "fire stroke", "phlegm stroke", "qi stroke", and divided into syndromes involving the collaterals, channels, fu organs, and zang organs based on severity and depth. For hemiplegia, despite various causes, it involves meridian disorders, often accompanied by facial deviation and slurred speech. Treatment should nourish blood, dispel wind, and unblock meridians, using Daqinjiao Decoction and Large or Small Huoluo Dan; for persistent cases, Renshen Zaizao Wan can be used, one pill daily. Acupuncture mainly uses Quchi and Yanglingquan, combined with Jianyu, Tianjing, Waiguan, Huaniao, Fengshi, and Zusanli.

Daqinjiao Decoction: Gentiana Macrophylla, Notopterygium, Pubescent Angelica, Saposhnikovia, Angelica Dahurica, Angelica, White Peony Root, Ligusticum, Raw Rehmannia, Asarum, Atractylodes, Poria, Scutellaria, Gypsum, Licorice

Da Huoluo Dan: White-bellied Rat Snake, Black Rat Snake, Clematis, Double-pointed Aconite, Wild Aconite, Gastrodia, Scorpion, Ephedra, Polygonum Multiflorum, Turtle Shell, Male Fern, Roasted Licorice, Notopterygium, Cinnamon, Agastache, Lindera, Coptis, Prepared Rehmannia, Rhubarb, Aucklandia, Agarwood, Asarum, Red Peony Root, Clove, Bombyx Batryticatus, Frankincense, Myrrh, Arisaema, Green Tangerine Peel, Drynaria, Benzoin, Cardamom, Aconite, Scutellaria, Poria, Cyperus, Scrophularia, Atractylodes, Ginseng, Saposhnikovia, Pueraria, Tiger Bone, Angelica, Earthworm, Rhinoceros Horn, Musk, Pine Resin, Dragon's Blood, Bezoar, Borneol (proprietary medicine).

Xiao Huoluo Dan: Sichuan Aconite, Wild Aconite, Arisaema, Earthworm, Frankincense, Myrrh (proprietary medicine)

Renshen Zaizao Wan: Ginseng, Angelica, Ligusticum, Coptis, Notopterygium, Saposhnikovia, Scrophularia, Agastache, Angelica Dahurica, Poria, Ephedra, Gastrodia, Dioscorea Collettii, Turmeric, Roasted Licorice, Cinnamon, Amomum Cardamomum, Alpinia Katsumadai, Polygonum Multiflorum, Amber, Astragalus, Rhubarb, Prepared Rehmannia, Male Rat Feces, Pangolin Scales, Benzoin, Agkistrodon, Scorpion, Clematis, Pueraria, Taxillus, Asarum, Red Peony

Root, Green Tangerine Peel, Atractylodes, Bombyx Batryticatus, Myrrh, Frankincense, Cinnabar, Drynaria, Cyperus, Bambusa Concretio Silicea, Typhonium Giganteum, Turtle Shell, Agarwood, Clove, Arisaema, Safflower, Rhinoceros Horn, Magnolia Officinalis, Earthworm, Colophony, Aucklandia, Borneol, Bezoar, Dragon's Blood, Tiger Bone (proprietary medicine)

X. Shoulder and Elbow Dislocation

Dislocation of the shoulder or elbow joint with inability to move, mostly caused by improper lifting of heavy objects; in children, often due to climbing, falling, or improper pulling by adults. The affected area is swollen and painful, with inability to lift; failure to treat early may lead to disability, requiring urgent treatment by traumatology.

XI. Knee Swelling and Pain

Swelling and pain in one or both knees, with unchanged skin color and no heat sensation, gradually accompanied by emaciation of the lower legs, shaped like a crane's knee, called "crane-knee wind". Mostly due to deficiency of the three yin meridians of the foot, with invasion of wind-dampness, treatment should promote blood circulation, nourish tendons, and manage wind-dampness, using Da Fangfeng Decoction or Shiquan Dabu Decoction plus Achyranthes, Notopterygium, and Pubescent Angelica. This disease is not easy to cure quickly; Yu Jiayan once said: "Crane-knee wind is wind-cold-dampness obstructing the knee. If the knee bone enlarges daily and the muscles above and below atrophy, it is not advisable to treat the knee first; instead, regulate qi and blood to gradually nourish the muscles, then treat the knee. This is similar to treating hemiplegia: urgently nourish the non-atrophied parts to restore qi and blood circulation. If one does not understand this and only uses wind-dispersing herbs like Ephedra and Saposhnikovia, it will rarely fail to cause complete atrophy. Thus, aggressively attacking the obstruction in crane-knee wind will inevitably lead to foot flaccidity and inability to use."

In children with crane-knee wind, due to congenital weakness and accumulation of yin cold in the knee, Liuwei Dihuang Wan is used to tonify the kidney, with deer antler to tonify the life gate fire, and Achyranthes to guide the herbs to the joints and strengthen the interior; ancient physicians regarded this as a fundamental treatment.

Pain radiating from one knee, with slight redness but not much swelling above and below, is "knee migrating wind", treated with Huangu Dan; swelling and pain on both sides of the knee, with chills and high fever, and the swollen area too hot to touch, is "xiyan du" (knee-eye toxin), treated with Xianfang Huoming Yin plus Achyranthes; if only the kneecap is swollen and painful with chills and fever, it is "knee abscess", treated as ordinary abscesses.

Da Fangfeng Decoction: Astragalus, Prepared Rehmannia, Angelica, White Peony Root, Eucommia, Saposhnikovia, Aconite, Ligusticum, Notopterygium, Ginseng, Achyranthes, Roasted Licorice, Atractylodes, Ginger, Jujube

Shiquan Dabu Decoction: Angelica, Prepared Rehmannia, White Peony Root, Ligusticum, Ginseng, Atractylodes, Poria, Licorice, Astragalus, Cinnamon

Liuwei Dihuang Decoction: Prepared Rehmannia, Cornus, Yam, Moutan Bark, Poria, Alisma

Huangu Dan: Angelica, Tiger Bone, Notopterygium, Pubescent Angelica, Saposhnikovia, Dioscorea Collettii, Achyranthes, Gentiana Macrophylla, Silkworm Feces, Wolfberry, Pine Knot, White Eggplant

Root, Atractylodes Lancea, Turtle Shell, White Wine

Xianfang Huoming Yin: Pangolin Scales, Angelica Dahurica, Saposhnikovia, Red Peony Root, Saponaria Thorn, Licorice, Angelica Tail, Fritillaria, Trichosanthes Root, Honeysuckle, Decoctionerine Peel, Frankincense, Myrrh, Yellow Rice Wine

XII. Groin Pain

Groin pain is rarely seen alone. If it occurs on one side, with stabbing pain like being pierced by an awl, inability to move, no external changes, no heat in the skin when pressed, a fixed tender point on heavy pressure, and alternating chills and fever, "bone-eating abscess" must be guarded against, treated with Wanling Dan internally. After a long time, it suppurates and erodes internally, with external appearance still hard to observe; a long needle can be used for probing. There is also one that occurs on the outer side of the thigh, without redness or heat, called "bone-attached abscess", with diffuse swelling, which is easier to diagnose.

Wanling Dan: Atractylodes Lancea, Ephedra, Notopterygium, Schizonepeta, Saposhnikovia, Asarum, Sichuan Aconite, Wild Aconite, Ligusticum, Angelica, Polygonum Multiflorum, Dendrobium, Scorpion, Licorice, Realgar (proprietary medicine)

XIII. Leg Swelling

Swelling of both shins, with heavy walking, is "beriberi" syndrome. Initially, there are no significant discomforts, but one feels weakness and stiffness in both feet, difficulty in moving, slight swelling of the dorsum of the feet, and later, especially swelling of both shins. Gradually developing, it can reach the lower abdomen and even the upper abdomen, showing fullness, but rarely affecting the whole body. In severe cases, there appear reversed qi with rapid panting, vomiting and inability to eat, polydipsia, palpitations in the chest, and even confusion, disordered speech, dull complexion, flaring nostrils and purple lips, called "beriberi attacking the heart", with very rapid death. The main cause is due to insufficient spleen yang, invasion of water-dampness pathogens into the meridians, blocking qi and blood from circulation, so it is also called "obstructive disease". *Outline of Beriberi* states: "Although this disease starts from the feet, the root is in the abdomen. Therefore, if the epigastrium is relaxed, even if other symptoms are severe, most are easy to cure; if the epigastrium is hard and full, it is difficult to treat. Therefore, those who want to treat this syndrome, regardless of the feet, must ask about the condition of the abdomen. Even if the swelling subsides and numbness is relieved, if the internal abdominal disease is not eliminated, it will recur." So most cases of beriberi have swelling not exceeding the knees; once it exceeds the knees, it is difficult to treat. The pulse should be slow rather than rapid. Treatment should focus on dredging, using Jiming Powder with added Atractylodes Lancea and Stephania, etc. This formula should be taken cold at dawn (slightly warm in winter); by daybreak, the stool should pass black fecal water, and meals should be taken a little later. A folk remedy uses peanuts and red beans boiled until soft, eaten with the soup, which can be used as auxiliary treatment. In addition, when traveling to a foreign place, those caused by acclimatization will gradually recover after returning home for rest.

XIV. Dry and Shriveled Legs

Dry and shriveled legs, rough skin, accompanied by pulling pain and numbness, decreased appetite, constipation, yellowish-red urine, restlessness, and occasional retching, are symptoms of "dry beriberi". The difference between dry beriberi and general "beriberi" is that the former has no swelling, while the latter mostly has swelling. Beriberi is due to stagnation of dampness; dry beriberi is due to excessive wind-heat, damaging fluid and blood. Therefore, if beriberi presents with a string-like rapid pulse and crimson tongue, it is mostly difficult to treat, using Jiawei Siwu decoction.

Jiawei Siwu Decoction: Raw Rehmannia, White Peony Root, Ligusticum, Angelica, Achyranthes, Papaya, Phellodendron

XV. Lower Limb Paralysis

Both lower limbs feel heavy and weak, difficult to move, or accompanied by numbness and radiating pain, while the upper limbs are generally normal, called "paraplegia", belonging to the category of "feng fei" (wind paralysis). Feng fei is a syndrome in "zhong feng" (stroke), essentially involving inability to voluntarily control the limbs, mainly with inability to move the lower limbs. Thus, Zhang Jingyue said: "Feng fei involves inability to control the limbs, flaccidity, numbness, difficulty in walking and grasping, even inability to walk." Use Dihuang Yinzi to warm and nourish the lower jiao's water and fire.

Attachment: The main symptoms of "myelitis" and "tabes dorsalis" in Western medical diagnosis also affect the lower limbs, manifesting as paralysis and weakness; mild cases have unsteady walking as if treading on cotton, severe cases have complete inability to move, muscle numbness with loss of pain and itching sensation, or formication, radiating bone and tendon pain, and coldness without warmth. Accompanied by urinary and fecal retention or dribbling urine, involuntary diarrhea, impotence, decreased libido, tightness in the waist and abdomen, soreness in the lower back, dizziness and tinnitus, pale tongue or red-tipped tongue with prickles, white greasy tongue coating, string-like tight or deep thready weak pulse, etc. All belong to deficiency of liver and kidney essence and blood, especially deficiency of both kidney yin and yang, thus causing tendons and bones to lose nourishment, accompanied by a series of deficiency manifestations such as impaired qi transformation and upward disturbance of deficient wind; Dihuang Yinzi with modifications is also used. Precisely because of primordial qi deficiency, using meridian-dredging, collateral-unblocking, diuretic, or intestine-astringing herbs has no effect.

Dihuang Yinzi: Prepared Rehmannia, Cornus, Dendrobium, Ophiopogon, Cistanche, Schisandra, Acorus, Polygala, Poria, Aconite, Cinnamon, Morinda

XVI. Red and Swollen Lower Limbs

Red patches on the lower limbs, slightly swollen and painful, burning to the touch, called "liu huo" (flowing fire), belonging to the category of "dan du" (erysipelas). Mild cases subside after seven days; severe cases are accompanied by chills, fever, headache, chest tightness, nausea, vomiting, constipation, and reddish urine. The cause is nothing more than internal accumulation of kidney fire and downward pouring of damp-heat. Use Bixie Huadu Decoction as the main formula, with appropriate additions of Honeysuckle, Phellodendron, Viola Herb, Rhubarb, Schizonepeta, Saposhnikovia; for external use, Jinhuang Powder mixed with chrysanthemum dew for application. A folk remedy uses thoroughly rinsed jellyfish skin for wrapping; the stone needle method can also be used to prick and release purple blood.

Bixie Huadu Decoction: Dioscorea Collettii, Angelica Tail, Moutan Bark, Achyranthes, Stephania, Papaya, Coix Seed, Gentiana Macrophylla

Jinhuang Powder: Arisaema, Tangerine Peel, Atractylodes Lancea, Phellodendron, Turmeric, Licorice, Angelica Dahurica, Trichosanthes Root, Magnolia Officinalis, Rhubarb (proprietary medicine)

XVII. Prominent Bluish Veins in Lower Limbs

Blue-green, earthworm-like varicose veins bulge along the calves, causing distending pain after prolonged standing or walking, and are commonly seen among laborers whose work requires them to remain on their feet. Commonly seen in laborers whose work requires long periods of standing. Due to disharmony of qi and blood and stagnation of collaterals, treatment should regulate nutrient and defensive qi, promote qi and harmonize blood, using herbs such as Angelica, White Peony Root, Raw Rehmannia, Astragalus, Cinnamon Twig, Dragon's Blood, Safflower, Papaya, Achyranthes; for long-standing cases, appropriately add Agkistrodon meat and Clematis.

Section 16 Hand and Foot Symptoms

Hands and feet belong to the limbs, being the extremities of the human body, called the four ends. However, the three yin and three yang meridians all converge at the fingertips and toe tips, so local symptoms in the hands and feet often reflect disharmony of qi and blood in the internal organs, such as finger numbness, hand tremors, fist-clenching, hand-drooping, sweating of hands and feet, and heat in the palms and soles.

I. Finger Numbness

Numbness in the fingers is a precursor to "zhong feng" (stroke). It starts with numbness in the ring finger, then the middle finger, then spreads to the other three fingers; some start with the index finger. Initially, it is only in the first segment of the fingers, gradually radiating upward to the arm. Xiqian Gao or Sangzhi Gao Wan should be taken for prevention.

In blood deficiency syndrome, due to disharmony of qi and blood, finger numbness often occurs along with other blood deficiency symptoms.

Xiqian Gao: Fresh Siegesbeckia herb juiced, decocted together with Raw Rehmannia and Licorice decoction, added with refined honey and concentrated into a paste.

Sangzhi Gao Wan: Polygonum Multiflorum, Wolfberry, Angelica Body, Black Sesame, Carbonized Chrysanthemum, Platycladi Seed, Tribulus Terrestris, made into pills with Mulberry Twig Paste

II. Finger Swelling

It is one of the symptoms of "edema". Fingers feel swollen in the morning, with difficulty in flexing and extending, which gradually relieves after activity, and is not treated as a main symptom. It can also be caused by disharmony of qi and blood in other diseases such as "stroke"; generally, drugs like Rhizoma Curcumae Longae, Siegesbeckia Herb, and Loofah Sponge are used to harmonize.

III. Finger Spasm

Fingers are spasmodically contracted and cannot straighten, while the area above the wrist moves as usual, commonly known as "chicken claw wind". Due to blood failing to nourish the tendons, combined with the contractive nature of wind-cold, Jiawei Jianghuang Powder is used.

If the arm or even the lower limbs are spasmodically contracted, it is the spasm syndrome; refer to the entry "Limb Spasm" in limb symptoms.

Jiawei Jianghuang Powder: Rhizoma Curcumae Longae, Notopterygium, Atractylodes Macrocephala, Angelica, White Paeony Root,

Licorice

IV. Sore between Fingers

Small, mustard-seed-like papules erupt in finger webs causes intolerable itching that intensifies with heat. When scratched, they bleed or ooze yellow exudate, forming dry crusts. Prolonged cases develop suppuration with concurrent itching and pain—a condition known as scabies. Scratching leads to bleeding or yellow fluid discharge, forming dry scabs, and in the long run, suppuration occurs with both itching and pain, called “scabies”. There are distinctions such as “dry scabies”, “wet scabies”, and “purulent scabies”, all caused by the transformation of wind-dampness accumulated toxins. Initially, it occurs between the fingers and gradually spreads all over the body, but rarely on the head and face. External treatment is the main approach: first, decoct three *qian* of Sichuan Pepper, five *qian* of Dried Alum, and 1 *liang* of Kochia Scoparia for soaking and washing, then apply Yisaoguang, once each morning and evening. Internal medicine can use Xiaofeng Powder to clear blood, dispel wind, and detoxify.

Yisaoguang: Sophora Flavescens, Phellodendron Amurense, Tobacco Resin, Dried Alum, Alum, Momordica Cochinchinensis, Gardenia, Cnidium Monnieri, Red Pepper, Camphor, Sulfur, Mercury, Calomel, White Arsenic, Cooked Lard (proprietary medicine)

Xiaofeng Powder: Schizonepeta, Saposhnikovia, Angelica, Raw Rehmannia, Sophora Flavescens, Atractylodes Lancea, Cicada Slough, Arctium Lappa, Sesame, Anemarrhena Asphodeloides, Gypsum, Licorice, Akebia

V. Hand Tremor

Trembling of both hands, often accompanied by head shaking, is due to the inability of the tendons to restrain, belonging to wind manifestations. *Standards of Diagnosis and Treatment* states: "The head is the meeting place of all yang. When wood qi rushes downward, the head moves alone while the hands and feet do not; when it spreads to the four extremities, the hands and feet move while the head does not." It also holds that: "This disease is rare in young adults, starts to occur after middle age, and is more common in the elderly." It is mainly due to insufficient yin and blood, unable to control wind and fire, so its occurrence in any syndrome is difficult to treat. Generally, nourish blood and eliminate wind, using Dingzhen Wan with modifications.

People who often drink cold wine are prone to hand tremor, which is also difficult to cure.

Dingzhen Wan: Raw Rehmannia, Prepared Rehmannia, Angelica, White Paeony Root, Ligusticum Chuanxiong, Astragalus, Saposhnikovia, Asarum, Gastrodia Elata, Gentiana Macrophylla, Scorpion, Schizonepeta, Atractylodes Macrocephala, Clematis Chinensis

VI. Hand Drooping

Hands hanging down, even the arms unable to move, is one of the collapse syndromes of "stroke"; refer to the entry "Coma" in visceral symptoms.

VII. Clenched Fist

Hands tightly clenched into fists, is one of the blockage syndromes of "stroke"; refer to the entry "Coma" in visceral symptoms.

VIII. Grasping the Air

Hands grasping at empty space, is one of the symptoms of confusion, mostly seen in warm diseases with pathogens invading the pericardium, accompanied by delirium. *Compendium of Medicine* states: "In the extreme stage of typhoid fever and febrile diseases, it is ominous if the hands follow the clothes, grasp the air, or touch the bed." Generally, symptoms such as grasping the air, pulling threads, following the clothes, and touching the bed belong to the same category and often appear simultaneously, mainly due to unclear consciousness and blurred vision, further development leads to coma and convulsions.

IX. Pulling Threads

Hands pulling at each other as if twisting silk threads, is one of the symptoms of confusion.

X. Following the Clothes

Hands touch the clothing and bedding as if seeing something is one of the symptoms of clouded consciousness. It is mostly due to liver heat, as stated in *Yixue Gangmu* (Outline of Medicine): "When a patient's hands seek the collar and randomly twist things, it is liver heat."

XI. Touching the Bed

Hands often touch the bed as if wanting to pick up something is one of the symptoms of clouded consciousness.

XII. Pale Nails

Pale and lusterless nails, often appearing together with pale lips and tongue, are symptoms of severe blood deficiency.

XIII. Cyanotic Nails

Bluish-purple nails, commonly seen in severe heat syndromes or deficient cold syndromes, are caused by qi and blood stagnation.

XIV. Dry and Thick Nails

Dry, thick, and stacked nails, commonly called "onychomycosis", form due to blood deficiency failing to nourish them, and are relatively difficult to cure.

Prolonged untreated "tinea manuum" can also cause nails to become dry and thick; a folk remedy involves covering the finger with a pig's gallbladder. Refer to the entry "Palmar Desquamation" in this section.

XV. Swollen and Painful Fingertips

Red, hot, swollen, and painful fingertips, later festering and breaking near the nail, with severe cases leading to complete nail loss, called "daizhi" (substitute finger), also known as "tianshetou chuang" (heavenly snake head sore). Use equal parts of dandelion and xanthium, ground into powder, decocted in strong vinegar for soaking and washing; alternatively: pound dandelion, mix with water, strain, and take the liquid. Apply the residue to the affected area.

Red, swollen, and painful fingertips, accompanied by numbness and itching, with rapid swelling spreading, pain affecting the heart, and a throbbing sensation, along with chills and fever, are mostly "dingdu" (nailhead furuncle toxin). Different names exist based on the location: Those on the tip of the finger are called "shetou ding" (snake head furuncle), those beside the nail "sheyan ding" (snake eye furuncle), those behind the nail "shebei ding" (snake back furuncle), those on the finger pad "shefu ding" (snake belly furuncle), those under the nail "yanzhua ding" (along the nail furuncle), and those between the finger joints "shejie ding" (snake joint furuncle), collectively called "zhiding" (finger furuncle). Caused by internal accumulation of fire toxin orwounded by an external object, treatment should clear heat and detoxify. Initially, use Wuwei Xiaodu Yin with added banzhilian (scutellaria barbata) and caoheche (rhizoma paridis), etc.; for severe cases, can add chansu wan (toad venom pill). During suppuration, use Wuwei Xiaodu Yin combined with Huanglian Jiedu Decoction, and can also add shigao (gypsum), lianqiao (forsythia), zhuye (bamboo leaf); for constipation, add dahuang (rhubarb) and xuanmingfen (sodium sulfate). Stop internal medication once pus drains, swelling subsides, and heat recedes. For external treatment, apply Qianchui Gao (thousand-hammer paste) initially; during suppuration, sprinkle Erbao Dan on the sore, cover with Qianchui Gao; once pus is exhausted and new tissue grows, switch to Shengji Powder (flesh-generating powder) and apply Taiyi Gao (supreme ointment). The above is the general treatment method for finger furuncles; note that this condition progresses rapidly and is extremely painful. Improper treatment can lead to spreading swelling, with severe "zouhuang" (running yellow) phenomena such as clouded consciousness, convulsions, and syncope. Additionally, suppuration times vary; those on the fingertip, fingerprint, and joints easily damage tendons and bones. If finger bones are damaged, the necrotic bone must be removed for healing, which should be handled by a surgeon.

Wuwei Xiaodu Yin: yinhua (honeysuckle), wild chrysanthemum, zihuadiding (viola philippica), tiankuizi (semiaquilegia adoxoides), pugongying (dandelion)

Chansu Wan: chansu (toad venom), qingfen (calomel), ku fan (dried alum), hanshuishi (calcite), ruxiang (frankincense), moyao (myrrh), tonglu (malachite), danfan (chalcanthite), shexiang (musk), xionghuang (realgar), woniu (snail), zhusha (cinnabar) (proprietary medicine)

Huanglian Jiedu Decoction: huanglian (coptis), huangbai (phellodendron), zhizi (gardenia), huangqin (scutellaria)

Qianchui Gao: songxiang (rosin), bima zi (castor bean), tonglu (malachite), xingren (apricot kernel), ercha (catechu), ruxiang (frankincense), moyao (myrrh), xuejie (dragon's blood), qingfen (calomel), zhenzhu (pearl), mayou (sesame oil) (proprietary medicine)

Erbao Dan: Eight *liang* of duanshigao (calcined gypsum), two *liang* of shengdan (elevated pellet), ground into fine powder

Shengji Powder: One *liang* each of hanshuishi (calcite), huashi (talc), longgu (dragon bone), wuzegu (cuttlefish bone); five *qian* each of dingfen (lead acetate), mituoseng (litharge), baifanhui (alum ash), ganyanzhi (dried carmine), ground into fine powder

Taiyi Gao: Scrophularia, Angelica Dahurica, Angelica Body, Cinnamon, Red Peony Root, Rhubarb, Raw Rehmannia, Momordica Cochinchinensis, Asafoetida, Calomel, Willow Twig, Pagoda Tree Twig, Human Hair, Lead Oxide, Frankincense, Myrrh, Sesame Oil (proprietary medicine)

XVI. Sunken Finger Pads

Referred to as "bi luo" (sunken pads), commonly seen in "cholera" with sudden loss of fluids, commonly called "bi luo sha" (a cholera-like syndrome with severe dehydration), one of the severe symptoms. Refer to the entry "Vomiting and Diarrhea" in visceral symptoms.

XVII. Palmar Desquamation

Dryness and itching of the palm, followed by white scales, with withered, dry, and cracked skin, spreading from the palm to the entire hand but not affecting the back of the hand, called "ezhangfeng" (goose palm wind). Due to blood dryness generating wind, it can cause nails to become dry and thick. Internally, take Qufeng Dihuang Wan; externally, apply Hongyou (red oil) or Runji Gao (moisturizing ointment). This condition lessens in hot weather and worsens in cold, being extremely stubborn. In hot weather, Xueshui (tinea liquid) can be used for soaking.

In the weak or ordinary people, peeling of hand skin in autumn is caused by blood deficiency and autumn dryness, requiring no treatment.

Qufeng Dihuang Wan: Raw Rehmannia, Prepared Rehmannia, Tribulus Terrestris, Sichuan Achyranthes, Anemarrhena, Phellodendron, Wolfberry, Cuscuta, Pubescent Angelica

Hongyou: One *qian* of red arsenic, one *liang* of sesame oil, fried until the arsenic is dry and fumes cease, remove the arsenic and retain the oil.

Runji Gao: Five *qian* of Angelica, one *liang* of Lithospermum, fried in four *liang* of sesame oil until the herbs are dry, strain the oil, reheat it, and add five *qian* of yellow wax to melt completely.

Xueshui: Stemona, Cnidium, Sulfur eight *liang* each, White Arsenic two *qian*, Blister Beetle two *liang*, Camphor, Calomel one *liang* and two *qian* each, Hibiscus Bark 10 *liang*, soaked in 20 *jin* of rice vinegar.

XVIII. Dorsal Foot Swelling

Due to spleen deficiency with downward flow of water-dampness, it is also the initial stage of "edema" disease. It often increases after activity and decreases after rest. Living in a humid place for a long time can cause dorsal foot swelling, with a heavy sensation when walking, which can also develop into "beriberi" swelling. For mild cases, use 3 *qian* each of raw and cooked Coix Seed soaked as a tea substitute; if it does not subside, use Guiling Cao Zao Decoction.

Guiling Cao Zao Decoction: Cinnamon Twig, Poria, Licorice, Jujube

XIX. Heel Pain

Heel pain without swelling or redness, inability to stand or walk for long is caused by deficiency of liver-kidney yin and blood. Though a minor illness, treatment should involve strong tonification, using Lujiaojiao Wan and Li'an Wan.

Lujiaojiao Wan: Deer Antler Glue, Deer Antler Frost, Prepared Rehmannia, Ginseng, Achyranthes, Poria, Cuscuta, Atractylodes, Eucommia, Turtle Shell, Angelica, Tiger Bone

Li'an Wan: Achyranthes, Eucommia, Psoralea, Phellodendron, Fennel

XX. Purple-Black Toes

The skin around the toes turns from purple to black, gradually spreading and decaying, oozing foul fluid. The flesh at the ulcerated area is dull in color, with an extremely foul odor and severe pain, worsening at night. As the decay spreads, it can affect all five toes one after another, gradually leading to necrosis of the affected joints, which may fall off on their own, leaving the wound unhealed for a long time. Mostly caused by accumulation of cold-dampness and wind, combined with blazing yin fire, the disease is called "tuoju" (gangrenous finger/toe), a dangerous external condition. *Nei Jing* (The Inner Canon) early on stated: "That which arises on the foot is called tuoyong (gangrenous abscess); if it appears red-black, it is incurable. If not red-black, it is not fatal; if it does not subside, promptly amputate it, otherwise death will follow." *Wai Ke Zheng Zong* (Orthodox External Medicine) also detailed the prognosis, considering it auspicious if initially appearing like hemp seeds, red-hot and painful, with swelling of the entire toe, a contracted base; after formation, the tip becomes necrotic without purple-black discoloration, pain occurring intermittently, swelling subsiding after pus discharge, and no foul odor. It is considered adverse if initially the flesh turns purple, with no swelling but stabbing pain, spreading black qi; after formation, the ulcer is shriveled, with black flesh and scorched skin, pain like knife cuts, toxin spreading to healthy toes, foul bloody discharge after ulceration, flesh and tendons rotting, and severe pain affecting the heart. Thus, treatment must emphasize both internal and external approaches, with internal formulas such as Yanghe Decoction, Simiao Yong'an Decoction, Yin-Yang Liangqi Dan, etc., used according to the syndrome. External treatment involves applying Hongling Dan; after decay, switch to Yuhong Gao, and concurrently use Hongling Jiu to rub the surrounding skin to promote blood circulation and relieve pain. If no improvement is seen, surgery should be performed before the spread continues.

Yanghe Decoction: Prepared Rehmannia, White Mustard Seed, Roasted Ginger, Licorice, Cinnamon, Deer Antler Glue, Ephedra

Simiao Yong'an Decoction: Scrophularia, Angelica, Honeysuckle, Licorice

Yin-Yang Liangqi Dan: Asparagus, Ophiopogon, Scrophularia, Schisandra, Human Urinary Calculus, Phellodendron, Licorice, Alisma, Dried Alum, Indigo Naturalis, Borneol

Hongling Dan: Realgar, Frankincense, Borax, Chlorite Schist, Myrrh, Borneol, Potassium Nitrate, Cinnabar, Musk (proprietary medicine)

Yuhong Gao: Angelica, Angelica Dahurica, White Wax, Calomel,

Licorice, Lithospermum, Dragon's Blood, Sesame Oil (proprietary medicine)

Hongling Jiu: Two *liang* each of Angelica and Cinnamon, one *liang* each of Safflower, Sichuan Pepper, and Dried Ginger, five *qian* each of Camphor and Asarum, soaked in two *jin* of alcohol for seven days

XXI. Web Space Dampness of the Foot

Downward flow of damp-heat, with fluid immersion, causing dampness in the toe webs, unbearable itching, often leading to rubbing until the skin breaks and pains, oozing blood and fluid, which temporarily relieves the itching but recurs the next day, persisting for years, commonly called "dampness". In severe cases, there is excruciating putrid pain, swollen toes, pus and fluid discharge, a foul odor, and difficulty walking, called "chou tianluo" (foul field snail), also "lan jiaoya" (rotten toe webs). Soak feet each night with a little alum in water, dry thoroughly after washing; apply Huanglian Gao for mild cases, and Sanshi Powder for severe breaks.

Huanglian Gao: Coptis, Angelica, Phellodendron, Raw Rehmannia, Turmeric, Yellow Wax, Sesame Oil (proprietary medicine)

Sanshi Powder: Three *liang* each of Calamine, Calcined Gypsum, and Red Halloysite, ground into powder

XXII. Plantar Corns

Due to wearing tight shoes for long walks or traversing rough roads, damaging blood vessels, hard calluses form on the feet, with roots embedded in the flesh, protruding as hard bumps, causing pain and hindering walking, called "rouci" (flesh thorn), commonly known as "corns". External treatment uses Qianjin Powder to corrode, but surgical removal is more straightforward.

Abrasions beside the heel, shaped like jujubes or chestnuts, swollen with shiny skin, which can suppurate, called "shangli" (upper chestnut), treated as ordinary external ulcers.

Qianjin Powder: Five *qian* each of Frankincense, Myrrh, Calomel, Cinnabar, Red Halloysite, Galla Chinensis, Realgar, and Ophicalcite, two *qian* of White Arsenic, ground into fine powder

XXIII. Ingrown Nails

Toenails grow into the flesh, with swelling beside the nails, pain when walking, which can cause breaking, prominent granulation tissue, and even pus invading under the nails; recovery can only occur after the nails fall off. The condition is called "jiaju" (nail abscess), commonly known as "embedded nail". First, use Pingnu Dan to corrode and flatten the granulation, then apply Shengji Powder to promote healing.

Pingnu Dan: 1.5 *qian* each of Dark Plum and Borax, five *fen* of Calomel, three *fen* of Borneol, ground into fine powder.

Shengji Powder: One *liang* each of Calcite, Talc, Dragon Bone, and Cuttlefish Bone; five *qian* each of Lead Acetate, Litharge, Alum Ash, and Dried Carmine, ground into fine powder.

XXIV. Dry and Cracked Skin

Dry, cracked, and painful skin on the palms and soles, called "junlie chuang" (cracked sore). It is more common in boatmen, cart pushers, fishermen, and dyers, caused by friction, pressure, trauma, and immersion. Decoct Cortex Lycii and Alum in water, soak the affected area until soft, then apply melted waxed sheep oil; if sheep oil is unavailable, lard can be used instead.

XXV. Cold Hands and Feet

There is a distinction between blood deficiency and yang deficiency, and it is also a precursor to reversal (cold limbs extending upward). Refer to the entry "Cold Limbs" in limb symptoms.

Persistent coldness in the hands, especially in winter, even difficulty warming up after sleep, although related to constitution, cannot be used as a diagnostic basis in general conditions.

XXVI. Heat in the Palms and Soles

Heat in the palms and soles, often with a desire to hold cold objects and extend hands and feet outside the quilt while sleeping; some have only heat in the palms or only in the soles. All are manifestations of insufficient yin blood and internal heat disturbance. If accompanied by irritable feverish sensation in the chest, it is called "five-center heat" (heat in the palms, soles, and chest). It is appropriate to add Cortex Lycii, Cynanchum atratum, etc., to yin-nourishing and blood-nourishing formulas.

For kidney deficiency with downward flow of damp-heat, heat in the soles, heat in the shins, and yellow-red urine, use Zhibai Bawei Wan with added Gentiana macrophylla.

Heat in the palms and soles is often accompanied by moist, sweaty palms and soles. Refer to the entry "Sweating of Hands and Feet" in this section.

Zhibai Bawei Wan: Raw Rehmannia, Cornus, Yam, Moutan Bark, Poria, Alisma, Phellodendron, Anemarrhena.

XXVII. Sweating of Hands and Feet

Sweating of hands and feet with heat in the palms and soles belongs to blood deficiency; sweating with cold hands and feet belongs to qi deficiency. Neither is treated as a main symptom. Appropriately add ingredients such as Jujube Seed, Floating Wheat, Ephedra Root, Calcined Oyster, and Dried Green Plum to the main formula.

For those with frequent excessive foot sweat, use five *qian* each of Alum and Pueraria, ground into powder, decocted in water for ten-odd boils, and soak the feet daily.

Section 17 Anterior Genital Symptoms

Due to physiological differences between men and women, anterior genital symptoms vary. This section includes impotence, genital retraction, coldness of the genitals, itching of the genitals, hernia, uterine prolapse, and corrosion of the genital area. In terms of etiology, they are mostly related to yang deficiency, qi sinking, liver fire, and damp-heat. Generally, the kidney is considered the innate foundation for men, and the liver for women; moreover, the Liver Meridian, Conception Vessel, and Governor Vessel all course through the genitals. Therefore, anterior genital symptoms are closely related to the liver, kidney, Conception Vessel, and Governor Vessel.

I. Impotence

In men who have not yet reached the period of sexual desire decline, the penis fails to erect, or erects but is not firm or lasting, which is called "yangwei" (impotence). It is mostly caused by excessive masturbation in adolescence, depletion of the life gate fire, deficiency and cold of essence and qi, as Zhang Jingyue put it, "cases of fire decline account for seven or eight out of ten". However, it is also closely related to excessive use of brain, overthinking, and damage to the heart and spleen. Generally, those with insufficient kidney qi are accompanied by symptoms of yang deficiency such as soreness and weakness of the waist and feet, and fear of cold; those with deficiency of the heart and spleen are mostly accompanied by symptoms of blood deficiency such as mental fatigue, palpitations, and insomnia. Common treatment formulas mostly tonify essence and blood, combined with warm and moist substances of animal origin, such as Banlong Wan, Erzhi Baibu Wan, Zanhua Xueyu Dan, Dabuyuan Jian, Qiangyang Zhuangjing Dan, etc., all of which can be selected. This disease is mostly partial to yang deficiency, so general treatment focuses on warm and hot substances, but it must be syndrome-specific, and fire-tonifying ingredients must be added to water-nourishing formulas; otherwise, it will take effect temporarily, damage the true yin, and lead to adverse consequences. At the same time, most patients with this syndrome are in a state of fear and mental distress, which also affects the curative effect, and they should be comforted.

Banlong Wan: Deer Antler Glue, Deer Antler Frost, Cuscuta, Platycladi Seed, Prepared Rehmannia

Erzhi Baibu Wan: Deer Antler Glue, Polygonatum, Wolfberry, Prepared Rehmannia, Cuscuta, Rosa Laevigata, Asparagus, Ophiopogon, Achyranthes, Broussonetia Fruit, Longan Aril, Deer Antler Frost, Ginseng, Astragalus, Poria, Raw Rehmannia, Cornus, Schisandra, Euryale, Yam, Anemarrhena

Zanhua Xueyu Dan: Carbonized Human Hair, Prepared Rehmannia, Wolfberry, Angelica, Deer Antler Glue, Cuscuta, Eucommia, Morinda, Fennel, Poria, Cistanche, Walnut, Polygonum Multiflorum, Ginseng

Dabuyuan Jian: Ginseng, Yam, Prepared Rehmannia, Eucommia,

Angelica, Cornus, Wolfberry, Roasted Licorice

Qiangyang Zhuangjing Dan: Prepared Rehmannia, Astragalus, Angelica, White Peony Root, Morinda, Ophiopogon, Wolfberry, Platycladi Seed, Rubus, Tiger Shank Bone, Deer Antler, Aconite, Cinnamon, honeyed pills

II. Easy Erection of the Penis

Frequent easy erection of the penis in daily life is mostly due to excessive ministerial fire, treated with Longdan Xiegan Decoction. Yin deficiency patients may also have easy erection during illness, which is due to water failing to control fire and reckless movement of deficient fire; bitter and cold substances to directly reduce fire are inappropriate, and Dabuyin Wan is used.

Longdan Xiegan Decoction: Gentiana, Gardenia, Scutellaria, Raw Rehmannia, Angelica, Plantago, Akebia, Bupleurum, Licorice, Alisma

Dabuyin Wan: Prepared Rehmannia, Turtle Shell, Phellodendron, Anemarrhena, Pig Spinal Cord

III. Prolonged Unretracted Penis

Referred to as "yinzong" (penile lengthening) in *Yixue Gangmu* (Outline of Medicine), caused by heat accumulation in the liver meridian, treated with Xiaochaihu Decoction plus Coptis and Phellodendron; for external use, loofah juice mixed with Galla Chinensis powder for application.

Xiaochaihu Decoction: Bupleurum, Scutellaria, Pinellia, Ginseng, Licorice, Ginger, Jujube

IV. Genital Coldness

Including coldness of the penis or scrotum without warmth, mostly due to decline of life gate fire or stagnation of cold qi in the kidney, treated with Shibu Wan. Women with coldness in the vagina, accompanied by a cold sensation in the abdomen, often affecting fertility due to deficiency and cold of the lower origin. Warming and nourishing methods are also used, and pills made of Cnidium and Evodia with musk added, wrapped in cotton, can be inserted into the vagina.

Shibu Wan: Aconite, Psoralea, Aucklandia, Morinda, Cinnamon, Sichuan Chinaberry, Corydalis, Cubeb, Fennel, Psoralea Corylifolia

V. Genital Swelling

Swelling of the scrotum or including the penile foreskin with a shiny appearance, without pain or itching, mostly caused by sitting on damp ground, more common in children, treated with 5 *qian* of Cicada Slough decocted for washing three times a day, and Sanshan Decoction taken internally.

Sudden swelling and pain of the female vulva, caused by strain to the blood aspect, treated with Qinjiao Decoction internally, and external fuming and washing with Artemisia Argyi, Saposhnikovia, and Euphorbia decoction.

In severe cases of "edema" with general swelling, including genital swelling, treatment is directed at the main symptom.

Sanshan Decoction: Plantago Seed, Fennel, Amomum, Scallion White

Qinjiao Decoction: Gentiana Macrophylla, Angelica, Acorus, Scallion White

VI. Genital Contraction

Contraction of the penis or scrotum can occur in both cold and heat syndromes; clinically, it is commonly seen as one of the critical signs of extreme deficiency of yin and yang.

Women can also experience genital contraction, i.e., the vulva drawing toward the lower abdomen, which is also a critical condition.

VII. Testicular Distension and Pain

Distending pain and sagging of the testicles, or radiating pain to the lower abdomen, is one of the symptoms of "shànqì" (hernia). There are many types of hernias; Zhang Zihe summarized them into seven types: "cold hernia", "water hernia", "fox hernia", "tendon hernia", "blood hernia", "large hernia", and "qi hernia", collectively called the seven hernias, all belonging to diseases of the scrotum and testicles with swelling or pain. Their characteristics are: Cold hernia is hard as stone, with pain radiating to the testicles; large hernia has a scrotum swollen like a bucket, without itching or pain; water hernia has a swollen scrotum with shiny skin and occasional genital sweating; fox hernia has painful swelling of the testicles, sagging when standing or walking, and retracting when lying down; blood hernia and tendon hernia are surgical conditions. Clinically, qi hernia is more common, also known as ordinary hernia, commonly called "small intestine qi". Due to failure of liver qi to circulate smoothly, or qi stagnation in the lower part from prolonged standing or long walking, treatment should focus on soothing the liver and regulating qi, using Jisheng Juhe Wan, Lixiang Powder; for persistent cases, Sanceng Huixiang Wan. However, if it recurs with exertion, due to qi deficiency failing to lift, Astragalus, Angelica, and Cimicifuga should be added; exclusive use of qi-moving and stagnation-dispersing herbs is inappropriate.

Excessive crying in children can also cause sagging pain of the testicles, commonly called “sag hernia”, treated similarly.

Jisheng Juhe Wan: Tangerine Seed, Sichuan Chinaberry, Magnolia Officinalis, Cinnamon, Corydalis, Immature Bitter Orange, Aucklandia, Akebia, Peach Kernel, Sargassum, Kelp, Sea Tangle

Lixiang Powder: Litchi Seed, Fennel

Sanceng Huixiang Wan: One *liang* each of Star Anise, Sichuan Chinaberry, Adenophora, Aucklandia, ground into powder, made into pills with rice paste, three *qian* each dose, three times a day – this is the first layer; after finishing the above, add one *liang* of Piper Longum and five *qian* of Areca, prepared and taken as before – this is the second layer; if still unhealed, add four *liang* of Poria and one *liang* of Aconite – this is the third layer. All are taken on an empty stomach with warm wine or light salt water.

VIII. Scrotal Itching

There are dry and wet types. The wet type has dampness and itching, or sores with peeling skin, which can spread to the feet causing sores and tinea, due to wind-damp toxin descending from deficiency; internally take Huoxue Qufeng Powder, externally dust with Jiaofen Powder. The dry type has scurf when scratched, with fluid oozing when broken, and burning pain like fire, due to blood deficiency generating dryness combined with liver meridian damp-heat, called “kidney sac wind”, commonly known as “hydrangea wind”; externally fume and wash with Shechuangzi Decoction, and apply Langdu Gao.

Huoxue Qufeng Powder: Tribulus Terrestris, Angelica, Ligusticum, Angelica Dahurica, Asarum, Peach Kernel, Pinellia, White Peony Root,

Trogopterus Dung, Raw Licorice, Atractylodes Lancea, Eucommia, Cinnamon, Coix Seed, Gastrodia, Tangerine Peel, Areca, Magnolia Officinalis, Aurantium

Jiaofen Powder: Ephedra Root, Male Fern, Cnidium, Sichuan Pepper, Angelica, Polyporus, Blister Beetle, Calomel, Safflower

Shechuangzi Decoction: Clematis, Cnidium, Angelica Tail, Amomum Shell, Rhubarb, Sophora Flavescens, Scallion White

Langdu Gao: Three *qian* each of Stellera, Sichuan Pepper, Sulfur, Areca, Clam Shell, Cnidium, Hydnocarpus, Dried Alum, ground into powder, mixed with one cup of sesame oil, boiled, and blended with one pig gallbladder.

IX. Anterior Genital Erosion

In both men and women, small blisters initially appear in the anterior genital area, gradually enlarging; after breaking, they start to erode, with bloody fluid dripping, the raised margins, and the middle corroded into a pit, oozing pus. All are caused by "syphilis" and called "gan chuang" (ulcerative sores). In men, they are classified as: those occurring under the glans are called "xia gan" (lower ulcer), those on the penis "zhu gan" (boring ulcer), those wrapped by the outer skin "xiu kou gan" (cuff ulcer), and those extensively eroded over time "la zhu gan" (candle ulcer). In women, they mostly occur on both sides of the vulva, also called "du jing chuang" (jealousy essence sore) and "chi chuang" (pubic sore).

"Yang mei chuang" (syphilitic sore) also starts in the genitals: those shaped like red beans embedded in the flesh are called "yang mei dou" (syphilitic beans), those itchy like wind rash "yang mei zhen" (syphilitic rash), and those starting with red halos followed by spots "yang mei ban" (syphilitic macules). In severe cases, there are bone and tendon pain, painful urination, and numerous sores on the hands and feet. After liberation, syphilis has been basically eradicated, and such syndromes are rarely seen clinically.

X. Pubic Lice

Eight-legged lice growing in the pubic hair of both men and women, causing unbearable itching, with redness after scratching, all transmitted through contact, called "yin shi chuang" (pubic lice sore). The lice heads burrow into the skin; a needle should be used to pick and remove the lice, followed by application of Yinxing Wuyou Powder.

Yinxing Wuyou Powder: One *qian* each of mercury, calomel, almond, aloe, realgar, and stellera, one *fen* of musk, ground into powder.

XI. Female Vulvar Itching

Itching in the female vagina is mostly caused by deficiency of liver and spleen qi with downward flow of damp-heat, accompanied by chest oppression, irritability, and scanty reddish urine, treated with Jiawei Xiaoyao Powder plus akebia and phellodendron. For unbearable itching and pain, frequent fluid discharge, and restlessness day and night, external fuming and washing with Shechuangzi Fang or Ta Yang Decoction is used.

Itchy lumps growing outside the vulva, due to small worms, called "yin shi" (vulvar erosion), also "yin chan", treated internally with Luhui Wan and externally with Ta Yang Decoction for fuming and washing.

Jiawei Xiaoyao Powder: angelica, white peony root, bupleurum, atractylodes, poria, licorice, mint, gardenia, moutan bark, ginger.

Shechuangzi Fang: cnidium, sichuan pepper, alum.

Ta Yang Decoction: carpesium, sophora flavescens, clematis, angelica tail, cnidium, eupatorium.

Luhui Wan: aloe, green tangerine peel, coptis, picrorhiza, thunder god vine, ulmus, carpesium, aucklandia, musk.

XII. Vaginal Flatulence

Vaginal flatulence in women, similar to passing flatus, called "yin chui" (vaginal flatus). Due to dryness of large intestine fluid and stagnation of food qi, Zhu Gao Fa Jian is used. However, for those with loose stools, He Li Le Powder from *Yi Zong Jin Jian* (Golden Mirror of Medical Orthodoxy) can be used.

Zhu Gao Fa Jian: lard, hair.

He Li Le Powder: terminalia, tangerine peel, magnolia officinalis.

XIII. Uterine Prolapse

Prolapse of the uterus or its protrusion outside the vagina, often with a sensation of lower abdominal sagging, called "yin zhong" (vaginal swelling), which is caused by insufficient rest after childbirth or excessive labor during menstruation, varying in degree but all due to qi and blood deficiency failing to contain, treated with Bu Zhong Yi Qi Decoction with increased cimicifuga.

Bu Zhong Yi Qi Decoction: astragalus, codonopsis, atractylodes, licorice, angelica, bupleurum, cimicifuga, tangerine peel, ginger, jujube.

Section 18 Posterior Genital Symptoms

The posterior genitalia refer to the anus; symptoms in this section include itching, pain, sagging, fissures, erosion, and sore toxins, all local disorders. Etiologically, they involve middle qi sinking and downward flow of damp-heat, closely related to internal organs. Therefore, some conditions require external treatment, which should be combined with internal medications for better effect.

I. Anal Itching

Anal itching is common in children with "pinworm disease"; the itching mostly occurs at night, with tiny worms crawling out. Use eight *qian* of quisqualis and one *qian* of raw rhubarb, ground into powder; administer one *fen* per year of age, with a maximum dose not exceeding two *qian* and two *fen*, for six consecutive days. Additionally, decoct one to two *liang* of stemona each night for retention enema.

II. Anal Prolapse

Protrusion of the anus, called "tuogang" (rectal prolapse), is more common in the elderly with insufficient middle qi, often occurring due to difficulty in defecation and prolapse after bowel movements. Use one *qian* of ginseng rhizome for decoction. It can also occur in cases of prolonged diarrhea or dysentery with qi deficiency and sinking. Ancient physicians once stated: "Heat leads to anal constriction, deficiency leads to anal prolapse." Therefore, the general treatment for this condition involves lifting and tonifying with herbs such as ginseng, atractylodes, cimicifuga, and pueraria, or nourishing blood and astringing with angelica, white peony root, gallnut, and red halloysite; promoting qi and breaking qi are contraindicated.

In patients with fistula, if the anus prolapses and bleeds after bowel movements, decoct five *qian* of gallnut, add one *qian* each of nitre and schizonepeta, and fumigate and wash with the hot decoction, then dust with gallnut powder.

III. Anal Fissure Pain

Anal fissure pain is referred to as "ganglie" (anal fissure) for short, characterized by pain and bleeding during bowel movements, or persistent pain after defecation. This condition is easily confused with "internal hemorrhoids". However, internal hemorrhoids generally do not cause pain during bowel movements and involve the most bleeding, making differentiation not difficult. It is advisable to administer Runchang Decoction internally and apply Shengji Powder externally.

In the early stage of anal fissure, the fissure is red in color; if it fails to heal for a long time, it turns grayish-white, with edges like a jar mouth, and small grains the size of mung beans or as large as a finger may grow near the fissure, forming external hemorrhoids. Refer to the entry "Anal Hemorrhoids" in this section.

Runchang Decoction: Angelica, Raw Rehmannia, Licorice, Hemp Seed, Peach Kernel

Shengji Powder: One *liang* each of calcite, talc, dragon bone, and cuttlefish bone; five *qian* each of lead acetate, litharge, alum ash, and dried carmine, ground into fine powder.

IV. Anal Erosion

In *Synopsis of the Golden Chamber*, it is pointed out in the "huhu" (fox bewilderment) disease that "erosion in the throat is called 'huo' (bewilderment), erosion in the genitals is called 'hu' (fox)". Its associated symptoms include a condition resembling typhoid fever, with quietness and a desire to sleep, inability to close the eyes, restlessness in lying and rising, loss of appetite, aversion to the smell of food, and the face alternating between red, black, and white. Internally, Gancao Xiexin

Decoction is administered, and external treatments include washing with sophora flavescens decoction and fumigating the anus with burning realgar.

Attachment: In Western medical diagnosis of "leukemia", there may be anal erosion, accompanied by white erosion in the throat, along with chills and fever, and a thready rapid pulse. The phenomena of yin deficiency with blazing fire and downward flow of damp-heat are relatively obvious; for internal formulas, Yangyin Qingfei Decoction and Duanxia Shenshi Decoction can be considered. Externally, Xilei Powder is insufflated into the throat, and Sanhuang Erxiang Powder is applied to the anus.

Gancao Xiexin Decoction: Licorice, Scutellaria, Dried Ginger, Coptis, Pinellia, Jujube

Yangyin Qingfei Decoction: Raw Rehmannia, Scrophularia, Ophiopogon, Fritillaria, Moutan Bark, White Peony Root, Licorice, Mint

Duanxia Shenshi Decoction: Phellodendron, Atractylodes Lancea, Ailanthus Root Bark, Sanguisorba, Hawthorn, Honeysuckle, Red Poria, Polyporus

Xilei Powder: Ivory Shavings, Pearl, Indigo Naturalis, Borneol, Spider Egg Case, Bezoar, Human Nail Clippings (proprietary medicine)

Sanhuang Erxiang Powder: One *liang* each of Coptis, Phellodendron, and Rhubarb; five *qian* each of Frankincense and Myrrh, ground into powder, mixed with sesame oil for application.

V. Anal Hemorrhoids

Small fleshy protrusions inside and outside the anus, resembling mounds, are collectively called "hemorrhoids". They are mostly caused by excessive consumption of greasy and spicy foods, prolonged sitting or standing, carrying heavy loads for long journeys, frequent constipation, physical weakness, and the invasion of wind-dryness, dampness-heat pathogens that accumulate due to deficiency. Those growing inside the anus are "internal hemorrhoids". Initially small and soft in texture, with a bright red or bluish-purple surface, they often bleed when scratched by stool but are not painful. Later, they gradually enlarge and may protrude outside the anus during bowel movements, retracting on their own afterward. In the late stage, they protrude not only during bowel movements but also when coughing or after prolonged standing, and are difficult to reset. At this time, their texture is slightly hard, the surface is slightly white, and they vary in shape and size (long, round, large, small). When hemorrhoids become incarcerated and cannot retract, they often cause swelling, pain, and ulceration, leading to secondary "anal fistula". Those growing outside the anus are called "external hemorrhoids", which are relatively hard to the touch, smooth in appearance, generally painless, and do not bleed. There are also cases where both internal and external hemorrhoids exist, called "internal and external hemorrhoids", which are often connected. They mostly occur at the left middle, right front, and right rear parts of the anus, especially the right front. There are many effective methods for treating hemorrhoids, such as internal treatment, acupuncture, moxibustion, ironing, fumigation and washing, external application, ligation, and hemorrhoid-curing (cauterization) methods. Among them, the hemorrhoid-curing method and ligation are radical treatments, but they require skilled operation and should be performed by experts. General internal treatment is suitable for initial hemorrhoids and elderly and weak patients: ① For pain, regardless of wind-dampness, dryness, or heat, use Zhitong Rushen Decoction; ② For bleeding, whether before or after defecation, if it is a wind-heat excess syndrome, use Liangxue Dihuang Decoction; if caused by alcohol-induced damp-toxin, use Kushen Dihuang Wan; ③ For protrusion, use Buzhong Yiqi

Decoction.

Zhitong Rushen Decoction: Gentiana Macrophylla, Peach Kernel, Gleditsia Seed, **Atractylodes Lancea, Saposhnikovia, Phellodendron, Angelica Tail, Alisma, Areca, Rhubarb**

Liangxue Dihuang Decoction: Raw Rehmannia, Angelica Tail, Red Peony Root, Coptis, Immature Bitter Orange, Scutellaria, Sophora Japonica, Sanguisorba, Schizonepeta, Cimicifuga, Trichosanthes Root, Licorice

Kushen Dihuang Wan: Sophora Flavescens, Raw Rehmannia

Buzhong Yiqi Decoction: Astragalus, Ginseng, Atractylodes, Licorice, Angelica Body, Tangerine Peel, Cimicifuga, Bupleurum

VI. Anal Sore Toxin

Abscesses occurring in the anus, mostly with a raised, red, swollen, and painful area on one side or around the anus, shaped like a peach or plum, accompanied by alternating chills and fever, constipation, and scanty reddish urine. In severe cases, there is a heavy, tight sensation in the anus, obstruction of qi downward, unbearable stabbing pain, and a slippery rapid pulse, with pus formation and rupture occurring in about three to five days. Among them, abscesses surrounding the anus are the most severe, called "zangdu" (visceral toxin); those forming pus on either the left or right side are milder, named "toufenshu" (stool-stealing rat); if pus discharges from both sides, it is more complex, named "gangmen yong" (anal abscess). These external conditions are mostly caused by excessive alcohol and rich foods leading to downward flow of dampness-heat. Treatment should clear heat, drain dampness, cool blood, and dispel stasis. Use Sanmiao Wan combined with Liangxue Dihuang Decction, removing Cimicifuga and Schizonepeta; for constipation, add

Rhubarb and Xuanmingfen; for scanty reddish urine, add Red Poria and Plantago; when pus is about to form, add Pangolin Scales and Gleditsia Thorns; for weak patients, use Ziyin Chushi Decoction, with external application of Jinhuang Powder. After rupture, internal medications can be stopped, and treatment follows that of ordinary ulcers.

Sanmiao Wan: Atractylodes Lancea, Phellodendron, Anemarrhena

Liangxue Dihuang Decoction: Raw Rehmannia, Angelica Tail, Red Peony Root, Coptis, Immature Bitter Orange, Scutellaria, Sophora Japonica, Sanguisorba, Schizonepeta, Cimicifuga, Trichosanthes Root, Licorice

Ziyin Chushi Decoction: Prepared Rehmannia, Angelica, White Peony Root, Ligusticum, Bupleurum, Scutellaria, Tangerine Peel, Anemarrhena, Fritillaria, Alisma, Cortex Lycii, Licorice, Ginger

Jinhuang Powder: Arisaema, Tangerine Peel, Atractylodes Lancea, Phellodendron, Turmeric, Licorice, Angelica Dahurica, Trichosanthes Root, Magnolia Officinalis, Rhubarb (proprietary medicine)

VII. Anal Pus Discharge

After hemorrhoids and anal abscesses rupture, with continuous pus discharge, or recurrent pus leakage after healing, accompanied by pain and itching, it is called "anal fistula". In addition to pus discharge, feces may sometimes come out of the fistula opening, and blood may flow from the orifice, often consuming qi and blood, causing the patient to become emaciated and develop consumptive conditions. The reason for persistent pus discharge in this condition is the formation of a tract within the sore; thus, for a radical cure, surgical methods such as incision and thread-drawing should be performed by surgeons. However, for weak patients, internal medications should first be used for conditioning to improve symptoms and enhance physical strength, preparing for surgery.

Section 19 Visceral Symptoms

All symptoms are related to the internal organs; even local conditions are mostly treated through the internal organs. This embodies the holistic approach of TCM in treating diseases. The visceral symptoms described in this section are all directly related to the internal organs, such as cough caused by upward reversal of lung qi, palpitations caused by restlessness of the heart spirit, and abnormal urination and defecation caused by disorders of the stomach, intestines, and bladder, etc. Since the occurrence of a symptom is not limited to one zang organ, and a disorder of one zang organ is not limited to one cause, when observing visceral symptoms, attention must be paid to the nature and functions of the viscera, their connections with other parts, as well as the relationship between symptoms and causes. Meanwhile, the internal organs are divided into the five *zang* and six fu organs, with each zang organ paired with a fu organ. Although diseases of the zang organs can transmit to the fu organs, and diseases of the fu organs can also transmit to the zang organs, in severe and chronic illnesses, more emphasis is usually placed on the five *zang* organs. Therefore, the basic theory of TCM takes the *zang-fu* organs as the core, with the five *zang* organs being the core of the core. Many conditions considered difficult to treat or incurable are judged based on the weakness of the five *zang* organs themselves and the depth of pathogenic invasion.

I. Cough

The syndrome of cough mainly occurs in the lung. The lung is a delicate organ, responsible for purification and descent; reversal of qi leads to cough. However, cough is often accompanied by phlegm turbidity, and phlegm is formed by the transformation of dampness, which arises from insufficient transportation and transformation of the spleen and stomach. *Nei Jing* (The Inner Canon) states: "It accumulates in the stomach and is related to the lung." Later generations also have the saying that "the spleen is the source of phlegm production, and the lung is the container of phlegm." There are two causes of this disease: One is external contraction, as the lung governs the skin and hair and is most susceptible to external pathogens, in accordance with its correspondence; the other is internal injury, mostly due to the influence of qi among mother-child zang organs, such as earth failing to generate metal, wood-fire insulting metal, and metal-water failing to mutually generate, etc.

External contraction coughs are commonly caused by wind-cold and internal heat. "Wind-cold cough" is characterized by profuse thin sputum; "wind-heat cough" by sticky, difficult-to-expectorate sputum, or dry cough without sputum. Both are accompanied by itchy throat, nasal congestion, and in more severe cases, chills, fever, headache, etc. Treatment should disperse and transform pathogens in the upper jiao: for the former, Xingsu Powder and Zhisou Powder are used; for the latter, Yinqiao Powder. San'ao Decoction can also be used as the main formula, with appropriate additions of burdock, cicada slough, fritillaria thunbergii, pinellia ternata, tangerine peel, boat-fruited sterculia, etc. When affected by autumn dryness pathogenic factors, there is mostly dry cough, nasal dryness, dry mouth, sore throat, and a slightly red tongue, treated with Qingzao Jiufei Decoction with modifications. In treating external contraction cough, it is inappropriate to use qi-lowering and cough-suppressing methods in the early stage, to avoid pathogen stagnation and transformation into other conditions. Moreover, since the upper jiao is like a feather, only light medications can reach it, so the use of light and agile herbs is valued.

Among internal injury coughs, common types include "damp-phlegm cough", with profuse, easily expectorated sputum, chest tightness, poor appetite, nausea, and a white greasy tongue coating, treated with Erchen Decoction. "Liver-fire cough" is characterized by expectoration of yellow sputum, chest and hypochondriac fullness with pulling pain, bitter taste in the mouth, and dry throat, treated with Qingqi Huatan Wan plus indigo naturalis. There is also "kidney-deficiency cough", caused by yin deficiency with deficient fire flaring upward.

with blood-streaked sputum, internal heat, dry throat, and a thready rapid pulse, treated with Baihe Gujin Decoction; due to yang deficiency with water overflowing to form phlegm, with salty-tasting sputum, coldness in the body, shortness of breath, and a deep thready weak pulse, treated with Jinkui Shenqi Wan. For external contraction cough, emphasis is placed on dispelling pathogens, but in cases of deficient body with excessive pathogens, both aspects should be considered. Internal injury cough also has deficiency and excess conditions, and one should not solely use tonifying and nourishing methods. Meanwhile, ancient physicians classified coughs into those of the five *zang* and six fu organs, such as "lung cough", "heart cough", "spleen cough", "liver cough", "kidney cough", "stomach cough", "bladder cough", etc., referring to the accompanying *zang-fu* symptoms caused by cough, with the main focus still on the lung. In other diseases such as "edema" which can also cause cough, it is due to the pathogenic factors affecting the lung, with the primary condition being the main concern.

Cough with expectoration of saliva and froth, shortness of breath on movement, emaciation, and a deficient rapid pulse is caused by heat damaging body fluids, leading to failure of the lung to be moistened, called "feiwei" (lung wilt). Treatment should focus on clearing and nourishing, with slight assistance in resolving phlegm, using Maimendong

Decoction. If prolonged without healing, it can cause injury to both qi and yin, dry skin and hair, tidal fever, and loss of voice, resembling consumption, which is difficult to treat. There is also a condition of expectorating saliva and froth without cough or thirst, frequent urination or enuresis, which is the deficient cold type of lung wilt. Due to declining lung qi failing to control the lower part, it is also difficult to treat, and warm and sweet nourishing methods are appropriate, using Gancao Ganjiang Decoction.

Cough with expectoration of foul-smelling thick sputum, accompanied by obvious chest pain, or fever, and a floating slippery rapid pulse, is the initial stage of "feiyong" (lung abscess). After pus formation and rupture, there is expectoration of pus and blood, or sputum like rice porridge, chest pain with fullness and restlessness, and a yellow greasy tongue coating. This condition is mostly a manifestation of excess heat, with heat binding blood to form an abscess; treatment should clear heat and transform turbidity, using Qianjin Caojing Decoction, with appropriate addition of Platycodon to expel pus and Lepidium to purge the lung. If pathogenic factors gradually subside, or if pus is not exhausted but healthy qi is deficient, clearing heat and nourishing yin is appropriate, using Jiegeng Xingren Jian or Jisheng Jiegeng Decoction.

Among coughs, there is one type with profuse thin white sputum mixed with foam, mostly occurring in the elderly, often triggered by sudden cold in autumn, worsening with severe cold in winter, and gradually subsiding in spring and summer. During attacks, there is asthma, preference for sleeping with a high pillow, and relief is felt when sputum is easily expectorated, called "tanyin cough". In mild cases, it is due to spleen yang deficiency; in severe cases, kidney yang is also deficient, leading to failure to transform water-dampness, which accumulates into fluid, ascending to soak the lung, resulting in cough and asthma. This is fundamentally different from ordinary cough. Treatment should use warm medicines to harmonize; mild cases treat the spleen with Linggui Zhugan Decoction, severe cases treat the kidney with Jinkui Shenqi Wan; when there is profuse sputum and severe cough and asthma, Linggui Wuwei Jiangxin Decoction or Sanzi Yangqin Decoction can also be used in combination. The formation of tanyin cough is mainly due to internal yang deficiency, so it is not easy to cure completely, treating the root (ben) and symptoms (biao) based on urgency. For example, if triggered by wind-cold, Xiaoqinglong Decoction can be used to dispel cold and transform fluid. Or if there is panting with head sweating, a sign of floating yang escaping outward, Heixi Dan can be used to dispel deep cold and recover yang qi, but neither should be used commonly or for a long time.

Xingsu Powder: Almond, Perilla, Platycodon, Peucedanum, Pinellia, Tangerine Peel, Poria, Aurantium, Licorice, Ginger, Jujube

Zhisou Powder: Schizonepeta, Aster, Platycodon, Stemona, Cynanchum, Tangerine Peel, Licorice

Yinqiao Powder: Honeysuckle, Forsythia, Schizonepeta, Fermented Soybean, Mint, Arctium, Platycodon, Bamboo Leaf, Licorice

San'ao Decoction: Ephedra, Almond, Licorice

Qingzao Jiufei Decoction: Mulberry Leaf, Gypsum, Almond, Ophiopogon, Ginseng, Licorice, Donkey-Hide Gelatin, Loquat Leaf, Black Sesame

Erchen Decoction: Pinellia, Tangerine Peel, Poria, Licorice

Qingqi Huatan Wan: Arisaema cum Bile, Pinellia, Tangerine Peel, Almond, Immature Bitter Orange, Trichosanthes, Scutellaria, Poria, Ginger Juice

Baihe Gujin Decoction: Lily, Raw Rehmannia, Prepared Rehmannia,

Scrophularia, Ophiopogon, Fritillaria, Platycodon, White Peony Root, Angelica, Licorice

Jinkui Shenqi Wan: Aconite, Cinnamon, Prepared Rehmannia, Cornus, Yam, Moutan Bark, Alisma, Poria

Maimendong Decoction: Ophiopogon, Pinellia, Ginseng, Licorice, Japonica Rice, Jujube

Gancao Ganjiang Decoction: Licorice, Dried Ginger

Qianjin Weijing Decoction: Reed Rhizome, Coix Seed, Peach Kernel, Winter Melon Seed

Jiegeng Xingren Jian: Platycodon, Almond, Licorice, Donkey-Hide Gelatin, Ophiopogon, Honeysuckle, Lily, Fritillaria, Forsythia, Aurantium, Spica Prunellae, Sargentodoxa

Jisheng Jiegeng Decoction: Mulberry Bark, Platycodon, Fritillaria, Angelica, Trichosanthes Peel, Astragalus, Lily, Schisandra, Aurantium, Licorice, Coix Seed, Stephania, Cortex Lycii, Anemarrhena, Almond, Lepidium

Linggui Zhugan Decoction: Poria, Cinnamon Twig, Atractylodes, Licorice

Linggui Wuwei Jiangxin Decoction: Poria, Cinnamon Twig, Schisandra, Dried Ginger, Asarum

Sanzi Yangqin Decoction: Perilla Seed, White Mustard Seed, Radish Seed

Xiaoqinglong Decoction: Ephedra, Cinnamon Twig, Asarum, White Peony Root, Dried Ginger, Schisandra, Pinellia, Licorice

Heixi Dan: Lead, Sulfur, Psoralea, Agarwood, Aconite, Cinnamon, Fennel, Psoralea Corylifolia, Nutmeg, Sichuan Chinaberry, Actinolite,

Aucklandia (proprietary medicine)

II. Dyspnea

Rapid breathing is called "qichuan" (qi dyspnea). The lung is the master of qi, and the kidney is the root of qi. The lung governs exhalation, and the kidney governs inspiration. When one organ is diseased or both are affected, there is abnormal ascent and descent, resulting in difficult breathing. Generally, dyspnea with chest fullness and loud voice, where the pathogen is in the lung, is excess dyspnea; dyspnea with long exhalation and short inhalation, where qi fails to return to the kidney, is deficiency dyspnea. Ye Tianshi once said: "When in the lung, it is excess; when in the kidney, it is deficiency." He also pointed out: "Unsmooth exhalation is a lung disease; noisy inhalation is a kidney disease." However, this condition mostly occurs in cough, edema, and consumptive diseases. In clinical syndrome differentiation, the cause and the condition should be considered together. Generally, excess dyspnea is mainly due to phlegm, often triggered by wind-cold and dryness-heat. For those due to wind-cold, accompanied by cough, chest fullness, aversion to cold or fever, white greasy tongue coating, and floating slippery pulse, Huagai Powder is used; for those due to dryness-heat, accompanied by fever, fullness with restlessness, sore throat, and thirst, Dingchuan Decoction is used. Deficiency dyspnea is mainly due to qi disorder; in lung deficiency, it is often accompanied by cough, weakness in speaking, or consumption of body fluids, mild fever, thirst, red tongue with peeled coating, treated with Shengmai Powder. In kidney deficiency, yang deficiency manifestations such as edema, aversion to coldness, and cold limbs are common, treated with Jinkui Shenqi Wan. Clinically encountered dyspnea can be severe and potentially dangerous; emergency measures should be taken when necessary. Generally, for resolving phlegm, Houzao Fen is used; for descending qi, Chenxiang Fen is used; for absorbing qi, ginseng and Gejie

Fen are used; for descending counterflow and recovering yang, Erwei Heixi Dan is used, taken with boiled water.

In children with "lung wind" and "measles" where the rash appears and suddenly fades, accompanied by shortness of breath, it is a severe syndrome of lung qi obstruction. Refer to the entries "Nasal Flaring" in nasal symptoms and "Measles" in systemic symptoms.

"Asthma" is a prominent syndrome among dyspneic conditions. Rapid breathing even to the point of opening the mouth and raising the shoulders is called "chuan" (dyspnea); noisy breathing with sounds in the throat during inhalation and exhalation is called "xiao" (wheezing). Asthma presents both syndromes, as stated in *Yixue Zhengchuan* (True Tradition of Medicine): "Chuan is described by the breath, xiao by the sound." This condition is more common in children, with folk classifications such as "salt asthma" and "sugar asthma", but the main types are "cold asthma" and "heat asthma", with cold asthma being particularly common. Cold asthma is caused by exposure to cold and eating/drinking in drafts, so it occurs upon exposure to cold. During an attack, there is chest and diaphragm fullness, rapid breathing, and phlegm sounds in the throat like the chirping of waterfowl, with a deep tight pulse and white slippery tongue coating. Shegan Mahuang Decoction or Lengxiao Wan is used. Heat asthma arises from chronic abundance of phlegm-heat and stagnated, unrelieved lung qi. During an attack, there is also throat noise, accompanied by restlessness and a slippery rapid pulse, treated with Yuxian Dan or Dingchuan Decoction. This condition is not easily cured completely; attention must be paid to diet and daily living, maintaining appropriate warmth, to prevent recurrence. *Zhangshi Yitong* (Zhang's Medical Compendium) mentions a white mustard application method for cold asthma: during the three hottest periods of summer (sanfu), use 1 *liang* of white mustard powder, five *qian* each of kansui and asarum, ground together into fine powder, add five *fen* of musk, pound and mix well with ginger juice, and apply to Feishu, Gaohuang, and Bailao acupoints. After application, there will be numbness and pain; do not remove it immediately, wait two hours before removing. Apply once ten days later, and repeat three times. In acupuncture and moxibustion, moxibustion is used for cold asthma and acupuncture for heat asthma, selecting acupoints such as Feishu, Gaohuang, Tiantu, Danzhong, Lieque, Zusanli, and Fenglong. Surgical cutting therapy also has effects.

Huagai Powder: Ephedra, Perilla, Almond, Mulberry Bark, Red Poria, Platycodon, Licorice

Dingchuan Decoction: Ephedra, Mulberry Bark, Ginkgo, Perilla Seed, Almond, Scutellaria, Coltsfoot, Pinellia, Licorice

Shengmai Powder: Ginseng, Ophiopogon, Schisandra

Jinkui Shenqi Wan: Aconite, Cinnamon, Prepared Rehmannia, Cornus, Yam, Moutan Bark, Alisma, Poria

Erwei Heixi Dan: Lead, Sulfur (proprietary medicine)

Shegan Mahuang Decoction: Belamcanda, Ephedra, Asarum, Pinellia, Aster, Coltsfoot, Schisandra, Ginger, Jujube

Lengxiao Wan: Ephedra, Almond, Asarum, Licorice, Arisaema cum Bile, Pinellia, Aconitum, Sichuan Pepper, Alum, Gleditsia, Aster, Coltsfoot, Medicated Leaven

Yuxian Dan: Slug, Fritillaria Thunbergii

III. Shortness of Qi

A subjective feeling of shortness of breath during inhalation and exhalation, with weakness in speaking, is due to deficient qi. As stated in *Nei Jing* (The Inner Canon): "Speaking in a weak voice, and repeating words throughout the day, this is qi exhaustion." It is common in chronic debilitating conditions, requiring tonification of the lung and spleen, using Sijunzi Decoction with added Astragalus; for dry throat, add Ophiopogon.

Sijunzi Decoction: Ginseng, Atractylodes, Poria, Licorice

IV. Sighing

Commonly known as sighing deeply, with a subjective feeling of breath obstruction and relief after exhaling, it is mostly seen in liver and stomach qi disorders. Refer to the entry "Chest Oppression" in chest and hypochondrium symptoms.

Unsmooth heart qi also leads to frequent sighing. *Nei Jing* states: "Anxiety and worry cause tightness in the heart's connection; tightness in the heart's connection leads to constriction of the qi tract; constriction causes obstruction, hence sighing to release it." Treatment should focus on nourishment.

V. Sneezing

It is one of the initial symptoms of a cold; frequent sneezing also occurs in the early stage of childhood "measles".

In chronic diseases with yang deficiency, sudden onset of sneezing indicates recovery of yang qi and a tendency toward improvement, as stated in *Nei Jing*: "When yang emerges from yin, there is sneezing."

VI. Yawning

Yawning fits often occur before the onset of malaria or during periods of mental fatigue. Nei Jing once said: "When yang enters yin, there is yawning." Thus, yawning in weak and chronic conditions is a sign of gradual decline of yang qi.

VII. Hematemesis

All cases of blood coming out of the mouth are generally referred to as hematemesis. Among them, blood originating from the lungs, often spat out in mouthfuls along with coughing, or with blood spots or streaks in the phlegm, is called “hemoptysis”; blood originating from the stomach, coming out with vomiting in large quantities (filling bowls or cups), is called “hematemesis”; blood originating from the larynx, which comes out as small blood clots with a single cough without prolonged coughing, is called “hemoptysis”.

Hemoptysis occurs due to coughing damaging the lung collaterals. A common cause is wind-heat invading the lung, accompanied by dry nose and mouth, and a floating rapid pulse, treated with Sangxing Decoction. If wood-fire insults metal, accompanied by hypochondriac pain and irritability, with a string-like rapid pulse, Daige Powder is used. For yin deficiency with internal heat, accompanied by tidal fever and shortness of breath, and a deficient rapid pulse, Baihe Gujin Decoction is used.

Hematemesis due to accumulated heat in the stomach, with vomited blood being a mixture of fresh and stagnant blood, accompanied by chest tightness with pain, epigastric upset and constipation, yellow greasy tongue coating, and a slippery rapid pulse, is treated with Dahuang Huanglian Xiexin Decoction combined with Sisheng Wan. This condition often presents with purple-black stools, which is due to downward movement of stagnant blood and does not require astringent stop-bleeding methods.

Hemoptysis is mostly caused by kidney deficiency with blazing fire, accompanied by diaphragmatic heat, flushed cheeks, dry throat, crimson tongue, and a thready rapid pulse. Initially, Qingyan Taiping Wan is used, followed by Qiwei Duqi Wan with added Ophiopogon and Achyranthes.

Women who experience hematemesis during each menstrual period are said to have "dao jing" (reversed menstruation). Refer to the entry "Menstrual Hematemesis" in gynecological symptoms.

Hematemesis is commonly seen in exogenous diseases and internal damage disorders, with extremely complex causes. *Leizheng Zhicai* (Classified Syndromes and Treatments) has briefly explained the medication principles for hematemesis: For exogenous pathogens in the lung defense, sweet-cool and clearing-descending herbs are appropriate, such as Adenophora, Ophiopogon, Fritillaria, and Trichosanthes Root; for pathogens in the heart nutrient level, light-clear and nourishing herbs are used, such as Raw Rehmannia, Scrophularia, Salvia, Forsythia, and Bamboo Leaf; for severe fire burning, bitter-cold herbs are added, such as Gardenia, Scutellaria, Anemarrhena, and Cortex Lycii. For wind-warmth, sweet-cool herbs are added, such as Mulberry Leaf, Reed Rhizome, and Sugarcane Juice; for summer heat consumption, clear-moistening herbs are added, such as Almond, Honeysuckle, Raw Rehmannia, and Rhinoceros Horn; for dry cough, purely sweet herbs are assisted, such as Asparagus, Donkey-Hide Gelatin, and Pear Juice. For internal heat with external cold, Mahuang Shenggou Decoction is appropriate. For internal damage hematemesis due to anger stirring liver fire, bitter-acrid and qi-descending herbs are used, such as Perilla Seed, Curcuma, Dalbergia, Moutan Bark, Gardenia, and Trichosanthes; for constrained damage to liver yin, sweet-sour and wind-calming herbs are used, such as Donkey-Hide Gelatin, White Peony Root, Raw Rehmannia, and Kumquat; for thought damaging the heart and spleen, sweet-warm and nutrient-benefiting herbs are used, such as Ginseng, Astragalus, Atractylodes, Angelica, and Tangerine Peel; for essence depletion and blood loss, essence-filling herbs are used, such as Ginseng, Sea Cucumber, Prepared Rehmannia, Wolfberry, and Placenta; for kidney deficiency with failure to absorb, water-strengthening and yang-subduing herbs are used, such as Prepared Rehmannia, Cornus, Schisandra, Achyranthes, and Lead; for yang deficiency with failure to contain, fire-guiding and origin-restoring herbs are used, such as Cinnamon Qiwei Wan with boy's urine. For hematemesis caused by neither internal nor external factors: for falls and injuries, guiding-downward herbs are first used, such as Raw Rehmannia, Angelica Tail, Peach Kernel, Rhubarb, and Pangolin Scales, followed by unblocking and tonifying herbs, such as Angelica, Curcuma, White Peony Root, Notoginseng, and Achyranthes; for strain damaging collaterals, nutrient-harmonizing and deficiency-regulating herbs are used, such as Inula, New Crocus, Angelica, White Peony Root, and Onion Tube; for tobacco and alcohol damaging the lung, sweet-cool and clear-moistening herbs are used, such as Moutan Bark, Ophiopogon, Rhinoceros Horn, Lotus Root Juice, and Pueraria Flower.

Medicines and formulas for emergency hemostasis include Shihui Wan, Huaruishi Powder, as well as Agrimonia pilosa, Carbonized Human Hair, Zicaozhu, etc. However, ancient physicians warned that "when seeing blood, do not rush to stop it." Miao Zhongchun more clearly pointed out: "There are three key points in treating hematemesis: It is appropriate to promote blood circulation rather than stop bleeding. When blood does not follow the meridians, it is due to qi counterflow and upward congestion. Promoting blood circulation allows it to follow the meridians, and bleeding will stop on its own. Stopping it will cause blood stasis; blood stasis will inevitably lead to fever, chest and hypochondriac pain, and the disease will become chronic. It is appropriate to tonify the liver rather than attack the liver. The liver is in charge of storing blood; in hematemesis, the liver fails to perform its function. Nourishing the liver will calm liver qi and allow blood to return to its proper place. Attacking the liver will cause liver deficiency, unable to store blood, leading to more uncontrollable bleeding. It is appropriate to descend qi rather than reduce fire. Excessive qi is fire; descending qi will cause fire to descend. When fire descends, qi will not rise upward, and blood, following qi, will not overflow from the upper orifices. Moreover, reducing fire necessarily involves cold and cool medicines, which will damage stomach qi. When stomach qi is damaged, the spleen cannot control blood, and blood will be even more unable to return to the meridians." Wu Jutong, considering qi as the commander of blood, advocated regulating the insubstantial qi. The clinical common use of methods to secure desertion and benefit qifurther proves the importance of treating qi in blood syndromes.

Sangxing Decoction: Mulberry Leaf, Almond, Adenophora, Fritillaria thunbergii, Fermented Soybean, Gardenia, Pear Peel

Daige Powder: Indigo Naturalis, Sea Clam Powder

Baihe Gujin Decoction: Raw Rehmannia, Prepared Rehmannia, Lily, Ophiopogon, Scrophularia, Angelica, White Peony Root, Fritillaria, Licorice, Platycodon

Dahuang Huanglian Xiexin decoction: Rhubarb, Coptis

Sisheng Wan: Platycladus orientalis Leaf, Artemisia argyi, Lotus Leaf, Raw Rehmannia

Qingyan Taiping Wan: Mint, Ligusticum chuanxiong, Saposhnikovia, Rhinoceros Horn, Persimmon Cream, Licorice, Platycodon

Qiwei Duqi Wan: Schisandra, Prepared Rehmannia, Cornus, Yam, Moutan Bark, Alisma, Poria

Mahuang Shenshao Decoction: Ephedra, Cinnamon Twig, Ginseng, Astragalus, Angelica, White Peony Root, Ophiopogon, Schisandra

Rougui Qiwei Wan: Cinnamon, Prepared Rehmannia, Cornus, Yam,

Moutan Bark, Alisma, Poria

Shihui Wan: Cirsium japonicum, Cephalanoplos segetum, Platycladus orientalis Leaf, Mint, Rubia cordifolia, Imperata cylindrica root, Gardenia, Rhubarb, Moutan Bark, Trachycarpus fortunei bark

Huaruishi Powder: Ophicalcite

VIII. Heart Palpitations

A subjective feeling of heart beating is called "xinji" (palpitations); in severe cases, it is called "zhengchong" (severe palpitations). Both belong to syndromes of restless heart spirit. Those caused by external factors, often due to hearing loud noises, seeing strange objects, or encountering danger, with panic and unease, are also called "jingji" (fright palpitations). Those caused by internal factors are mainly due to insufficient heart blood, where the heart fails to be nourished and the spirit cannot settle, often accompanied by feelings of panic and timidity. Therefore, external causes result in temporary and superficial illness, while internal causes develop gradually and are more profound. However, fright can cause palpitations, and palpitations make one prone to fright; the two are often connected. Generally, palpitations from fright stop when the spirit calms, requiring no treatment. If they persist for many days, with mental restlessness, inability to sit or lie peacefully, disturbed sleep with dreams, and poor appetite, it is mostly related to hyperactivity of liver and heart fire or deficiency of liver and gallbladder qi. Zhusha Anshen Wan, Wendan Decoction, and Ruizhu Wan can be used for treatment. For heart blood deficiency, nourishing blood and calming the spirit is appropriate, using Zaoren Decoction or Yangxin Decoction. For irregular pulses (intermittent or skipped beats), assisted by acrid and moistening herbs, Zhigancao Decoction is used.

Upward counterflow of water qi can also cause palpitations, called "water qi attacking the heart." Symptoms include dizziness, chest tightness, thirst without desire to drink, scanty urine, and a deep tight pulse. This syndrome is mainly due to insufficient heart yang; promoting yang and draining water is appropriate, with no need for spirit-calming herbs, using Fuling Gancao Decoction.

This syndrome often occurs together with dizziness, blurred vision, insomnia, poor memory, tinnitus, spontaneous sweating, fatigue, etc., forming a deficient syndrome, treated with Zhenxin Dan without cinnamon.

Zhusha Anshen Wan: Raw Rehmannia, Angelica, Coptis, Cinnabar, Licorice

Wendan Decoction: Pinellia, Tangerine Peel, Poria, Licorice, Immature Bitter Orange, Bamboo Shavings

Ruizhu Wan: Cinnabar, Indigo, Pig Heart Blood

Zaoren Decoction: Ginseng, Astragalus, Angelica, Poria, Fushen, Jujube Seed, Polygala, Tangerine Peel, Licorice, Lotus Seed, Ginger, Jujube

Yangxin Decoction: Astragalus, Angelica, Poria, Fushen, Ligusticum, Pinellia, Platycladi Seed, Jujube Seed, Polygala, Schisandra, Ginseng, Cinnamon, Roasted Licorice

Zhigancao Decoction: Roasted Licorice, Ginseng, Cinnamon Twig, Donkey-Hide Gelatin, Raw Rehmannia, Hemp Seed, Ginger, Jujube

Fuling Gancao Decoction: Poria, Cinnamon Twig, Licorice, Ginger

Zhenxin Dan: Jujube Seed, Ophiopogon, Asparagus, Schisandra, Poria, Fushen, Dragon's Tooth, Ginseng, Prepared Rehmannia, Yam, Cinnamon, Plantago Seed, Polygala, Cinnabar

IX. Insomnia

Difficulty falling asleep or tossing and turning all night, generally referred to as insomnia. It is mostly caused by excessive thinking and worry, overstrain, blood deficiency of the heart and spleen, or qi and blood weakness after illness or childbirth in women. Accompanied by sallow complexion, physical fatigue, dizziness, heavy eyes, pale tongue, and thready weak pulse, treatment should mainly nourish the heart and spleen, using Guipi Decoction. Blood deficiency insomnia often leads to hyperactivity of heart fire, irritability, excessive sweating, dry mouth and tongue, treated with Tianwang Buxin Dan or Zhusha Anshen Wan. It may also cause hyperactivity of liver yang, dizziness, distending headache, palpitations, treated with Hupo Duomei Wan. If kidney yin deficiency with excessive heart fire causes insomnia, known as disharmony between the heart and kidney, Huanglian Ejiao Decoction or Jiaotai Wan is used. For acupuncture treatment, for heart blood deficiency, select Shenmen and Sanyinjiao; for disharmony between the heart and kidney, add Xinshu, Shenshu, Zhaohai, and Yongquan; for liver fire hyperactivity, add Ganshu, Danshu, and Taichong. Treatment is best performed two hours before bedtime for better results

Food stagnation and phlegm-fire obstruction can also cause insomnia, as stated in *Nei Jing*: "When the stomach is disharmonious, sleep is restless." Accompanied by profuse phlegm, chest tightness, difficulty in urination and defecation, greasy tongue coating, and slippery pulse, Wendan Decoction and Banxia Shumi Decoction are used. Zhang Jingyue said: "Sleep is rooted in yin, with the spirit as its master. When the spirit is calm, there is sleep; when the spirit is restless, there is insomnia. The reasons for restlessness are, on the one hand, disturbance by pathogenic factors, and on the other hand, insufficiency of nutrient qi." Here, insufficiency of nutrient qi generally refers to blood deficiency, and disturbance by pathogenic factors refers to such factors as phlegm-fire and food retention. Therefore, treating insomnia cannot be achieved solely by tonification and tranquilization.

Guipi Decoction: Ginseng, Atractylodes, Fushen, Jujube Seed, Astragalus, Angelica Body, Polygala, Aucklandia, Roasted Licorice, Longan, Ginger, Jujube

Tianwang Buxin Dan: Raw Rehmannia, Ginseng, Scrophularia, Salvia, Asparagus, Ophiopogon, Angelica, Schisandra, Poria, Platycodon, Polygala, Jujube Seed, Platycladi Seed

Zhusha Anshen Wan: Raw Rehmannia, Angelica, Coptis, Licorice, Cinnabar

Hupo Duomei Wan: Amber, Codonopsis, Poria, Polygala, Antelope Horn, Licorice

Huanglian Ejiao Decoction: Coptis, Scutellaria, White Peony Root, Donkey-Hide Gelatin, Egg Yolk

Jiaotai Wan: Coptis, Cinnamon

Wendan Decoction: Pinellia, Tangerine Peel, Poria, Licorice, Immature Bitter Orange, Bamboo Shavings

Banxia Shumi Decoction: Pinellia, Millet

X. Easy Awakening

Easy awakening during sleep, mostly due to being frightened or inherent timidity of the heart and gallbladder, resulting in muddled consciousness during sleep and easy awakeness, should be treated from the liver meridian, using Suanzao Ren Decoction with added White Peony Root and Oyster.

Suanzao Ren Decoction: Jujube Seed, Anemarrhena, Ligusticum,

Poria, Licorice

XI. Drowsiness

Drowsiness is mostly seen in phlegm-damp syndromes. Internal obstruction of phlegm-dampness leads to tiredness of middle qi and mental fatigue, accompanied by chest tightness, poor appetite, and white greasy tongue coating, treated with Pingwei Powder plus Acorus. This syndrome is more common during the rainy season in the south, commonly called "damp obstruction"; Agastache, Pinellia, Amomum, and Coix Seed can be added.

Drowsiness and desire to sleep after eating, due to spleen weakness with insufficient transportation, mostly with normal pulse and tongue, treated with Liujunzi Decoction.

Yang deficiency symptoms include mental fatigue with desire to sleep, aversion to cold and huddled sleeping, suitable for warming and tonifying shaoyin, using Fuzi Lizhong Decoction.

After illness, deep sleep often occurs, with refreshment upon waking, which is not a pathological sign and should not be disturbed.

Pingwei Powder: Atractylodes lancea, Magnolia officinalis, Tangerine peel, Licorice

Liujunzi Decoction: Ginseng, Atractylodes, Poria, Licorice, Pinellia, Tangerine peel

Fuzi Lizhong Decoction: Aconite, Ginseng, Atractylodes, Roasted ginger, Licorice

XII. Infantile Night Crying

Infants' crying with fright at night is called "night crying". It is mostly due to heat accumulation in the liver and heart meridians. Decoct Zhudengxin (cinnabar-coated rush), bamboo leaves, and Uncaria for oral administration; for severe cases, use Anshen Zhenjing Wan.

Anshen Zhenjing Wan: Bambusa concretio silicea, Fushen, Arisaema cum bile, Jujube seed, Ophiopogon, Red peony root, Angelica, Mint, Coptis, Cinnabar, Bezoar, Gardenia, Akebia, Dragon bone, Indigo naturalis

XIII. Dreaminess

Restless sleep with numerous disturbing dreams, mostly of frightening, terrifying, or strange events is commonly seen in blood deficiency syndromes, mainly due to restless heart spirit. *Synopsis of the Golden Chamber* states: "Those with insufficient qi and blood pertain to the heart; those with heart deficiency are prone to fear, desire to sleep when closing the eyes, dream of traveling far, with scattered spirit and reckless movement of the ethereal soul and corporeal soul." Use Yiqi Anshen Decoction.

Yiqi Anshen Decoction: Angelica, Fushen, Raw rehmannia, Ophiopogon, Jujube seed, Polygala, Ginseng, Astragalus, Arisaema cum bile, Bamboo leaves, Coptis, Licorice

XIV. Irritability and Restlessness

Heat in the chest with unease is "fan" (irritability); heat in the hands and feet with restlessness is "zao" (restlessness). Although "fanzao" (irritability and restlessness) is often mentioned together, they are actually two syndromes. *Leizheng Zhicai* (Classified Syndromes and Treatments) says: "Internal heat is fan, external heat is zao. Fan arises from the lung, zao arises from the kidney. When heat transmits to the lung and kidney, both fan and zao occur." It also says: "Fan is yang, belonging to fire with a root, so cases with only fan without zao or fan preceding zao are all easy to treat; zao is yin, belonging to fire without a root, so cases with only zao without fan or zao preceding fan are all difficult to treat." When this syndrome appears in febrile diseases, Zhizi Chi Decoction is used for fan, and Sini Decoction for zao. If there is fan with cold feet and a deep faint pulse, it also belongs to yin syndrome, treated with Shenfu Decoction. For residual heat after illness with deficient fan and unease, Zhuru Decoction is used.

In internal damage disorders, fan is more common than zao, often seen in yin deficiency with fire stirring, worse at night, treated with Shengmai Powder plus Raw Rehmannia, Jujube Seed, and Fushen. There are also cases of fan with vomiting, treated with Jupi Decoction; fan with difficult urination, treated with Zhuling Decoction.

Zhizi Chi Decoction: Gardenia, Fermented soybean

Sini Decoction: Aconite, Dried ginger, Licorice

Shenfu Decoction: Ginseng, Aconite

Zhuru Decoction: Ginseng, Ophiopogon, Bamboo shavings, Pinellia, Poria, Licorice, Floating wheat

Shengmai Powder: Ginseng, Ophiopogon, Schisandra

Jupi Decoction: Tangerine peel, Ginger

Zhuling Decoction: Polyporus, Poria, Donkey-hide gelatin, Talc, Alisma

XV. Amnesia

Amnesia is also called "shanwang" (prone to forgetting) and "xiwang" (fond of forgetting). Due to excessive thinking and exhaustion of mental power, treatment should nourish and tonify the heart and kidney. Lin

Xitong said: "A person's spirit resides in the heart; the essence of the heart depends on the kidney; and the brain is the residence of the original spirit and the sea of essence and marrow, which is indeed the basis of memory." Wang Ren'an also said: "Treating amnesia must harmonize the heart and kidney, so that the spirit of the heart communicates downward with the kidney, and the essence of the kidney ascends upward to the brain. Essence can generate qi, qi can generate spirit; when the spirit is calm and qi is clear, there will naturally be few forgetting episodes." Formulas such as Kongsheng Zhenzhong Dan, Zhuque Wan, and Anshen Dingzhi Wan can be appropriately selected.

Kongsheng Zhenzhong Dan: Turtle shell, Dragon bone, Polygala, Acorus

Zhuque Wan: Agarwood, Fushen, Ginseng

Anshen Dingzhi Wan: Ginseng, Atractylodes, Poria, Fushen, Acorus, Polygala, Ophiopogon, Jujube Seed, Bezoar, Cinnabar, Longan

XVI. Coma

Unconsciousness or confused awareness is called coma. It is mostly caused by pathogenic factors blocking the clear orifices and clouding the spirit, occurring in both exogenous and internal injury diseases, and is one of the severe symptoms. Generally, exogenous diseases progress gradually to coma, while internal injury disorders can have sudden onset. Treatment involves emergency measures, focusing on opening the orifices. Commonly used Chinese patentmedicines, such as Suhexiang Wan, Zhibao Dan, Zixue Dan, Angong Niuhuang Wan, Niuhuang Qingxin Wan, and Yushu Dan are commonly used proprietary medicines. Additionally, Tongguan Powder is blown into the nose to induce sneezing, and Kaiguan Powder is applied to the teeth to open tightly closed jaws, promoting awakening to facilitate medicine administration.

Coma in exogenous diseases mostly occurs when heat transforms in typhoid or warm diseases, with pathogenic factors transmitting to the pericardium. Initially, there is mania and delirium, with a red crimson tip of the tongue, gradually progressing to picking at empty space, pulling threads, and groping for clothes or the bed. Opening the orifices and clearing heat is appropriate, using emergency medicines such as Angong Niuhuang Wan, Zixue Dan, and Zhibao Dan. Among these three proprietary medicines, Niuhuang is the coolest, followed by Zixue, then Zhibao. Their main indications are somewhat similar but each has its strengths. For patients with stubborn constipation, the 'extracting-firewood-from-cauldron-base' method can be applied by administering Major Drastic Purgative Decoction (Da Chengqi Decoction) or Fluid-Increasing Decoction for Purgation (Zengye Chengqi Decoction)." When exogenous diseases progress to the coma stage, there is mostly persistent high fever, worsening in the afternoon, restlessness, and occasional delirium; Qinggong Decoction should be used first. In damp-warm syndrome, where damp-heat steams the chest, coma often occurs during the stage of macular eruption, but it is mostly a state of semi-consciousness. For mild cases, Ganlu Xiaodu Dan is used; for severe cases, Shenxi Dan.

Affected by summerheat-warmth, with restless sleep, irritable thirst, crimson tongue, occasional delirium, eyes open and not closing, or preferring to keep them closed, these are premonitory signs of coma, treated with Qingying Decoction. For those already in coma, Angong Niuhuang Wan is used. If suddenly collapsing while working or walking under the scorching sun, it is called "heatstroke"; Suhexiang Wan is used urgently, or juice of chopped green onions and garlic mixed with water for administration.

Among internal injury disorders, "wind stroke" is the most critical cause of coma, with sudden collapse, loss of consciousness, accompanied by snoring, deviated mouth and eyes, and hemiplegia. Differentiation between yin and yang, blockage and desertion is necessary for treatment. Cases with clenched fists, tightly closed jaws, sawing-like sounds, red face, rough breathing, rapid string-like forceful pulse, and yellow greasy tongue coating are yang patterns of blockage syndrome, treated with Jufang Niuhuang Qingxin Wan. Those with calmness without irritability, snoring, deep slow pulse, and white greasy slippery tongue coating are yin patterns of blockage syndrome, treated with Suhexiang Wan, with bloodletting at Twelve Well Points or Ten Diffusion Points, and acupuncture at Baihui and Shuigou Points. Cases with closed eyes, open mouth, snoring, flaccid hands, enuresis, or even a flushed face like makeup, oily sweating, cold extremities, and a faint thready pulse on the verge of extinction are desertion syndrome, treated with Shenfu Decoction plus Dragon Bone and Oyster, and moxibustion at Shenque, Qihai, and Guanyuan until awakening. There are also cases showing both desertion and excessive phlegm blocking the internal orifices, called "internal blockage with external desertion", treating with Sansheng Yin plus Ginseng to secure desertion and open blockage.

"Jue syndrome" involves temporary coma, unconsciousness, and cold extremities, but without hemiplegia, making it easy to differentiate from wind stroke. When occurring due to sudden anger causing qi counterflow, with unconscious collapse, locked jaw, and clenched fists, it is "qi jue", treated with Wumo Yin. Those with a history of phlegm turbidity, sudden upward congestion blocking qi, with phlegm sounds in the throat, have "phlegm jue", treated with Daotan Decoction. If coma occurs due to undigested food stagnation with abdominal distension, it is "food jue", treated with Baohe Wan. For the initial stage of these jue syndromes, Suhexiang Wan or Yushu Dan can be used for emergency treatment, along with methods to open the orifices and jaws.

Suddenly dizziness with collapse, pale complexion, spontaneous sweating, and loss of consciousness is called "faint". Due to deficiency of both liver blood and kidney yin, with wind-yang disturbing upward, mild cases regain consciousness naturally within a few minutes, and after awakening, Lingyangjiao Decoction is used for conditioning. Severe cases with incessant sweating, cold limbs, and hidden pulse can lead to collapse, requiring strong decoction of ginseng in large amounts for administration.

"Epilepsy" has a history of attacks, characterized by sudden collapse, accompanied by convulsions of limbs, clenched jaws, salivation from the mouth, and abnormal sounds like the braying of pigs or sheep. Consciousness is regained shortly after, with short-term dizziness, headache, and mental fatigue after waking. The attacks occur at irregular intervals, ranging from several times a day, once every few days, once every few months, to once every few years. It is mostly caused by fright damaging the liver and kidney, fire scorching body fluids to form phlegm, internally disturbing the spirit and externally blocking the meridians. Calming the spirit and resolving phlegm is appropriate, using Dingxian Wan and Xianzheng Zhenxin Dan, and acupuncture at Fengchi, Xinshu, Ganshu, Yaoqi, Jiuwei, Zhongwan, Jianshi, Shenmen, etc.

Infantile "acute infantile convulsions" have a rapid onset, with symptoms including staring eyes, clenched jaws, stiff neck, opisthotonos, floating tight string-like rapid pulse, and purple-blue fingerprint. Before these symptoms appear, there is high fever first, followed by convulsions after three to several days, crying without tears, and then transitioning into a coma. The causes include fright, wind, phlegm, and heat, with their characteristics as follows: due to fright, there are first panic with cold limbs, fear and restlessness, and clouded consciousness; due to wind, there are first twitching of hands and feet, body trembling, clenched jaws, and rolling eyes; due to phlegm, there are first cough with phlegm congestion and shortness of breath, and gurgling sounds in the throat; due to heat, there are first confusion and delirium, red eyes and lips, constipation, and reddish urine. However, these four cannot be completely separated and often appear together, mainly due to external pathogens transforming into heat, heat excess generating wind and phlegm, phlegm-heat congestion and blockage, and then sudden convulsions upon accidental contact with foreign objects or hearing strange sounds. The treatment first focuses on eliminating phlegm to open the orifices, clearing heat and calming fright, using Niuhuang Qingxin Wan or Huichun Dan dissolved for administration, followed by Qingre Huatan Decoction or Gouteng Yin. Acute infantile convulsions are a dangerous syndrome, requiring first aid with proprietary medicines; Zixue Dan, Zhibao Dan, Hupo Baolong Wan, etc., can be chosen, and Tongguan Powder can be blown into the nose to induce sneezing, along with acupuncture at Shixuan (to bleed), Renzhong, Yintang, Dazhui, Hegu, Yongquan, Xingjian, etc. If symptoms such as flaccid hands, closed eyes, open mouth, bulging fontanelle, and enuresis appear, the prognosis is poor, and even if not fatal, sequelae such as paralysis and dementia often occur.

"Malaria with confusion" easily leads to coma; for heat malaria with confusion, Zixue Dan is used, and for cold malaria with confusion, Suhexiang Wan is used, combined with decoctions for emergency treatment.

In the late stage of "tympanites", with obstruction of urine and stool, or hematemesis, nose and mouth bleeding, accompanied by clouded consciousness, it is an incurable sign.

Suhexiang Wan: Clove, Benzoin, Aucklandia, Sandalwood, Storax, Loulu Xiang (probably a misnomer, possibly another aromatic herb), Frankincense, Agarwood, Piper Longum, Terminalia, Rhinoceros Horn,

Cinnabar, Borneol, Atractylodes, Aconite (proprietary medicine)

Zhibao Dan: Rhinoceros Horn, Amber, Cinnabar, Bezoar, Hawksbill Turtle Shell, Musk (proprietary medicine)

Zixue Dan: Talc, Gypsum, Calcite, Magnetite, Antelope Horn, Aucklandia, Rhinoceros Horn, Agarwood, Clove, Cimicifuga, Scrophularia, Roasted Licorice, Glauber's Salt, Nitre, Cinnabar, Musk (proprietary medicine)

Angong Niuhuang Wan: Bezoar, Turmeric, Rhinoceros Horn, Coptis, Cinnabar, Borneol, Musk, Pearl Powder, Gardenia, Realgar, Scutellaria, Gold Foil (proprietary medicine)

Niuhuang Qingxin Wan: Bezoar, Musk, Borneol, White Peony Root, Ophiopogon, Scutellaria, Angelica, Saposhnikovia, Atractylodes, Bupleurum, Platycodon, Ligusticum, Poria, Almond, Medicated Leaven, Cattail Pollen, Ginseng, Rhinoceros Horn, Antelope Horn, Cinnamon, Fermented Soybean Sprout, Donkey-Hide Gelatin, Ampelopsis, Dried Ginger, Realgar, Yam, Licorice, Gold Foil, Jujube (proprietary medicine)

Yushu Dan: Omitted (proprietary medicine)

Tongguan Powder: Arisaema, Gleditsia, Musk, Centipede, Stiff Silkworm (proprietary medicine)

Kaiguan Powder: Arisaema, Borneol, Dark Plum (proprietary medicine)

Dachengqi Decoction: Rhubarb, Sodium Sulfate, Magnolia Officinalis, Immature Bitter Orange

Zengye Chengqi Decoction: Raw Rehmannia, Scrophularia, Ophiopogon, Rhubarb, Sodium Sulfate

Qinggong Decoction: Scrophularia, Lotus Plumule, Coiled Bamboo

Leaves, Forsythia Plumule, Rhinoceros Horn

Ganlu Xiaodu Dan: Talc, Capillary Wormwood, Scutellaria, Acorus, Fritillaria, Akebia, Agastache, Belamcanda, Forsythia, Mint, Amomum, Medicated Leaven

Shenxi Dan: Rhinoceros Horn, Acorus, Scutellaria, Raw Rehmannia, Honeysuckle, Golden Juice, Forsythia, Isatis Root, Fermented Soybean, Scrophularia, Trichosanthes Root, Lithospermum (proprietary medicine)

Qingying Decoction: Rhinoceros Horn, Raw Rehmannia, Scrophularia, Bamboo Leaf Plumule, Ophiopogon, Salvia, Coptis, Honeysuckle, Forsythia

Shenfu Decoction: Ginseng, Aconite

Sansheng Yin: Aconitum, Aconite, Arisaema, Aucklandia

Wumo Yin: Areca, Aucklandia, Agarwood, Lindera, Immature Bitter Orange

Daotan Decoction: Pinellia, Poria, Tangerine Peel, Licorice, Arisaema, Immature Bitter Orange

Baohe Wan: Hawthorn, Medicated Leaven, Raphani Seed, Poria, Pinellia, Tangerine Peel, Forsythia

Lingyangjiao Decoction: Antelope Horn, Turtle Shell, Raw Rehmannia, Moutan Bark, White Peony Root, Bupleurum, Mint, Cicada Slough, Chrysanthemum, Spica Prunellae, Abalone Shell

Dingxian Wan: Gastrodia, Fritillaria, Arisaema cum Bile, Pinellia, Tangerine Peel, Poria, Fushen, Salvia, Ophiopogon, Acorus, Polygala, Scorpion, Stiff Silkworm, Amber, Cinnabar, Bamboo Sap, Ginger Juice, Licorice

Xianzheng Zhenxin Dan: Bezoar, Rhinoceros Horn, Pearl Powder,

Cinnabar, Polygala, Licorice, Arisaema cum Bile, Ophiopogon, Coptis, Fushen, Acorus, Jujube Seed, Gold Foil

Huichun Dan: Fritillaria, Bambusa Concretio Silicea, Arisaema cum Bile, Typhonium, Saposhnikovia, Gastrodia, Notopterygium, Cinnabar, Bezoar, Realgar, Snake Stone, Stiff Silkworm, Scorpion, Musk, Borneol (proprietary medicine)

Qingre Huatan Decoction: Fritillaria, Trichosanthes Root, Immature Bitter Orange, Scutellaria, Coptis, Scrophularia, Cimicifuga, Licorice

Gouteng Yin: Antelope Horn, Uncaria, Gastrodia, Scorpion, Ginseng, Licorice

Hupo Baolong Wan: Amber, Cinnabar, Fushen, Sandalwood, Bambusa Concretio Silicea, Arisaema cum Bile, Immature Bitter Orange, Immature Bitter Orange, Ginseng, Yam, Licorice, Gold Foil (proprietary medicine)

XVII. Dementia

Mental confusion, alternating laughter and crying, incoherent speech, or silence, or painful groaning is called "dian syndrome", commonly known as "wenchi" (literary dementia). Before the onset, it is mostly due to unrelieved mental stimulation, manifested as emotional distress, dull consciousness, preference for quietness and sleep, refusal to eat or drink, with a thready string-like pulse. Treatment should regulate qi and relieve depression, using Xiaoyao Powder; for cases with phlegm, supplemented with Baijin Wan. If the disease persists without healing, due to hidden consumption of yin and blood and transformation of qi stagnation into fire, it can also turn into mania, with a poor prognosis, as stated in *Nei Jing*: "In dian disease, if attacks are like mania, it is incurable."

There are also cases with dull eyes, slow speech, clumsy limb movements, slow pulse, accompanied by dizziness, excessive sweating, palpitations, and insomnia, which is one of the symptoms of internal wind. Nourishing the liver and extinguishing wind is appropriate, using Zhenzhumu Wan with added whole scorpion; blood-activating and collaterals-unblocking herbs are contraindicated.

Xiaoyao Powder: Angelica, White Peony Root, Bupleurum, Atractylodes, Poria, Licorice, Mint

Baijin Wan: Alum, Turmeric

Zhenzhumu Wan: Pearl Shell, Raw Rehmannia, Prepared Rehmannia, Codonopsis, Angelica, Platycladi Seed, Jujube Seed, Fushen, Dragon's Tooth, Agarwood

XVIII. Mania

Mania is mostly a heat syndrome, as stated in *Nei Jing*: "All restlessness, mania, and excess belong to heat." When occurring in febrile diseases, it is often due to persistent high fever, constipation, and pathogenic factors invading the pericardium. Treatment involves clearing the heart or purging the bowels; refer to the entry "Coma" in this section.

Initially, there is irritability and anger, reduced sleep and food intake, followed by cursing and shouting, disregard for relatives and strangers, and even holding knives or sticks, discarding clothes and being naked, climbing walls and roofs, with strength greater than usual, red face, bright eyes, and a string-like slippery rapid pulse. This is called "kuang disease", commonly known as "wuchi" (martial dementia), caused by reversed flow of liver and gallbladder qi transforming into fire, clouding the clear orifices, treated with Jiawei Shengtieluo Yin or Huqing Wan.

Mania and depression are mostly caused by emotional suppression.

Generally speaking, diseases caused by emotions are quite complex. Zhu Danxi said: "When qiand blood is harmonious, no disease arises; once there is suppression, various diseases occur." He believed that qi stagnation comes first, followed by stagnation of dampness, phlegm, heat, blood, and food, establishing the theory of six stagnations, with Yueju Wan as the main formula. However, clinically, due to transformation of qi stagnation into fire, and excessive fire generating wind, a series of syndromes such as liver qi, liver fire, and liver wind often appear. *Leizheng Zhicai* pointed out: "All ascending qi comes from the liver; the liver tends to ascend and disperse, not tolerating stagnation. Stagnation causes reversal of meridian qi, leading to belching, distension, vomitting, violent anger with hypochondriac pain, chest fullness with anorexia, diarrhea, and hernia, all due to reckless liver qi. Stagnation of ministerial fire in wood transforms into fire, causing acid regurgitation, hypochondriac pain, mania, flaccidity, syncope, abdominal mass, hiccup, and bleeding, all due to liver fire rushing upward. Wind depends on wood; wood stagnation transforms into wind, causing dizziness, vertigo, tongue numbness, tinnitus, convulsions, impediment, and stroke-like conditions, all due to liver fire stirring." Therefore, in the initial stage, they are generally called "stagnation syndrome", mainly treated by soothing, purging, and calming the liver, using Huagan Jian, Jiegan Jian, Xiaoyao Powder, etc. When fire and wind are generated, the treatment mainly focuses on clearing, purging, and softening the liver, using Huoyu Decoction, Xieqing Wan, Yiguan Jian, Sanjia Fumai Decoction, etc.

Jiawei Shengtieluo Yin: Iron Filings, Scrophularia, Salvia, Ophiopogon, Cinnabar, Uncaria, Trichosanthes Root, Fritillaria, Arisaema cum Bile, Forsythia, Polygala, Acorus, Poria, Fushen

Huqing Wan: One *liang* each of Rhinoceros Horn and Rhubarb, 5 *qian* each of raw Gardenia and raw Polygala, one pair of tiger eyes, ground into powder, made into pills with white honey, coated with Cinnabar.

Yueju Wan: Cyperus, Atractylodes lancea, Ligusticum, Gardenia, Medicated Leaven

Huagan Jian: White Peony Root, Green Tangerine Peel, Tangerine Peel, Fritillaria, Moutan Bark, Gardenia, Alisma

Jiegan Jian: Perilla Leaf, White Peony Root, Tangerine Peel, Pinellia, Poria, Magnolia officinalis, Amomum

Xiaoyao Powder: Angelica, White Peony Root, Bupleurum, Atractylodes, Poria, Licorice, Mint, Ginger

Huoyu Decoction: Scutellaria, Forsythia, Turmeric, Ophiopogon, Mint, Trichosanthes, Peach Kernel, Bamboo Leaf, Licorice

Xieqing Wan: Gentiana, Gardenia, Rhubarb, Angelica, Ligusticum, Notopterygium, Saposhnikovia

Yiguan Jian: Adenophora, Ophiopogon, Raw Rehmannia, Angelica Body, Wolfberry, Sichuan Chinaberry

Sanjia Fumai Decoction: Oyster, Turtle Shell, Turtle Plate, Raw Rehmannia, White Peony Root, Donkey-Hide Gelatin, Ophiopogon, Hemp Seed, Licorice

XIX. Hiccups

Hiccuping repeatedly with short and frequent sounds is called "e ni" (hiccups). Occasional attacks are often caused by drinking cold beverages or inhaling cold air; measures such as irritating the nose to induce sneezing, holding the breath, or focusing one's thoughts to divert attention can all stop it. If it persists, a small amount of ginger can be chewed and taken with boiled water. However, when it appears during illness, especially in the elderly and those with chronic weak conditions, it often becomes a severe symptom. Therefore, this condition should be differentiated into excess and deficiency: In excess syndrome, the hiccup sounds are loud, with a slippery large pulse; in deficiency syndrome, the hiccup sounds are faint, with weak physique and qi. The general treatment method is to harmonize the stomach and descend counterflow, with Dingxiang Shidi Decoction as the main formula, and cloves and persimmon calyx as the key herbs for this condition. However, cloves and persimmon calyx have different properties and flavors; since hiccups are mostly due to intermingling of cold and heat with conflict between the two qi, the treatment often combines cold and heat herbs. For excess syndrome, ginseng should be removed; for severe cold, cinnamon can be used; for severe phlegm-dampness, add pinellia, tangerine peel, and magnolia bark; for heat complicated cases, appropriately reduce cloves and add bamboo shavings and loquat leaves; for deficiency syndrome, it can be combined with Xuanfu Daizheshi Decoction.

Dingxiang Shidi Decoction: Cloves, Persimmon Calyx, Ginseng, Ginger

Xuanfu Daizheshi Decoction: Inula, Haematite, Ginseng, Licorice, Pinellia, Ginger, Jujube

XX. Dysphagia and Regurgitation

Difficulty in swallowing food, often feeling a blockage in the throat and chest, especially for dry foods which are harder to pass down, is called "ye ge" (dysphagia and regurgitation). Ancient physicians classified it into five types based on causes: "qige" (qi blockage), "xue ge" (blood blockage), "tan ge" (phlegm blockage), "huo ge" (fire blockage), and "shi ge" (food blockage). However, the main causes are nothing more than qi stagnation due to worry and thought, and damage to yin from alcohol and sexual indulgence. Zhang Jingyue stated: “The syndrome of dysphagia and regurgitation is necessarily caused by excessive worry, anxiety, accumulated overwork and depression, or excessive alcohol and sexual activity damaging yin. Yin damage leads to depletion of essence and blood; failure of qi to move causes dysphagia and regurgitation in the upper part, while depletion of essence and blood causes dryness and constipation in the lower part.” Therefore, in the initial stage of the disease, it tends to be qi stagnation, first feeling obstruction in the esophagus, then developing qi dysphagia, often worsening with mental depression and alleviating when in a good mood. Gradually worsening, blood stasis appears: Water and drinks can be taken, but grain food is hard to swallow, and even if swallowed, it is regurgitated; there is occasional pain in the chest and epigastrium, or vomiting blood and bloody stools, or vomiting fluid like red bean juice, or difficult defecation with stool as hard as sheep dung. At this time, body fluids are extremely exhausted, the body becomes emaciated, and eventually, even drops of water and drinks cannot be swallowed, with stomach qi exhausted. The prognosis of this disease is mostly poor, especially in the elderly and weak, which is even harder to treat. In the initial stage, relieving stagnation and moistening dryness is appropriate, using Qige Powder; for long-term blood stasis, use Tongyou Decoction minus cimicifuga plus curcuma; after opening, use Wuzhi Anzhong Yin for conditioning. Wind disease, consumption, tympanites, and dysphagia and regurgitation are called the four major syndromes; the general treatment methods include regulating qi, resolving phlegm, dispelling stasis, generating fluids, strengthening the spleen, and moistening the intestines, etc. However, acrid-dry and dissipating agents must be used with caution to prevent damaging qi and yin, and moistening and nourishing yin agents should also be cautious of affecting digestion and transportation.

Qige Powder: Adenophora, Salvia, Poria, Fritillaria, Curcuma, Amomum Shell, Lotus Stalk, Rice Bran

Tongyou Decoction: Raw Rehmannia, Prepared Rehmannia, Peach Kernel, Safflower, Angelica, Licorice, Cimicifuga

Wuzhi Anzhong Yin: Chive Juice, Milk, Ginger Juice, Pear Juice, Lotus Root Juice

XXI. Belching

Belching is common in patients with stomach diseases and weak spleen and stomach, due to qi stagnation in the middle jiao, chest and diaphragm fullness, and relief after belching. It is generally not treated as a main symptom, and appropriate additions can be made to the prescription such as magnolia bark, tangerine peel, cloves, sandalwood, amomum, and agastache. If due to spleen yang weakness and indigestion, with frequent belching after meals, Jianpi Powder is used.

Belching is often accompanied by passing flatus; generally, qi stagnation in the stomach mostly goes upward, and qi stagnation in the intestines mostly goes downward, so medications should be differentiated accordingly.

Jianpi Powder: Ginseng, Atractylodes, Clove, Agastache, Amomum, Nutmeg, Medicated Leaven, Roasted Licorice, Ginger, Jujube

XXII. Acid Regurgitation

Regurgitation of acid from the stomach with a burning sensation and discomfort is mostly due to liver qi invading the stomach. Generally, Zuojin Wan is used; cuttlefish bone and calcined Concha Arcae can also be used to stop it. Zuojin Wan is mainly composed of Coptis and Evodia in a ratio of six to one. However, acid regurgitation can be differentiated into heat-biased and cold-biased types. For heat-biased cases, bamboo shavings and charred gardenia can be added to the formula; for cold-biased cases, the dosages of Coptis and Evodia can be appropriately adjusted, with addition of clove and fresh ginger.

Zuojin Wan: Coptis, Evodia

XXIII. Nausea

It is one of the symptoms of phlegm-dampness. A feeling of rising in the chest with a desire to vomit but no vomiting occurs; appropriate additions such as Pinellia, Poria, fresh ginger, and optionally Fructus Aurantii, bamboo shavings, etc., can be made to the prescription.

Liver yang dizziness can also cause nausea, which is not treated as a main symptom. When liver yang is subdued, stomach qi will naturally harmonize; Fructus Aurantii and bamboo shavings can also be added to the formula for temporary relief.

In pregnant women, aversions to objects and nausea are called "e zu" (morning sickness). Refer to the entry "Pregnancy Vomiting" in gynecological symptoms.

XXIV. Vomiting

Vomiting occurs because the stomach fails to properly descend and instead rebels upward. Ancient physicians distinguished "ou" (vomiting with sound but no content) from "tu" (vomiting with both sound and content); in reality, they often occur simultaneously and are difficult to separate. Diagnosis and treatment are generally based on accompanying symptoms and the nature of the vomitus. If there is a sour sensation before vomiting, with more clear fluid, preference for heat and aversion to cold, white greasy tongue coating, and excessive saliva in the mouth after vomiting with a continued desire to retch, it belongs to stomach cold, treated with Banxia Ganjiang Decoction or Wuzhuyu Decoction. If the vomitus is a mixture of sour and bitter fluids, with a foul odor in the mouth, preference for cold and aversion to heat, and vomiting often occurring right after eating, with yellow greasy tongue coating, it belongs to stomach heat, treated with Zhuru Decoction. If there is chest and epigastric fullness before vomiting, belching and acid regurgitation, and the vomitus consists mostly of sour, rotten undigested food, with a feeling of relief after vomiting, it indicates food stagnation in the stomach, treated with Shengjiang Jupi Decoction plus Medicated Leaven, Millet Sprout, and Barley Sprout. Those with a history of phlegm turbidity, chest tightness, dizziness, palpitations, and vomiting of sticky phlegm have phlegm-fluid in the stomach, treated with Xiao Banxia Decoction plus Poria. There are also cases of intermingled cold and heat, with chest and diaphragm stuffiness, intermittent vomiting, slippery pulse, and yellow greasy tongue coating, treated with Banxia Xiexin Decoction. This method of pungent opening and bitter descending is relatively commonly used in vomiting syndromes, but ginseng and jujube in the formula can be adjusted as appropriate. For cases with extremely severe damp-heat phlegm turbidity, thick greasy tongue coating, frequent vomiting and nausea, and immediate vomiting upon drinking water, which is difficult to stop, two-three *fen* of Yushu Dan can be taken with boiled water.

When food is ingested but vomited out after a day and a half, with the vomitus mostly undigested, it is called "fan wei" (regurgitation) due to stomach cold and spleen weakness. *Synopsis of the Golden Chamber* states: "When the spleen is injured, it fails to transform; food eaten in the morning is vomited in the evening, and food eaten in the evening is vomited in the morning, named stomach reversal." Wang Bing also said: "Food entering and being vomited out indicates absence of fire."

Treatment should warm the middle and strengthen the middle jiao, using Dingxiang Touge Powder. For long-term cases with deficient nutrient blood, mental fatigue, thready pulse, and constipation, Da Banxia Decoction is used.

In infants, the spilling and vomiting of milk after feeding is called "xian ru" (milk regurgitation), commonly known as "milk reflux". It is mostly due to overfeeding; occasional occurrences require no treatment. For frequent occurrences with sour, rotten milk or sour-smelling stools, Xiaoru Wan is used.

Banxia Ganjiang Decoction: Pinellia, Dried Ginger

Wuzhuyu Decoction: Evodia, Ginseng, Ginger, Jujube

Zhuru Decoction: Bamboo Shavings, Licorice, Pinellia, Tangerine Peel, Gardenia, Loquat Leaf, Ginger, Jujube

Shengjiang Jupi Decoction: Fresh Ginger, Tangerine Peel

Xiao Banxia Decoction: Pinellia, Fresh Ginger

Banxia Xiexin Decoction: Pinellia, Scutellaria, Dried Ginger, Ginseng, Roasted Licorice, Coptis, Jujube

Yushu Dan: Omitted (proprietary medicine)

Dingxiang Touge Powder: Clove, Ginseng, Atractylodes, Cyperus, Amomum, Cardamom, Malt, Aucklandia, Agarwood, Green Tangerine Peel, Tangerine Peel, Magnolia officinalis, Agastache, Pinellia, Roasted Licorice

Da Banxia Decoction: Pinellia, Ginseng, White Honey

Xiaoru Wan: Cyperus, Medicated Leaven, Malt, Tangerine Peel, Amomum, Roasted Licorice

XXV. Vomiting and Diarrhea

Chest and epigastric stuffiness, abdominal pain, vomiting followed by diarrhea, foul-smelling qi, subsequent chills and fever, greasy tongue coating, and slippery rapid pulse, which is mostly caused by food stagnation injuring the middle jiao or concurrent external pathogenic invasion; treatment should disperse, transform, and guide out stagnation, using Huoxiang Zhengqi Powder. This syndrome is more common in children; although it comes on acutely, recovery is also rapid.

Suddenly, there is gurgling in the abdomen or cramping pain, with incessant vomiting and diarrhea, watery diarrhea, followed by collapse, sunken eyes, shrunken collarbones, leg cramps, and a faint deep hidden pulse. This is the severe "huoluan" (cholera) syndrome, commonly known as "fasha" (sha qi onset) or "shaqi" (sha qi), which can cause death within hours, hence other colloquial names such as "bieluo sha" (shriveled snail sha), "diaojiao sha" (hanging foot sha), and "ziwu sha" (noon/midnight sha). This disease often occurs in summer and autumn, is contagious, mainly due to unclean diet, exposure to cold, disharmony of the intestines and stomach, and failure to separate clear and turbid. *Nei Jing* states: "When clear and turbid interfere with each other, disturbing the intestines and stomach, it becomes cholera." Due to the critical condition forcing sudden depletion of yang qi and body fluids, timely treatment is essential. First, take Chansu Wan orally, fill the navel with salt and moxibustion, perform acupuncture and moxibustion at Zhongwan, Tianshu, Guanyuan, Zusanli, etc., and administer Sini decoction, Dashun Powder, etc., internally to recover yang.

Vomiting and diarrhea occurring together, with foul-smelling vomitus and diarrhea, accompanied by fever, restlessness, limb pain, thirst with desire to drink, scanty dark urine, yellow greasy tongue coating, and soft slippery or soft rapid pulse. This is summerheat-dampness accumulated in the intestines and stomach, similar to cholera but different in nature. Thus, ancient physicians distinguished true and false cholera, referring to true cholera as "cold cholera" and false cholera as "heat cholera". Treatment should clear and transform with bitter-cold herbs, using Ranzhao Decoction or Canshi Decoction, and acupuncture at Quze, Weizhong, Quchi, Neiguan, Chengshan, etc.

Folk medicine has a scraping method for cholera: use copper coins or magnetic spoons dipped in sesame oil or vegetable oil, scrape downward from top to bottom on the shoulders, neck, back, chest and hypochondria, and the crooks of the arms and knees until the skin turns reddish-purple. Zhang Jingyue once said: "For deep-seated toxins, scraping the back is essential." This method is considered to promote smooth flow of qi and blood, alleviating symptoms, and is one of the effective first-aid measures.

Huoxiang Zhengqi Powder: Agastache, Perilla, Magnolia officinalis, Tangerine Peel, Angelica dahurica, Areca Peel, Atractylodes, Poria, Pinellia 曲, Platycodon, Licorice, Ginger, Jujube

Chansu Wan: Toad Venom, Cinnabar, Realgar, Atractylodes, Clove, Gleditsia, Musk (proprietary medicine)

Sini Decoction: Aconite, Dried Ginger, Licorice

Dashun Powder: Aconite, Cinnamon, Almond, Licorice

Ranzhao decoction: Talc, Gardenia, Fermented Soybean, Scutellaria, Eupatorium, Magnolia officinalis, Pinellia, Amomum

Canshi Decoction: Silkworm Feces, Papaya, Coix Seed, Fermented Soybean Sprout, Coptis, Pinellia, Scutellaria, Evodia, Gardenia, Tetrapanax

XXVI. Upward Reversal and Downward Obstruction

Upward reversal with vomiting, inability to take food, and downward obstruction with inability to urinate, or obstruction of both urine and stool, is called "guange" (block and repulsion). *Treatise on Febrile Diseases* states: "The cun pulse is floating and large; floating indicates deficiency, large indicates excess. At the chi position, it is guan (block), and at the cun position, it is ge (repulsion). Guan leads to inability to urinate, ge leads to vomiting and reversal." First, use acrid-aromatic, orifice-opening, and descending herbs to treat the upper, such as agarwood, clove, agastache, storax, amomum, and ginger; then use bitter-cold, qi-circulating, and downward-draining herbs to unblock the lower, such as rhubarb, phellodendron, akebia, talc, plantain seed, etc. There are also cases with cold in the upper and heat in the lower, treated with Huanglian Decoction, replacing cinnamon twig with cinnamon.

Huanglian Decoction: Coptis, dried ginger, cinnamon twig, ginseng, licorice, pinellia, jujube

XXVII. Poor Appetite

The stomach governs reception, and the spleen is in charge of transportation and transformation; together they are the root of postnatal reproduction and transformation, and the source of middle qi. Therefore, poor appetite includes lack of desire to eat, feeling hungry but unable to eat, easy satiety, difficulty in digesting after eating, as well as tastelessness in food and aversion to greasy foods, all reflecting disharmony between the spleen and stomach. Generally, if the disease is in the stomach but not the spleen, there is hunger but inability to eat, easy satiety, tastelessness, and aversion to greasy; if the disease is in the spleen but not the stomach, there is no feeling of hunger and difficulty in digesting after eating; if both the spleen and stomach are diseased, there is neither hunger nor desire to eat. The main factors causing this disease are, first, damp turbidity, and second, deficiency of middle qi. Internal obstruction of damp turbidity leads to dysfunction of transportation and transformation, accompanied by white greasy or thick greasy tongue coating; treatment should aromatically harmonize the middle, using Hewei Erchen Jian or Da Hezhong Yin. Deficiency of middle qi results in weak digestive capacity, with mostly clean tongue coating; treatment should tonify qi and strengthen the middle, using Yigong Powder or Shenling Baizhu Powder. There are also cases where middle qi is trapped due to retained dampness, or damp turbidity fails to transform due to insufficient middle qi, requiring consideration of both aspects. In addition, qi stagnation, cold, phlegm, food retention, and internal accumulation of damp-heat can all affect appetite, each treated according to syndrome differentiation. This syndrome can appear in general diseases and is rarely treated as a main symptom, but since the spleen and stomach are the postnatal foundation, clinical attention should be extremely paid to it, and this is often taken into account in prescriptions.

Reduced food intake in severe or chronic diseases, gradually leading to loss of desire to eat, indicates deterioration of postnatal vitality, as stated in *Nei Jing*: "Those who take grain thrive, those who stop grain perish," with a mostly poor prognosis.

Hewei Erchen Jian: Pinellia, tangerine peel, poria, licorice, amomum, ginger, jujube

Da Hezhong Yin: Aucklandia, magnolia officinalis, fructus aurantii, pinellia, tangerine peel, dried ginger, alisma, hawthorn, malt, amomum

Yigong Powder: Ginseng, atractylodes, poria, tangerine peel, licorice

Shenling Baizhu Powder: Ginseng, atractylodes, poria, yam, hyacinth bean, coix seed, amomum, tangerine peel, lotus seed, platycodon

XXVIII. Polyphagia and Easy Hunger

Able to eat, easily hungry, and thirsty, without gaining muscle, with hard stools, is due to stomach dryness and heat, a characteristic of "zhongxiao" (middle consumption) in wasting-thirst syndrome. Clearing heat and generating fluids is appropriate, using Taiqing Yin or Xiaoke Fang. The main symptoms of wasting-thirst are polydipsia, polyphagia, polyuria, i.e., thirst with desire to drink, polyphagia with emaciation, frequent and copious urination, which often vary in severity. There may be obvious polydipsia with the other two less prominent, or polyphagia as the main symptom with the other two secondary, or polyuria as the main symptom with the other two mild. Ancient physicians classified it into upper, middle, and lower consumption based on the prominence of these three, but treatment should not be absolutely divided.

A sudden desire to eat and ability to eat during febrile diseases is not necessarily a normal state; "chuzhong" (central elimination, a critical sign) must be guarded against. *Treatise on Febrile Diseases* states: "In cases of syncope with diarrhea, the patient should be unable to eat; if they can eat instead, it is feared to be 'chuzhong' (central elimination). Give them noodle cakes; if there is no fever, it indicates that stomach qi is still present, and recovery is certain." It also says: "The abdomen should be cold, and the patient should be unable to eat; if they can eat instead, this is called 'chuzhong', and death is certain." "Chuzhong" means the elimination of middle qi, which can be understood as the deterioration of stomach qi, thus indicating an incurable condition.

In children with polyphagia and a craving for tea leaves, soil, etc., it is a syndrome of "worm accumulation". Refer to the entry "Abdominal Pain" in abdominal and umbilical symptoms.

Taiqing Yin: Anemarrhena, Dendrobium, Ophiopogon, Akebia, Gypsum

Xiaoke Fang: Coptis, Trichosanthes Root, Raw Rehmannia, Lotus Root Juice, Cow's Milk

XXIX. Loose Stools

Unformed stools, loose and thin like sauce or duck droppings, are called "tangxie" (pastry diarrhea), also known as "wuxie" (duck-stool diarrhea). It is mostly due to spleen deficiency failing to transport and transform. *Jinkui Yi* (Supplements to the Golden Chamber) states: "The spleen is responsible for transporting the stomach's fluids. When spleen qi is weak and unable to distribute them, fluids and waste together rush down through the same orifice." *Synopsis of the Golden Chamber* refers to "spleen qi decline leading to duck-like loose stools." During diarrhea, there is borborygmus and dull abdominal pain, often with an urge to defecate immediately after eating. Persisting for a long time, middle qi becomes more deficient, with mental fatigue, reduced appetite, sallow complexion, and a soft weak pulse, treated with Xiangsha Liujunzi Decoction plus Nutmeg. Patients with normally loose stools or unformed stools after improper diet all show signs of spleen deficiency.

Damp-heat pouring downward can also cause loose stools, with abdominal pain and incomplete evacuation during diarrhea, a burning sensation in the anus, dark yellow feces, scanty dark urine, and a yellow greasy tongue coating. It is more common between summer and autumn, with initial accompanying chills and fever, treated with Ruling Decoction.

Hyperactivity of liver fire, spleen deficiency with accumulated dampness, abdominal distension and pain, loose stools, frequent flatulence, irritable temperament, string-like slippery pulse, yellow greasy tongue coating, and relatively red tongue body are treated with Tongxie Yaofang.

In this formula, Saposhnikovia combined with Atractylodes enters the spleen and stomach meridians, dispelling wind and dampness, and dissipating stagnant qi, different from relieving the exterior.

Loose stools with black color are a sign of bleeding. Refer to the entry "Hematochezia" in this section.

Xiangsha Liujunzi Decoction: Aucklandia, Amomum, Codonopsis, Atractylodes, Poria, Licorice

Ruling Decoction: Elsholtzia, Polyporus, Red Poria, Alisma, Atractylodes, Coptis, Hyacinth Bean, Magnolia officinalis, Licorice

Tongxie Yaofang: Atractylodes, Saposhnikovia, White Peony Root, Tangerine Peel

XXX. Watery Diarrhea

Diarrhea with watery stools and undigested food is called "shuixie" (watery diarrhea), also known as "ruixie" (dampness diarrhea) or "sunxie" (indigestion diarrhea). It is mostly caused by cold exposure and retained dampness, with a sudden onset, abdominal pain, borborygmus, unbearable discomfort, and can cause chills and fever, accompanied by headache and body aches, white slippery tongue coating, treated with Huoxiang Zhengqi Powder. For diarrhea caused solely by cold pathogens injuring the interior, warming the middle and dispelling cold is appropriate, using Lingjiang Zhugui Decoction; or for diarrhea due to excessive dampness, resolving dampness and promoting diuresis is appropriate, using Weiling Decoction.

Improper diet can also easily cause diarrhea, characterized by abdominal pain followed by diarrhea, extremely foul odor, and relief of pain after diarrhea, accompanied by chest tightness, fetid belching, anorexia, etc., treated with Zhishi Daozhi Wan minus Rhubarb plus Raphani Seed.

Abdominal pain with borborygmus, alternating pain and diarrhea, burning sensation in the anus, dark and scanty urine, resembling dysentery but without tenesmus, is called "huoxie" (fire-heat diarrhea), treated with Da Fenqing Yin.

Watery diarrhea caused by internal injury is commonly due to spleen-kidney yang deficiency. Food is likely to pass down immediately after ingestion, with undigested food, and dull, lingering abdominal pain. Mild cases involve the spleen, severe cases involve the kidney, collectively called "xuxie" (deficiency-type diarrhea). There are also cases of diarrhea occurring once at dawn, called "chenxie" (morning diarrhea), commonly known as "wugengxie" (fifth-watch diarrhea), also caused by insufficient kidney yang. For spleen diarrhea, Lizhong Decoction or Shenling Baizhu Powder is used; for kidney diarrhea, Sishen Wan or Jiaofu Wan is used.

Diarrhea syndrome is relatively complex and must be differentiated into deficiency and excess, cold and heat, severity, as well as pathogenic factors and internal organs. *Yizong Bidu* (Essential Readings for Medical Professionals) once proposed nine major methods: ① Diluting and permeating, to expel dampness through urine, such as Silin Powder; ② Raising and lifting, to stimulate the upward movement of stomach qi, such as Shengyang Chushi Decoction; ③ Clearing and cooling, using bitter-cold to purge heat, such as Gegen Qinlian Decoction; ④ Dispersing and resolving, to eliminate phlegm accumulation, qi stagnation, food retention, and water stagnation, such as Huoxiang Zhengqi Powder; ⑤ Sweet and moderating, for incessant diarrhea, such as Shenling Baizhu Powder; ⑥ Sour and astringing, for prolonged diarrhea with qi dissipation, such as Wumei Wan; ⑦ Drying the spleen, for spleen deficiency with inability to separate water and grains, such as Lizhong Decoction; ⑧ Warming the kidney, for fire deficiency failing to generate earth (spleen), such as Sishen Wan; ⑨ Astringing, for prolapse of the large intestine, such as Chishizhi Yuyuliang Decoction. *Leizheng Zhicai* also proposed a general formula for diarrhea, using Atractylodes, Poria, Tangerine Peel, Licorice, Alisma, Amomum, Medicated Leaven, Malt; adding Aucklandia and roasted Ginger for cold; adding Scutellaria and White Peony Root for heat; adding Atractylodes lancea and Pinellia for dampness; adding Nutmeg and Terminalia for uncontrollable diarrhea; adding Ginseng, Astragalus, and Cimicifuga for prolonged cases.

Huoxiang Zhengqi Powder: Agastache, Perilla, Magnolia officinalis, Tangerine Peel, Areca Peel, Angelica dahurica, Poria, Atractylodes, Fermented Pinellia, Platycodon, Licorice, Ginger, Jujube

Lingjiang Zhugui Decoction: Poria, Fresh Ginger, Atractylodes, Cinnamon Twig

Weiling Decoction: Atractylodes lancea, Atractylodes, Magnolia officinalis, Tangerine Peel, Alisma, Polyporus, Poria, Licorice

Zhishi Daozhi Wan: Fructus Aurantii Immaturus, Atractylodes, Poria, Scutellaria, Coptis, Rhubarb, Alisma, Medicated Leaven

Da Fenqing Yin: Poria, Polyporus, Alisma, Akebia, Gardenia, Fructus Aurantii, Plantain Seed

Lizhong Decoction: Ginseng, Atractylodes, Poria, Roasted Ginger

Shenling Baizhu Powder: Ginseng, Poria, Atractylodes, Tangerine Peel, Yam, Licorice, Hyacinth Bean, Lotus Seed, Amomum, Coix Seed, Platycodon

Sishen Wan: Nutmeg, Psoralea, Schisandra, Evodia

Jiaofu Wan: Sichuan Pepper, Aconite, Cornus, Mantidis Ootheca, Pilose Antler, Dragon Bone

Silin Powder: Atractylodes, Alisma, Red Poria, Polyporus

Shengyang Chushi Decoction: Atractylodes lancea, Notopterygium, Saposhnikovia, Cimicifuga, Bupleurum, Licorice, Medicated Leaven, Polyporus, Alisma, Tangerine Peel, Malt

Gegen Qinlian Decoction: Pueraria, Scutellaria, Coptis, Licorice

Wumei Wan: Dark Plum, Asarum, Cinnamon Twig, Aconite, Ginseng, Coptis, Dried Ginger, Phellodendron, Sichuan Pepper, Angelica

Chishizhi Yuyuliang Decoction: Red Halloysite, Limonite

XXXI. Frequent Bowel Movements

Having bowel movements two or three times a day, with normal stool and no discomfort, is a sign of insufficient middle qi. If this is a habit, it is not considered a pathological symptom.

XXXII. Fecal Incontinence

It is common in prolonged unresolved diarrhea with prolapse of the large intestine, and astringents should be used; refer to the entry "Watery Diarrhea" in this section.

Kidney yang deficiency unable to control the two excretions (urine and feces), with both fecal incontinence and enuresis, which are unconscious or difficult to control even when sensed. Treatment should warm and nourish the kidney and life gate; astringents alone cannot be effective. Conversely, kidney deficiency with insufficient qi transformation can cause obstruction of urine and feces, which should also be treated mainly by warming and nourishing the kidney and life gate, without using purgative methods. Therefore, the general treatment principle is to unblock for obstruction of urine and feces, and to stop for incontinence, while also considering the spleen according to *Nei Jing*'s statement that "insufficient middle qi leads to changes in urination and defecation", and further considering qi transformation based on "the kidney governing the two excretions".

XXXIII. Constipation

Constipation is short for "dry constipation". When it appears in the course of typhoid fever, warm diseases, etc., it is mostly a heat syndrome, due to internal heat and intestinal dryness, making the stool unable to pass smoothly. At the same time, because of constipation, pathogenic heat cannot descend; in the lower part, there is abdominal fullness and pain; in the upper part, there is restlessness, and even coma and delirium. Accompanied by high fever, spontaneous sweating, thirst, a slippery rapid pulse, a yellow greasy or dry rough tongue coating with little fluid, the treatment adopts urgent purgation, using Da Chengqi Decoction and Xiao Chengqi Decoction. Generally, excessive heat with constipation is most likely to damage yin, causing symptoms such as sore throat, so it is also called urgent purgation to preserve yin. However, in cases of inherent fluid deficiency or after yin has been damaged, the purgative method alone is inappropriate; Biyue Marin Pills and Zengye Chengqi Decoction can be selected, and sometimes only Zengye Decoction is used, as Wu Jutong put it, "using the nature of tonic medicines as purgatives". Using purgatives for heat syndrome constipation is a common method, but when unnecessary, purgation is not the main treatment, and only moistening medicines such as hemp seed, trichosanthes seed, and plum seed can be added to the prescription. For cases with both exterior and interior syndromes, Liangge Powder can be used to resolve both exterior and interior. For more complex cases, *Wenbiao Tiaobian* (Systematic Differentiation of Warm Diseases) points out: "If purgation is missed when it should be applied, and healthy qi cannot transport the medicine, failure to transport the medicine leads to death, and Xinjia Huanglong Decoction is the main treatment; for dyspnea and restlessness, phlegm congestion, a full large pulse on the right cun, and failure of lung qi to descend, Xuanbai Chengqi Decoction is the main treatment; for a firm pulse on the left chi, red and painful urination, frequent severe thirst, Daochi Chengqi Decoction is the main treatment." This shows that the treatment of constipation in febrile diseases should be combined with specific conditions to achieve better results.

Constipation that appears in miscellaneous syndromes or simple habitual constipation has four types: "heat constipation", "qi constipation", "deficiency constipation", and "cold constipation". Generally, bowel movements occur once every three to four days or five to six days, with difficulty in excretion, and different accompanying symptoms due to different causes. For example: Heat constipation is accompanied by bad breath and red urine; qi constipation by chest and hypochondriac fullness; deficiency constipation by dizziness, dry throat, fatigue after defecation, shortness of breath and sweating; cold constipation is more common in the elderly, accompanied by mild abdominal pain that is relieved by warmth and a deep slow pulse. Treatment methods: Heat constipation should clear, moisten, and purge with bitterness, using Biyue Marin Pills and Gengyi Pills; qi constipation should smooth qi and promote stagnation, using Liu Mo Yin; deficiency constipation should nourish yin and moisten dryness or benefit qi and moisten the intestines, using Wuren Pills and Huangqi Decoction; cold constipation should warm, unblock, and dispel yin, using Banliu Pills and Congrong Runchang Pills.

Patients with habitual constipation often develop hemorrhoids and anal fissures due to dry stool, with blood during defecation, which should be distinguished from "hematochezia".

Postpartum women often have difficulty in defecation; refer to the entry “Postpartum Constipation” in gynecological symptoms.

Newborn infants with constipation, accompanied by red face, abdominal distension, refusal to nurse, and frequent crying, mostly due to heat toxin accumulation, are treated with three-four *fen* of Sanhuang Wan mixed with honey for administration.

Da Chengqi Decoction: Rhubarb, Fructus Aurantii Immaturus, Magnolia officinalis, Sodium Sulfate

Xiao Chengqi Decoction: Rhubarb, Fructus Aurantii Immaturus, Magnolia officinalis

Biyue Marin Pills: Hemp Seed, Almond, White Peony Root, Rhubarb, Fructus Aurantii, Magnolia officinalis

Zengye Chengqi Decoction: Scrophularia, Ophiopogon, Raw Rehmannia, Rhubarb, Sodium Sulfate

Zengye Decoction: Scrophularia, Ophiopogon, Raw Rehmannia

Liangge Powder: Rhubarb, Sodium Sulfate, Gardenia, Forsythia, Scutellaria, Mint, Bamboo Leaf, Licorice

Xinjia Huanglong Decoction: Raw Rehmannia, Licorice, Ginseng, Scrophularia, Angelica, Ophiopogon, Sea Cucumber, Rhubarb, Sodium Sulfate, Ginger

Xuanbai Chengqi Decoction: Gypsum, Rhubarb, Almond, Trichosanthes Peel

Daochi Chengqi Decoction: Raw Rehmannia, Red Peony Root, Coptis, Phellodendron, Rhubarb, Sodium Sulfate

Gengyi Pills: Aloe, Cinnabar

Liu Mo Yin: Agarwood, Aucklandia, Areca, Lindera, Fructus Aurantii Immaturus, Rhubarb

Wuren Pills: Peach Seed, Almond, Pine Nut, Platycladi Seed, Plum Seed

Huangqi Decoction: Astragalus, Tangerine Peel, Hemp Seed

Banliu Wan: Pinellia, Sulfur (proprietary medicine)

Congrong Runchang Wan: Cistanche, Agarwood, Hemp Seed

Sanhuang Wan: Rhubarb, Coptis, Scutellaria

XXXIV. Pellet-like Stools

Stools in pellets, like chestnuts or jujubes, due to intestinal dryness and heat, are called "zaoshi" (stercoroma). The method to identify dry feces is stated in *Treatise on Febrile Diseases*: "If a patient has not had a bowel movement for five or six days, with pain around the umbilicus, restlessness, and paroxysmal symptoms, there is dry feces, which causes the inability to defecate." It also says: "After severe purgation, no bowel movement for six or seven days, unresolved restlessness, and abdominal fullness and pain indicate dry feces; the reason is the presence of retained food." Generally, dry feces in the abdomen should be purged, but after purging, further purgation is inappropriate.

In the late stage of "yege" (dysphagia), with spitting of white foam and sheep-dung-like pellet stools, it indicates desiccation of the stomach and intestines, which is difficult to treat. Ancient physicians used Yizhiren (Alpinia oxyphylla), Jiuzhi (Allium tuberosum seeds), and Banxia (Pinellia) decocted, taken with ginger juice, almond paste, white honey, and cow's milk.

XXXV. Flatulence (Passing Gas)

Passing gas through the anus is called "shiqi" (flatus), commonly known as "xugong" (borborygmus). It is mostly due to indigestion or liver-stomach qi stagnation; relief after passing gas requires no treatment. However, frequent gas passing or inability to pass gas with abdominal distension and discomfort should be treated with Aucklandia, Cyperus, Green Tangerine Peel, etc., to dispel stagnation. This syndrome often occurs with belching, but the former is in the intestines and the latter in the stomach; refer to the entry "Belching" in this section.

Treatise on Febrile Diseases points out: "If there is no bowel movement for six or seven days, fear of dry feces; to determine, give a small amount of Xiao Chengqi Decoction. If gas passes after the decoction enters the abdomen, there is dry feces, and purgation is permissible; if no gas passes, the stool is only hard at the beginning, and purgation must not be performed later." Thus, passing gas is used as a diagnostic method.

XXXVI. Mucus in Stool

Passing mucus in stools, either red, white, or mixed red and white, accompanied by abdominal pain, tenesmus, occurring seven to eight times a day or even dozens of times, is the main symptom of "dysentery". Because the mucus is passed with difficulty, it is also called "changpi" (dysentery) or "zhixia" (stagnant diarrhea), and classified into "bai li" (white dysentery) and "chi li" (red dysentery) based on mucus color. The disease mostly occurs in summer and autumn, caused by external contraction of summerheat-dampness, internal injury from raw and cold food, accumulated stagnation, and dysfunction of transportation and transformation; it may also be complicated by epidemic toxins, leading to more severe conditions. Generally, it is divided into damp-heat dysentery and cold-damp dysentery. Cold-damp dysentery initially contains feces, later only white mucus and foam, with dull abdominal pain, white greasy tongue coating, and soft slow pulse, treated with Buhuanjin Zhengqi Powder, with Aucklandia and Cinnamon added for severe cases.

Damp-heat dysentery mostly has red and white pus and mucus, accompanied by chills and fever, yellow greasy tongue coating, and slippery rapid pulse, treated with Muxiang Binlang Wan, Zhishi Daozhi Wan, or Shaoyao Decoction. When dysentery gradually eases, harmonizing the middle and draining heat is appropriate, using Xianglian Wan; for persistent abdominal pain, Wuji Wan is used. Treating dysentery should not stop diarrhea too early, nor should excessive purgation or diuresis be used. Besides clearing and resolving damp-heat and eliminating stagnation, regulating qi and harmonizing blood must be supplemented, as Yi Lao (a physician) said: "Regulating qi relieves tenesmus; harmonizing blood heals pus in stools."

Dysentery with retching, inability to take food, is called "jinkou li" (fasting dysentery). Manifesting with a red tongue, yellow dry rough coating, and thready rapid pulse, it is treated with Kaijin Powder. Intermittent attacks with prolonged duration are called "xiuxi li" (intermittent dysentery), treated with Da Duanxia Decoction. Stools with mixed yellow, red, black, and white mucus are called "wuse li" (multicolored dysentery), treated with Zhenren Yangzang Decoction. For severe heat patterns with bloody pus, unresolved fever, Baitouweng Decoction is used; for prolonged dysentery with qi and blood deficiency, cold, and incontinence, Taohua Decoction is used. All these are severe syndromes.

Ni Hanchu has three formulas for dysentery, treating general diarrhea. ① Initial stage formula: Coptis, Scutellaria, White Peony Root, Hawthorn each 1.5 *qian*; Fructus Aurantii, Magnolia officinalis, Areca, Green Tangerine Peel each 0.8 *qian*; Angelica, Sanguisorba, Roasted Licorice each 0.5 *qian*; Safflower 0.3 *qian*; Aucklandia 0.2 *qian*; Peach Kernel 1 *qian*. For purely white dysentery, remove Sanguisorba and Peach Kernel, add Tangerine Red 0.4 *qian* and Aucklandia 0.3 *qian*; for severe stagnation, add wine-fried Rhubarb 2 *qian*, halved for young children. Decoct and take on an empty stomach, suitable for red-white dysentery with tenesmus, fever, and abdominal pain. Most effective within 3-5 days, also effective within 10 days, and the modified formula is used after half a month. ② Modified formula: Wine-fried Coptis, Wine-fried Scutellaria, Wine-fried White Peony Root, Peach Kernel each 0.6 *qian*; Hawthorn 1 *qian*; Tangerine Red, Green Tangerine Peel, Betel Nut, Sanguisorba each 0.4 *qian*; Roasted Licorice, Safflower each 0.3 *qian*; Angelica 0.5 *qian*; Aucklandia 0.2 *qian*, decocted for oral administration. For cases lasting over a month with spleen-stomach weakness and slippery diarrhea, tonifying and regulating are needed. ③ Tonifying and regulating formula: Wine-fried Coptis, Angelica, Ginseng, Atractylodes, Roasted Licorice each 0.5 *qian*; Wine-fried Scutellaria, Tangerine Red each 0.6 *qian*; Wine-fried White Peony Root 0.4 *qian*, decocted for oral administration. For pregnant women, remove Peach Kernel, Safflower, and Areca from the above three formulas. In addition, folk remedies include 1 *liang* of fresh Portulaca oleracea, decocted with brown and white sugar; and 15 shelled Brucea javanica seeds wrapped in longan aril, taken with boiled water three times a day.

Buhuanjin Zhengqi Powder: Agastache, Magnolia officinalis, Tangerine Peel, Pinellia, Atractylodes lancea, Licorice, Ginger, Jujube

Muxiang Binlang Wan: Aucklandia, Areca, Green Tangerine Peel, Tangerine Peel, Cyperus, Fructus Aurantii, Black Morning Glory Seed, Coptis, Phellodendron, Sparganium, Curcuma zedoaria, Rhubarb, Sodium Sulfate

Zhishi Daozhi Wan: Fructus Aurantii Immaturus, Rhubarb, Atractylodes, Poria, Coptis, Scutellaria, Alisma, Medicated Leaven

Shaoyao Decoction: White Peony Root, Scutellaria, Coptis,

Angelica, Cinnamon, Licorice, Areca, Aucklandia, Rhubarb

Xianglian Wan: Aucklandia, Coptis

Wuji Wan: White Peony Root, Evodia, Coptis

Kaijin Powder: Ginseng, Coptis, Acorus, Salvia, Semen Nelumbinis, Poria, Tangerine Peel, Wax Gourd Peel, Old Rice, Lotus Stalk

Da Duanxia Decoction: Roasted Ginger, Asarum, Galangal, Aconite, Dragon Bone, Oyster, Dried Alum, Nutmeg, Terminalia, Red Halloysite, Pomegranate Peel

Zhenren Yangzang Decoction: Terminalia, Nutmeg, Angelica, Atractylodes, White Peony Root, Ginseng, Aucklandia, Cinnamon, Poppy Shell, Licorice

Baitouweng Decoction: Pulsatilla, Ash Bark, Coptis, Phellodendron

Taohua Decoction: Red Halloysite, Dried Ginger, Japonica Rice

XXXVII. Hematochezia

For blood in the stool, it is necessary to distinguish between fresh and dark blood, and whether the blood appears before or after the stool. Blood before stool is called "jinxue" (proximal bleeding) in *Synopsis of the Golden Chamber*; Zhang Jingyue stated that it "may be in the rectum or anus", with bright red blood, and sometimes blood spattering down, named "changfeng" (intestinal wind), all due to downward rushing of damp-heat, treated with Chixiaodou Danggui Powder, Huaihua Powder; for severe dampness, Cangzhu Diyu Decoction is used. Blood after stool is called "yuanxue" (distal bleeding) in *Synopsis of the Golden Chamber*; Zhang Jingyue stated that it "may be in the small intestine or the stomach", with dark purple blood, accompanied by mental fatigue, sallow complexion, and pale tongue, treated with Huangtu Decoction.

Hematochezia is often related to "hemorrhoids and fistulas"; it is necessary to ask about anal discomfort, refer to the entry "Anal Hemorrhoids" in this section.

Dark black stools in deficient cold stomach pain are a sign of bleeding. Refer to the entry "Epigastric Pain" in abdominal and umbilical symptoms.

Chixiaodou Danggui Powder: Adzuki Bean, Angelica

Huaihua Powder: Sophora Flower, Platycladus Leaf, Stir-fried Schizonepeta, Fructus Aurantii

Cangzhu Diyu Decoction: Atractylodes lancea, Sanguisorba

Huangtu Decoction: Atractylodes, Aconite, Licorice, Rehmannia, Donkey-Hide Gelatin, Scutellaria, Furnace Heart Soil

XXXVIII. Scanty and Yellow Urine

When it appears in general conditions, it is due to internal heat and internal accumulation of damp heat, as stated in *Nei Jing*: "Yellow urine indicates heat in the lower abdomen." It is not treated as a main symptom, and appropriate additions such as talc, coix seed, red poria, and tetrapanax can be made to the prescription.

Dark and thick yellow urine that stains clothes is one of the symptoms of "jaundice"; refer to the entry "Yellow Skin Color" in systemic symptoms.

XXXIX. Clear and Profuse Urine

Its appearance in general conditions indicates no internal heat; its appearance in deficient conditions is a sign of lower origin deficiency and cold, as stated in *Nei Jing*: "All water fluids in diseases that are clear and cold belong to cold."

XL. Frequent Urination

Frequent urination accompanied by dry mouth and tongue, unquenchable thirst, and normal bowel movements is "shangxiao" (upper consumption) syndrome; drinking one part and urinating one part, or even excessive urination with urine volume exceeding intake, or urine like grease, is "xiaoxiao" (lower consumption) syndrome, collectively called "xiaoke" (wasting-thirst). Ancient physicians divided wasting-thirst into upper, middle, and lower consumption: Upper consumption belongs to lung heat, treated with Tianhuafen Powder; lower consumption belongs to kidney yin deficiency, treated with modified Dihuang Wan. However, in this disease, dryness-heat and yin deficiency often interact as cause and effect—more deficient yin leads to more intense heat, and more intense heat leads to more deficient yin. Thus, *Linzheng Zhinan* (Guide to Clinical Practice) states: "The syndrome of three consumptions, though divided into upper, middle, and lower, essentially involves nothing more than yin deficiency with yang hyperactivity, and fluid exhaustion with heat excess." This indicates that heat in wasting-thirst mostly arises from dryness, and bitter-cold herbs that directly subdue heat should not be used to damage vitality. Meanwhile, upper consumption can also have cold patterns due to failure of water to transform into qi, as stated in *Nei Jing*: "Heart transferring cold to the lung results in lung consumption, with drinking one part and urinating two parts, incurable." In lower consumption, there can also be yang deficiency failing to nourish the source of transformation, so *Synopsis of the Golden Chamber* states: "In men with wasting-thirst, urine is excessive instead, drinking one dou and urinating one dou, with Shenqi Wan as the main treatment." Upper and lower consumption can transform into "lung atrophy", "hemiplegia", and abscesses, hence there are many prepared formulas such as Huangqi Zhuye Decoction, Shengjin Yin, Ouzhi Gao Yin, Yuantu Wan, and Shuangbu Wan, which can be modified according to specific conditions.

Frequent urination in general conditions and the elderly is one of the kidney deficiency syndromes.

Frequent urination or persistent low-grade fever in children in summer is due to contraction of summerheat, with heat accumulating in the bladder, treated with Jisu Powder soaked as a tea substitute.

Frequent urination in women with small volume, urgency, and abdominal distension is mostly due to liver qi stagnation failing to disperse; dispersing qi and mild diuresis are appropriate, and astringents should not be used, treated with Xiaoyao Powder plus plantain seed.

Tianhuafen Powder: Trichosanthes Root, Raw Rehmannia, Ophiopogon, Pueraria, Schisandra, Licorice, Japonica Rice

Modified Dihuang Wan: Prepared Rehmannia, Yam, Cornus, Moutan Bark, Schisandra, Bailao Jian

Shenqi Wan: Prepared Rehmannia, Cornus, Yam, Aconite, Cinnamon, Alisma, Poria, Moutan Bar

Huangqi Zhuye Decoction: Ginseng, Astragalus, Angelica, White Peony Root, Raw Rehmannia, Ophiopogon, Ligusticum, Poria, Licorice, Gypsum, Bamboo Leaves

Shengjin Yin: Asparagus, Ophiopogon, Raw Rehmannia, Prepared Rehmannia, Angelica, Schisandra, Trichosanthes, Trichosanthes Root, Licorice, Hemp Seed

Ouzhi Gao Yin: One cup each of human milk, raw rehmannia juice, and lotus root juice, 5 *qian* of coptis, 1 *liang* of trichosanthes root, ground into powder and simmered together, then added with ginger juice and white honey to make a paste.

Yuantu Wan: Cuscuta, Schisandra, Poria, Lotus Seed, Yam

Shuangbu Wan (shuangpu pill: Deer Horn Glue, Ginseng, Poria, Coix Seed, Prepared Rehmannia, Cistanche, Angelica, Dendrobium, Astragalus, Papaya, Schisandra, Cuscuta, Raspberry, Agarwood, Alisma, Musk

Jisu Powder: Talc, Licorice, Mint

Xiaoyao Powder: Angelica, White Peony Root, Bupleurum, Atractylodes, Poria, Licorice, Mint, Ginger

XLI. Dribbling After Urination

Difficulty in urination with incessant dribbling after urination, common in the elderly with kidney qi weakness, insufficient qi transformation, and inability of the bladder to control, treated with Da Tusizi Wan.

Da Tusizi Wan: Cuscuta, Pilose Antler, Cinnamon, Aconite, Dendrobium, Prepared Rehmannia, Ranunculus sceleratus, Poria, Alisma, Achyranthes, Cornus, Dipsacus, Cistanche, Eucommia, Saposhnikovia, Psoralea, Cubeb, Agarwood, Morinda, Fennel, Ligusticum, Schisandra, Mantidis Ootheca, Raspberry

XLII. Painful Urination

Painful and difficult urination is called "lin syndrome" (stranguria), mostly caused by damp-heat in the kidney and bladder. *Chaoshi Bingyuan* (The Origin of Diseases by Chao) states: "Kidney deficiency leads to frequent urination; bladder heat causes rough flow of urine; frequent and rough urination with dribbling and obstruction is called stranguria." The urine is mostly yellow, with lower abdominal urgency, or accompanied by low back pain, and can also cause fever. Treatment should clear and promote diuresis, using Bazheng Powder.

Stranguria with blood is "blood stranguria". In the initial stage with red-purple blood and a rapid forceful pulse, it is excess heat, and clearing heat and cooling blood is appropriate, using Xiaoji Yinzi. For prolonged cases with pale red blood, mild pain, and a deficient rapid pulse, nourishing yin and stopping bleeding is appropriate, using Qiangen Powder.

Difficulty in urination with unbearable pain, yellow-red turbid urine with sand or stones, and slight relief after urination is called "sha lin" (sand stranguria) or "shi lin" (stone stranguria). Ershen Powder is used, and Lysimachia christinae (2 to 4 *liang*) can be decocted for regular administration. For all stranguria syndromes, tonifying methods are contraindicated, as qi becomes more distended when tonified, blood becomes more stagnant when tonified, and heat becomes more intense when tonified; sweating is also contraindicated for fear of stirring blood.

In general exogenous fever and yin deficiency internal heat syndromes, there may also be a burning slight pain during urination with scanty yellow urine, which is not regarded as stranguria. If it appears during high fever, talc and tetrapanax can be added to the prescription; for damp-warm syndrome, add artemisia capillaris and plantain; for yin deficiency syndrome, add raw rehmannia and anemarrhena.

Bazheng Powder: Polygonum aviculare, Akebia, Dianthus superbus, Gardenia, Licorice, Plantain, Rhubarb, Talc

Xiaoji Yinzi: Cephalanoplos segetum, Stir-fried Cattail Pollen, Lotus Rhizome Node, Talc, Akebia, Raw Rehmannia, Angelica, Licorice, Gardenia, Bamboo Leaf

Qiangen Powder: Rubia cordifolia, Scutellaria, Donkey-Hide Gelatin, Platycladus Leaf, Raw Rehmannia, Licorice

Ershen Powder: Lygodium japonicum, Talc, Akebia, Ophiopogon, Plantain

XLIII. Dysuria

Stagnant urination with only dripping, and distending discomfort in the lower abdomen is called "dysuria". It may be due to failure of qi transformation in the upper jiao, accompanied by dry throat, restlessness, shortness of breath and other lung heat symptoms, treated with HuangqinQingfei Yin plus bamboo leaf and tetrapanax; for dryness of the water source, add asparagus and ophiopogon, almond. It may be due to failure of qi transformation in the middle jiao, accompanied by body fatigue, shortness of breath, mental exhaustion and other spleen deficiency symptoms, treated with Chunze Decoction; for severe deficiency with sinking of middle qi, add astragalus and cimicifuga. It may be due to failure of qi transformation in the lower jiao, accompanied by mental decline, fear of cold, low back pain and other life gate yang deficiency symptoms, treated with Xiangrong Wan; for cases with concurrent yin deficiency, securing yin and promoting qi is appropriate, using Zishen Tongguan Wan.

Complete inability to pass urine, even a single drop, is called "long zheng" (dyssuria), which is one of the severe syndromes. It can occur suddenly or be caused by swelling, etc. The patient has the urge to urinate but cannot expel urine, with unbearable distension in the lower abdomen, requiring urgent treatment. Zhang Jingyue said: "If the water passage is blocked, it will invade the spleen and stomach upward causing distension, invade the muscles externally causing swelling, spread to the middle jiao causing vomiting, and attack the upper jiao causing dyspnea. If blocked for several days, the suffering will be unbearable, leading to danger." Therefore, *Nei Jing* instructs that "when urination and defecation are impaired, treat the branch symptoms" (where "small and large" refer to urine and stool). Although ancient treatment methods distinguish between cold, heat, deficiency, and excess, in emergency management, diuresis is the main approach, using Wuling Powder with added Plantain, Akebia, Crickets, etc. The emetic method can also be used: after taking medicine, use a goose feather to stimulate the throat; vomiting can make qi rise, and when qi rises, the lower jiao becomes unobstructed. Or external treatments: stir-fry half a *jin* of salt until hot, wrap in cloth and apply to the lower abdomen; or mash one garlic clove and three raw Gardenias and apply to the navel. Acupuncture at Zhongji, Bladder Shu, Sanyinjiao, etc., are also syndrome-specific treatments.

Conditions such as "edema" and "water tympanites" all involve dysuria, gradually progressing to anuria, which can easily lead to coma. It is more severe if accompanied by a floating large pulse or string-taut rapid pulse, and a red tongue with little fluid.

Dysuria in pregnant women is called "zhuan bao" (vesical dysuria), affected by fetal qi. Refer to the entry "Dysuria During Pregnancy" in gynecological symptoms.

HuangqinQingfei Yin: Scutellaria, Gardenia

Chunze Decoction: Poria, Atractylodes, Polyporus, Alisma, Ginseng, Cinnamon Twig

Xiangrong Wan: Pilose Antler, Musk, Aconite, Cistanche, Prepared Rehmannia, Psoralea, Agarwood, Angelica

Zishen Tongguan Wan: Anemarrhena, Phellodendron, Cinnamon

Wuling Powder: Atractylodes, Poria, Polyporus, Alisma, Cinnamon Twig

XLIV. Urinary Incontinence

Inability to control urination is called "yi niao" (enuresis). It is mostly a deficiency syndrome due to the bladder's failure to restrain. *Nei Jing* states: "Incontinence is due to the bladder's failure to restrain." It also says: "Failure to store urine is due to the bladder's failure to contain it." Since the kidney and bladder are internally-externally related, kidney deficiency and cold lead to inability to control water. Treatment mainly focuses on tonifying the kidney and securing retention, using Suoquan Wan or Gongdi Wan. For urinary urgency and incontinence after exertion, mostly due to qi deficiency, Gupu Decoction is used.

Women with liver qi stagnation, unable to disperse, experiencing abdominal distension with frequent urge to urinate, inability to hold back, or even involuntary urination with small volume, should be treated mainly by soothing the liver. Refer to the entry "Frequent Urination" in this section.

Enuresis in children during sleep, commonly known as "bedwetting", is treated with Biquan Wan. Acupuncture at Shenshu, Pangguangshu, Guanyuan, Qihai, Zhongji, Sanyinjiao, etc., can be used. This condition is extremely stubborn, sometimes persisting until the age of ten or more. One *liang* of Fennel can be placed in a pig bladder, baked dry, crushed, divided into six portions, and one portion steeped for drinking daily.

Enuresis in "apoplexy" is one of the collapse syndromes. Enuresis accompanied by coma and staring eyes in typhoid fever, febrile diseases, and miscellaneous diseases is difficult to treat.

Suoquan Wan: Alpinia oxyphylla, Lindera, Yam

Gongdi Wan: Prepared Rehmannia, Cuscuta, Schisandra, Alpinia oxyphylla, Psoralea, Aconite, Atractylodes, Poria, Allium tuberosum seeds, Yam

Gupu Decoction: Astragalus, Astragalus complanatus, Mantidis Ootheca, Cornus, Angelica, Fushen, Motherwort, White Peony Root, Cimicifuga, Sheep Bladder

Biquan Wan: Alpinia oxyphylla, Poria, Atractylodes, Ampelopsis, Stir-fried Gardenia, White Peony Root

XLV. Frequent Night Urination

Day is yang, night is yin. Frequent urination at night, ranging from two to three times to five or six times, is one of the kidney deficiency syndromes. It is often interdependent with insomnia—insomnia leads to the urge to urinate, and urination further affects sleep. It is mainly due to insecurity of the lower origin, and thus Mantidis Ootheca, Raspberry, Schisandra, etc., should be added to tranquilizing prescriptions.

XLVI. Urinary Bleeding

Blood passing with urine, bright red without pain or with extremely slight pain, is called "niaoxue" (hematuri). It is mostly caused by fire in the heart and small intestine forcing blood to move erratically, so *Yixue Rumen* (Introduction to Medicine) states: "Urinary bleeding is due to the heart transferring heat to the small intestine." It is often accompanied by dry mouth, oral ulcers, and a red sharp-tipped tongue, treated with Daochi Powder plus Scrophularia and Cogon Grass Rhizome.

Urinary bleeding with dribbling and pain is "blood stranguria"; refer to the entry "Painful Urination" in this section.

Daochi Powder: Raw Rehmannia, Akebia, Bamboo Leaf, Licorice

XLVII. Turbid Urine

Turbid substances like pus discharged from the urethra, mixed with blood, are called red turbidity; without blood, it is called white turbidity. More is discharged before urination, with no pain during urination, mostly due to insufficient heart qi, reckless movement of ministerial fire, and downward pouring of damp-heat. Initially, Zhzhuo Guben Wan is used, later Bixie Fenqing Yin.

Those with a history of promiscuous sexual activities often have it accompanied by stranguria, with pain during urination, treated with Bazheng Powder plus Smilax glabra and Bixie.

Yellow and turbid urine is more common in heat syndromes, as stated in *Nei Jing*: "Turbidity of water fluids all belongs to fire." Treatment should appropriately add talc and akebia to the prescription for clearing and promoting diuresis. If it appears in miscellaneous diseases, with not very yellow color and powdery sediment after clarification, it is mostly due to insufficient middle qi, treated with Baoyuan Decoction plus Euryale and Cimicifuga.

Zhuzhuo Guben Wan: Phellodendron, Coptis, Poria, Polyporus, Pinellia, Amomum, Alpinia oxyphylla, Licorice, Lotus Stamen

Bixie Fenqing Yin: Bixie, Acorus, Lindera, Alpinia oxyphylla, Poria, Licorice

Bazheng Powder: Polygonum aviculare, Akebia, Dianthus superbus, Gardenia, Licorice, Plantain, Rhubarb, Talc

Baoyuan Decoction: Astragalus, Ginseng, Licorice, Cinnamon

XLVIII. Urine with Semen

Semen threads discharged after urination, without pain, and in the long run, low back pain, due to the kidney's failure to store and consolidate, treated with Tusizi Wan combined with Jujing Wan.

Tusizi Wan: Cuscuta, Poria, Yam, Lotus Seed, Wolfberry

Jujing Wan: Isinglass, Astragalus complanatus

XLIX. Seminal Emission

In men with seminal emission, emission during dream intercourse is called "mengyi" (dream emission), and emission without dream intercourse is called "huajing" (involuntary emission). Generally, dream emission is attributed to hyperactivity of the monarch and ministerial fire, tending to excess, while involuntary emission is attributed to the kidney's failure to contain, tending to deficiency. There is also the saying that "dream emission is a heart disease, non-dream emission is a kidney disease". Therefore, in treatment, the former often uses Ziyin Jianghuo Decoction and Longdan Xiegan Decoction, the latter uses Jujing Wan and Sangpiaoxiao Powder, etc. However, seminal emission is related to the heart, liver, and kidney. As Zhu Danxi said: "The kidney is in charge of storage, the liver is in charge of discharge; both have ministerial fire, and their system is connected to the heart. The heart is the monarch fire; it is easily moved when affected by things. When the heart moves, the ministerial fire moves; when it moves, semen flows out. Even without intercourse, the ministerial fire can rise suddenly, leading to involuntary discharge." Thus, dream emission does not necessarily mean no kidney yin deficiency, and involuntary emission can also stir up heart and liver fire; they cannot be completely separated. In particular, prolonged seminal emission can lead to both yin and yang deficiency. If tonic medicines such as Banlong Wan and Gujing Wan are often taken, they may stir up ministerial fire. Therefore, the treatment of seminal emission should not be too biased. Shuilu Erxian Dan and Jinsuo Gujing Wan, which focus on mild astringency, have certain significance.

Severe seminal emission can lead to failure of the sperm gate to contain, with semen discharge upon seeing sexual stimuli or after urination, called "baiyin" (spermaturia). *Yixue Rumen* (Introduction to Medicine) states: "Or hearing of sexual matters, or seeing beautiful faces, or having endless thoughts, unfulfilled desires, or excessive sexual intercourse, leading to relaxation of the ancestral muscles, resulting in muscle atrophy and spontaneous semen emission, which is called white turbidity." It also says: "As soon as the desire arises, semen follows the thought; prolonged stagnation causes itching and pain in the penis, often as if needing to urinate, either discharged with urine or flowing spontaneously without urine, which is worse than dream emission." Treatment should focus on astringency, using Qianshi Wan, and Gujing Wan or Jinsuo Gujing Wan can also be used.

Not all seminal emissions are pathological. Occasional emission in unmarried adults or married individuals who are away from sexual activity is not considered a disease. As for frequent seminal emission caused by self-indulgence, leading to dizziness, low back pain, and mental fatigue, one must exercise self-restraint and cannot rely solely on medication.

Ziyin Jianghuo Decoction: Raw Rehmannia, Angelica, White Peony Root, Scrophularia, Ligusticum, Anemarrhena, Phellodendron

Longdan Xiegan Decoction: Gentiana, Raw Rehmannia, Gardenia, Scutellaria, Angelica, Akebia, Bupleurum, Licorice, Plantain Seed, Alisma

Jujing Wan: Isinglass, Astragalus complanatus

Sangpiaoxiao Powder: Ginseng, Fushen, Acorus, Polygala, Mantidis Ootheca, Dragon Bone, Turtle Shell, Angelica

Banlong Wan: Prepared Rehmannia, Cuscuta, Psoralea, Platycladi Seed, Fushen, Deer Horn Glue

Gujing Wan: Cuscuta, Allium tuberosum seeds, Oyster, Dragon Bone, Schisandra, Mantidis Ootheca, White Halloysite, Poria

Shuilu Erxian Dan: Cherokee Rose Fruit, Euryale

Jinsuo Gujing Wan: Astragalus complanatus, Euryale, Dragon Bone, Oyster, Lotus Stamen, Lotus Seed

Qianshi Wan: Euryale, Lotus Stamen, Yam, Tribulus terrestris, Raspberry, Dragon Bone

L. Infertility

Infertility is also called "wusi" (sterility) and concerns both men and women. For men without specific symptoms, ancient physicians mostly treated it from the perspective of deficient and cold essence and qi. *Yixue Rumen* states: "In men with yang depletion, impotence, and cold, thin semen." *Mai Jing* (The Pulse Classic) also says: "A weak and hesitant pulse in men indicates infertility, due to cold essence and qi." Treatment focuses on tonifying the kidney, using Wuzi Yanzong Wan, Xusi Dan, and Changchun Guangsizi Wan.

Clinically, patients with no sperm detected in laboratory tests, who are unable to conceive, can also take Wuzi Yanzong Wan and other formulas for a long time.

Wuzi Yanzong Wan: Wolfberry, Raspberry, Cuscuta, Plantain Seed, Schisandra

Xusi Dan: Cornus, Asparagus, Ophiopogon, Psoralea, Cuscuta, Wolfberry, Raspberry, Cnidium, Morinda, Prepared Rehmannia, Allium tuberosum seeds, Astragalus, Dragon Bone, Oyster, Yam, Angelica, Cynomorium, Ginseng, Atractylodes, Tangerine Peel, Yellow Dog Kidney, Placenta

Changchun Guangsizi Wan: Ginseng, Raw Rehmannia, Cornus, Asparagus, Ophiopogon, Yam, Wolfberry, Cuscuta, Achyranthes, Eucommia, Poria, Schisandra, Platycladi Seed, Angelica Body, Morinda, Psoralea, Lotus Stamen, Cistanche, Astragalus complanatus, Raspberry, Deer Horn Glue, Turtle Shell, Tiger Bone Glue, Isinglass, Pig Spinal Cord, Yellow Beef, Mutton, Black Dog Meat, Donkey Whip, Dog Kidney, Silkworm Moth, Placenta

Section 20 Gynecological Symptoms

The symptoms recorded in this section are limited to the four aspects of menstruation, leukorrhea, pregnancy, and childbirth. Breast diseases and disorders of the external genitals are scattered in other sections. Ancient physicians attached great importance to the liver as the congenital foundation in gynecological diseases and also valued the extraordinary meridians of Chong, Ren, Du, and Dai. Primarily, the liver is in charge of storing blood, and in women's diseases, regulating menstruation is the priority. The Du Meridian starts from the lower pole; the Ren Meridian starts below the middle pole and ascends along the abdomen to Guanyuan; the Chong Meridian starts from Qichong, runs upward alongside the navel; the Dai Meridian starts from the hypochondriac region and constrains all meridians, which are closely related to the physiological characteristics of women. However, in treatment, it still starts from the whole body, basically the same as internal medicine, and external treatment methods for breast ulcers, etc., are also consistent with surgery. Therefore, it is necessary to pay attention to the particularity of gynecology and also understand its generality in order to better apply the principles, methods, formulas, and medicines.

1. Advanced Menstruation

The menstrual cycle is based on one month. If it comes more than six or seven days in advance every month, or even twice a month, it is called "advanced menstruation". Generally, it is due to indulging in spicy food, excessive liver fire, or invasion of pathogenic heat. Blood becomes reckless under heat. The menstrual flow is heavy, dark red or purple-black in color with clots, thick and sticky in texture, with a fishy smell, accompanied by irritability, a slippery and rapid or string-like and rapid pulse. The treatment should cool the blood and clear heat, using Qinlian Siwu Decoction or Qingjing decoction. For those with yin deficiency and internal heat, menstruation is often advanced, with a small amount, red color without clots, accompanied by dizziness, insomnia, five heart heat, and a thready and rapid pulse. FuQingzhu said, "It is mainly heat with insufficient fluid", and Liangdi Decoction is used. There are also cases of qi deficiency failing to control blood, with advanced menstruation, heavy flow, light color, thin texture, weak waist and legs, empty and sagging lower abdomen, and prolonged dripping. Buqi Gujing Wan is used. If this condition occurs occasionally in advance, it is mostly treated as heat; if it is often advanced, there are both deficiency and excess, and the constitution should also be considered.

Qinlian Siwu Decoction: Scutellaria baicalensis, Coptis chinensis, Rehmannia glutinosa, Angelica sinensis, Ligusticum chuanxiong, Paeonia lactiflora

Qingjing Decoction: Paeonia suffruticosa, Lycium chinense, Paeonia lactiflora, Rehmannia glutinosa, Artemisia annua, Poria cocos, Phellodendron chinense

Liangdi Decoction: Rehmannia glutinosa, Lycium chinense, Scrophularia ningpoensis, Paeonia lactiflora, Ophiopogon japonicus, Asini Corii Colla

Buqi Gujing Wan: Codonopsis pilosula, Poria cocos, Atractylodes macrocephala, Astragalus membranaceus, Amomum villosum

2. Delayed Menstruation

If the menstrual period is delayed by more than six or seven days each time, up to forty or fifty days, it is called "delayed menstruation". When it comes, the amount is small, light red and not thick, accompanied by dizziness, palpitations, and a thready and weak pulse, mostly due to blood deficiency in Chong and Ren Meridians, and Renshen Yangying Decoction is used. There are also cases of deficiency and cold in Chong and Ren Meridians, with frequent delays, continuous abdominal pain, cold body and limbs, scanty menstrual flow, light color or dark black, using Jiaoai Siwu Decoction.

The menstrual period is usually regular, but occasionally delayed, mostly due to cold exposure and qi stagnation. The former, such as indulging in raw and cold food or being exposed to cold pathogens, causes cold in Chong and Ren Meridians and blood stasis, often with lower abdominal pain, purple and dark menstrual color with clots, using Yanhusuo Powder. The latter, primarily caused by liver qi stagnation due to anger and emotional constraint, manifests as blood stasis with symptoms including distending pain in the lower abdomen and purplish menstrual flow with dark clots. The formula Tiaojing Yin is prescribed to regulate menstruation and resolve stasis. Generally, for treating menstruation and its absence, peach kernel, safflower, motherwort fruit, cattail pollen, and lycopus lucidus are commonly used to promote menstruation, which can be added as appropriate, but the cause must be considered, and one cannot rely solely on attacking stasis.

If menstruation is normal but suddenly delayed, with symptoms such as anorexia, nausea, drowsiness, deficiency cold and deficiency heat, and a moderate and smooth pulse, pregnancy must be guarded against. *Huangdi Neijing* says: "How to know that a woman is going to give birth? She has a disease but no pathogenic pulse."

Renshen Yangying Decoction: Ginseng, Astragalus membranaceus, Angelica sinensis, Paeonia lactiflora, Cinnamomum cassia, Atractylodes macrocephala, Glycyrrhiza uralensis, Citrus reticulata, Rehmannia glutinosa, Schisandra chinensis, Poria cocos, Polygala tenuifolia, Ginger, Jujube

Jiaoai Siwu Decoction: Donkey-Hide Gelatin, Artemisia argyi, Prepared Rehmannia, Angelica, Ligusticum, White Peony Root

Yanhusuo Powder: Corydalis, Angelica, Ligusticum, Frankincense, Myrrh, Cattail Pollen, Cinnamon

Tiaojing Yin: Angelica, Achyranthes, Cyperus, Poria, Green Tangerine Peel, Charred Hawthorn

3. Irregular Menstrual Cycle

Menstruation occurring 7 or more days earlier or later for at least 3 consecutive cycles, without fixed regularity, is termed irregular menstrual cycle. It is mostly due to liver qi stagnation affecting the kidney, with menstrual flow either heavy or scanty, purple color with clots, abdominal and lumbar pain, and should be treated by soothing the liver and harmonizing blood, using Dingjing Decoction.

Women's menstruation ceases around the age of forty-eight or forty-nine. Before cessation, the cycle is often irregular, commonly known as "menstrual disorder", and in cases with heavy flow like flooding, Zixue Decoction with modifications is used.

Dingjing Decoction: Prepared Rehmannia, Angelica, White Peony Root, Cuscuta, Yam, Poria, Charred Schizonepeta, Bupleurum

Zixue Decoction: Ginseng, Astragalus, Scutellaria, Cornus,

Ligusticum, Prepared Rehmannia

4. Amenorrhea

Absence of menstruation for two or three months is called "jingzu" (amenorrhea due to stagnation) or "jingbi" (amenorrhea). It is mainly caused by blood depletion and blood stagnation. Although there are many causes for blood depletion and blood stagnation, after they form, treatment focuses on nourishing blood and breaking stasis. For amenorrhea due to blood depletion, symptoms include emaciation, pale complexion, palpitations, shortness of breath, dizziness, blurred vision, weak lower back and legs, general fatigue, poor appetite, and in severe cases, tidal fever, night sweats, flushing cheeks, hair loss, dry cough with hemoptysis, loose stools, etc., which are consumptive symptoms, commonly called "ganxue lao" (consumptive disease with amenorrhea). Treatment should nourish and tonify the Chong and Ren Meridians while regulating the five *zang* organs, selecting Xiaoying Jian, Jielao Powder, Dabuyuan Jian, or Guilu Erxian Jiao. For amenorrhea due to blood stagnation, symptoms often include abdominal distension and pain, worse on pressure, chest and diaphragm fullness, mental depression, dry mouth without desire to drink. Due to stagnant old blood preventing new blood production, deficiency signs such as blurred vision, dizziness, and dry scaly skin may also appear. Treatment should promote blood circulation and dispel stasis, using Zelan Decoction, Niuxi Powder, or Dahuang Zhechong Wan. The deficiency and excess in this syndrome are distinct, so careful examination of the pulse, tongue, and consideration of healthy qi are necessary. Generally, for blood depletion, the pulse is mostly deficient, thready, and hesitant; if blood deficiency generates heat, the pulse is deficient, rapid, and restless; the tongue is mostly pale, or the tip is delicate red, with a thin coating or no coating. For blood stagnation, the pulse is mostly deep, string-like, and hesitant, or deep, thready, and tight; the tongue is dark red or has purple spots. The general treatment principles are: for mild blood depletion, nourish and regulate the liver and spleen; for severe cases, nourish and tonify the liver and kidney; for mild blood stagnation, promote and regulate blood vessels; for severe cases, use stasis-dispelling methods.

After a woman's first menstruation, it often comes again after several months; if there are no disease signs, no treatment is needed.

Some women, due to unique constitutional endowment, have regular menstruation every two months, three months, or even once a year, called "bingyue" (bimonthly menstruation), "jujing" (seasonal menstruation), and "bienian" (yearly menstruation) respectively, and should not be treated as amenorrhea.

Xiaoying Jian: Angelica, Prepared Rehmannia, White Peony Root, Wolfberry, Yam, Roasted Licorice, Fushen, Ziziphus Seed

Jielao Powder: White Peony Root, Astragalus, Prepared Rehmannia, Licorice, Angelica, Adenophora, Pinellia, Poria, Schisandra, Donkey-Hide Gelatin

Dabuyuan Jian: Ginseng, Prepared Rehmannia, Yam, Wolfberry, Cornus, Angelica, Roasted Licorice, Eucommia

Guilu Erxian Jiao: Turtle Shell Glue, Deer Horn Glue, Ginseng, Wolfberry (proprietary medicine)

Zelan Decoction: Lycopus, Angelica, White Peony Root, Licorice

Niuxi Powder: Achyranthes, Angelica, White Peony Root, Cinnamon Twig, Moutan Bark, Peach Kernel, Corydalis, Aucklandia

Dahuang Zhechong Wan: Rhubarb, Scutellaria, Licorice, Peach Kernel, Almond, White Peony Root, Raw Rehmannia, Dry Lacquer, Ground Beetle, Leech, Grub, Horsefly (proprietary medicine)

5. Excessive Menstrual Flow

Menstrual flow exceeding the normal amount, or lasting for more days than usual, is generally called "excessive menstruation". It is commonly seen in the syndrome of advanced menstruation, and may also occur again one or two days after the menstruation has ended. Both are caused by blood heat, and Gujing Wan can be used.

Heavy bleeding or continuous bleeding during or outside the menstrual period is called "benglou" (collapse and leakage). "Beng" (collapse) refers to a sudden and profuse flow like a flood; "lou" (leakage) refers to a slower and continuous dripping. However, leakage can turn into collapse, and collapse is often followed by leakage, so they cannot be absolutely distinguished. There are many causes for this syndrome. Generally, sudden onset is mostly due to yin deficiency and blood heat, with dark red blood, accompanied by restlessness, irritability, poor sleep, and a slippery rapid pulse, treated with Qingre Gujing Decoction. If the patient is inherently weak with heavy menstrual flow leading to continuous dripping, it is mostly due to qi failing to contain blood, with light red blood, accompanied by fatigue, shortness of breath, a thin moist tongue coating, and a large empty pulse, treated with Buzhong Yiqi Decoction. Prolonged benglou not only severely depletes nutrient blood but also weakens qi; qi deficiency is more likely to lead to yang deficiency, so in the end, it often results in damage to both qi and blood, yin and yang, and cannot be treated from a single aspect. Meanwhile, benglou is an acute syndrome; massive blood loss can cause syncope and collapse, so while treating the root cause, the branch symptoms must be addressed, and when necessary, treating the branch may be the main focus. Although the disease may be cured, it is prone to recurrence, and medication should still be taken to nourish and regulate after the bleeding stops. In FuQing*zhu Nvke* (FuQingzhu's Gynecology), formulas for uterine bleeding such as

Guben Zhibeng Decoction, Modified Danggui Buxue Decoction, and Qinghai Wan can be selected. Attention should be paid to cases occurring in elderly women, those with unrecuperated postnatal strength, and those during pregnancy, which is often a precursor to miscarriage.

Gujing Wan: Turtle Shell, Phellodendron, Ailanthus Bark, Cyperus, Scutellaria, White Peony Root

Qingre Gujing Decoction: Turtle Shell, Oyster, Donkey-Hide Gelatin, Raw Rehmannia, Wolfberry Bark, Charred Gardenia, Scutellaria, Sanguisorba, Palm Charcoal, Lotus Rhizome Node, Licorice

Buzhong Yiqi Decoction: Astragalus, Codonopsis, Atractylodes, Angelica, Licorice, Tangerine Peel, Cimicifuga, Bupleurum, Ginger, Jujube

Guben Zhibeng Decoction: Prepared Rehmannia, Atractylodes, Astragalus, Angelica, Roasted Ginger, Ginseng

Modified Danggui Buxue Decoction: Angelica, Astragalus, Notoginseng, Mulberry Leaf

Qinghai Wan: Prepared Rehmannia, Cornus, Yam, Moutan Bark, Schisandra, Ophiopogon, Atractylodes, White Peony Root, Dragon Bone, Wolfberry Bark, Mulberry Leaf, Scrophularia, Adenophora, Dendrobium

6. Scanty Menstrual Flow

Menstrual flow less than normal or with a short duration is called "scanty menstruation". It is more common in the syndrome of delayed menstruation. The constitution and cause should be considered, and one should not casually use attacking methods just because the flow is scanty.

7. Continuous Menstruation

Women over fifty years old whose menstruation continues when it should have stopped, except for those with no abnormalities compared to usual, if the flow is heavy, should be on guard against the development of "benglou".

8. Resumed Menstruation after Cessation

Elderly women with resumed menstruation after cessation, with mostly purple blood clots, FuQingzhu believed it is due to yin essence depletion, blazing dragon thunder fire, and failure of the liver and spleen to govern and store, treated with Anlao Decoction.

Anlao Decoction: Ginseng, Astragalus, Prepared Rehmannia, Atractylodes, Angelica, Cornus, Donkey-Hide Gelatin, Charred Schizonepeta, Licorice, Cyperus

9. Pale Menstrual Color

Pale red menstrual blood is mostly a sign of blood deficiency; if accompanied by thin texture, it indicates qi and blood deficiency; if it is as pale as rice water with no menstrual blood color, it indicates extreme deficiency of true yang, but it must be combined with other symptoms.

10. Dark Purple Menstrual Color

Dark purple menstrual blood: If it is thick with clots, it belongs to blood heat; if not thick, it belongs to cold; even with clots, it is due to cold congelation and qistagnation; if it is dark with scanty flow like bean paste, it is blood deficiency with cold.

11. Menstruation with Clots

Menstruation with clots is generally referred to as "stasis". Stasis syndrome is often accompanied by abdominal pain, which eases after the clots are discharged. Clots formed due to cold are dark and non-sticky, and the pain is relieved by warmth; those formed due to heat are mostly purplish-red, with abdominal pain that worsens upon pressure. Commonly used stasis-resolving formulas include Xiongui Decoction, Taohong Siwu Decoction, Danggui Powder, etc., or Yimu Gao taken mixed with water.

However, menstrual clots are different from internal blood stasis; treatment should focus on resolving stasis and must be combined with regulating menstruation, not solely on aggressive elimination.

Xiongui Decoction: Ligusticum, Angelic

Taohong Siwu Decoction: Peach Kernel, Safflower, Angelica, Rehmannia, Ligusticum, Peony

Danggui Powder: Angelica, Peony, Herba Artemisiae Anomalae, Fructus Aurantii, Corydalis, Myrrh

Yimu Gao: Motherwort, Brown Sugar (proprietary medicine)

XII. Abdominal Pain During Menstruation

Generally, there is discomfort or slight soreness and pain in the lower back and abdomen during menstruation, which is a normal phenomenon. If there is severe abdominal pain with each menstruation, it is called “dysmenorrhea”, also known as “menstrual pain”. The causes of dysmenorrhea include deficiency, excess, cold, heat, qi stagnation, and blood stasis. Generally, pain that worsens upon pressure is excess; pain that is relieved by pressure is deficiency. For delayed menstruation, pain relieved by pressure is due to cold; for advanced menstruation, pain that worsens upon pressure is due to heat. Cramping or colicky pain is due to cold obstruction; intermittent or stabbing pain is due to blood stasis. Dull, continuous pain is deficiency; pain with a sinking sensation is qi deficiency; pain with distension is qi stagnation. Clinically, it is mainly divided into three types: pain before menstruation, pain during menstruation, and pain after menstruation. Pain in the lower abdomen and small abdomen, or radiating to the hypochondria and breasts with distension, starting 3-4 days to 7-8 days before menstruation and gradually subsiding after menstruation begins, is premenstrual pain. Severe pain in the lower abdomen when menstruation is about to start, with scanty, difficult flow, and the pain decreasing as the flow increases until it stops completely after menstruation ends, is pain during menstruation. No abdominal pain before or during menstruation, but pain in the lower abdomen starting when menstruation is about to end, with a sinking sensation, dull and vague pain, and soreness and fatigue in the lower back, is postmenstrual pain. The location of these three types of menstrual pain is mainly the lower abdomen. The differences are: premenstrual pain often involves the lower abdomen with distension; pain during menstruation is concentrated in the lower abdomen, like cramping or stabbing; postmenstrual pain is not severe, with a sinking sensation. Regarding their causes and treatments, both premenstrual pain and pain during menstruation are due to internal blood stasis, but premenstrual pain is accompanied by qi stagnation, and pain during menstruation by cold obstruction. Modified Tiaojing Yin and Yanhusuo Powder are used, and qi-regulating, cold-dispelling, blood-activating, and stasis-resolving medicines such as Bupleurum, Lindera, Safflower, Peach Kernel, Roasted Ginger, Artemisia argyi, and Trogopterus Dung can be appropriately used. Postmenstrual pain is due to deficiency of both qi and blood, with failure of the Chong and Ren Meridians to contain; Jiaoai Siwu Decoction with added Astragalus and Codonopsis to benefit qi, or with added Dragon Bone, Oyster, and Cimicifuga for astringing and lifting, can be used. Heat syndrome is less common in this condition; even if there is stagnant heat in premenstrual pain, Shengxue Qingre Fang from *Wanbing Huichun* is preferred. For acupuncture treatment, for excess pain, select Qihai, Hegu, and Sanyinjiao; for deficiency pain, select Shenshu, Guanyuan, Zusanli, and Sanyinjiao. Generally, needles are used for excess conditions, and moxibustion for deficiency conditions.

Tiaojing Yin: Angelica, Achyranthes, Cyperus, Poria, Green

Tangerine Peel, Charred Hawthorn

Yanhusuo Powder: Corydalis, Angelica, Ligusticum, Frankincense, Myrrh, Cattail Pollen, Cinnamon

Jiaoai Siwu Decoction: Donkey-Hide Gelatin, Artemisia argyi, Prepared Rehmannia, Angelica, Ligusticum, White Peony Root

Shengxue Qingre Fang: Angelica, Ligusticum, White Peony Root, Raw Rehmannia, Moutan Bark, Peach Kernel, Safflower, Aucklandia, Cyperus, Corydalis, Licorice

XIII. Low Back Pain During Menstruation

Low back soreness during menstruation is mostly due to weakness and insufficient liver and kidney. Eucommia and Dipsacus can be added to menstruation-regulating formulas for concurrent treatment; it is not treated as a main symptom.

XIV. Body Pain During Menstruation

It is mostly caused by blood deficiency; regulating menstruation will stop the pain. If body pain with contracture is accompanied by wind-cold, appropriately add Cinnamon Twig and Notopterygium.

XV. Breast Distension During Menstruation

It is due to liver qi stagnation, mostly seen in the syndrome of "dysmenorrhea". In severe cases, there are lumps in the breasts, and nipple pain is unbearable to touch, which heals spontaneously after menstruation ends. Refer to the entry "Abdominal Pain During Menstruation" in this section.

XVI. Fever During Menstruation

During menstruation, a slight fever is often felt, due to disharmony of qi and blood or internal stagnation of qi-fire. A small amount of Bupleurum can be added to the menstruation-regulating formula to harmonize it. If it occurs for a long time in the syndrome of amenorrhea, it is consumptive fever due to blood depletion. Refer to the entry “Amenorrhea” in this section.

XVII. Hematemesis During Menstruation

Vomiting of blood in mouthfuls with purple clots, often accompanied by nosebleeds, one or two days before menstruation or during menstruation, is called “hematemesis during menstruation”. Since oral and nasal bleeding often leads to reduced or stopped menstrual flow, as if the blood flows backward, it is commonly known as “reverse menstruation” or “abnormal menstruation”. It is mostly due to excessive liver fire and reckless movement of blood heat. Patients often have an irritable temperament and like to eat spicy foods such as pepper and ginger. It is accompanied by lower abdominal pain, hypochondriac distension, headache, restlessness, and poor sleep, with a string-like and rapid pulse. FuQingzhu said, “Hematemesis in various meridians is caused by internal injury; hematemesis due to reversed menstruation is caused by internal overflow and agitation. The symptoms are quite different, but the qi reversal is the same.” Treatment should soothe the liver, smooth qi, and guide blood downward, using Shunjing Decoction with added Achyranthes.

Shunjing Decoction: Raw Rehmannia, Angelica, White Peony Root, Moutan Bark, Adenophora, Charred Schizonepeta

XVIII. Hematochezia During Menstruation

Recurrent hematochezia occurring 1-2 days prior to menstrual onset, accompanied by decreased menstrual flow, is termed menstrual hematochezia. Since menstrual blood does not follow the normal path, it is also called "aberrant menstruation". It is mostly caused by deficiency of the liver, spleen, and kidney, accompanied by pale complexion, dizziness, blurred vision, palpitations, fear, shortness of breath, mental fatigue, soreness and weakness of the waist and feet, loose stools, frequent urination, pale red tongue, and a deficient and thready pulse. Use Buxue Decoction or Shunjing Liang'an Decoction.

Buxue Decoction: Raw and Prepared Rehmannia, Astragalus, Angelica Body, White Peony Root, Atractylodes, Eucommia, Charred Schizonepeta, Charred Roasted Ginger, Charred Cyrtomium

Shunjing Liang'an Decoction: Angelica, White Peony Root, Prepared Rehmannia, Cornus, Ginseng, Atractylodes, Ophiopogon, Morinda, Charred Schizonepeta, Cimicifuga

XIX. Leukorrhea with Red or White Discharge

White mucus flowing from the vagina continuously like a belt, or in large quantities with dripping, like nasal discharge or saliva, is called "white leukorrhea"; if white leukorrhea is mixed with blood, with clear separation of red and white, it is called "red and white leukorrhea"; if it is simply light red, thick and sticky, like blood but not blood, it is called "red leukorrhea". In addition, there are leukorrhea with colors of green, yellow, grayish-black, and a mixture of five colors, hence the names "green leukorrhea", "yellow leukorrhea", "black leukorrhea", and "five-color leukorrhea", which are relatively rare and collectively called "leukorrhea". The occurrence of this disease is mainly due to the failure of the Dai Meridian to constrain and the Ren Meridian to consolidate, combined with factors such as spleen deficiency and liver depression, leading to downward pouring of damp turbidity and damp-heat pathogens. Syndrome differentiation and treatment focus on color, smell, and clarity. All cases of white leukorrhea, sticky, thin, with little foul smell, accompanied by backache, mental fatigue, poor appetite, inability to bear labor (with increased leukorrhea after labor), mostly belong to spleen deficiency with damp turbidity, treated with Wan dai Decoction. Red or red-white mixed leukorrhea, thick and sticky, with a fishy smell, accompanied by dry mouth, bitter taste, yellow urine, and increased leukorrhea around menstruation, mostly belong to liver depression with damp-heat, treated with modified Xiaoyao Powder and Qinggan Zhilin Decoction.

Elderly women or those with congenital deficiencies and weakness after illness, with clear and profuse leukorrhea like pouring, cold and sore waist, cold limbs, dizziness, blurred vision, and a deep, weak pulse, is called "white collapse", which is extreme deficiency of the extraordinary meridians and requires strong tonification, using Neibu Wan.

Wandai Decoction: Atractylodes lancea, Atractylodes macrocephala, Yam, Ginseng, White Peony Root, Tangerine Peel, Licorice, Charred Schizonepeta, Bupleurum, Plantain Seed

Modified Xiaoyao Powder: White Peony Root, Bupleurum, Artemisia capillaris, Poria, Licorice, Tangerine Peel, Gardenia

Qinggan Zhilin Decoction: White Peony Root, Angelica, Raw Rehmannia, Donkey-Hide Gelatin, Moutan Bark, Phellodendron, Achyranthes, Cyperus, Black Bean, Jujube

Neibu Wan: Pilose Antler, Cuscuta, Astragalus complanatus, Astragalus, Cinnamon, Aster, Mantidis Ootheca, Cistanche, Aconite, Tribulus terrestris

XX. Bleeding During Pregnancy

Vaginal bleeding during pregnancy, dripping down, is called “tailou” (threatened abortion). This bleeding occurs intermittently without regularity, with no other symptoms except slight fatigue. However, continuous bleeding can cause restlessness of the fetus or a feeling of fetal descent, and frequent urination. Due to qi and blood deficiency, with the Chong and Ren Meridians failing to constrain, Zhuqi Bulou Decoction is used, and rest is advisable to prevent increased bleeding.

Zhuqi Bulou Decoction: Ginseng, Atractylodes, Scutellaria, Raw Rehmannia, Motherwort, Dipsacus, Licorice

XXI. Nausea and Vomiting During Pregnancy

In the second or third month of pregnancy, aversion to food, preference for sour and salty foods, nausea and vomiting, called “ezu” (morning sickness), is one of the early pregnancy symptoms. It is affected by fetal qi and disappears naturally after three months, generally requiring no treatment. In severe cases, with frequent vomiting and mental exhaustion, Jupi Zhuru Decoction is used, sipped slowly. There is a saying that Pinellia can affect the fetus, but ancient physicians often used it for pre-natal diseases, and it is also commonly used now with no adverse reactions observed.

Jupi Zhuru Decoction: Ginseng, Tangerine Peel, Bamboo Shavings, Pinellia, Ophiopogon, Red Poria, Loquat Leaf, Ginger, Jujube

XXII. Abdominal Pain During Pregnancy

Abdominal pain during pregnancy is called “baozu” (gestational abdominal pain). *Synopsis of the Golden Chamber* points out: “In a woman who is six or seven months pregnant, with a string-like pulse and fever, the fetus becomes more distended, abdominal pain and chills, with the lower abdomen feeling like being fanned; the reason is that the uterus is open, and Fuzi Decoction should be used to warm the uterus." It also says: "If a pregnant woman has abdominal pain, it is baozu, treated with Jiaoai Decoction." And: "A woman with severe abdominal pain during pregnancy is treated with Danggui Shaoyao Powder." This indicates that abdominal pain during pregnancy can be caused by uterine deficiency and cold, qi stagnation, blood deficiency, etc. However, treatment generally focuses on regulating qi and stabilizing the fetus, using modified Xiaoyao Powder; excessive use of pungent, warm, aromatic, and dry medicines that promote blood circulation and consume qi should be avoided to prevent damage to the fetal origin.

Fuzi Decoction: Aconite, Poria, Ginseng, Atractylodes, White Peony Root

Jiaoai Decoction: Donkey-Hide Gelatin, Artemisia argyi, Ligusticum, Rehmannia, White Peony Root, Licorice

Danggui Shaoyao Powder: Angelica, White Peony Root, Ligusticum, Atractylodes, Poria, Alisma

Xiaoyao Powder: Angelica, White Peony Root, Bupleurum, Atractylodes, Poria, Licorice, Mint, Ginger

XXIII. Edema During Pregnancy

Between the fifth and seventh months of pregnancy, swelling starting from both feet and gradually spreading to the head, face, and the whole body is called "zizhong" (gestational edema). It is mainly caused by spleen and lung qi deficiency, with qi failing to transform dampness, which soaks the muscles, treated with Quansheng Baizhu Powder. Q*ianjin Yaofang* (Essential Prescriptions for Emergencies) includes the method of Liyu Decoction: five *qian* of Atractylodes, four *qian* of Poria, three *qian* each of Angelica and White Peony Root, ground into coarse powder; then one carp, scaled and gutted, boiled to make juice; two cups of the juice, five *qian* of the medicinal powder, a little tangerine peel, and seven slices of ginger are added and decocted for oral administration.

Quansheng Baizhu Powder: Atractylodes, Ginger Peel, Areca Peel, Poria Peel, Tangerine Peel

XXIV. Distension and Oppression During Pregnancy

Chest and diaphragm fullness, hypochondriac distension, and restlessness of the fetus during pregnancy are called “zixuan” (feeling of suffocation in pregnancy). Caused by emotional depression and phlegm-qi congestion, Zisu Yin is used. FuQingzhu treated it from the liver and spleen with Jieyu Decoction, which can be modified as appropriate.

Zisu Yin: Perilla Leaf, Areca Peel, Angelica, White Peony Root, Ligusticum, Tangerine Peel, Ginseng, Licorice

Jieyu Decoction: Ginseng, Atractylodes, Poria, Angelica, White Peony Root, Fructus Aurantii, Amomum, Gardenia, Mint

XXV. Cough During Pregnancy

Cough during pregnancy is called “zisou” (gestational cough). Due to upward reversal of fetal fire and failure of the lung to clear and downbear, Baihe Powder is used.

Baihe Powder: Lily, Aster, Ophiopogon, Platycodon, Mulberry Bark, Licorice, Bamboo Shavings

XXVI. Irritability During Pregnancy

Restlessness and palpitations with timidity after pregnancy are called “zifan” (gestational dysphoria). Caused by unsmooth heart qi and upward disturbance of fetal heat. Treatment should distinguish between presence and absence of phlegm: for cases without phlegm, clear heat and relieve restlessness with Jiawei Zhuye Decoction; for cases with phlegm, add Bambusa Concretio Silicea and Tangerine Red.

Jiawei Zhuye Decoction: Ginseng, Scutellaria, Bamboo Leaf, Ophiopogon, Red Poria, Japonica Rice

XXVII. Convulsions During Pregnancy

After six or seven months of pregnancy, or during childbirth, sudden convulsions of the limbs, locked jaws, staring eyes, loss of consciousness, and even general spasms with opisthotonos. Regaining consciousness after a short time and recurring, similar to epilepsy, is called "zixian" (eclampsia). Mainly due to insufficient yin and blood with internal stirring of deficient wind, Gouteng Decoction and Lingyang Jiao Powder are used depending on the severity. This disease is quite serious among pregnancy disorders; severe cases with long duration and frequent attacks can cause death of the mother and fetus. However, before the onset, there are generally prodromal symptoms such as headache, dizziness, general fatigue, palpitations, shortness of breath, nausea, vomiting, and fullness in the middle epigastrium, which can be used for diagnosis and prevention.

Gouteng Decoction: Uncaria, Angelica, Poria, Ginseng, Platycodon, Taxillus

Lingyang Jiao Powder: Antelope Horn, Angelica Pubescens, Saposhnikovia, Uncaria, Angelica, Ziziphus Seed, Fushen, Almond, Acanthopanax Bark, Coix Seed, Aucklandia, Jujube

XXVIII. Fainting During Pregnancy

Dizziness, fainting, and locked jaws with inability to speak during pregnancy are called "ziyun" (gestational vertigo). Mostly due to liver yang with phlegm turbidity ascending counterflow, treated with Sangju Huangqin Decoction plus Pinellia, Fructus Aurantii, and Bamboo Shavings.

Sangju Huangqin Decoction: Mulberry Leaf, Chrysanthemum, Scutellaria, White Peony Root, Licorice, Uncaria, Vitex, Abalone Shell

XXIX. Hoarseness During Pregnancy

Hoarseness or loss of voice during pregnancy is called "zian" (gestational aphonia). *Nei Jing* states: "A woman with child, becoming hoarse in the ninth month, this is due to blockage of the uterine collateral vessels. The uterine collateral vessels are connected to the kidney; the Shaoyin vessel passes through the kidney and connects to the root of the tongue, and it will recover in the tenth month." Thus, this condition may not require treatment. When treated, it is appropriate to tonify lung and kidney qi to nourish the fetus, using Shengmai Powder decocted to deliver Liuwei Dihuang Wan. Be cautious not to use methods that promote orifices and disperse.

Shengmai Powder: Ginseng, Ophiopogon, Schisandra

Liuwei Dihuang Wan: Prepared Rehmannia, Cornus, Yam, Moutan Bark, Poria, Alisma

XXX. Dysuria During Pregnancy

There are two types of dysuria during pregnancy: One is frequent urination with dripping, painful and rough urination, called "zilin" (gestational strangury), mostly due to binding of fetal fire and damp-heat. Although similar to general stranguria, treatment should not overly promote diuresis to prevent damaging fetal qi and causing miscarriage; it is appropriate to clear, moisten, and promote diuresis with Zilin Decoction. The other type occurs in the seventh or eighth month of pregnancy, with normal appetite but inability to urinate, urgent lower abdominal distension, and restlessness, called "zhuanbao" (gestational urinary retention), also mostly due to downward pouring of damp-heat, treated with Sanbu Wan. There is also cases where fetal qi descends, compressing the bladder, causing anuria, often triggered by overeating, exertion, or holding urine while lifting weights; treatment should promote lifting, using Jutai Siwu Decoction. Zhu Danxi once used Shenzhu Yin, followed by emetic stimulation after ingestion to lift qi, which is an emergency method.

Zilin Decoction: Raw Rehmannia, Donkey-Hide Gelatin, Scutellaria, Gardenia, Akebia, Licorice

Sanbu Wan: Coptis, Scutellaria, Phellodendron, Talc

Jutai Siwu Decoction: Angelica, White Peony Root, Prepared Rehmannia, Ligusticum, Ginseng, Atractylodes, Tangerine Peel, Cimicifuga

Shenzhu Yin: Ginseng, Atractylodes, Tangerine Peel, Licorice, Pinellia, Prepared Rehmannia, Angelica, White Peony Root, Ligusticum, Ginger, Jujube

XXXI. Diarrhea During Pregnancy

Diarrhea with red and white mucus during pregnancy, accompanied by paroxysmal abdominal pain, can easily cause miscarriage and is one of the severe syndromes, differing from general treatment methods. *Zhang's Medical Manual* points out that there are three prohibitions and five assessments for diarrhea during pregnancy. The three prohibitions are: First, prohibiting purging the intestines and stomach, which can cause the fetal qi to descend; second, prohibiting promoting diuresis in the bladder, which can cause depletion of yin fluid; third, prohibiting astringing and stagnating qi, which can worsen tenesmus. The five assessments are: First, assessing whether the patient can take food or not; second, assessing whether urination is smooth or not; third, assessing whether there is abdominal pain or not; fourth, assessing whether there is tenesmus or not; fifth, assessing whether there is fever or not. It is also believed that after clarifying the five assessments and not violating the three prohibitions, then observe the thickness of the accumulation and the freshness of the color for separate treatment. The formulas used include Juyuan Jian, Houpo Decoction, Houjiang Shengan Banxia Decoction, Qinshao Decoction, Xianglian Wan, Sanwu Jiaoai Decoction, Zhuche Wan, etc., which can be selected based on syndrome differentiation.

Juyuan Jian: Ginseng, Astragalus, Atractylodes, Licorice, Cimicifuga, Ginger, Jujube

Houpo Decoction: Magnolia officinalis, Tangerine Peel, Atractylodes, Licorice, Fructus Aurantii Immaturus, Fermented Pinellia, Ginger, Jujube

Houjiang Shengan Banxia Decoction: Magnolia officinalis, Ginseng, Licorice, Pinellia, Ginger, Jujube

Qinshao Decoction: Scutellaria, White Peony Root, Licorice

Xianglian Wan: Coptis, Aucklandia

Sanwu Jiaoai Decoction: Donkey-Hide Gelatin, Artemisia argyi, Pomegranate Peel

Zhuche Wan: Coptis, Donkey-Hide Gelatin, Angelica, Dried Ginger

XXXII. Threatened Miscarriage

A small amount of vaginal bleeding, accompanied by mild cramping pain in the lower abdomen and back or a sensation of pelvic heaviness, are characteristic symptoms of threatened miscarriage. If the symptoms persist and bleeding increases, it can lead to miscarriage. Generally, it is treated as fetal heat, using modified Antai Powder.

If the mother is ill and the fetus cannot be nourished, it can also cause threatened miscarriage; but treating the mother's illness will make the fetus safe on its own.

Antai Powder: Raw Rehmannia, White Peony Root, Angelica, Ligusticum, Donkey-Hide Gelatin, Artemisia argyi, Astragalus, Licorice, Sanguisorba, Ginger, Jujube

XXXIII. Fetal Loss

Loss of the fetus within three months of pregnancy, when the fetus is not yet fully formed, is called "abortion". Loss after three months, when the fetus is already formed, is called "miscarriage", also known as "half delivery". If after abortion or miscarriage, the next pregnancy is lost at the same time, it is called "habitual abortion". There are many causes for abortion and miscarriage: due to qi deficiency failing to contain the fetus, accompanied by chills and abdominal pain, Huangqi Buqi Decoction is used. Due to blood heat causing the fetus to be unstable, accompanied by thirst, restlessness, and dry stool, modified Siwu Decoction is used. Due to falls or sprains damaging the fetus, Liqi Sanyu Decoction is used. Due to unregulated sexual activity damaging the fetus, Guqi Tianjing Decoction is used. Before fetal loss, there are generally symptoms of fetal movement, abdominal pain, and bleeding, so timely fetus protection is necessary; if there is soreness and distension in the lower back, the fetus is mostly difficult to preserve, and early preparation should be advised. For those with habitual abortion, they should rest well after conception and appropriately take medicines for regulation and tonification.

Huangqi Buqi Decoction: Astragalus, Angelica, Cinnamon

Modified Siwu Decoction: Prepared Rehmannia, White Peony Root, Angelica, Ligusticum, Gardenia, Cornus, Yam, Moutan Bark

Liqi Sanyu Decoction: Ginseng, Astragalus, Angelica, Poria, Safflower, Moutan Bark, Charred Roasted Ginger

Guqi Tianjing Decoction: Ginseng, Astragalus, Atractylodes, Prepared Rehmannia, Angelica, Notoginseng, Charred Schizonepeta

XXXIV. Postpartum Blood Stasis

After childbirth, the residual blood stasis and serous fluid in the uterine cavity are called "lochia", which must be discharged from the body. Otherwise, stagnant blood can form blood stasis, which is most likely to leave behind symptoms such as abdominal pain and masses. Folk custom of decocting motherwort with brown sugar for drinking after childbirth has certain significance. The causes of retained lochia may be qi stagnation or cold exposure, and Shenghua Decoction or modified Niuxi Powder is used.

Within 20 days after childbirth, the lochia should be exhausted; if it persists beyond the period, it is generally called "prolonged lochia". However, there are cases where the lochia has already been exhausted, but there is continuous dripping due to qi deficiency failing to contain blood, characterized by a pale color, no fishy smell, lower back pain, a feeling of lower abdominal sagging from time to time, mental fatigue, dizziness, blurred vision, a pale tongue, and a slow and weak or deficient and thready pulse, treated with Shengju Dabu Decoction. Prolonged persistence can lead to "bloody collapse".

Shenghua Decoction: Angelica, Ligusticum, Peach Kernel, Roasted Ginger, Roasted Licorice, Yellow Wine, Children's Urine

Niuxi Powder: Cyathula, Cinnamon, Red Paeony Root, Peach Kernel, Angelica, Aucklandia, Moutan Bark

Shengju Dabu Decoction: Astragalus, Ginseng, Atractylodes, Licorice, Angelica, Prepared Rehmannia, Ophiopogon, Ligusticum, Tangerine Peel, Cimicifuga, Angelica Dahurica, Coptis, Charred Schizonepeta

XXXV. Postpartum Abdominal Pain

Postpartum abdominal pain is mostly caused by scanty and stagnant lochia with internal accumulation of blood stasis, commonly known as "baby pillow pain", treated with Shixiao Powder. FuQingzhu once said: "When blood circulates smoothly, stasis will naturally be eliminated; when blood is stagnant, stasis will cause trouble. If one does not tonify blood but instead dispels blood, although blood stasis can be eliminated, consumption is inevitable. It is better to use the method of promoting blood circulation and removing stasis while tonifying blood, so that qi and blood are not consumed and stasis is completely eliminated." Sanjie Dingteng Decoction can be used. If abdominal pain is due to excessive blood loss and emptiness of the blood chamber, it is often accompanied by cold signs, with continuous vague pain that is relieved by warmth, treated with Danggui Shengjiang Yangrou Decoction; replacing mutton with deer horn glue or donkey-hide gelatin is also good.

Shixiao Powder: Cattail Pollen, Trogopterus Dung

Sanjie Dingteng Decoction: Angelica, Ligusticum, Moutan Bark, Motherwort, Charred Schizonepeta, Frankincense, Charred Hawthorn, Peach Kernel

Danggui Shengjiang Yangrou Decoction: Angelica, Ginger, Mutton

XXXVI. Postpartum Dizziness

Sudden dizziness, blurred vision, inability to sit up, or chest fullness, nausea, vomiting, and even locked jaws, coma, and loss of consciousness after childbirth are called "yumo" (depressive clouding). It is one of the severe postpartum syndromes, and can lead to sudden collapse if not rescued in time. Mainly due to blood deficiency of the heart and liver, with the spirit having no abode, immediately prick the center of the eyebrow with a silver needle to let blood, and decoct and administer Danggui Buxue Decoction. There are also cases where blood stasis rushes upward, confusing the mind, commonly known as "blood syncope", and immediately administer 2 *qian* of Duxing Powder mixed with warm wine. At this time, there is a deficiency type and an excess type, with significant differences in treatment, which must be clearly distinguished: in the deficiency type, the lochia is abundant, with prior palpitations and confusion, and during syncope, the mouth is open, hands are flaccid, limbs are cold, cold sweat drips, and the pulse is large and empty or extremely thready and faint; In excess syndrome, lochia is scanty, preceded by abdominal pain, epigastric fullness and urgency, coarse breathing with panting, locked jaw and clenched fists during syncope.

Danggui Buxue Decoction: Astragalus, Angelica

Duxing Powder: Trogopterus Dung, half raw and half stir-fried, ground into powder

XXXVII. Postpartum Fever

Postpartum blood deficiency with excessive sweating makes one susceptible to external pathogens, triggering chills and fever, and treatment should address both the root and the branch, using Zhuye Decoction. In this syndrome, due to blood deficiency failing to nourish all vessels, plus wind pathogen invasion and meridian constriction, it can easily develop into limb convulsions, stiff neck and back, and even locked jaws and opisthotonos, as stated in *Synopsis of the Golden Chamber*: "Newly delivered women with blood deficiency and excessive sweating, prone to wind attack, thus developing convulsions." Zirong Huoluo Decoction is used.

Blood deficiency generating heat can also cause fever. Its symptoms include slight fever, spontaneous sweating, dizziness, tinnitus, palpitations, a pale tongue, and a large, hollow pulse. If it persists for a long time, the body becomes emaciated, the fever worsens in the afternoon, accompanied by night sweats, flushed cheeks, and a dry cough, developing into a consumptive disease called "ruluo" (puerperal consumptive disease), treated with modified Digupi Yin. Empirical formulas include recuperative methods using hen soup and pork kidney soup: take one hen, simmer to make a clear broth; grind 3 *qian* each of Angelica, Prepared Rehmannia, Astragalus, Atractylodes, and Cinnamon into coarse powder; use one bowl of the hen broth to decoct 4 *qian* of the medicinal powder, take three times a day. Or take 1 *liang* each of Angelica and White Peony Root (stir-fried with wine), decoct and strain; cut one pair of pig kidneys into dice-sized pieces, add 1 he of japonica rice, 1 *qian* of fermented soybean, a little green onion, ginger, and salt, and cook together for consumption.

Zhuye Decoction: Bamboo Leaf, Pueraria, Saposhnikovia, Platycodon, Cinnamon Twig, Ginseng, Licorice, Ginger, Jujube

Zirong Huoluo Decoction: Ligusticum, Angelica, Prepared Rehmannia, Ginseng, Astragalus, Fushen, Gastrodia, Roasted Licorice, Tangerine Peel, Schizonepeta, Saposhnikovia, Notopterygium, Coptis

Digupi Yin: Prepared Rehmannia, Angelica, Ligusticum, White Peony Root, Wolfberry Bark, Moutan Bark

XXXVIII. Postpartum Constipation

Synopsis of the Golden Chamber states: "Newly delivered women suffer from three diseases: first, convulsions, second, depressive clouding, third, difficulty in defecation." The general cause is mostly blood deficiency. Blood deficiency leads to depletion of body fluids, which fail to moisten the intestines, resulting in constipation, a common postpartum symptom. Treatment should focus on moistening purgation, adding hemp seed, platycladi seed, etc., to blood-nourishing formulas.

XXXIX. Postpartum Frequent Urination

Increased frequency of urination after childbirth, even dozens of times a day and night, with inability to control and dripping incontinence, are mostly due to qi and blood depletion, and should be treated with nourishing, tonifying, and astringing, using Gupu Decoction.

Gupu Decoction: Mantidis Ootheca, Astragalus, Astragalus complanatus, Cornus, Angelica, Fushen, Motherwort, White Peony Root, Cimicifuga, one sheep bladder (decocted to replace water)

XL. Postpartum Scanty Lactation

Scanty or no lactation after childbirth, with no distending pain in the breasts, is due to qi and blood deficiency failing to generate and transform, treated with Tongru Dan. If the breasts are distended and painful, hard on pressure, with scanty and rough lactation, it is due to qi stagnation and blocked breast collaterals, and treatment should promote smooth flow, using Yongquan Powder. If distension and pain cause low-grade fever, remove pig's trotters and add Bupleurum and Dandelion.

Tongru Dan: Codonopsis, Astragalus, Angelica, Ziziphus Seed, Akebia, Platycodon, Pig's Trotters

Yongquan Powder: Vaccaria, Clove, Stemona, Trichosanthes Root, Bombyx Batryticatus, Pangolin (equal parts ground into powder), 4 pills each time, taken with pig's trotter decoction.

XLI. Infertility

Women who have been married for more than two years, with the husband being healthy but failing to conceive, or who have given birth to one or two children but have not conceived for several years, are all called "infertility syndrome". The causes of infertility include congenital and acquired pathological factors. Acquired factors include deficiency-cold, phlegm-dampness, and stagnant heat. Infertility due to deficiency-cold, caused by improper care during menstruation, excessive consumption of raw and cold foods, exposure to wind to seek coolness, prolonged sitting on damp ground, and wind-cold invading the uterus, often accompanied by cold abdomen with occasional pain, delayed menstruation, pale and scanty flow, decreased libido, weak waist and legs, a deep weak or deep hesitant pulse, treated with Aifu Nuangong Wan, Yulin Zhu, or Wenbao Yin. Infertility due to phlegm-dampness, more common in obese women who indulge in rich foods, with profuse thick leukorrhea and pale menstrual blood, treated with Qigong Wan. Infertility due to stagnant heat, mostly caused by liver qi stagnation transforming into fire, or blood deficiency generating heat, latent in the Chong and Ren Meridians, more common in thin individuals, with chest and hypochondriac distension, dizziness, palmar heat, irregular menstruation or scanty purple flow, a thready string-like rapid pulse, treated with Kaiyu Zhongyu Decoction or Qinggu Zishen Decoction.

Aifu Nuangong Wan: Artemisia argyi, Cyperus, Angelica, Dipsacus, Evodia, Ligusticum, White Peony Root, Astragalus, Raw Rehmannia, Cinnamon

Yulin Zhu: Atractylodes, Poria, White Peony Root, Ligusticum, Roasted Licorice, Angelica, Prepared Rehmannia, Cuscuta, Eucommia, Deer Antler Frost, Sichuan Pepper

Wenbao Yin: Atractylodes, Morinda, Ginseng, Eucommia, Cuscuta, Yam, Euryale, Cinnamon, Aconite, Psoralea

Qigong Wan: Pinellia, Atractylodes lancea, Cyperus, Medicated Leaven, Poria, Tangerine Peel, Ligusticum

Kaiyu Zhongyu Decoction: Angelica, White Peony Root, Atractylodes, Poria, Moutan Bark, Cyperus, Trichosanthes Root

Qinggu Zishen Decoction: Wolfberry Bark, Moutan Bark, Ophiopogon, Scrophularia, Adenophora, Atractylodes, Dendrobium, Schisandra

Appendix

A Brief Explanation of Syndrome Differentiation and Treatment

Syndrome differentiation and treatment is both the process and the fundamental method of treating diseases in TCM. In summary, the content of syndrome differentiation and treatment includes a set of principles involving theory, method, formula, and medicine. To correctly apply this method, one must have a certain level of theoretical knowledge and possess various basic knowledge as a foundation. This book provides some reference materials for each common symptom, which is certainly not comprehensive, especially in clinical practice where flexible application based on specific circumstances is required. Therefore, let's further discuss the essence and spirit of syndrome differentiation and treatment, as well as preliminary opinions on its specific application.

I. Let's start with the character "证" (zheng).

The correct writing of "证" should be "證". Originally, "证" and "證" were two different characters with different meanings. Customarily, they are often used interchangeably for simplification, and here we also follow the general habit of using "证" instead of "證". It is also written as "症", which is a folk variant of "證". This character is not found in the *Kangxi Dictionary*, and the *Cihai* notes that "症 is a folk variant of 證". It can be seen that the characters "證", "证", and "症" used in current TCM actually refer to the same thing and have the same meaning. The correct writing is "證", the simplified form is "证", and the folk variant is "症". That is, "证" refers to syndrome, and "症" refers to symptom. As for the meaning of

"证" in medicine, it only represents clinical manifestations. Generally, an individual "证" is called a symptom, and when several symptoms are combined to form a disease condition, it is called a syndrome. For example, headache is a symptom; if combined with fever, body pain, and a floating pulse, it becomes an exogenous syndrome. In clinical practice, various symptoms are analyzed and synthesized to explore the etiology and determine the syndrome, just like handling a case where evidence must be collected, the background must be clarified, and then appropriate handling is given. Therefore, syndrome differentiation is about how to understand the disease, and treatment is about how to determine the treatment method. It is the specific application and embodiment of TCM theory in clinical practice. It includes theory, principles, and is related to formulas and medicines. These four elements are closely integrated and indispensable; the lack of any one will make it impossible to be correct. Meanwhile, syndrome differentiation and treatment is based on a comprehensive analysis of symptoms through the four diagnostic methods and eight principles to explore the occurrence and development laws of the disease, thereby formulating a treatment policy and giving appropriate treatment. If symptoms are not carefully differentiated or are considered in isolation, it is impossible to see the essence of the disease and make a correct conclusion, and thus the treatment method, prescription, and medication cannot be appropriate.

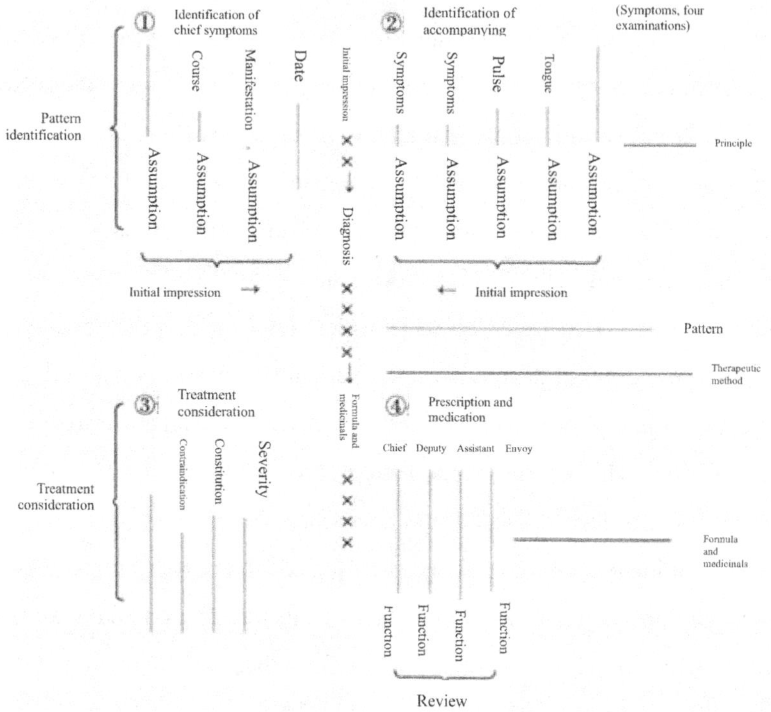

To facilitate the clinical mastery and application of the principle of syndrome differentiation and treatment, the following chart is proposed for discussion.

The method of using this chart is as follows: every disease has a main symptom. After listening to the patient's chief complaint and understanding the general condition, first grasp the main symptom and inquire about it. When asking, one should have a plan in mind: Why ask this way? What is the purpose of such a question? Then, comprehensively study the obtained information to form a preliminary impression. Of course, this is not definitive and may be revised. Secondly, distinguish the accompanying symptoms described by the patient and those that need to be understood, including pulse, tongue, complexion, etc. The differentiation of accompanying symptoms should be done with as careful inquiry as the main symptom to form a preliminary impression. Then, combine the preliminary impressions from both aspects to make an overall diagnosis, i.e., the syndrome. The preliminary impressions from these two aspects may be partially consistent and partially inconsistent, but it will be clear which are primary and which are secondary. This is the first step. Based on the diagnosis, formulate a treatment policy, that is, the therapeutic method. The therapeutic method determined here is only a principle; to prescribe based on it, considerations such as the severity of the disease, contraindications, the patient's constitution, and the medication history are also needed, which is the stage of treatment determination. This is the second step. From the result of treatment determination, select formulas and medicines, distinguish the roles of sovereign, minister, assistant, and guide drugs, and draw up a prescription. This is the third step. At this point, syndrome differentiation and treatment are completed, which is the entire process from diagnosis to treatment of a disease. These three steps: The first step is the theory, the second step is the method, and the third step is the formulas and medicines. Therefore, it can be said that syndrome differentiation and treatment is based on theory, method, formulas, and medicines.

Several issues should be clarified: ① Clarifying the main symptom can lead to a preliminary impression, but relying solely on the main symptom is insufficient. It is necessary to further observe the accompanying symptoms, including the pulse and tongue, to see if they are related to the main symptom. If they arise from the main symptom, the correctness of the preliminary impression is confirmed; otherwise, reconsideration is needed. For example, sudden fever is mostly due to exogenous pathogenic factors, which are often accompanied by fear of cold. If the patient reports feeling cold, the preliminary impression of the main symptom would be wind-cold cold. Further checking the accompanying symptoms such as itchy throat, nasal congestion, and cough can confirm wind-cold affecting the lung. If sudden chills and fever are accompanied by vomiting, diarrhea, etc., one must consider causes like cold attacking the intestines and stomach or dietary impairment. How to diagnose cold in the intestines and stomach? When differentiating accompanying symptoms, there should be phenomena such as vomiting clear water, diarrhea with undigested food, stomach pain, abdominal pain, borborygmus, thin white tongue coating, and no thirst. How to diagnose food stagnation? There should be symptoms like vomiting sour and foul matter, foul-smelling diarrhea, chest and abdominal distension, relief after vomiting and diarrhea, sticky mouth, and thick greasy tongue coating. Therefore, syndrome differentiation is meticulous and progressively in-depth, mainly involving comprehensive analysis and induction. ② Based on the results of syndrome differentiation for treatment, first, focus on the main symptom, determine the main therapeutic method according to the primary cause of the disease, and then take other accompanying symptoms into account. Attention to accompanying symptoms should be appropriately given under the main treatment; using medications merely following symptoms regardless of the main treatment will lead to loss of direction and make the prescription scattered and disorganized. ③ Syndrome differentiation changes with the progression of the disease; it is not a fixed conclusion after the first differentiation for a disease. In acute illnesses, the results of syndrome differentiation and treatment may be completely different today from yesterday. For example, in a fever syndrome, there may be fear of cold without sweating yesterday, but today there is sweating, no fear of cold, but instead aversion to heat—one is an exterior syndrome, the other an interior syndrome. Of course, some chronic intractable syndromes do not change much, so there is no need for daily re-differentiation and re-evaluation. However, the condition is always changing; if there is improvement or no obvious effect after a period, repeated examination is necessary, and one cannot insist on "not changing the prescription if it is effective" just because it is effective or stable. ④ How to grasp the main symptom? Generally, systemic symptoms, particularly severe symptoms, or symptoms that cause the patient the most suffering are taken as the standard, such as fever, rash, coma, massive bleeding, edema, diarrhea, abdominal pain, etc., which can all be main symptoms. The main symptom of a disease is not fixed; it is determined by the changes in the condition. For example, in exogenous fever with cough, fever is the main symptom; when the fever subsides but the cough persists, cough becomes the main symptom. Even if an accompanying symptom is mistakenly taken as the main symptom, as long as the syndrome differentiation is correct, the same conclusion can be drawn. For instance, in exogenous fever with cough, if cough (instead of fever) is taken as the main symptom, during the differentiation of cough, symptoms like itchy throat and thin white sputum are observed, and during the differentiation of accompanying symptoms, phenomena such as chills and fever, head distension, nasal congestion, floating slippery rapid pulse, and thin white tongue coating are found, the final conclusion will naturally be exogenous affection, with the therapeutic method focusing on relieving the exterior, and it will also be recognized that fever should be the main symptom. Of course, this does not mean arbitrarily taking a symptom as the main symptom during syndrome differentiation, but rather that different main symptoms may be identified from different perspectives. The key is that syndrome differentiation is comprehensive; as long as the overall condition is considered without isolating symptoms, consistent diagnostic results can be obtained.

In clinical practice, as long as there are symptoms to differentiate, no matter how many or how complex they are, this method can be applied. If there are truly no symptoms at all, then there is no basis for differentiation.

Can differentiation be made through the four diagnostic methods when there are no symptoms? Of course, it can. Ancient physicians used pulse diagnosis to determine life and death, and there is the saying of "disregarding symptoms and following the pulse". However, disregarding symptoms does not mean there are no symptoms; it mainly refers to relying on pulse diagnosis when there is a contradiction between pulse and symptoms. Similarly, there is also the saying of "disregarding the pulse and following symptoms". This shows that the four diagnostic methods are the diagnostic methods of TCM and must be combined with each other, especially with symptoms. One-sided emphasis on any single aspect is inappropriate. Precisely because of this, only through such syndrome differentiation can a relatively clear diagnosis be made, and a prognosis can be judged based on the developmental trend of the condition. After prescribing a formula, rechecking the main symptoms and accompanying symptoms can help more clearly see whether the medication is delicate and appropriate. Here are two specific cases illustrating the application of this method. These two cases have both commonalities and particularities, which can be compared.

Case 1: A female patient surnamed Li, 51 years old, with nephritis.

Case 2: A female patient surnamed Tian, 65 years old, with pneumonia.

Both are female, relatively old, with fever as the main symptom. The duration of fever is the same, and the fever occurs in the afternoon, with the temperature ranging between 38°C and 39°C. Through examination, the nephritis patient in Case 1 has no obvious edema, only some puffiness on the face. She feels chilly before the fever, and after sweating, the fever gradually decreases but does not subside completely. She also has nausea, even vomiting, no thirst, and yellowish-red urine. The pneumonia patient in Case 2 has basically improved inflammation, only slight cough with sticky sputum. She does not feel cold before the fever, is thirsty and drinks a lot when feverish, sweats a lot, and the fever subsides completely after sweating. She also has severe low back pain. In terms of pulse and tongue, the pulse of Case 1 is slippery and rapid, the tongue is slightly crimson, with a white and greasy coating; the pulse of Case 2 is thready, rapid, and string-like, the front half of the tongue coating is peeled, and the root has a thin yellow coating. After understanding the condition, analysis and research using the above chart lead to the following conclusions: The fever in the nephritis patient of Case 1 is due to external pathogens transmitting inward, resulting in dampness obstructing and heat lurking, similar to the syndrome of dampness-warmth where pathogens accumulate in the middle jiao and cannot be released. The fever in the pneumonia patient of Case 2 may also be caused by external pathogens, but there is no longer an exterior syndrome, and body fluids are severely damaged, forming yin deficiency with internal heat, similar to the deficiency of both qi and yin in the late stage of pulmonary consumption. In general, the fever in the nephritis patient is an excess syndrome, while the fever in the pneumonia patient is a deficiency syndrome, so the treatment methods and prescriptions are completely different.

Identification of accompanying symptoms

- Red tongue with white greasy — Dampness obstructing with latent heat
- Slippery and rapid pulse — Stomach heat
- Dark yellow urine — Stomach heat
- No thirst — Stomach dampness
- Nausea, even vomiting — Stomach dampness
- History of edema, currently mild facial puffiness — Spleen dampness

→ Damp-heat in the stomach

[Chief symptom] Fever → (Diagnosis) External pathogen transmitting inward, damp-heat accumulating in the stomach, unable to disperse and discharge → (Treatmentprinciple)Clearand

Identification of chief

- Persistent fever despite — External pathogen
- Initially afraid of cold — External pathogen
- Fever in the afternoon — Yangming heat
- Illness duration of half a month — Not an exterior syndrome

→ External pathogen transmitting to Yangming

Prescription and medication

Eupatorium, red poria, rice-paper plant pith, etc.

- Modifications — Pinellia, dried tangerine peel
- Bitter orange, bamboo shavings — Harmonize the stomach
- Talc, coix seed — Transform dampness with mild diuresis
- Magnolia bark, cardamom — Clear heat
- Agastache rugosa — Aromatic to expel pathogen

Treatment consideration

- Dampness in the middle burner, suitable for transformation rather than diuresis
- Heat in Yangming, suitable for clearing the stomach
- Sweating present, no need to induce sweating to reduce fever
- Pathogen lurking internally, still suitable for dispersion and promotion of outward transmission

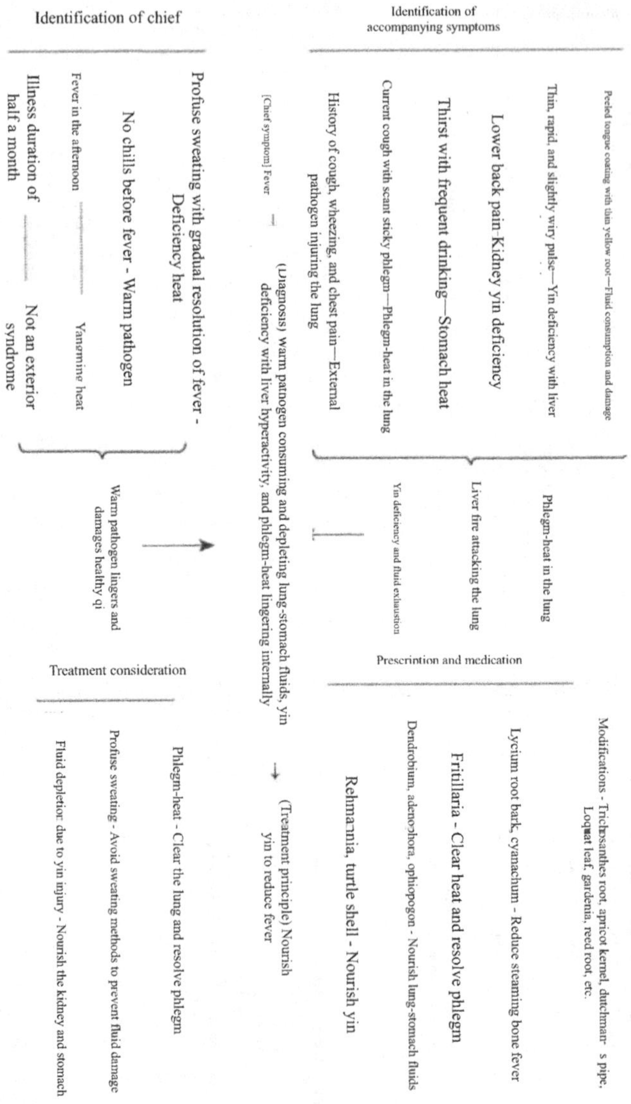

Appendix Table 2:

It should be pointed out that nephritis and pneumonia are disease names diagnosed in Western medicine. When using the method of syndrome differentiation and treatment in TCM, it is necessary to conduct a comprehensive analysis objectively based on actual symptoms in accordance with TCM theories and principles. If one subjectively holds preconceived notions, it is inevitable to feel confused about why such nephritis can cause fever and why the fever persists after the pneumonia has subsided, making it difficult to proceed with treatment. Meanwhile, using this chart for syndrome differentiation and treatment mainly aims to illustrate how to combine the main symptom with accompanying symptoms, how to make a confirmed diagnosis based on preliminary impressions, how to determine the treatment method based on etiology and pathogenesis, and how to prescribe medications according to the treatment method. With such a framework, when encountering complex and difficult conditions, it can serve as a basis for analysis and research. As for simple conditions, although the syndrome differentiation process does not need to be so complicated, the way of thinking in the mind is still the same. Because only through comprehensive consideration can a correct prescription be made, and one can judge whether others' prescriptions are correct. For example, in a case of wind-cold, a 3.5-year-old boy had a fever (38.5°C) without sweating for four days, with continuous cough day and night, a hoarse voice, a slippery and rapid pulse, a thin and greasy tongue coating, and normal diet and bowel movements. This is a common syndrome, which can be easily diagnosed as wind-cold stagnating in the upper jiao, with lung qi failing to disperse and penetrate, without heat transformation and transmission to the interior, and without accompanying symptoms of intestinal and stomach food stagnation. San'ao Decoction plus cicada slough, burdock, platycodon, tangerine red, and sterculia lychnophora was used. After one dose, slight sweating occurred, the fever subsided, and the cough became sparse. However, he had taken three doses of Chinese medicine before, and the last prescription contained as many as fifteen ingredients, including mulberry leaves, chrysanthemums, schizonepeta, saposhnikovia, honeysuckle, forsythia, platycodon, licorice, almonds, thunberg fritillary, pinellia, tangerine peel, aster, folium isatidis, and reed rhizome, which seemed somewhat mixed. To explain this issue, the above method can also be used for analysis.

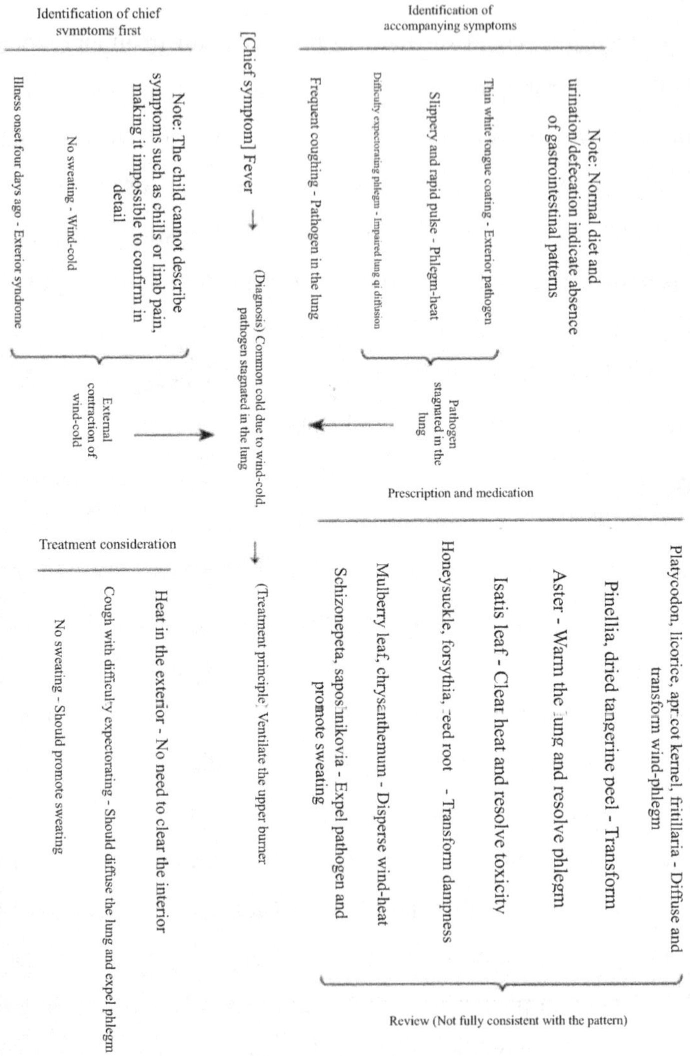

From the chart, it can be seen that syndrome differentiation is for confirming the diagnosis, and treatment determination is for prescribing medications. The theories, methods, formulas, and medicines are consistent. It also shows that syndrome differentiation is important, and treatment determination is equally important. Syndromes must be differentiated, and treatments must be determined, while prescribing medications still requires careful consideration. Yu Jiayan emphasized "first discussing the disease, then discussing the medicine". Discussing the disease is syndrome differentiation, and discussing the medicine is treatment determination. Both the disease and the medicine must go through "discussion", that is, "differentiation" and "discussion" must never be neglected.

II. After understanding the method of syndrome differentiation and treatment, it is necessary to further understand why differentiation is needed and why discussion is needed. Without solving this fundamental problem, it is impossible to conduct in-depth and detailed work. Let's first talk about syndrome differentiation.

The main basis for syndrome differentiation is symptoms, which are reflections of internal organ disorders. Some symptoms may be the same, but the underlying internal organ disorders are different. For example, fever is a common symptom: it can occur in exogenous diseases as well as internal injuries; in exogenous diseases, it can be seen in cold damage, warm diseases, etc., and in internal injuries, it can be caused by lung diseases, liver diseases, etc. This requires careful syndrome differentiation to distinguish them. How to differentiate? There are certain steps. Starting with the fever itself: Whether there is fear of cold, whether there is sweating, whether the fever subsides after sweating (and if so, whether it subsides completely), whether the fever persists throughout the day, whether there are differences between morning and afternoon, or if it only occurs in the afternoon, or if there are several episodes of irregular fever in a day, whether the fever is high or low-grade and indistinct, etc. These various conditions, including exogenous factors, internal injuries, and other causes of illness, must first be clarified to form a preliminary impression. Further, connecting with accompanying symptoms: Whether there is headache, body pain, dysphoria with heat, palm heat, dry mouth, desire to drink water, as well as whether there is flushed cheeks, cold feet, nasal congestion, cough, vomiting, diarrhea, sweating with chills, clouded consciousness, stiff neck and back, convulsions of hands and feet, and then combining with pulse condition, tongue coating, facial complexion, and the duration of the illness. Through multi-faceted examination, a deeper understanding can be achieved to make a correct diagnosis and determine the treatment method. It is obvious that the symptoms related to fever mentioned above include a variety of different syndromes. For example:

Fever, fear of cold, headache, general pain, absence of sweating, pulse floating-tight and rapid – initial stage of cold damage (Taiyang syndrome).

Fever, absence of fear of cold but instead aversion to heat after sweating, thirst with desire to drink cold water, yellow greasy tongue coating, pulse large-slippery and rapid – Yangming syndrome of cold damage.

Fever, fear of cold, recurrent episodes throughout the day, nausea and vomiting, bitter taste in the mouth, pulse string-like and rapid – Shaoyang syndrome of cold damage.

Fever, worsening in the late afternoon, steaming sweating, abdominal distension, constipation, yellow greasy and dry rough tongue coating – stomach excess syndrome of cold damage.

Fever, fear of cold, headache, sweating, dry mouth, cough, pulse floating and rapid – wind-warm syndrome.

Fever, dry mouth, restlessness, clouded consciousness, crimson tip of the tongue – syndrome of warm disease with heat invading the pericardium.

Fever, dry mouth, clouded consciousness with delirium, convulsions of hands and feet, pulse thready and rapid – convulsion syndrome of warm disease.

Fever, fear of cold, headache, stiff neck and back, opisthotonos, pulse string-like and tight – convulsion disease.

Fever, cold feet, dry mouth without desire to drink, chest tightness with nausea and vomiting, scanty yellow urine, dull facial complexion, yellow greasy tongue coating – damp-warm syndrome.

Fever, fear of cold, headache, nasal congestion, cough, thin white tongue coating – wind-cold syndrome.

Fever, epigastric and abdominal distension with pain, vomiting of sour and foul matter, diarrhea, thick greasy tongue coating – food stagnation syndrome.

Fever, mostly in the afternoon, shortness of breath, dry cough, sticky sputum with blood, excessive sweating, pulse deficient-thready and rapid – syndrome of deficiency of both qi and yin in the lung.

Fever, mostly in the afternoon, mild in intensity, heat in the palms and soles, night sweats, flushed cheeks, pulse thready and rapid – syndrome of liver-kidney yin deficiency.

Fever, profuse sweating, fever subsiding but instead fear of cold, spasms in the limbs, pulse floating and weak – yang depletion syndrome.

From the syndromes listed above, some syndromes are originally exterior or cold syndromes, but due to differences in one or two symptoms, they transform into interior or heat syndromes. This shows the significance of syndrome differentiation and the importance of being meticulous in it.

Once syndrome differentiation is clear, treatment determination follows, which is still complex and meticulous. It can also be divided into two steps: First, determine the general method, such as using the diaphoretic method for exterior syndromes, and the clearing method for heat syndromes; then, combine with specific conditions: for exterior syndromes due to wind-cold, use pungent-warm diaphoresis; for those due to wind-heat, use pungent-cool diaphoresis; for heat syndromes in the stomach, if there is heat without excess, clear the stomach; if there is heat with excess, use purgation. Following this method to handle the above-listed fever syndromes, there are:

Pungent-warm diaphoretic method (Taiyang syndrome)

Pungent-cold stomach-clearing method (Yangming syndrome)

Harmonizing the pivot method (Shaoyang syndrome)

Heat-clearing and purgative method (stomach excess syndrome)

Pungent-cool exterior-releasing method (wind-warm syndrome)

Nutrient-clearing and orifice-opening method (syndrome of heat invading the pericardium)

Blood-cooling and wind-extinguishing method (convulsion syndrome)

Fluid-generating and muscle-relaxing method (convulsion disease)

Heat-clearing and dampness-transforming method (damp-warm syndrome)

Lung-dispersing and wind-dispelling method (wind-cold syndrome)

Food-eliminating and middle-harmonizing method (food stagnation syndrome)

Heat-clearing and lung-yin-nourishing method (syndrome of deficiency of both qi and yin in the lung)

Yin-nourishing and steaming-reducing method (syndrome of liver-kidney yin deficiency)

Yang-restoring and exterior-consolidating method (yang depletion syndrome)

With a clear treatment principle, there is a direction for selecting formulas and medications. However, prescriptions vary in potency and must be determined based on the severity of the condition, the patient's age, constitution, etc. Therefore, prescriptions for the same syndrome often differ from person to person. It should be noted, though, that the treatment policy remains consistent. TCM has a vast array of medicines and formulas, and it is difficult to restrict specific ones for the same syndrome. As long as the treatment policy is consistent, there is basically no major discrepancy. Regarding the prescription of medicines themselves, there is a set of principles including the seven formulas, ten preparations, and the roles of sovereign, minister, assistant, and guide drugs, which mainly target the etiology, disease location, and symptoms. Etiology and disease location are the root causes of the disease, while symptoms are the manifestations of pathological changes; once the root causes are eliminated, symptoms will naturally disappear. Hence, comprehensive symptoms are emphasized during diagnosis, and treatment methods are emphasized in prescribing rather than using medicines for each symptom individually, as stated in *Huangdi Neijing*: "In treating diseases, one must seek their root." However, the patient's suffering and mental distress often change with the severity and fluctuation of symptoms, so it is necessary to appropriately address certain symptoms. For instance, in cases of massive bleeding or severe abdominal pain, stopping bleeding or relieving pain is sometimes an urgent task. Nevertheless, whether for general purposes or emergency treatment, the use of medicines still considers the location and cause of the disease. In summary, the general basis for prescribing medicines is combining the disease location and etiology with symptoms.

For example, a cold is caused by wind pathogens attacking the lung; thus, the disease location is the lung, the etiology is wind, and the treatment policy is to disperse lung qi and expel wind. Symptoms of a cold may include aversion to wind, fever, presence or absence of sweating, headache, general pain, hoarseness, itchy throat, cough, profuse or scanty sputum, easy or difficult expectoration, nasal congestion with runny nose, dry mouth or not, thin or thick tongue coating, etc. When prescribing medicines, under the principle of dispersing lung qi and expelling wind, symptoms can be appropriately addressed. Commonly used medicines for dispersing lung qi and expelling wind include schizonepeta, saposhnikovia, mint, ephedra, perilla, fermented soybean, mulberry leaf, etc. These medicines vary in nature, some being slightly warm and others slightly cool, and are used according to different etiologies (such as wind-cold, wind-warm, etc.). In short, they dispel pathogens and release the exterior through the lung. Therefore, after using these medicines, there is no need to separately consider symptoms like aversion to wind or absence of sweating; on the contrary, sweating should be appropriately controlled if present. Also, since aversion to wind usually disappears after profuse sweating and fever subsides accordingly, low-grade fever is rarely considered separately. Only when the fever is severe or there is a tendency of heat transforming and spreading inward are heat-clearing medicines such as charred gardenia, forsythia, honeysuckle, scutellaria, and artemisia annua used. Other medicines effective for individual symptoms, such as chrysanthemum and vitex for headache, gentiana macrophylla, notopterygium, mulberry twig, and loofah sponge for body pain, cicada slough and sterculia lychnophora for hoarseness and itchy throat, almond, thunberg fritillary, pinellia, and tangerine peel for cough, arctium and platycodon for difficult expectoration, xanthium and magnolia flower for nasal congestion and runny nose, trichosanthes peel and reed rhizome for dry mouth, etc., are not all used. When used, they are added in appropriate amounts based on the severity of symptoms. Especially when a single medicine can address multiple aspects, there is no need to mechanically use one medicine for each symptom, creating redundancy. Precisely because the basic principle for treating colds is to disperse lung qi and expel wind, any added medicines for symptoms must conform to this principle. As a result, many medicines for reducing fever, relieving cough, resolving phlegm, quenching thirst, and treating headache or body pain are not selected. It is easy to understand why formulas for treating colds, such as Congchi Decoction (Scallion and Fermented Soybean Decoction) which uses only scallion white and fermented soybean, San'ao Decoction (Three-Aversion Decoction) which uses only ephedra, almond, and licorice, Yinqiao Powder (Honeysuckle and Forsythia Powder) and Xingsu Powder (Apricot and Perilla Powder) which are more complex, and even Erchen Decoction (Two-Chen Decoction) and Xanthii Powder which are not originally for treating colds but are often cited, vary in complexity and combination for this reason. If a patient is frail and easily catches colds, or if a cold lingers and fails to resolve for a long time, the aspect of physical weakness must be considered. Ancient physicians used ginseng (as in Shensu Yin) and astragalus, atractylodes (as in Yupingfeng Powder) for exogenous diseases, but these are not routine methods.

In prescribing medications, it is essential to distinguish between primary and secondary factors, with the primary focus being on identifying the direct underlying cause as the original etiology. During the course of a disease, the original etiology is not fixed and often changes its role due to other factors, so one cannot mechanically treat the original etiology as the primary cause. The etiology referred to in TCM is closely related to pathogenesis: On the one hand, pathogenesis is observed through the primary cause, and on the other hand, etiology is determined through pathogenesis. If one overemphasizes the primary cause while ignoring other factors, not only will the prescription be rigid, but it may also lead to errors. For example, the formation of phlegm-fluid retention, in mild cases, is due to spleen yang deficiency, and in severe cases, due to kidney yang deficiency, hence the saying that "external fluid retention is treated by regulating the spleen, and internal fluid retention by regulating the kidney." But is the primary cause phlegm-fluid retention itself, or spleen-kidney yang deficiency? How to determine the treatment principle? Understanding the relationship between etiology and pathogenesis makes it easy to see that phlegm-fluid retention arises from spleen-kidney yang deficiency and is a product of the pathological process; it is certainly not the original etiology, but once it forms, it becomes a pathogenic factor causing cough and asthma, thus phlegm-fluid retention should be regarded as the primary cause. Clearly, simple spleen-kidney yang deficiency alone would not result in symptoms of profuse phlegm, cough, and asthma. However, in treatment, because phlegm-fluid retention fundamentally stems from spleen-kidney yang deficiency, unlike ordinary cough and asthma, warm-transforming medicines such as dried ginger, schisandra, asarum, pinellia, and poria are commonly used. Additionally, since phlegm-fluid retention is often triggered by wind-cold, accompanied by chills and fever, Xiaoqinglong Decoction is also used. The formulation of Xiaoqinglong Decoction actually adds ginger, pinellia, asarum, and schisandra to the base of ephedra and cinnamon. In the absence of wind-cold and with mild cough and asthma, Linggui Ganzhu Decoction and Shenqi Wan are generally used for root-level nourishment. Of course, for types of phlegm-fluid retention such as hanging fluid retention and branch fluid retention, purgative methods are also used, as these syndromes all arise from phlegm-fluid retention, which must be treated as the primary focus, with different approaches for different conditions, essentially within this framework. This is Zhang Zhongjing's principle for treating phlegm-fluid retention: His clarity in distinguishing disease location and etiology led to a set of rules for prescribing medications. For the same phlegm-fluid retention disorder, methods such as warm transformation, dispersion transformation, warm nourishment, or purgation may be used, with not only different means but also different purposes, demonstrating that prescription of medications is guided by theory. The so-called flexible application refers to formulating specific treatments based on concrete conditions under established principles, not subjective speculation.

III. To correctly apply the method of syndrome differentiation and treatment, one must first master the basic skills, and then continuously become proficient through clinical practice. If the basic skills are poor, one tends to be superficial and unsubstantial; without clinical practice, it is difficult to adapt to changes and achieve depth and meticulousness. Meanwhile, reading previous physicians' medical records is highly helpful and inspiring. Medical records are records of clinical practice in TCM and concrete manifestations of syndrome differentiation and treatment. Some are detailed, others are relatively concise, but they generally include four aspects: symptoms, etiology, pulse and tongue conditions, and treatment methods, with a close integration of theory and practice. The number of medicines in prescriptions, and even the addition or subtraction of one or two ingredients, can reveal the principles of using established formulas.

Hua Xiuyun stated in the "General Remarks" of *Linzheng Zhinan Yi'an* (Guide to Clinical Practice: Medical Records): "The art of medicine lies in recognizing syndromes, establishing methods, and using formulas—these are the three key elements. A hasty approach in any of these makes one unfit to be a healer. There are often cases where a syndrome is recognized, yet a good method cannot be established; or a method is established, yet an appropriate formula cannot be chosen. This is due to incomplete learning. Among these three, recognizing syndromes is particularly crucial. Methods and formulas can be mastered by memorizing more from books in daily study; but recognizing syndromes requires extensive reference to the essence of ancient sages' teachings, going from breadth to conciseness, so that one can have clear and firm insights in clinical practice. If syndrome recognition is unclear, even the initial steps will be wrong." This explains the characteristics of medical records and their relationship with syndrome differentiation and treatment. He further said: "One must know how to read these records. For a single category, observe the differences in the patient's condition, symptoms, and pulse; then one will understand that although the disease name is the same, its origin may differ. Note what method is used in this record, what other method in that record, what formula for this method, what other formula in that case—carefully study the intricate changes. Further, carefully relate the sovereign, minister, assistant, and guide medicines in the formulas to the disease origin; especially pay attention to the addition or subtraction of one or two ingredients from ancient formulas. Mark the parts where syndromes are differentiated and methods are established, and everything will become clear. Do not read through them hastily; merely grasping the superficial without understanding the essence will ultimately be of no benefit. However, to understand these records, one must be a person with clear reasoning, an open and flexible mind, and who has studied *Ling Shu*, *Su Wen*, and the works of previous sages—only then can one appreciate the insights within." This refers to the way of reading medical records and also illustrates the importance of learning syndrome differentiation and treatment from medical records and mastering basic skills.

The writing style of previous physicians' medical records differs from modern medical records. They mainly start from actual symptoms and focus on key points, so they are not as comprehensive as medical records, but their indicators are very clear. Moreover, since syndrome differentiation has certain theoretical foundations, in some places only syndromes are mentioned without describing symptoms. For example, writing "yang jaundice" refers to a series of damp-heat jaundice symptoms such as yellow eyes, yellow urine, and bright yellow skin. Sometimes, symptoms that do not appear are also mentioned, which are of great significance in syndrome differentiation—such as pointing out "urine not yellow" or "stools not loose" to indicate the absence of internal heat or spleen deficiency, serving as a basis for medication. Additionally, common treatments for ordinary diseases that have become standard methods are relatively rarely recorded in medical records; most records are of difficult, complex, severe cases, or those with particularities among ordinary ones. Therefore, the case notes often include a reminder, repeated explanations, or citations of evidence. These instances of conciseness are not omissions, and details are not redundancies; on the contrary, they all explain the issues and are key points worthy of attention. Here, several selections from *Linzheng Zhinan Yi'an* are included, along with preliminary understandings as examples.

Case 1: Hemiplegia on the left side, blood deficiency failing to nourish the tendons and bones, internal wind attacking the collaterals, left pulse slow and large.

Prepared Polygonum multiflorum four *liang*, Lycium barbarum two *liang*, Angelica sinensis (body) two *liang*, Achyranthes bidentata (steamed) two *liang*, Rhizoma Gastrodiae (roasted) two *liang*, Sesamum indicum two *liang*. Grind into powder. Use Chrysanthemum morifolium three *liang*, Dendrobium nobile four *liang*, black soybean hulls four *liang*, decoct to make juice. Add honey, form into extremely fine pills. Take four *qian* in the morning with boiling water. (From the section on wind stroke)

[Note] In terms of symptoms, this case only mentions "hemiplegia on the left side". Hemiplegia refers to hemiparesis. Since the left side is associated with blood and the right with qi in TCM, the specific mention of left-sided hemiplegia indicates it belongs to wind stroke, which may be accompanied by syncope, deviation of the mouth and eyes, etc. These are not listed in the case, indicating it is a sequela of wind stroke with other symptoms no longer present. Therefore, considering only left-sided hemiplegia, combined with a slow and large pulse, it is diagnosed as "blood deficiency failing to nourish the tendons and bones, internal wind attacking the collaterals" due to deficiency of liver and kidney yin and blood, with restless internal wind. Although the treatment method is not explicitly stated, nourishing blood and extinguishing wind is implied. Since the liver governs tendons and the kidney governs bones, emphasis should be placed on nourishing the lower jiao. Thus, the formula uses Polygonum multiflorum, Lycium barbarum, Angelica sinensis, Sesamum indicum, and black soybeans to tonify the liver and kidney, with a focus on nourishing blood. Dendrobium can also nourish the kidney and clear deficient heat, following the principle that "to treat wind, first treat blood; when blood circulates, wind subsides". Assisted by Gastrodia elata and Chrysanthemum to extinguish wind, and Achyranthes bidentata to strengthen tendons and bones, while Sesamum indicum and Dendrobium can also treat wind-damp impediment and weak legs, forming a formula that both treats the root and the branch. Therefore, Xu Lingtai analyzed the blood-nourishing and wind-extinguishing medicines in this formula and commented, " This formula provides mild tonification without the risk of heat production from tonification.

Case 2: Chronic blood loss has long injured yin qi. Further suffering from worry, sorrow, and depression, yang qi, accompanied by internal wind, has caused severe dizziness. The blood residence is empty, qi invades the left side, resulting in deviation of the mouth, numbness of the limbs, slurred speech (inability to speak), and flaccid feet unable to walk. Clearly, the liver and kidney are deficient and weak, yin qi fails to ascend, so we heavily cultivate the lower jiao, hoping to calm the wind. We propose using Hejian's method.

Rehmannia glutinosa (processed) 4 *liang*, Achyranthes bidentata 1.5 *liang*, Cornus officinalis 2 *liang*, Polygala tenuifolia (stir-fried black) 1.5 *liang*, Lycium barbarum 2 *liang*, Chrysanthemum morifolium (stir-fried) 2 *liang*, Schisandra chinensis 1.5 *liang*, Dendrobium nobile 2.4 *liang*, Poria cocos (with wood) 2 *liang*, Cistanche deserticola (light) 1.2 *liang*. Add honey to make pills, take 4 *qian*. (From the section on wind stroke)

[Note] This is also a wind stroke syndrome of blood deficiency failing to nourish the tendons and bones, with internal wind attacking the collaterals, but with left-sided limb numbness not reaching the level of hemiplegia. The main symptoms are wind disturbing the upper body causing deviation of the mouth and slurred speech, and yin deficiency in the lower body causing flaccid feet and weakness. Thus, from the root causes of the disease such as blood loss and depression, it is diagnosed as liver and kidney yin deficiency failing to ascend. It is advocated to heavily cultivate the lower jiao to calm the wind. The syndrome belongs to aphasia, syncope, and wind-induced weakness. Liu Hejian's Dihuang Yinzi (Rehmannia Drink) is adopted. Since there are no signs of yang deficiency, Aconitum carmichaelii, Cinnamomum cassia, and Morinda officinalis are removed. Also, due to yin deficiency with wind movement, Acorus calamus (with its pungent and penetrating nature) is removed, and Lycium barbarum and Chrysanthemum are added to nourish blood and extinguish wind, along with Achyranthes bidentata to descend and treat flaccid feet.

Case 3: The pulse is thready and rapid; thready indicates deficiency of zang yin, rapid indicates consumption of nutrient fluid. Illness in the summer and autumn of last year caused injury, further aggravated by failure to store in warm winter. In spring, the earth qi rises, liver wood wind stirs, resulting in right-sided limb paralysis, stiffness of the tongue collaterals with slurred speech. It is clearly a syndrome of deficient root foundation. Vulgar methods of reducing qi, descending phlegm, diffusing, and attacking wind further rob genuine yin, gradually leading to muddled spirit like drowsiness. If syncope occurs, how can it be treated? We propose using Zhongjing's Fumai Decoction method.

Fumai Decoction minus Zingiber officinale and Cinnamomum cassia. (From the section on wind stroke)

【Note】 This case is also a wind stroke. From the combination of etiology and symptoms, it is a deficiency of both qi and blood, but due to incorrect treatment, genuine yin is further damaged, especially manifested as a muddled spirit like drowsiness and a thready rapid pulse, indicating extreme deficiency of the heart. The heart generates blood, stores the spirit, and governs the pulse; impaired circulation of the meridians will inevitably exacerbate hemiplegia, and syncope should be prevented.

Therefore, Fumai Decoction is used to first treat the heart. Fumai Decoction originally nourishes heart fluid, benefits heart qi, and unblocks heart yang; due to the thready and rapid pulse, ginger and cinnamon (pungent and hot) are removed, turning it into a gentle and moistening formula. Later, Wu Jutong, based on this method, established the Modified Fumai Decoction in *Systematic Differentiation of Warm Diseases* as the main formula to rescue yin fluid when warm pathogens enter the lower jiao. Ancient physicians' application of established formulas, such as this formula and Dihuang Yinzi in the previous case, although deviating from the original intent, also demonstrates quick wit and dexterity, which is worthy of learning.

Case 4: Warm pathogens attack externally, causing cough and head distension; clear the upper jiao.

Apricot kernel, mulberry bark, platycodon, thunberg fritillary, akebia, reed rhizome. (Cough section)

【Note】 Based solely on the two symptoms of cough and head distension, it is difficult to make a confirmed diagnosis. However, it has been diagnosed as "external attack by warm pathogens", so there must be symptoms of wind-warm. Citing Ye Tianshi's *Exogenous Warm Heat*: "Warm pathogens attacking externally first invade the lung" and "The lung governs qi, and its correspondence is with the skin and hair, so it is said to be in the exterior. In the initial stage of the exterior, lightly pungent and cool formulas are used; if accompanied by wind, add mint, arctium, etc.; if accompanied by dampness, add reed rhizome, talc, etc., either expelling wind outside the heat or draining dampness below the heat, so that they do not bind with heat, and the pathogen is bound to be isolated." It can be seen that in this case, with cough as the main symptom, there should be accompanying symptoms such as headache, difficult expectoration, dry mouth, scanty yellow urine, etc. The pulse and tongue are not mentioned, but they should generally be slippery rapid and yellow greasy. Therefore, the formula uses apricot kernel, thunberg fritillary, and platycodon to dispel wind-phlegm, mulberry bark to clear heat, all focusing on the lung, plus akebia and reed rhizome to clear heat and gently drain, also dispelling dampness.

Case 5: Yin deficiency with attack by warm pathogens, cough and head distension; use gentle medicines.

Mulberry leaf, apricot kernel, tendrilled fritillary, white adenophora, raw licorice, sweet pear peel. (Cough section)

【Note】 This case has the same symptoms and etiology as the previous case. Due to inherent yin deficiency and no signs of accompanying wind or dampness, mulberry leaf, apricot kernel, and tendrilled fritillary are used to clear and transform upper jiao phlegm-heat, along with adenophora, licorice, and pear peel for clearing and moistening. The "gentle medicines" mentioned here refer to the principle that "the upper jiao is like a feather, only gentle medicines can reach it", not referring to the dosage.

Case 6: Cough subsiding, tidal fever; in a young person, due to yin deficiency and qi heat.

Wolfberry bark three *qian*, artemisia annua one *qian*, anemarrhena one *qian*, raw licorice three *fen*, southern adenophora one *qian*, dendrobium three *qian*. (Cough section)

【Note】 This case also involves cough with lung heat and yin deficiency, but the presence of tidal fever indicates a more advanced stage of yin deficiency. Persistent heat will inevitably further consume qi and yin, hence it is specifically noted. In addition to using adenophora, licorice, and dendrobium to moisten the lung, wolfberry bark, artemisia annua, and anemarrhena are added to clear heat and reduce steaming. The "subsiding" in "cough subsiding" indicates the disease has lasted for a long time and the cough is no longer frequent, so apricot kernel, fritillary, etc., are not used.

The above examples are, of course, not comprehensive or in-depth, nor are they representative. They mainly illustrate the different writing styles of ancient medical records and provide a glimpse into the methods of studying them. Through careful study, they can be of certain help in syndrome differentiation and treatment. Facts have proven that Xu Lingtai, a renowned physician of his time, made appropriate comments on Ye Tianshi's medical records, and Hua Xiuyun, Shao Xinfu, etc., explored a set of rules from Ye Tianshi's experiences, all of which required great efforts. In short, medical records are a fine tradition of TCM. There are many passed down from ancient physicians, each with their own strengths. One should absorb the essence from various sources like a bee making honey, enriching one's own knowledge to improve medical skills.

Finally, it must be stated that treating diseases focuses on syndrome differentiation. All measures such as treatment methods, prescriptions, and medications are based on syndrome differentiation. Therefore, with correct syndrome differentiation, reasonable treatment can be carried out. Generally, syndrome differentiation and treatment is also referred to as syndrome differentiation "implementation" of treatment. In fact, the purpose of syndrome differentiation is for treatment. However, it should be understood that "implementation" of treatment does not mean nofurther consideration. Under correct syndrome differentiation, to ensure that the prescribed medications are closely tailored to the specific condition and that the dosage is appropriate, a process of discussion is still necessary. If one mistakenly believes that syndrome differentiation and treatment only requires syndrome differentiation without the need for treatment planning, it is easy to mechanically apply established formulas with little consideration of dosage, thereby reducing the therapeutic effect. For this reason, in this article and this book, "syndrome differentiation and treatment" is used consistently, mainly to indicate that consideration is necessary during treatment implementation, and its meaning is basically the same.

New Principles of Treatment

Introduction

As early as the 1930s, Mr. Qin Bowei was inspired by *Yixue Xinwu* (Insights into Medical Studies), which states: "Diseases of the human body are not separated from internal injuries and external contractions. Wind, cold, summer heat, dampness, dryness, and fire are external contractions; joy, anger, worry, thought, sadness, fear, shock, yin deficiency, and dietary injury are internal injuries. In total, there are nineteen characters, from which all the ever-changing diseases arise." and Mo Meishi's *Yanjing Yan* (Discourses on Studying the Classics) which says: "The causes of all diseases are eight: first, pathogenic qi; second, water dampness; third, ghosts and spirits; fourth, insects and beasts; fifth, objects; sixth, diet; seventh, medicinal stones; eighth, human affairs." He believed that the treatment rules of TCM were complex and scattered, and it was necessary to summarize and extract their essence. On the basis of Cheng and Mo's theories, combined with clinical practice, he adjusted and modified them into thirteen major treatment principles: wind, cold, summer heat, dampness, dryness, fire, qi, blood, phlegm, deficiency, food, insects, and pestilence.

"Principle" here refers to norms and rules. These principles govern the selection of treatment methods, the application of formulas, the administration of medicines, and their modifications. They adapt to syndromes and change accordingly, with flexible methods generating thousands of formulas and methods to respond to various diseases. There are fifty-six principles, subordinate to the thirteen major categories. They include classical formulas and contemporary formulas, encompass cold damage and warm diseases, cover external contractions and internal injuries, and are not restricted to *zang-fu* organs or meridians. They integrate the treatment principles of various schools, hence named *New*

Principles of Treatment.

Section 1 Wind

Wind is light, active, and can penetrate without trace. It easily invades the human body and causes diseases rapidly. When wind invades the exterior, mild cases present with nasal congestion, heavy voice, sneezing with clear nasal discharge, cough with spontaneous sweating, headache, and fever; severe cases may have phlegm congestion, asthma, hoarseness, and dry throat. When wind invades the interior, it affects different levels. Invading the muscle interstices, it causes finger numbness, muscle insensitivity, and deviation of the mouth and eyes, called "attacking the collaterals"; when nutrient blood is deficient and wind invades the meridians, leading to heavy body sensation and difficulty in walking, it is called "attacking the channels"; further deep invasion with upward congestion of phlegm, blocking the clear orifices, resulting in unconsciousness, is called "attacking the fu-organs"; when the spirit is scattered, with salivation, and loss of control over urination and defecation, it is called "attacking the *zang*-organs".

The treatment of wind syndromes should distinguish between external and internal wind. External wind should be dispersed and released from the exterior; internal wind should be extinguished and yang should be settled. Wind-like syndromes are not true wind; one must identify the pathogenic factor, and treat according to the syndrome. For phlegm-induced stroke, eliminate phlegm; for fire-induced stroke, reduce fire; for qi-induced stroke, smooth qi; for blood stasis, break blood; for food accumulation, unblock the fu-organs.

The treatment principles for wind are categorized into the following three.

1. Disperse Wind and Release the Exterior Principle

〔Principle Indications〕 Applicable to mild cases of wind cold.

Wind invades from outside, first attacking the exterior, affecting the lung defense system, with slight fear of wind, mild fever, unclear head and eyes, general discomfort, sneezing, itchy throat, or mild cough.

〔Medications〕 Schizonepeta spike, light Saposhnikovia, mint leaf, winter mulberry leaf, light fermented soybean, Hangzhou chrysanthemum, scallion white.

〔Explanation〕 Wind pathogen is neutral in nature; if not combined with cold or warm pathogens, only pungent-neutral wind-dispersing and exterior-releasing methods are needed. For minor illnesses, minor treatment is sufficient; there is no need to make a fuss. The above medicines are mild, gentle, and light, guiding wind pathogens to exit through the defense level.

If there is nasal congestion, add Xanthium and Magnolia flower; for cough, add bitter apricot kernel and Zhejiang fritillary; for head distension, increase Hangzhou chrysanthemum and add Vitex. Do not use overly pungent-warm substances such as Ligusticum, Notopterygium, or Angelica pubescens.

2. Harmonize Nutrient and Defense Principle

〔Principle Indications〕 Applicable to disharmony of nutrient and defense, susceptibility to wind pathogens, or wind invading blood collaterals. Where pathogens gather, qi must be deficient; disharmony of nutrient and defense indicates impaired bodily functions, differing from the previous principle which dispels pathogens. When wind invades the collaterals, causing skin insensitivity and deviation of the mouth and eyes, harmonizing nutrient and defense is also appropriate to dispel wind pathogens in the collaterals.

〔Medications〕 Sichuan cinnamon twig, large white peony root,

Chinese angelica tail, light Saposhnikovia, tender mulberry branch, fresh ginger slice, large red date.

〔Explanation〕 Medicines are divided into three groups. First, cinnamon twig and white peony root, the basic group for harmonizing nutrient and defense. Second, Chinese angelica tail, Saposhnikovia, and mulberry branch to dispel wind, activate blood, and unblock collaterals. Third, fresh ginger and red date to support healthy qi for harmonization.

3. Chase Wind and Expel Pathogens Principle

〔Principle Indications〕 Applicable to true wind stroke. Wind pathogens enter the *zang-fu* organs; attacking the fu-organs causes disorientation and limb disability; attacking the *zang*-organs causes inability to speak, and drooling.

〔Medications〕 Roasted ephedra, Sichuan cinnamon twig, Notopterygium, Angelica pubescens, Sichuan asarum, roasted Bombyx batryticatus, simmered Gastrodia, Acorus calamus

〔Explanation〕 Wind pathogens have deeply entered the *zang-fu* organs, so the formula focuses on penetration and expulsion. Ephedra penetrates pathogens in the muscle interstices; cinnamon twig reaches pathogens in the blood collaterals. Notopterygium disperses wind in the Taiyang channel; Angelica pubescens dispels wind in the Shaoyin channel. Asarum enters both Taiyang and Shaoyin. Bombyx batryticatus dispels wind-phlegm; Gastrodia eliminates phlegm and extinguishes wind; Acorus calamus awakens the spleen and opens the orifices.

〔Interpretation〕 For diseases caused by wind pathogens, only wind-dispelling is needed. Pathogens enter at different levels and transform with varying depths, so treating wind must distinguish the location: Wind in the muscle exterior is dispersed and released; wind in the nutrient and defense, with slightly deeper location and involvement of muscle interstices and meridians, requires harmonizing nutrient and defense to dispel pathogenic factors in the meridians; wind entering the *zang-fu* organs, mostly seen in people with kidney deficiency, should be treated with consideration of Shaoyang and Shaoyin.

Section 2 Cold

Cold is yin-cold in nature, but once it invades the human body, it often transforms into heat due to yang. The exterior is yang; when cold invades the exterior, there is fever, aversion to cold, absence of sweating, headache, stiff neck, general joint pain, and a floating-tight pulse. The interior is yin; when cold invades the interior, there is severe spasm, locked jaws with inability to speak, trembling limbs, chilly sensation, cold skin without sweating, profuse diarrhea with inability to control, and a deep-tight pulse.

Treating cold should use warm medicines, following the common principle in *Neijing* that "cold is treated with heat". When cold invades the body, the location differs, and the warming methods vary. Cold in the exterior is treated with warm release. Cold in the spleen is treated with warm movement. Cold in the kidney is treated with warm tonification. Cold in the liver is treated with warm downward-draining. For cold in both exterior and interior, treat each separately.

1. Disperse Cold Principle

〔Indications〕 Applicable to the initial stage of exogenous cold pathogen invasion. Cold pathogen-induced diseases occur in all seasons, most commonly in winter. In mild cases, it injures the exterior, presenting with symptoms such as chills, fever, and the fever may subside after sweating. This is what is referred to as "when the body is as hot as a burning charcoal, sweating will dispel the heat".

〔Medications〕 Light fermented soybean, scallion white, fragrant perilla, Sichuan notopterygium, roasted ephedra, Sichuan cinnamon twig, bitter platycodon

〔Explanation〕 Since cold is yin in nature, pungent-warm medicines are used for treatment. This differs from the use of pungent-neutral medicines for wind pathogens and pungent-cool medicines for wind-warm pathogens. Depending on the severity of the invading cold pathogen, the medications are classified into mild, moderate, and severe. For mild cases, fermented soybean and scallion white are used, as in Congchi Decoction. For moderate cases, perilla and notopterygium are used. For severe cases, ephedra and cinnamon twig are used, following the idea of Mahuang Decoction.

If there is cough, add arctium, bitter apricot kernel, and Zhejiang fritillary. If there is profuse phlegm, use pungent-warm phlegm-resolving medicines such as tangerine red and pinellia.

2. Warm and Move the Middle Palace Principle

〔Indications〕 Applicable to cold invading the spleen and stomach, with deficiency-cold in the middle jiao. Symptoms include abdominal pain, spontaneous diarrhea, fatigue, poor appetite, cold limbs, extreme aversion to draft, no thirst, and a deep-weak pulse.

〔Medications〕 Light dried ginger, superior codonopsis, raw atractylodes, simmered aucklandia, large amomum, broad tangerine peel, refined pinellia

〔Explanation〕 Cold pathogen invading the interior mostly affects the spleen and stomach, suppressing yang qi. Treatment involves warming the middle and dispelling cold. Dried ginger warms the middle, staying in place without moving. Codonopsis and atractylodes warmly tonify spleen yang. Aucklandia and amomum warmly move qi activity, awakening the spleen and regulating the stomach.

If caused by external invasion of cold pathogen, add perilla and saposhnikovia to dispel cold with pungent-warm properties, warm the middle and transform turbidity. If caused by internal injury from raw and cold foods, add fresh ginger.

3.Warm the Lower Jiao Principle

〔Indications〕 Applicable to cold invading Shaoyin. Symptoms include cold body with aversion to cold, cold limbs, abdominal pain relieved by pressure, borborygmus with diarrhea, and a deep pulse.

〔Medications〕 Raw aconite root, light dried ginger, roasted licorice, scallion white, cinnamon heart, trigonella, poria

〔Explanation〕 When cold pathogen invades deeply, pungent-hot medicines are appropriate. Aconite, dried ginger, and roasted licorice constitute Sini Decoction. If cold pathogen is overwhelming and yang is on the verge of depletion, dispel cold and unblock yang simultaneously by adding scallion white to aconite and dried ginger, forming Baitong Decoction. Aconite warmly dispels cold pathogen in the qi aspect; cinnamon warmly unblocks cold pathogen in the blood aspect. If kidney yang and vital fire are affected, trigonella and simmered nutmeg should be used to warmly tonify the fire of the lower jiao. Atractylodes and poria, which strengthen the spleen and warm the middle, can all be selected.

4.Warm and Downbear Jueyin Principle

〔Indications〕 Applicable to liver-stomach deficiency-cold with upward counterflow of turbid yin. The Jueyin channel wraps around the stomach and belongs to the liver. Liver-stomach deficiency-cold presents with epigastric and abdominal pain, relieved by warmth and pressure. When the stomach fails to harmonize and downbear, turbid yin qi counterflows upward, causing desire to vomit after eating, acid regurgitation with heartburn, and vomiting of cold saliva. Cold pathogen invading the middle earth, with failure of clear yang to ascend, leads to diarrhea. Deficiency of yang qi failing to reach the limbs results in cold hands and feet. Yin cold invading the Jueyin collaterals causes cold lower abdomen and testicular spasm pain.

〔Medications〕Evodia, fresh ginger slices, stir-fried Sichuan pepper, fennel, combined lindera, cinnamon heart, corydalis

〔Explanation〕 Evodia is pungent-hot, entering the liver and stomach channels, lowering qi and counterflow. Nausea, vomiting, and acid regurgitation are due to upward counterflow of cold turbid yin qi in the stomach. Fresh ginger, with stronger qi than flavor, pungently disperses, warms the stomach, and stops vomiting. Dried ginger is not used because of its weak ability to downbear counterflow; charred ginger is not used as it lacks ascending function. Sichuan pepper, fennel, lindera, and cinnamon all warm the liver and stomach, downbearing counterflow and calming upward surges. Corydalis, toosendan fruit, lychee seed, and tangerine seed, which relieve pain and spasm, can all be used.

5.Warm and Disperse Exterior and Interior Principle

〔Indications〕 Applicable to constitutional yang deficiency with cold pathogen invading Taiyang and Shaoyin channels, having both the root of yang deficiency and the branch of cold invasion, thus presenting with severe aversion to cold, mild fever, and a deep pulse.

〔Medications〕 Processed aconite root, Sichuan cinnamon twig, light dried ginger, roasted ephedra, fragrant perilla, light saposhnikovia, northern asarum

〔Explanation〕 Treating both root and branch: One aspect is supporting deficient yang qi with aconite, cinnamon twig, dried ginger, or fresh ginger. Aconite acts internally, invigorating yang qi to drive out pathogens, and can consolidate defense, preventing yang depletion from sweating caused by ephedra and cinnamon twig. The other aspect is dispersing exterior cold with ephedra, perilla, and saposhnikovia. Ephedra acts externally, promoting yang qi, opening and releasing to dispel cold, along with asarum, a superficial medicine of the kidney channel, which penetrates both exterior and interior.

〔Interpretation〕 Zhang Zhongjing's *Treatise on Cold Damage* is the criterion for treating cold in later generations. Among the six channels in cold damage, Yangming involves cold pathogen transforming into heat, and Shaoyang involves alternating cold and heat, neither being pure cold syndromes. Thus, cold syndromes in the exterior only belong to Taiyang. For severe cases, ephedra and cinnamon twig are used; for mild cases, schizonepeta, saposhnikovia, notopterygium, and angelica pubescens. Cold syndromes in the interior are treated based on differentiation of the three yin channels.

Section 3 Summer Heat

Among the six excess pathogens, although each season is said to be dominated by one—wind in spring, cold in winter, dryness in autumn, dampness in late summer—they can actually occur throughout the year. Only summer heat pathogen occurs exclusively in summer. Summer heat must be accompanied by dampness, thus differing from warm heat; summer heat invading directly also differs from damp heat. When summer heat invades the body, it causes dizziness, fever, sweating with asthma, polydipsia with excessive talking, fatigue with shortness of breath, chest tightness with nausea and vomiting, and in severe cases, bleeding, jaundice, and hidden rashes. Reverse transmission to the pericardium, causing syncope, convulsions, and unconsciousness, is called summer heat syncope, which is life-threatening if not urgently treated. The key to treating summer heat is prioritizing clearing and resolving. A surging, rapid pulse indicates yang summer heat, suitable for dispersing summer heat and clearing; a large weak or soft thin pulse indicates yin summer heat, suitable for benefiting qi, nourishing yang, and simultaneous clearing and resolving. There are two principles for treating summer heat, differentiating between mild and severe cases.

1. Disperse Heat and Expel Summer Heat Principle

〔Indications〕 Applicable to syndromes of summer heat attack occurring immediately in summer. In summer, the environment is humid and steaming, so summer heat must be accompanied by dampness. Symptoms include fever without sweating, polydipsia with facial griminess, fatigue with listlessness, dizziness and head distension, nausea and vomiting, and a deficient soft pulse.

〔Medications〕 Fresh agastache, fresh eupatorium, fresh lotus leaf, light bamboo shavings, Liuyi Powder, light akebia, forsythia fruit

〔Explanation〕 Agastache, eupatorium, lotus leaf, and bamboo shavings are aromatic, awakening the spleen, expelling summer heat, and clearing heat—they are the main medicines for treating summer heat, with fresh ones being better. Liuyi Powder and akebia clear heat and drain dampness, enabling summer heat-dampness pathogens in the exterior, interior, and triple jiao to be discharged through the lower jiao. Forsythia fruit clears and penetrates summer heat in the defense level. Others such as aurantium, amomum, and cardamom, which regulate qi and stimulate appetite, can also be selected as appropriate.

2. Clear the Heart and Eliminate Summer Heat Principle

〔Indications〕 Applicable to severe summer heat stroke. Symptoms include sudden heat with collapse, faintness and unconsciousness, profuse sweating, red face, fever, and delirium.

〔Medications〕 Clean forsythia, Sichuan coptis, blackened gardenia, artemisia annua stem, powdered talc, light akebia, Zixue Dan

〔Explanation〕 Forsythia, coptis, and gardenia clear heat and eliminate summer heat. Artemisia annua, pungent and aromatic, eliminates summer heat and clears deficient heat. Talc and akebia clear heat and drain dampness. In cases of high fever with unconsciousness and blocked orifices, Zixue Dan or Zhibao Dan are used to clear heat, open orifices, and awaken consciousness.

For those with a weak constitution, summer heat stroke is more common; or those with a non-weak constitution, due to summer heat pathogen, suffering from profuse sweating with collapse and injury to both qi and fluid, ginseng (or American ginseng), ophiopogon, and schisandra—i.e., Shengmai Powder—are used to benefit qi, generate fluid, and astringe yin to stop sweating.

〔Interpretation〕 Summer heat is a heat pathogen, so warm-hot medicines are contraindicated; summer heat must be accompanied by dampness, so aromatic, penetrating, light, and clear-resolving substances such as agastache, eupatorium, bamboo leaves, and talc are appropriate. For exogenous diseases in summer, many are adept at using Xiangru Yin (Elsholtzia Decoction). Examining closely: Elsholtzia is a pungent-warm diaphoretic, how can it skillfully treat summer heat? The formula comes from *Heji Jufang* (Formulas of the Bureau of Compilation) for treating summer cases of indulging in cold and drinking cold beverages, where yang qi is constrained by yin cold, presenting with chilly aversion to cold, steaming heat on the skin, heavy head without sweating, abdominal pain, vomiting, and diarrhea—obviously treating summer cold damage, unrelated to summer heat. Scholars must clearly distinguish this.

Section 4 Dampness

Dampness pathogen is heavy, turbid, sticky, and stagnant. Its manifestations are heaviness, stagnation, lingering, and gloominess. Its origins are external, such as mountain mists and miasmas, rainy damp steaming, long journeys through water, prolonged residence in damp places, sweat-soaked clothes; and internal, such as rich and greasy foods, roasted and fried foods, raw cold and sweet greasy foods. Damp syndromes mostly arise from spleen yang deficiency or depression and exhaustion; treatment should first regulate spleen yang. Spreading and permeating, it affects all bones and five *zang*-organs: In the upper part, it presents with heavy head, yellow eyes, nasal congestion, and heavy voice; in the middle part, stuffiness and discomfort; in the lower part, swelling of the shins and feet; in the meridians, afternoon fever, aching muscles and bones, lower back pain with inability to turn, flaccid and aching limbs; in the muscles, swelling and fullness, feeling like mud when pressed; in the joints, stiff flexion and extension; in the collaterals, fixed heaviness; in the skin, numbness and insensitivity; in qi and blood, fatigue and lack of strength; in the lung, asthma, fullness, and cough; in the spleen, phlegm, saliva, and swelling; in the liver, hypochondriac fullness and hernia; in the kidney, lower back pain and genital sweating; entering the fu-organs, borborygmus, vomiting, strangury with turbidity, diarrhea with tenesmus, painful rough yellow-red urine; entering the *zang*-organs, unconsciousness, staring eyes, and inability to speak.

In treating dampness: For upper parts, sweating is appropriate; for lower parts, draining is appropriate; for interior deficiency, strengthening the spleen is appropriate; for accompanied wind, resolving the muscles is appropriate; for yang deficiency, supplementing fire is appropriate; for yin deficiency, enriching water is appropriate; dampness with heat is treated with bitter-cold drying; dampness with cold is treated with pungent-hot elimination. All methods of dispelling dampness involve using wind medicines to overcome dampness, promoting urination to move dampness, purging the bowels to expel dampness, and eliminating phlegm to dispel dampness.

The specific principles for treating damp syndromes are six.

1. Aromatic Transform Dampness Principle

〔Indications〕 Applicable to those with damp turbidity invasion and spleen-stomach disharmony. The spleen governs dampness, so damp syndromes prioritize treating the spleen. External dampness invasion is mostly due to rain and water immersion; internal dampness stagnation is mostly due to excessive consumption of raw cold fruits, rich greasy foods, and irregular diet. The stomach is the exterior of the spleen; when dampness pathogen first attacks, it first invades the stomach, presenting with chest tightness, epigastric stuffiness, poor appetite, stickyand greasy in mouth, nausea, and even vomiting. Treatment focuses on aromatic transformation, penetrating dampness, and harmonizing stomach qi. Retention of dampness pathogen causes qi stagnation, further promoting dampness retention; aromatic qi-regulating and dampness-transforming is the initial stage of treating dampness.

〔Medications〕 Agastache stem, eupatorium leaf, white cardamom, amomum shell, fingered citron, refined pinellia, stir-fried coix seed

〔Explanation〕 Agastache and eupatorium act on the upper, exterior, and outer parts, using aroma to disperse and penetrate dampness;

amomum, cardamom, tangerine peel, fingered citron, and pinellia act on the middle, aromatically regulating qi and transforming dampness; coix seed acts on the lower part, promoting diuresis with sweet-bland herbs to drain dampness without leading pathogens into the stomach. Agastache uses stems not leaves because agastache stem's aroma tends to regulate qi, broaden the chest, and transform dampness; agastache leaf tends to release the exterior. Amomum and cardamom use shells not seeds, focusing on penetration. Tangerine peel, fingered citron, and pinellia are essential medicines for treating dampness, needing no further explanation. Coix seed also unblocks meridians and treats impediment and flaccidity; Coix Seed (Yiyiren) dredges meridians and treats impediment/wilting syndromes; for discharging pus and reducing swelling, it should be used raw.

2. Warm and Dry Damp Turbidity Principle

〔Indications〕Turbid dampness entrenched in the middle jiao, leading to dysfunction of the spleen in transportation. Stomach dampness and spleen dampness are essentially the same, but due to the different natures of the spleen and stomach, stomach dampness is mostly caused by initial obstruction of damp turbidity, which can be resolved by aromatic transformation and dispersing; Dampness encumbering the spleen manifests as epigastric fullness, poor appetite, sluggish digestion, abdominal distension with loose stool, and a white greasy tongue coating. In short, for mild damp turbidity syndrome, when it is biased toward the stomach, aromatic dampness transformation is appropriate; for severe damp turbidity, when it is biased toward the spleen, warming and drying damp turbidity is suitable.

〔Medications〕Atractylodes lancea, Atractylodes macrocephala, Magnolia officinalis, green tangerine peel, tangerine peel, stir-fried Aurantium, white cardamom, dried Acorus calamus, medicated leaven

〔Explanation〕 Atractylodes lancea is bitter and warm, a powerful medicine for drying dampness, used when damp pathogen occupies the spleen. Compared with Atractylodes macrocephala, Atractylodes macrocephala mainly strengthens the spleen and secondarily dries dampness, used when middle yang is weak and unable to transport. Magnolia officinalis is aromatic, dry, and regulates qi, relieving chest and epigastric fullness; its dampness-drying power is inferior to Atractylodes lancea, but its ability to relieve fullness is superior. Tangerine peel is aromatic and regulates qi to assist in transforming dampness; green tangerine peel dredges liver qi, used when there are liver meridian symptoms such as costal distension. Acorus calamus is pungent and aromatic, awakening the spleen, used when dampness alone strands the spleen, spleen fails to transport, appetite is poor, mouth is sticky, and middle epigastrium is stuffy. Medicated leaven is a good medicine for strengthening the spleen and stomach and promoting digestion, used as an auxiliary according to the syndrome.

Prolonged stagnation of dampness often transforms into heat, just like grain piling up, generating heat after long stagnation; Coptis chinensis and Phellodendron amurense can be added to clear heat and dry dampness.

3. Downward Leading and Draining Dampness Principle

〔Indications〕 Applicable to water-damp stagnation in the lower jiao, with heaviness below the waist, lower limb edema, difficulty in urination, red and astringent urine, etc. The above two principles are applicable to damp turbidity stagnation in the middle jiao, one biased toward the stomach and one toward the spleen; this method allows water-damp in the lower jiao to be discharged through diuresis. The treatment principles in *Neijing* such as "for those in the lower part, lead and exhaust them" and "purify the bladder" refer to this. Li Dongyuan said: "Treating dampness without promoting urination is not the correct treatment." More precisely, it should be: Treating dampness stagnation in the lower jiao without promoting urination is not the correct treatment. This is a common method for treating dampness.

〔Medications〕 Plantago seed, Alisma orientalis, Stephania tetrandra, Phaseolus calcaratus, Poria cocos peel, Benincasa hispida peel, Areca catechu peel

〔Explanation〕 The medicines are divided into two groups: One group includes Plantago seed, Alisma orientalis, Stephania tetrandra, and Benincasa hispida peel promotes diuresis with its bland nature and drains dampness by facilitating urination.

The other group includes Poria cocos peel, Phaseolus calcaratus, and Areca catechu peel, which strengthen the spleen, move qi, and assist in dampness elimination.

4. Expel Dampness and Promote Diuresis Principle

〔Indications〕 Applicable to accumulated water-damp that cannot be eliminated, in cases of excess constitution and excess syndrome; once accumulated into water, it cannot be eliminated without aggressive expulsion. "Expel" is a step further than "drain"; the syndrome not only presents with lower limb edema but also swelling of the head, face, and limbs, and abdominal distension. There is not only difficulty in urination but also retention of both urine and feces. Generally, treating water-damp should promote urination; aggressive expulsion is used only when edema is severe and diuresis is ineffective. This method is drastic, expelling water pathogen through both the anterior and posterior yin. Expelling water is an expedient measure, not a common method, and should be used cautiously. Fei Boxiong said: "Those whose water is expelled through the anterior yin survive; those through the posterior yin die," further pointing out its severity.

〔Medications〕 Pharbitis seed (black and white), Lepidium apetalum, processed Euphorbia kansui, Phytolacca acinosa root, Gryllulus chinensis, Gryllotalpa africana, Areca catechu

〔Explanation〕 Pharbitis seed and Lepidium apetalum are powerful medicines for promoting diuresis; Pharbitis seed also has the function of moving qi, breaking qi to promote water circulation; Lepidium apetalum opens the lung to promote water circulation. Euphorbia kansui and Phytolacca acinosa are drastic water-expelling medicines, but both are toxic, and their dosage and administration methods should be carefully considered. Insect medicines such as Gryllulus chinensis and Gryllotalpa africana search and clear collaterals, capable of moving water-damp in deep collaterals. Areca catechu moves qi, promotes diuresis, and reduces swelling as an auxiliary.

5. Induce Sweating to Eliminate Dampness Principle

〔Indications〕 Applicable to dampness invading the skin and muscles, similar to the patterns of wind-water, skin-water, and overflowing fluid in the *Golden Chamber*. It is caused by dampness pathogen attacking the Taiyang channel; although it is an exogenous condition, it differs from common cold. There are mild exterior symptoms: chills and fever without sweating, or headache (but a heavy distension rather than severe pain), or cough (but with a weak cough sound), general heaviness and fatigue, oppressive joint pain, edema, a thin white and greasy tongue coating, and a floating and soft pulse. Treatment should disperse and penetrate dampness in the Taiyang channel, which is what the *Inner Canon* refers to as "opening the ghost gate".

〔Medications〕 Roasted ephedra, purple duckweed, light saposhnikovia, notopterygium, angelica pubescens, fresh ginger peel, atractylodes peel, astragalus peel

〔Explanation〕 Ephedra, duckweed, and fresh ginger are pungent-warm to induce sweating, disperse dampness, promote diuresis, and reduce edema; saposhnikovia and notopterygium dispel wind to overcome dampness. For general edema, both notopterygium and angelica pubescens are used together. Since water-dampness is in the skin, "peel medicines treat the skin": fresh ginger peel, atractylodes peel, and astragalus peel are selected. Astragalus strengthens defensive qi, expels dampness, induce sweating to eliminate dampness without injuring healthy qi. For internal water-dampness, alisma, plantago seed, and stephania can be used as appropriate to promote diuresis.

6. Clear and Transform Damp-Heat Principle

〔Indications〕 Dampness is a yin pathogen, heat is a yang pathogen; the combination of dampness and heat presents various characteristic symptoms. In addition to general warm-heat symptoms, there are chest tightness, nausea, heavy body pain, indistinct fever, cold hands and feet, scanty urine, loose stools, a thick greasy tongue coating, etc. Wu Jutong once said: "Dampness is a yin pathogen, coming in late summer; it comes gradually, and its nature is stagnant and sticky, unlike cold pathogen which is resolved with a sweat, or warm-heat which subsides with cooling, so it is difficult to resolve quickly." Therefore, damp-warm syndrome is only suitable for gentle clearing and penetrating transformation, i.e., simultaneously clearing heat and penetrating dampness, with more emphasis on qi movement—when qi transforms, dampness also transforms. However, due to the varying degrees of dampness and heat, treatment may focus more on clearing or more on transforming. This principle is also a method for treating damp-warm syndrome.

〔Medications〕 Smooth apricot kernel, white cardamom, raw coix seed, refined pinellia, powdered talc, light akebia, fresh bamboo shavings

〔Explanation〕 Damp-warm pathogen pervades the triple jiao; treatment should start from the triple jiao: Apricot kernel is used in the upper jiao to open lung qi and disperse dampness; white cardamom in the middle jiao to awaken the spleen and transform dampness; coix seed in the lower jiao to promote diuresis and drain dampness. This follows the idea of Sanren Decoction. It is further assisted by talc for clearing and draining, akebia for gentle dispersion, magnolia bark for aromatic transformation, and bamboo shavings for clearing and penetrating.

In the initial stage of damp-warm syndrome, when it is biased toward the upper jiao, germinated soybean is used; if the pathogen enters the interior with chest and diaphragm fullness, restlessness and oppression, light fermented soybean is used for its pungent aroma to penetrate the pathogen and release the stagnant qi in the middle jiao.

〔Interpretation〕 The six principles for eliminating dampness are: aromatic transformation, warm drying, downward draining, aggressive expulsion, sweating, and clear transformation. Briefly summarized, they are transformation, drying, draining, and expulsion. Transformation includes aromatic transformation and clear transformation, using light medicines focusing on the upper jiao; treating dampness mostly uses warm medicines, and wind medicines to overcome dampness are often categorized here; draining is a major method for treating dampness, allowing dampness an exit with quick effects; when draining is ineffective, aggressive expulsion and drastic methods are used—these medicines are powerful, and when used appropriately, can eliminate stubborn water, but when used improperly, disaster strikes instantly.

Section 5 Dryness

Dryness corresponds to the season of autumn, but in the human body, it must manifest as depletion of yin fluids. The formation of dryness syndrome occurs in two ways: One is when the lung is scorched by fire, with depletion of fluids in the upper part, failing to nourish the hundreds of vessels and bones, resulting in withered hair, dry skin externally, and insufficient moisture in the internal organs; Severe illness causing severe depletion, combined with misuse of Yang-tonifying drying formulas, alcoholic drinks, roasted meats, pungent-heat foods and greasy flavors, all of which abnormally fuel pathogenic fire, damage genuine yin, gradually depleting bodily fluids until yin-fluid exhaustion occurs." The external manifestations of dryness syndrome include: chapped skin when affecting the exterior; dry throat and nose when in the upper part; irritable thirst with desire to drink when in the middle part; dryness-induced constipation and absence of menstruation when in the lower part; dry cough with phlegm clots when affecting the lung; a tendency to grieve and cry when affecting the heart; flaccidity and weakness in the hands and feet. The pulse in dryness syndrome is mostly thready, astringent, and weak.

In the treatment of dryness, moistening comes first. For moistening substances, sweet-cold ones are preferred to nourish the fluids of the lung and stomach; followed by salty-cold ones to nourish the essence of the liver and kidney. Pungent-hot, bitter-cold, bland-draining, aromatic medicines, and formulas for purging excess are all excluded.

The treatment of dryness is divided into three principles for the upper, middle, and lower parts.

1. Moisten the Upper and Clear Dryness Principle

〔Indications〕 Applicable to dryness affecting the heart and lung. The lung is a delicate organ, and fire-heat easily scorches the metal (lung). Symptoms include dry cough with no phlegm, dry mouth, irritable thirst, red dry tongue with little coating, and a deficient rapid pulse.

〔Medications〕 Northern adenophora, barley, trichosanthes root, sweet apricot kernel, tendrilled fritillary, raw pear peel, smoked plum flesh

〔Explanation〕 Adenophora, ophiopogon, and trichosanthes generate fluids and nourish liquids, clearing deficient heat due to fluid deficiency in the upper jiao. Sweet apricot kernel moistens the lung and large intestine, stopping cough. Tendrilled fritillary moistens the lung and relieves cough. Pear peel, bamboo leaf, and imperata root are sweet-cold, clearing heat and generating fluids. Bitter-cold medicines are not used here because bitterness can transform into dryness and rob fluids. Smoked plum is an excellent substance for generating fluids, suitable for dryness syndromes in the upper, middle, and lower jiao, especially effective for the upper and middle jiao.

2. Moisten the Middle and Clear Dryness Principle

〔Indications〕 Applicable to dryness affecting the middle jiao, especially dominated by dryness and depletion of stomach fluids. The most prominent symptom is polyphagia with easy hunger, along with heat vexation, sweating, and emaciation.

〔Medications〕 Fresh rehmannia, fresh dendrobium, trichosanthes root, plump polygonatum, sugarcane juice, plump anemarrhena, fresh reed rhizome

〔Explanation〕 Rehmannia nourishes yin, clears stomach heat to moisten dryness. Dendrobium, trichosanthes, and polygonatum are excellent for generating fluids. For severe excessive hunger with rapid digestion, polygonatum is used in large doses. Sugarcane juice is known as "heavenly dew drink", benefiting the large intestine and draining heat. Anemarrhena and reed rhizome are sweet-cold, generating fluids.

3. Moisten the Lower and Clear Dryness Principle

〔Indications〕 Applicable to dryness affecting the lower jiao (liver, kidney, and large intestine), with symptoms such as difficult and dry constipation, emaciation, dry skin with poor luster, flaccid and weak legs, red tongue with little fluid, and a thready weak pulse.

〔Medications〕 Beijing scrophularia, fine rehmannia, large asparagus, light cistanche, raw white peony root, hemp seed, whole trichosanthes fruit

〔Explanation〕 The treatment principle is "increasing water to move the boat", addressing "boat stagnation due to lack of water". Scrophularia is used in large doses to nourish yin and generate fluids, moisten dryness and clear heat; rehmannia nourishes yin and clears heat; asparagus nourishes fluids and moistens dryness; raw white peony root nourishes yin and astringes yin; hemp seed, a fatty nut, moistens the lower part; trichosanthes moistens the lung and large intestine, descends lung qi, and unblocks the bowels. These medicines, with the nature of tonics, function as purgatives, capable of attacking excess while preventing deficiency.

〔Interpretation〕 The three principles for treating dryness mentioned above are all formulated for dryness and depletion of body fluids. As for autumn dryness disease, it refers to wind-warm syndrome suffered in autumn. Although named after dryness, it is actually an exogenous warm disease, presenting with chills and fever, headache, cough with choking, dry mouth, dry lips, and difficult expectoration. Treatment involves adding one or two light sweet-cold moistening medicines to wind-warm formulas, such as reed rhizome, adenophora, ophiopogon, pear peel, watermelon rind, etc. There are also terms like cool dryness and warm dryness, which refer to tendencies toward wind-warm or wind-cold, and can be treated with integrated methods.

Section 6 Fire

Fire, heat, warmth, and toxin have the same nature but different names, so they are often referred to interchangeably. Fire is the entity of heat, and heat is the function of fire. Warmth is mild heat, and heat is intense warmth. Fire is the entity of toxin, and toxin is extreme fire. The physiological fire, latent and gentle, warms and nourishes the viscera and every limb, securing a person's allotted span of life; the pathological fire, by contrast, scorches the yin-fluids, plunders and injures the original qi, and rots the very fabric of the body. The five *zang*-organs govern the five emotions; excessive five emotions can all transform into fire. Diet, sexual overexertion, and excessive clothing can also cause fire. Qi stagnation leads to fire arising from the lung; anger leads to fire arising from the liver; excessive drinking leads to fire arising from the spleen; anxiety leads to fire arising from the heart; sexual overexertion leads to fire arising from the kidney. Various fire syndromes occur: Toothache with bleeding gums, swelling of the cheeks and jaw are stomach fire; yellow eyes with bitter taste, restlessness in sitting and lying are gallbladder fire; tongue erosion with throat pain, constipation are large intestine fire; urinary retention with dribbling, red and white vaginal discharge are small intestine fire; lower abdominal pain with scanty urine are bladder fire; dizziness with fatigue, heat in the palms and soles are triple jiao fire. Fire syndromes also have many complicated variations. Accompanied by damp turbidity, there is cough with thick phlegm, even pus and blood; heat lingering in the lower jiao leads to turbid urine with dribbling, lower abdominal pain and distension; extreme heat causing extreme cold, fire transforming into cold, presents with chills and shivering, hidden pulse in the limbs—this must be carefully observed.

The treatment of fire follows the clear teachings in *Neijing*: Excess fire is purged, deficient fire is nourished, stagnant fire is dispersed, yang fire is directly suppressed, yin fire is warmed and guided.

Fire tends to flame upward; upward-rising heat is fire, and internal unmanifested heat is heat. Treating heat only requires clearing, while treating fire must involve descending.

The five principles for treating fire are as follows.

1. Calm the Sovereign Fire Principle

〔Indications〕 Applicable to hyperactivity of heart fire, or heart transferring heat to the small intestine. Symptoms include heart vexation, insomnia, palm heat, tongue erosion with swollen tongue, red and astringent urine.

〔Medications〕 Fine rehmannia, light bamboo leaf, cinnabar lampwick, clean forsythia, Sichuan coptis, blackened gardenia, clean rhinoceros horn

〔Explanation〕 Rehmannia is sweet-bitter-cold, entering the heart to clear heat and cool blood, entering the kidney to nourish yin and generate fluids. When kidney water is sufficient, heart fire is subdued, making it especially suitable for heat in the heart channel with mild yin injury. Light bamboo leaf and cinnabar lampwick are sweet-light-cold, clearing the heart and relieving vexation, guiding heat downward to be excreted through urine. For more severe heart fire, forsythia, coptis, and gardenia (bitter-cold) clear the heart and purge fire. Rhinoceros horn is a superior medicine for cooling the heart, but due to its high price, it is used only when necessary.

For hyperactivity of heart fire with clouded consciousness and delirium, add Zixue Dan. For heat damaging blood and forcing reckless bleeding, add moutan bark.

2. Bitterly Drain Ministerial Fire Principle

〔Indications〕 Applicable to hyperactivity of liver-gallbladder dragon-thunder fire, or downward pouring of liver channel damp-heat. Symptoms include irritability and easy anger, chest and hypochondriac fullness and pain, head distension and headache, red eyes and ear pain, bitter taste and dry throat, nocturnal emission with turbid discharge, persistent penile erection.

〔Medications〕 Gentiana scabra, light scutellaria, Prunella vulgaris, Tongguan akebia, fine rehmannia, Sichuan phellodendron, Beijing paeonia rubra

〔Explanation〕 Gentiana scabra is extremely bitter and cold, purging fire and eliminating dampness, serving as a powerful medicine for cooling the liver. Scutellaria and Prunella vulgaris clear Shaoyang (upper part), while Phellodendron drains Jueyin (lower part); these three bitter-cold medicines purge excess fire in the liver and gallbladder channels. Since damp-heat pathogens are stagnant in the lower jiao, akebia, plantago seed, alisma, and the like are used to guide them out through the kidney and bladder, providing an exit for the pathogens. However, the liver is the organ that stores blood; excess fire in the liver channel easily injures yin and blood, and the medicines used here are bitter-drying, draining, and damaging to yin. Thus, rehmannia and paeonia rubra are used to nourish blood and benefit yin, cooling and softening the liver.

3. Subdue and Control Excess Fire Principle

〔Indications〕 Applicable to tangible heat accumulation stagnating in the Yangming stomach and intestines. Symptoms include abdominal fullness and pain, hard as stone when pressed, constipation or heat accumulation with side flow, fever, dry mouth and tongue, and even irritability and delirium.

〔Medications〕 Raw Sichuan rhubarb, mirabilite, Jiangzhi shi (immature bitter orange), raw licorice, honeysuckle, clean forsythia, charred gardenia

〔Explanation〕 Rhubarb is extremely bitter and cold, purging heat and promoting bowel movement, eliminating excess accumulation, activating blood and resolving stasis, with the power of a "general" breaking through barriers; its potency is sharper when used raw. Mirabilite, salty and cold, increases fluids, purges heat, softens hardness, and moistens dryness. Zhi shi descends qi and relieves distension, assisting the downward movement of stagnation. Raw licorice clears heat and purges fire, and also harmonizes other medicines. For heat filling the triple jiao, honeysuckle, forsythia, and gardenia are used as assistants.

4. Diffuse and Release Stagnant Fire Principle

〔Indications〕 Applicable to liver-gallbladder stagnant fire. Symptoms include distending pain in the head and eyes, chest and hypochondriac restlessness and fullness, red and swollen painful gums, irritability and easy anger.

〔Medications〕 Soft bupleurum, stir-fried mint, winter mulberry leaf, Hangzhou chrysanthemum, light yellow tea, tender uncaria, kudingcha (Ilex kudingcha)

〔Explanation〕 Stagnant fire should be released. Stagnant fire cannot be descended or purged, only suitable for pungent-cool dispersion and drainage. Bupleurum is pungent and neutral, mint is pungent and cool, both soothing the liver and resolving depression. Mulberry leaf, chrysanthemum, scutellaria, uncaria, and kudingcha gently clear and cool the liver.

5. Settle and Nourish Deficient Fire Principle

〔Indications〕 Applicable to yin deficiency with heat and deficient fire flaring upward. The disease location is in the liver and kidney, especially the kidney. Symptoms include tidal fever, heat in the palms and soles, night sweats, and even deficient fire attacking upward with red face and eyes, sore throat, tooth pain, sleeplessness, headache, and cold lower limbs.

〔Medications〕 Fresh rehmannia, large white peony root, Beijing scrophularia, raw abalone shell, raw oyster, roasted turtle shell, superior cinnamon

〔Explanation〕 First, nourish the lower origin: Rehmannia and white peony root nourish the liver and blood; scrophularia, salty and cold, nourishes the kidney to absorb and settle fire. Second, settle and descend deficient fire: Raw abalone shell and raw oyster are heavy in nature and descending in tendency; turtle shell is salty, neutral, and heavy, nourishing yin and filling essence, strengthening water to reduce fire. When deficient fire is severe, a small amount of cinnamon is used to lead fire back to its origin

〔Interpretation〕 The five principles for treating fire—calming, bitter draining, subduing, diffusing, and settling—are applied respectively to hyperactive heart fire, blazing liver-gallbladder fire, accumulated stomach-intestinal fire, stagnant liver fire, and upward-floating kidney fire. In short, they address only two aspects: Excess and deficiency. Excess fire is treated with clearing, descending, and draining; deficient fire with settling, nourishing, and absorbing. Among them, "releasing stagnant fire" though called diffusion, is completely different from diffusing wind-cold attacking the exterior. Pungent-warm and ascending-dispersing substances are strictly avoided; only bupleurum, mint, mulberry leaf, etc.—pungent-neutral or pungent-cool to penetrate and disperse—are needed, along with cooling substances like gypsum, coptis, forsythia, scutellaria, and chrysanthemum to cool the fire. In cases of stagnant fire, knowing only pungent dispersion without cooling penetration will lead to failure.

Section 7 Qi

Qi in the body flows everywhere; qi disorders can occur anywhere, hence the saying: "Hundreds of diseases arise from qi." The treatment of qi disorders may seem scattered and disorderly, but for those who understand its essentials, it is systematic and orderly.

Qi transforms into seven conditions: Anger causes vomiting blood, chest fullness with hypochondriac pain, jianjue (fire-induced reversal) and bojue (qi reversal); Excessive joy drives one to wild, unceasing laughter—the yang qi can no longer be contained;sorrow results in blurred vision, nasal acidity, uterine bleeding, flaccid pulse, and shortness of breath; fear brings bone soreness, flaccid reversal, broken hollows, and yin impotence; shock causes salivation, rolled eyes, open mouth, madness, stiffness, and unconsciousness; overstrain leads to panting, coughing blood, lower back pain, bone flaccidity, lung rales, scanty essence, and amenorrhea; pensiveness results in loss of appetite, drowsiness, confusion, middle jiao distension, and blockage of the triple jiao.

Although the syndromes are numerous, the treatment principles are no more than calming its rebellion, dispersing its accumulation, descending its floating, soothing its stagnation, containing its dispersion, and settling its chaos. Briefly summarized, they are regulating, settling and descending, and lifting and raising.

1. Soothe and Benefit Qi Stagnation Principle

〔Indications〕 Applicable to anger, melancholy, and unsmooth qi. Qi disorders first affect the liver; the liver belongs to wood and easily overacts on earth (spleen/stomach), thus often affecting the spleen and stomach leading to liver-stomach disharmony. Symptoms include chest and hypochondriac depression, epigastric and abdominal distension and pain, unsmooth bowel movements, and relief after belching or passing gas. Treatment involves regulating qi, soothing qi, rectifying qi, benefiting qi, and moving qi. Different names denote varying degrees of severity, but overall they all regulate qi, as stated in *Neijing*: "Soothe qi to make it harmonious."

〔Medications〕 Tribulus terrestris, broad curcuma, processed cyperus, Jiang aurantium, stir-fried green tangerine peel, whole angelica, Fu ligusticum

〔Explanation〕 Tribulus terrestris soothes the liver and regulates qi, dispels wind and unblocks collaterals—it is the first choice for soothing the liver, especially suitable for head and eye symptoms; in cases of lower deficiency and upper excess, white and brown tribulus can be used together. Cyperus regulates qi of the triple jiao, focusing on the liver and stomach; aurantium regulates qi of the intestines, liver, and gallbladder; green tangerine peel enters the liver and also regulates the intestines and stomach. Curcuma regulates qi in the blood; the liver takes blood as its substance and qi as its function, with a close relationship between substance and function, often combined with yang medicines in the blood such as angelica and ligusticum—angelica nourishes and harmonizes blood, ligusticum invigorates blood, regulates qi, and relieves pain.

For cold bias, add galangal which can enter the liver's blood collaterals to dispel cold in the liver collaterals; used with cyperus, it forms Liangfu Pills to regulate liver qi and warm liver collaterals. For stomach disharmony with belching, add dried fingered citron; for liver yin injury, add rose flower; for stomach yin injury, add kumquat cake.

2. Calm and Settle Qi Floating Principle

〔Indications〕 Applicable to floating and erratic heart qi, wandering spirit, palpitations, and severe palpitations. The heart governs the spirit; spirit unrest involves the heart. The liver and heart have a mother-child relationship—heart unrest leads to liver yang hyperactivity; spirit unrest causes heart-kidney disharmony. Heart fire should descend and be contained, kidney water should ascend and nourish; heart-kidney disharmony with spirit unrest should also consider the liver and kidney.

〔Medications〕 Ziziphus spinosa, platycladus seed, longan aril, cinnabar poria with wood, green dragon's teeth, left oyster, magnetite

〔Explanation〕 Medicines can be divided into two aspects: One is tonifying and nourishing the heart, such as ziziphus spinosa, platycladus seed, and longan aril; the other is sedative and tranquilizing medicines—dragon's teeth enter the heart as the main heavy settling and descending medicine; cinnabar poria with wood is a sedative that tonifies the heart and spleen; oyster enters the liver to assist; magnetite assists the kidney in containing.

3. Lift and Raise Qi Sinking Principle

〔Indications〕 Applicable to middle qi sinking. The spleen governs middle qi; middle qi sinking is also spleen qi sinking, with symptoms including fatigue, limb tiredness, lassitude with shortness of breath, persistent loose stools, prolapse of the anus, uterine bleeding, and incessant leukorrhea. The stomach governs descending, the spleen governs ascending; tonifying the spleen promotes lifting.

〔Medications〕 Roasted astragalus, stir-fried codonopsis, roasted cimicifuga, soft bupleurum, raw atractylodes, clear roasted licorice, stir-fried tangerine peel

〔Explanation〕 Astragalus and codonopsis reinforce qi and tonify the middle jiao, complementing each other. However, the former tends to lift and raise the middle qi, while the latter tends to tonify the middle qi. For those with ascending deficient fire, astragalus is not used; for those with chest and epigastric stuffiness, codonopsis is not used. These two medicines form the material basis. Cimicifuga and bupleurum, which ascend upward, provide the driving force. These two medicines are bitter, neutral, and thin in flavor, belonging to yang within yin, and can guide the tonifying effects of astragalus and codonopsis upward. Lifting and raising the middle qi must be based on tonifying the spleen and stomach, achieving the purpose of lifting through cimicifuga and bupleurum. Atractylodes and licorice reinforce qi, strengthen the spleen, and regulate dampness. When qi is deficient, its movement becomes sluggish; thus, aromatic and spleen-awakening tangerine peel is added to promote its flow.

〔Interpretation〕 In treating qi disorders, three key pivot points should be grasped: Stagnated and accumulated qi should be regulated; rebellious, floating, scattered, and chaotic qi should be settled and astringed; sunken and depressed qi should be lifted and raised. Regulation mainly targets the liver and stomach; settling and astringing mainly targets the heart, with consideration of the liver and kidney; lifting and raising mainly targets the spleen, with consideration of the lung and kidney. The method of reinforcing qi is included in the principle of tonifying deficiency.

Section 8 Blood

Blood is derived from the refined essence of food and water. Improper daily life, excessive emotions, overstrain, sexual indulgence, and irregular diet are all sufficient to stir fire and damage qi. Stirred fire drives hot blood to move recklessly; damaged qi leads to blood losing its attachment, either exiting through the upper orifices, lower orifices, overflowing into the muscles, or stagnating in the meridians, *zang-fu* organs. Reckless movement upward results in vomiting blood and nosebleeds; flowing downward causes blood in urine and stool; stagnation in the meridians leads to abscesses; stagnation in the intestines and viscera forms masses; blood may combine with wind-heat to become macules and rashes; or stagnate with yin cold to cause pain and impediment. Although blood syndromes have various manifestations, each has specific characteristics in syndrome differentiation. Heat accumulating in the lung and stomach presents with chest fullness and a forceful pulse; violent anger with qi rebellion presents with a red face and a string-like pulse; yang deficiency with blood escaping externally presents with coldness and aversion to cold; yin deficiency with upward hyperactivity of fire presents with cough, asthma, and internal heat; overstrain of the heart failing to generate blood presents with vexation and restlessness; overstrain of physical labor failing to contain blood presents with spontaneous sweating and fatigue; stagnation damaging the spleen presents with melancholy and poor appetite; overstrain damaging lung qi presents with prolonged cough without phlegm; qi failing to govern blood presents with scattered bleeding; accumulated stasis presents with blood clots; stagnation in the upper part presents with purple blood; deficient fire in the lower part presents with fresh blood; blood congealed by cold presents with dark black blood; lung abscess presents with blood mixed with pus; intense phlegm-fire presents with phlegm followed by blood; rampant yin deficiency fire presents with blood followed by phlegm; food damaging the stomach presents with stuffiness and vomiting blood; excessive drinking leading to intoxication presents with vomiting of sour and putrid blood.

The key principles in treating blood syndromes are: Promoting blood circulation is preferable to stopping bleeding; descending qi is preferable to using cold to reduce fire. For blood syndromes of various *zang*-organs, different approaches are applied: The lung should be cleared and descended, not ascended and dispersed; the heart should be nourished, not consumed and scattered; the spleen should be warmed, not treated with sour and cold; the liver should be soothed, benefited, and gently harmonized, not constricted; the kidney should be tonified with water and nourished with yin, not attacked.

Blood syndromes can be treated with six principles.

1. Clear and Cool Hot Blood Principle

〔Indications〕 Applicable to reckless movement of hot blood with bleeding from the upper orifices. Caused by either external pathogen invasion or internal injury from the five emotions, with hyperactivity of liver fire and heat in the blood aspect, differing from general excess heat syndromes which are intense in the qi aspect. Reckless movement of hot blood leads to bleeding, mostly vomiting blood and nosebleeds—the so-called “injury to the yang collaterals causes blood to move upward”—with bright red blood.

〔Medications〕 Fresh rehmannia, large white peony root, moutan bark, blackened gardenia, carbonized honeysuckle, carbonized scutellaria, carbonized lotus root nodes...

〔Explanation〕 First, nourish yin to treat the root cause: Fresh rehmannia clears heat, nourishes yin, cools blood, and stops bleeding; white peony root nourishes yin and astringes the nutrient aspect, and when used raw, cools blood and calms blood. For heat in the blood with blood stasis, red peony root can be used, or both red and white peony roots together. Nourishing yin is the foundation of this principle, and it should be done with clear, gentle, and light substances, avoiding greasy ones, so rehmannia preparata and polygonum multiflorum are unsuitable. Second, cool the blood: Moutan bark is the first choice for cooling blood, as it cools blood to stop bleeding and can resolve stasis; gardenia clears heat in the triple jiao—charred gardenia enters the blood aspect, while raw gardenia enters the qi aspect. The above address the root cause. Carbonized honeysuckle, carbonized scutellaria, and carbonized lotus root nodes clear heat, astringe, and stop bleeding to address the branch symptoms. Warm diseases are most likely to stir blood, often requiring cooling blood to stop bleeding, as seen in the modifications of formulas like Sangju Yin and Yinqiao Powder in *Systematic Differentiation of Warm Diseases*. Modifications to Sangju Yin: "When the pathogen first enters the nutrient aspect, add scrophularia and rhinoceros horn. In the blood aspect, remove mentha and reed rhizome, add ophiopogon, rehmannia, polygonatum, and moutan bark." Modifications to Yinqiao Powder state: "For nosebleeds, remove schizonepeta and fermented soybean, add imperata root, carbonized platycladus, and blackened gardenia."

When using hemostatic medicines, attention must also be paid to the bleeding site—for example, add cogongrass flower for nosebleeds; add celosia for red eyes or even bleeding; use platycladus leaf and rubia more for coughing blood.

2. Warm and Harmonize Blood Principle

〔Indications〕 Applicable to cold in the blood aspect with congealed and stagnant blood. Cold invasion leading to blood stasis is more common in women, presenting with cold lower abdominal pain, delayed menstruation, painful menstruation, or even amenorrhea.

〔Medications〕 Stir-fried angelica, large ligusticum, wine-fried white peony root, cinnamon heart, carbonized ginger, artemisia argyi wool, dalbergia odorifera

〔Explanation〕 Blood flows when warmed, so qi-activating, blood-circulating, and warming medicines should be used. Based on Siwu Decoction: Angelica and ligusticum are yang medicines in the blood, warming and nourishing blood, moving qi and relieving pain; white peony root is a yin medicine in the blood, its cold nature transformed to warm through wine processing, regulating blood and relieving pain gently; rehmannia raw (bitter-cold) and rehmannia preparata (greasy) are not included; cinnamon heart warms and nourishes heart blood, tending to act on the heart-liver blood aspect. Dried ginger and aconite are not used because their dryness and harshness are unsuitable for the blood aspect. Carbonized ginger, being charred, can enter the blood; artemisia argyi warms and unblocks blood vessels; dalbergia odorifera warms qi movement to assist blood circulation.

3. Unblock Channels and Disperse Stasis Principle

〔Indications〕 Indicated for static blood that has stagnated and coalesced into tangible masses. Symptoms include dark-colored menstrual flow, amenorrhea with abdominal pain, and lower abdominal masses. Stasis is the main issue, with cold and heat often not prominent; blood stasis here is more severe than in the previous principle.

〔Medications〕 Whole angelica, large ligusticum, stir-fried red peony root, spatholobus stem, Leonurus japonicus fruit, processed cyperus, toosendan fruit

〔Explanation〕 Still based on Siwu Decoction, white peony root is replaced with red peony root to enhance blood circulation and stasis dispersion. Spatholobus stem circulates freely, nourishes and activates blood, unblocks channels and dispels stasis, nourishing blood without causing stagnation and dispelling stasis without injuring healthy qi, and can be used in larger doses. Leonurus japonicus fruit enters the blood aspect, regulates liver channels, unblocks the thoroughfare and conception vessels, making it an excellent medicine for dispelling stasis and unblocking channels. Qi is the commander of blood, and among qi-regulating medicines in blood-activating formulas, cyperus is most frequently used. Ancient physicians once used it alone in powder form to treat miscellaneous syndromes caused by blood stasis and qi stagnation, calling it Dusheng Wan (Sole Victory Pill). Ye Tianshi once used Xiaoyao Powder minus atractylodes plus cyperus to target the key issue. Toosendan fruit and corydalis (i.e., Jinlingzi Powder) assist in activating blood, moving qi, and relieving pain.

3. Attack and Break Blood Accumulation Principle

〔Indications〕 Applicable to blood masses and lumps. Blood stasis, stagnation, and accumulation into masses is a gradual process, and treatment must distinguish the stages.

〔Medications〕 Salvia miltiorrhiza, angelica tail, Carthamus tinctorius, peach kernel paste, Sparganium stoloniferum, Curcuma zedoaria, Lycopus lucidus leaf

〔Explanation〕 The single herb salvia is said to have the same effect as Siwu Decoction, praised for both nourishing blood and activating blood circulation, thus regarded as the main herb. The entire formula still focuses on nourishing blood, promoting blood circulation on the basis of nourishing blood, and dispelling stasis on the basis of promoting blood circulation. This is a principle. Wang Qingren was skilled in using stasis-dispelling methods, also focusing on promoting blood circulation. Angelica tail nourishes blood and breaks up stagnant blood. Peach kernel and safflower activate blood and dispel stasis. Since masses have already formed, sparganium and zedoaria break up blood and expel stasis. However, attention must be paid to dosage and timing. Lycopus assists in activating blood and unblocking channels.

Furthermore, considering the causes of stasis obstruction: for cold congelation, add cinnamon, charred ginger, and aged artemisia; for qi stagnation, add cyperus and green tangerine peel; for deep-seated stasis, add insects like eupolyphaga and tabanus, which can penetrate deeply.

4. Benefit Qi and Disperse Stasis Principle

〔Indications〕 Applicable to qi stagnation and blood stasis in the upper jiao, with stabbing pain in the chest and hypochondria, or a feeling of "constantly wanting to press on the chest"—similar to "liver retention" in the *Golden Chamber*—or difficult expectoration of blood, chest impediment with qi obstruction.

〔Medications〕 Stir-fried red peony root, peach kernel paste, roasted frankincense and myrrh, Sichuan curcuma, genuine fresh jiangxiang (purple ginger), loofah sponge, platycladus leaf

〔Explanation〕 Red peony root moves stasis in the meridians; peach kernel moves stasis in the *zang-fu* organs. Frankincense and myrrh are qi medicines in the blood, activating qi and blood to relieve pain. Curcuma, a blood medicine in qi, has excellent pain-relieving effects. Aurantium regulates the liver and soothes qi. Fresh jiangxiang enhances penetrating power; in the absence of jiangxiang, safflower can be substituted, with saffron being optimal but expensive and hard to find. Loofah sponge and tangerine pith can guide medicines into the collaterals. Platycladus leaf cools blood and stops bleeding, used when bleeding occurs.

5. Benefit Qi and Contain Blood Principle

〔Indications〕 Applicable to qi failing to contain blood, with slow bleeding. Qi here refers to middle qi, also called spleen qi. When the spleen fails to govern blood, bleeding is slow and oozing, with dark blood color, mostly from the lower parts—such as abdominal pain with bloody stool, gynecological metrorrhagia, or even severe uterine bleeding with fainting. It is accompanied by middle qi deficiency symptoms such as shortness of breath, poor appetite, fatigue with movement, and a deficient thready pulse. Blood depletion leads to qi depletion; in severe cases, collapse phenomena like rapid breathing, sweating on the head, and palpitations may occur, requiring urgent qi stabilization.

〔Medications〕 Clear roasted astragalus, stir-fried codonopsis, raw atractylodes, calcined dragon bone, calcined oyster, ass-hide gelatin pearls, terra flava ustulata

〔Explanation〕 Astragalus, codonopsis, and atractylodes are sweet-warm, benefiting qi and strengthening the spleen to contain blood. Astragalus is used for defensive qi deficiency, atractylodes for middle qi deficiency, codonopsis for heart qi deficiency, and ginseng for collapse. Calcined dragon bone and oyster astringe and stop bleeding. Ass-hide gelatin tonifies blood and stops bleeding. Terra flava ustulata is sweet-warm, strengthening the middle, used to treat incessant bloody stool.

For persistent uterine bleeding, add charred Trachycarpus fortunei (Chen Zong Tan); in severe hemoptysis or hematemesis, use charred Rehmannia glutinosa root (Sheng Di Tan); during the convalescent stage of hematemesis when yin-blood is already depleted, use charred prepared Rehmannia (Shu Di Tan) or add Bletilla striata (Bai Ji) to astringe and stanch the bleeding.

〔Interpretation〕 The six principles for treating blood are cooling, warming, activating, breaking, dispersing, and astringing. In short, they are circulation and stopping. Warming, activating, breaking, and dispersing all promote blood circulation to invigorate blood; cooling and astringing calm blood to stop bleeding. Only the blood-activating and stasis-dispelling principle uses circulation as tonification and movement as stopping, thus combining both circulation and stopping.

Section 9 Phlegm

Phlegm is a term in Chinese medicine referring to pathological products and syndromes. In Chinese medicine, besides phlegm syndromes in cough and asthma, it has a broader meaning. Treating from the perspective of phlegm has unexpected effects on many diseases (including some refractory ones), hence the ancient saying: “Strange diseases are all caused by phlegm.” Treating phlegm is a characteristic therapeutic approach in Chinese medicine.

All kinds of phlegm syndromes are caused by exogenous pathogenic factors such as wind-cold and the six excesses, or internal injuries from the seven emotions and improper diet, which lead to qi counterflow, turbid fluids, and stagnation and condensation of body fluids. Where phlegm resides, it follows qi to reach everywhere. It may stagnate in the lung, accumulate in the stomach and intestines, block the chest and diaphragm, or lodge in the limbs, meridians, and collaterals, and all parts of the body. It manifests as cough, asthma, vomiting, nausea, stuffiness and obstruction in the chest and diaphragm, heartburn and palpitations, dizziness, heart palpitations, mania, chills and fever, and swelling with pain. The manifestations of phlegm have quite specific characteristics, such as gurgling sounds in the chest and diaphragm, a constant cold feeling at one point on the back, a creeping sensation all over the body like insects crawling, a feeling of two qi intertwining in the chest, nodules under the skin and between the membranes that are neither red nor swollen, lumps on the neck that are like scrofula but not scrofula, obstruction in the throat like a plum stone, expectoration like peach gum, hard swelling and numbness of the limbs, mass formation at the tip of the ribs, stabbing pain in the bones and joints that is irregular, soreness and weakness in the waist and legs, vomiting of cold saliva, green water, or black juice, dreams of fireworks, swords and halberds clustering, diarrhea with mucus, urine like thick juice, and other conditions such as blockage and obstruction, 走马 throat impediment, toothache and tinnitus, consumption and paralysis, amenorrhea and leukorrhea in women, convulsions in children, and even seeing ghosts for no reason, with a consciousness that is neither clear nor asleep. All these can be treated from the perspective of phlegm with careful differentiation.

The formation of phlegm must have its root causes. Therefore, in treating phlegm syndromes, it is necessary to treat the etiology and pathogenesis of phlegm production, while also taking into account resolving phlegm, thus resulting in various principles for treating phlegm.

1. Diffuse the Lung and Resolve Phlegm Principle

〔Indications〕 Applicable to exogenous wind-cold, cough with excessive phlegm. In exogenous cough, the pathogenic factor is on the exterior, and the disease location is in the lung. Treatment should focus on dispelling exogenous pathogenic factors. Since the pathogen is wind-cold, using pungent-warm to diffuse the lung, release the exterior, and stop cough, combined with resolving phlegm, forms the diffuse the lung and resolve phlegm principle.

〔Medications〕 Schizonepeta spike, closed saposhnikovia, mint leaf, perilla leaf, bitter apricot kernel, elephantopus scaber, bitter platycodon

〔Explanation〕 Schizonepeta, saposhnikovia, mint, and perilla leaf dispel wind and release the exterior. Apricot kernel and elephantopus scaber open the lung, regulate qi, and resolve phlegm. Platycodon acts on the upper part, which can assist in dispelling wind and has the effect of stopping cough and resolving phlegm.

If wind-cold is severe, with nausea and white phlegm with much foam, add fresh ginger; if cough with upward qi is severe, add peucedanum to descend counterflow; if there is chest and diaphragm fullness, nausea and qi counterflow, remove elephantopus scaber and add aster, as aster and platycodon, one ascending and one descending, arc more coordinated; if the throat is itchy, add sterculia lychnophora and cicada slough; if there is head distension or pain, add chrysanthemum.

2. Clear Heat and Resolve Phlegm Principle

〔Indications〕 Applicable to phlegm-heat in the lung, thirst and dry throat. Phlegm-heat is mostly caused by wind-warm. Therefore, in the initial stage, treatment should focus on clearing and diffusing. If heat is severe after a long time, clearing and purging the lung can be used, or combined with cooling and resolving phlegm, thus forming the clear heat and resolve phlegm principle.

〔Medications〕 Frosted mulberry leaf, bitter apricot kernel, tendrilled fritillary, trichosanthes peel, loquat leaf, morus bark, lycium bark

〔Explanation〕 Mulberry leaf is an excellent medicine for dispelling wind-heat and clearing heat; apricot kernel clears the lung and resolves phlegm, and must be added when there is much phlegm; in the later stage of cough, when lung yin is consumed, sweet apricot kernel is used; fritillary resolves phlegm, elephantopus scaber is suitable when there is an exterior syndrome, and tendrilled fritillary is used when heat is severe without an exterior syndrome; trichosanthes peel clears heat, resolves phlegm, generates fluids, and also unblocks the large intestine to benefit lung qi; loquat leaf resolves phlegm, and is not used in the initial stage of exogenous diseases because loquat leaf has the disadvantage of retaining pathogens (nowadays, "loquat syrup" is used in clinical practice for coughs of any nature without syndrome differentiation, which is probably inappropriate); morus bark and lycium bark, which are the components of Xiebai Powder, have the functions of clearing heat, purging the lung, stopping cough and relieving asthma.

As mentioned earlier, if there are head and eye symptoms, add chrysanthemum; if cough is severe, add peucedanum; if exogenous pathogens have been resolved, stemona can be used; for cough with sore throat and difficulty in expectorating phlegm, add water chestnut.

3. Downbear Qi and Transform Phlegm Principle

〔Indications〕 Applicable to lung cold with phlegm coagulation, phlegm asthma with upward qi. The lung governs purification and descent; lung cold with phlegm coagulation will inevitably lead to upward qi. Urgently dispel qi and diffuse, and warm-transform cold phlegm that counterflows upward. It is essential to focus on both downbearing qi and warm transformation.

〔Medications〕 Inula flower, refined pinellia, perilla seed, citrus red, white mustard seed, radish seed, medicated leaven

〔Explanation〕 All medicinals in the formula are warm in nature. Inula flower, perilla seed, white mustard seed, and radish seed have good effects in downbearing qi, but they are not suitable for severe exogenous symptoms, or perilla seed can be replaced with perilla leaf. The root cause is phlegm, so pinellia and citrus red are most appropriate; however, if dampness is severe, ginger juice-fried pinellia and medicated leaven can be used.

For phlegm coagulation, add pumice and sea clam shell; for severe lung cold, add aster and coltsfoot flower; for severe dampness requiring drainage, add coix seed and wax gourd seed.

4. Dry Dampness and Resolve Phlegm Principle

〔Indications〕 Applicable to damp accumulation with phlegm coagulation, cough with nausea. Lung cold with phlegm coagulation, caused by lung cold, is treated by warming the lung; damp phlegm coagulation, located in the spleen and stomach, is treated by drying dampness. Generally, phlegm-resolving medicines focus on the lung, while damp phlegm is located in the spleen and stomach. In addition to cough, the main manifestations include nausea, hiccups, chest tightness, and poor appetite. Therefore, treating damp phlegm should take into account three aspects: drying dampness, regulating qi, and resolving phlegm.

〔Medications〕 Processed atractylodes, ginger pinellia, processed magnolia bark, citrus red, stir-fried coix seed, light dried ginger, stir-fried aurantium

〔Explanation〕 Atractylodes is an excellent medicine for drying dampness; for severe external dampness, use a large amount of atractylodes; for severe internal dampness, which is treated by strengthening the spleen, rice-processed atractylodes can be used; magnolia bark warms and transforms the middle jiao to promote qi movement; ginger pinellia is pungent-warm to resolve phlegm; citrus red regulates qi and resolves phlegm, with stronger dampness-drying and qi-regulating effects than tangerine peel; for severe external dampness, use a large amount of fresh ginger; coix seed strengthens the spleen and regulates dampness, and stir-fried coix seed enhances the dampness-drying effect; aurantium relieves qi stagnation in the middle jiao to assist in transforming dampness.

For decline of life gate fire, warm the kidney, add cinnamon.

5. Warm and Transform Phlegm-Fluids Principle

〔Indications〕 Applicable to spleen-kidney cold with upward overflow of phlegm-fluids, urgent panting and cough. Phlegm-fluids is a special syndrome among phlegm syndromes. Its main location is in the middle jiao, caused by middle yang deficiency, and the pathogen is a yin pathogen, so treatment should focus on strengthening the spleen and supporting yang. Zhang Zhongjing's statement that "phlegm-fluids should be treated with warm medicines to harmonize" refers to this.

〔Medications〕 Poria, cinnamon twig, stir-fried atractylodes, roasted licorice, light dried ginger, schisandra, refined pinellia

〔Explanation〕 Linggui Zhugan Decoction is the basic formula for treating phlegm-fluids. Cinnamon twig supports yang, atractylodes strengthens the spleen, poria drains dampness, and licorice tonifies the middle, with the main effect of warming and moving spleen yang. Dried ginger, schisandra, and pinellia are pungent-warm to transform fluids, which are essential medicines for eliminating fluids in Zhang Zhongjing's works.

For severe external cold, add ephedra; for severe internal fluids, add asarum; for regulating qi and resolving phlegm, add tangerine peel; for water-hen sound in the throat, add stalactite.

6. Clear and Downbear Phlegm-Heat Principle

〔Indications〕 Applicable to upward rushing of heat-phlegm, clouded consciousness and qi stagnation. The first to fifth principles mainly target the lung and spleen, thus mainly manifesting as cough, asthma, phlegm-fluids, etc. This principle involves upward rushing of phlegm-heat, disturbing the head and eyes (the residence of spirit). Treatment should clear and downbear phlegm-heat.

〔Medications〕 Roasted morus bark, bile arisaema, bamboo yellow, light bamboo juice, acorus, trichosanthes seed, Jiang aurantium

〔Explanation〕 Morus bark and bile arisaema are agile and smooth, purging phlegm-heat; bamboo yellow and light bamboo juice cool and descend phlegm-heat; aurantium and trichosanthes benefit the large intestine to clear phlegm-heat. Aurantium can also descend qi, and when qi descends, phlegm also descends; acorus is volatile in nature, good at transforming damp turbidity, with the function of resolving phlegm and dispersing stagnation.

For qi stagnation, add curcuma; for gurgling phlegm sounds, add tendrilled fritillary; for blocked meridians, add loofah sponge.

7. Attack and Expel Phlegm Accumulation Principle

〔Indications〕 Applicable to stagnation of phlegm-fluids, hanging fluids and branch fluids. For stubborn phlegm stagnation that cannot be transformed or dissipated, aggressive expulsion is used. Mild cases use medicines like Mengshi Guntan Pills; severe cases use medicines like Kongxian Dan. For mild phlegm-fluids, Tingli Xiefei Decoction is used; for severe cases, Shizao Decoction. Although the formulas vary in potency, they are all aggressive and drastic agents, not suitable for frequent or prolonged use, and should be used with greater caution in those with weak constitution.

〔Medications〕 Lepidium seed, Jiang aurantium, wax gourd seed, genkwa flower, euphorbia kansui, Alisma orientalis, Kongxian Dan

〔Explanation〕 The first six medicines are selected from the above formulas. Lepidium has a strong descending and purging effect, unsuitable for those without excessive lung excess; bamboo juice lubricates the bowels to benefit the lung; wax gourd seed benefits the lung; alisma promotes diuresis, allowing fluid pathogens to exit through urine; euphorbia kansui and genkwa flower are powerful agents for expelling fluids; if necessary, knoxia and veronicastrum can be added. Kongxian Dan is a prepared medicine, very effective in attacking and expelling stubborn phlegm and hanging fluids.

8. Dissolve and Reduce Phlegm Nodules Principle

〔Indications〕 Applicable to phlegm-qi coagulation, goiter, scrofula. Scrofula is caused by stagnation of phlegm turbidity combined with liver-gallbladder qi stagnation. Treatment mainly uses softening and reducing methods, and more importantly, soothing the liver and regulating qi—phlegm nodules are the branch, while liver-gallbladder qi-fire is the root, so both root and branch should be addressed.

〔Medications〕 Large fritillary, white silkworm, appendiculate cremastra, sargassum, kelp, refined pinellia, citrus red

〔Explanation〕 Fritillary and cremastra resolve phlegm; silkworm resolves phlegm and unblocks collaterals; sargassum and kelp soften hardness and disperse nodules; pinellia and citrus red mainly treat phlegm coagulation.

For liver stagnation, add bupleurum; for liver fire, add prunella; for blood deficiency, add angelica and white peony root.

〔Interpretation〕 The eight principles for treating phlegm are diffusing, transforming, downbearing, drying dampness, warm transforming, clear descending, attacking, and dissolving. For phlegm itself, they come down to four words: clearing, descending, moistening, and resolving. For the *zang*-organs, the main focuses are protecting the lung and nourishing fluids, cultivating the spleen and transforming fluids, and tonifying the kidney to return [phlegm] to the viscera. Grasping these essentials allows mastery over all kinds of phlegm syndromes.

Section 10 Deficiency

Deficiency has various etiologies: either external injury from alcohol and sexual indulgence, internal injury from the seven emotions, injury from diet and overstrain, or excessive desires. Alcohol injures the lung, with damp-heat steaming, consuming lung yin; sexual indulgence injures the kidney, emptying the essence chamber, leaving ministerial fire unchecked; anxiety injures the heart, depleting blood, making fire prone to flare upward; overstrain injures the spleen, generating fire internally, damaging genuine yin; anger injures the liver, causing liver fire to blaze upward, scorching blood and leading to bleeding.

Recognizing deficiency, once one grasps the subtleties, is not difficult. Red cheeks and crimson lips indicate yin deficiency below forcing yang upward; dry mouth and excessive thirst result from insufficient kidney yin, prompting the body to seek water for self-rescue; hoarse voice and difficulty speaking signal declining kidney qi; Rapid, labored breathing with mouth agape and raised shoulders signals a yin-deficient, desiccated lung in which qi has lost its anchorage; parched throat and sore pharynx reveal a waning of true water below, allowing vacuous fire to blaze above; sleeplessness and mental drift arise when blood fails to nourish the heart and the spirit can no longer settle within; frequent restlessness reflects yang lacking yin, with softness failing to balance hardness; tense, aching tendons and irritability arise from water deficiency and wood dryness, depriving the liver of nourishment; food losing its flavor and muscles wasting away mark the collapse of the spleen's primal vitality and the daily decline of its transformative power; the throbbing beneath the left breast, with palpitations and anxious heart, reveal qi's failure to return to and be housed within essence; night sweats have two causes—with fire, yin cannot contain; without fire, yang cannot consolidate; profuse, clear, frothy phlegm results from spleen deficiency failing to control water, which overflows as phlegm; bone pain like fractures signifies exhausted true yin; hot pain in the lower back and ribs indicates liver-kidney deficiency; cold below the knees reflects declining life gate fire and weak true yang; dribbling, yellow, astringent, painful urination stems from depleted true yin where qi cannot transform fire; burning soles result from deficient fire drying yin and exhausted fountain (kidney) essence; chills in the skin with cough and frothy sputum indicate defensive aspect weakness; cough with internal heat and bloody sputum reflects nutrient aspect depletion; blood and essence loss signifies devastated liver and kidney; blood stasis with dry cough comes from stagnant fire scorching; reduced appetite, cough, and diarrhea after long treatment indicate medicinal damage to the spleen and stomach.

Treating deficiency prioritizes tonification—the classics state, "Deficiency requires tonification"—yet one must not tonify blindly. First, clarify the location of deficiency: which *zang-fu* organs? Second, determine the nature of deficiency: First distinguish yin and yang. Essence, blood, fluids, and nutrients all belong to yin; qi and defense belong to yang. Following this principle will rarely go astray.

Deficiency treatment principles are summarized into eight.

1. Tonify the Lung and Nourish Yin Principle

〔Indications〕 Applicable to deficiency of both qi and yin in the lung. The lung has a yin substance and yang function: governing respiration, controlling the skin and hair, circulating fluids, and irrigating all vessels. Prolonged illness damages the lung, withering its lobes, impairing distribution and transformation, preventing qi and fluid circulation—either yin deficiency affecting qi or qi deficiency affecting yin. Symptoms include cough with shortness of breath; when the interstices of skin and hair are insecure, there is profuse sweating and aversion to wind. Sputum is scant or the cough is dry and non-productive; in severe cases the sputum may be streaked with blood. The voice is weak and timid, the throat dry and lacking moisture.

〔Medications〕 American ginseng, northern adenophora, barley ophiopogon, sweet apricot kernel, tendrilled fritillary, roasted aristolochia, imperata root

〔Explanation〕 American ginseng is cool yet tonifying, suitable for qi-yin deficiency with fire. For those needing ginseng but intolerant of its warm nature, this is optimal—though expensive, pseudostellaria can substitute, albeit inferior. Adenophora and ophiopogon gently nourish lung-stomach yin, moistening dryness and generating fluids. Sweet apricot kernel moistens the lung and stops cough, suitable for consumptive dyspnea; bitter apricot kernel is bitter, cooling, dispersing, and slightly toxic, inappropriate here. Tendrilled fritillary is highly moistening, able to moisten lung dryness; Zhejiang fritillary is bitter-cold, descending and draining, suitable for exogenous wind, phlegm-heat stagnating the lung. Aristolochia clears and descends lung and intestinal heat, stopping cough and asthma. Imperata Rhizoma acts primarily in the blood phase, excelling at clearing blood-level heat to cool and regulate the blood; it is especially suitable for cases of blood-streaked sputum.

2. Tonify and Strengthen the Middle Principle

〔Indications〕 Applicable to weak spleen and stomach. Caused by internal injury from diet/overstrain or congenital deficiency, resulting in postprandial abdominal distension, bland taste with reduced appetite, loose stools, along with sallow complexion, fatigued limbs, weak voice, and soft, soggy pulse.

〔Medications〕 Stir-fried codonopsis, poria, raw atractylodes, clear-roasted licorice, yam, stir-fried hyacinth bean, stir-fried millet sprout

〔Explanation〕 Codonopsis, poria, atractylodes, and roasted licorice constitute the Sijunzi Decoction, which reinforces qi and tonifies the middle, strengthens the spleen, and nourishes the stomach. Yam is sweet and neutral, both reinforcing qi and nourishing yin, with astringent properties, and can strengthen the spleen to stop diarrhea. Hyacinth bean is less effective in tonification than atractylodes and yam, but it is neither dry nor greasy, making it an excellent medicine for strengthening the spleen and eliminating dampness. When the spleen and stomach are weak and their transportation function is impaired, even a little food can easily cause distension, so a small amount of millet sprout, etc., is added to aid digestion. However, the variety should not be many, and the dosage should not be large; otherwise, it would overshadow the main ingredients, putting the cart before the horse.

3. Tonify Defense and Secure the Exterior Principle

〔Indications〕 Applicable to deficient constitution with unconsolidated defensive yang. Symptoms include spontaneous sweating, aversion to wind, and susceptibility to colds.

〔Medications〕 Cotton astragalus peel, ginseng fibrous root, stir-fried atractylodes, processed aconite slice, floating wheat, glutinous rice root, large red dates

〔Explanation〕 Ginseng, astragalus, and atractylodes are the main medicines for reinforcing qi. The combined use of these three medicines can enhance the therapeutic effect. However, no medicine is better than astragalus in securing the exterior and stopping sweating. Cotton astragalus peel is used because the peel acts on the skin. Defensive qi originates from the lower jiao, so processed aconite slice, which is extremely pungent and hot, is used to powerfully tonify the primordial yang of the lower jiao. Floating wheat enters the heart meridian and is good at stopping sweating. Glutinous rice root astringes to arrest sweating. Red dates are sweet and moderate, harmonizing the middle, preventing the medicines from having adverse effects.

4. Generate Fluids and Nourish Liquids Principle

〔Indications〕 Applicable to insufficient fluids and internal injury dryness syndrome. It is mostly caused by constitutional yin deficiency and fluid depletion, or fluid depletion in the elderly and weak, or consumption of fluids and blood after childbirth, or consumption of fluids in the later stage of febrile diseases, leading to depletion of stomach fluids and intestinal dysfunction. Symptoms include difficulty in swallowing food, difficulty in digesting food after ingestion, or even reduced food intake with dysphagia, dry and hard stools, or like sheep feces, which are difficult to excrete.

〔Medications〕 Fresh rehmannia, fresh dendrobium, trichosanthes root, large white peony root, hemp seed, plump anemarrhena, fresh reed rhizome

〔Explanation〕 Fresh rehmannia is sweet and cold, moistening, treating insufficient yin fluids. Fresh dendrobium nourishes the stomach and generates fluids. When these two medicines are used fresh, their ability to generate fluids and clear heat is stronger. Trichosanthes root is sweet and sour, generating fluids, relieving thirst, and moistening dryness. White peony root tonifies blood and astringes yin. Hemp seed is sweet and neutral, oily and moistening, having the function of moistening dryness and lubricating the intestines, and also being able to tonify deficiency. For severe heat, anemarrhena is added to nourish yin, reduce fire, moisten dryness, and lubricate the intestines. Reed rhizome is light and not greasy, generating fluids without the disadvantage of retaining pathogens.

5. Nourish Nutrients and Tonify Blood Principle

〔Indications〕 Applicable to insufficient source of production, liver blood deficiency, or consumption of essence and blood due to prolonged illness, or caused by excessive blood loss. Symptoms include dizziness, palpitations, blurred vision, dizziness, tinnitus, deficiency vexation, insomnia, sallow complexion, pale lips and nails, scanty and light-colored menstruation or amenorrhea in women.

〔Medications〕 Processed polygonum multiflorum, angelica body, stir-fried white peony root, ass-hide gelatin pearls, longan aril, dodder cake, astragalus complanatus seed

〔Explanation〕 Polygonum multiflorum tonifies the liver and kidney, benefits essence and blood, and is neither cold, dry nor greasy. Angelica and white peony root tonify blood and nourish nutrients. Ass-hide gelatin is an essential medicine for nourishing yin, tonifying blood, and stopping bleeding, and is most suitable for blood deficiency, dizziness, palpitations, and insomnia. Dodder and T astragalus complanatus seed are not dry or greasy, nourishing the liver and kidney. The liver and kidney share the same origin; to tonify liver blood, it is necessary to nourish kidney essence. Longan aril tonifies the heart and spleen, reinforcing qi. If the spirit is restless, platycladus seed and ziziphus seed can be added.

I often use this principle in treating blood diseases such as leukemia, aplastic anemia, and hemophilia, which is in line with the idea of Jingyue's Great Dodder Drink.

6. Nourish Yin and Fill the Kidney Principle

〔Indications〕 Applicable to depletion of kidney essence. This syndrome is caused by internal injury from sexual overindulgence, or prolonged illness affecting the kidney, or extreme heat damaging yin in the later stage of febrile diseases. Symptoms include soreness and weakness of the waist and knees, heel pain, spermatorrhea, dizziness, tinnitus and other kidney deficiency symptoms, along with five-center heat, night sweats, dry throat and other yin deficiency symptoms.

〔Medications〕 Large rehmannia preparata, cornus, ripe ligustrum, lycium fruit, black sesame, roasted turtle shell, thick eucommia

〔Explanation〕 Rehmannia preparata is an essential medicine for tonifying the liver and kidney, not only nourishing yin and blood, but also generating essence and replenishing marrow, suitable for all syndromes of yin deficiency, blood deficiency, and essence depletion. Cornus is sour and warm, astringing and absorbing, nourishing essence and blood. Ligustrum and lycium fruit both tonify yin and yang; ligustrum benefits yin without greasiness, and lycium fruit is neutral and strengthens the kidney. Black sesame benefits essence and blood. When yin deficiency with excessive heat, turtle shell is used to nourish yin and clear heat. Eucommia tonifies the liver and kidney, strengthens muscles and bones, and is most suitable for kidney deficiency with low back and waist pain.

7. Consolidate and Contain the Essence Gate Principle

〔Indications〕 Applicable to unclosed essence gate, nocturnal emission without dreams, seminal emission with impotence, or even seminal flow at the sight of sexual stimuli, or semen discharge after urination, with a thready and weak pulse. "The kidney governs storage, the root of sealing and storing"; the root of the disease is in the kidney, and the pathogenesis is consumptive disease failing to contain and consolidate. It is completely different from seminal emission and spermatorrhea due to damp-fire in the lower jiao with a string-like pulse and yellow tongue coating, and must not be confused.

〔Medications〕 Large rehmannia preparata, cornus, schisandra, rosa laevigata, mantis egg case, calcined dragon bone and oyster, Jianlian stamen

〔Explanation〕 Nourishing the kidney and filling essence, and consolidating and astringing are treated together. Rehmannia preparata, cornus, and schisandra nourish and consolidate the essence gate to strengthen the root. Rosa laevigata, mantis egg case, lotus stamen, calcined dragon bone and oyster—all astringent and consolidating medicines—treat the branch.

8. Warm and Tonify the Lower Origin Principle

〔Indications〕 Applicable to kidney yang deficiency with cold, declining life gate fire. The life gate is the source of transformation for the whole body; declining life gate fire presents with aversion to cold, cold limbs, cold and sore lower back, worsening in winter, frequent and incontinent urination, impotence, premature ejaculation in men, etc.

〔Medications〕 Raw aconite block, Biezhi ginseng, deer antler slice, psoralea, large rehmannia preparata, alpinia oxyphylla, walnut meat

〔Explanation〕 Aconite, a powerful medicine for supplementing fire, is used as the sovereign, combined with ginseng, forming Shenfu Decoction. Deer antler is salty and warm, supplementing fire and invigorating yang. The kidney is the abode of water and fire; invigorating yang and nourishing yin must be considered together, otherwise excessive fire will scorch yin and further damage essence and qi. Zhang Jiebin said: "Those who are good at supplementing yang must seek yang within yin, so that yang receives yin assistance and generates endlessly." Psoralea, rehmannia preparata, alpinia oxyphylla, and walnut are all used for this purpose.

〔Interpretation〕 All principles for deficiency syndromes use tonification, as mentioned above, distinguishing yin and yang, differentiating *zang-fu* organs, with clear context. To simplify, it comes down to two words: warm and cool. Warm medicines assist yang, supplementing qi, defense, and lower origin life gate fire; cool medicines benefit yin, nourishing the lung, stomach, and liver-kidney nutrients, fluids, and essence; there is also consolidation, with indistinct cold and heat but slightly warm medicinal properties, which belongs to yang supplementation.

Section 11 Food

Food is paramount to the people. Food must undergo digestion and transportation by the spleen and stomach to be transformed into essence. Thus, food stagnation has both external and internal causes. External causes are irregular diet; internal causes are the spleen and stomach's inability to digest, leading to chest and diaphragm stuffiness, vomiting, acid regurgitation, belching with egg-like odor, anorexia, and headache.

Diagnosing food stagnation is relatively easy, with a clear cause, mostly after overeating. However, its pulse condition is worth studying. For general food accumulation, the pulse is normal with floating and large at the cun and guan positions, but astringent when pressed; slippery, rapid, and forceful or slippery, strong, and deep pulse indicates retained food;

tight and deep pulse indicates cold food with stagnation; deep, tight, and thready pulse indicates cold food damaging the spleen; blurred and indistinct pulse indicates sticky retained food with stagnant stomach qi; slow and stagnant pulse indicates spleen deficiency failing to promote essence and stomach deficiency failing to ripen food.

Treatment principles for food stagnation should clarify duration, depth, location in the stomach or intestines, and excess or deficiency tendency, which can be summarized into the following three.

1. Digest Food Accumulation Principle

〔Explanation〕 Applicable to all cases of food stagnation with epigastric stuffiness and anorexia. Zhang Zhongjing said: "Water can carry a boat, and it can also capsize it." Diet is originally the main source of nutrition for the human body, but stagnation caused by irregular diet becomes a disease. The disease location is in the stomach; treatment uses dispersing and guiding, focusing on two aspects: One is to disperse food accumulation, and the other is to strengthen the stomach and regulate qi. Emphasis can be placed on either of the two.

〔Medications〕 Charred hawthorn, charred medicated leaven, stir-fried malt, radish seed, chicken's gizzard-membrane, stir-fried aurantium, broad tangerine peel

〔Explanation〕 The first several medicines disperse food accumulation; chicken's gizzard-membrane promotes digestion and strengthens the stomach; aurantium and tangerine peel strengthen the stomach and regulate qi.

For cold-induced nausea, add fresh ginger; for heat-induced nausea, add bamboo shavings; for abdominal distension and fullness, add magnolia bark; for infantile food accumulation, add grain worms; for qi distension in both hypochondria, use green tangerine peel.

2. Attack and Downbear Food Accumulation Principle

〔Indications〕 Applicable to food stagnation in the intestines with abdominal pain and constipation. Long-standing food accumulation presents with nausea, abdominal pain, distension, constipation, etc. At this point, the disease is in the intestines rather than the stomach; simple dispersion is no longer sufficient, so treatment should focus on dispersing and attacking, assisted by descending qi to relieve fullness.

〔Medications〕 Brocade rhubarb, senna leaf, Jiang aurantium, mirabilite, stir-fried medicated leaven, stir-fried malt, charred hawthorn

〔Explanation〕 Rhubarb and senna leaf attack and disperse; radish seed promotes digestion and descends qi; the charred three immortals (hawthorn, leaven, malt) disperse accumulation.

For severe abdominal distension and fullness, add areca nut and areca peel; for qifullness with loss of appetite, add costus root and tangerine peel.

3. Assist the Spleen and Promote Digestion Principle

〔Indications〕 Applicable to spleen-stomach weakness with difficulty in digesting food after ingestion. The first two principles target excess syndromes, one in the stomach and one in the intestines, so the treatment principle is to eliminate excess. In this principle, spleen deficiency is the root cause, with symptoms such as poor appetite, lack of hunger, stagnation even after eating a little, and difficulty in digesting food. The disease location is in the spleen; first, tonify the spleen, but since food stagnation has already formed, assist with dispersing agents that do not damage qi.

〔Medications〕 Stir-fried atractylodes, stir-fried aurantium, amomum fruit, pinellia leaven, areca peel, Xinhui tangerine peel, chicken's gizzard-membrane

〔Explanation〕 The above medicines strengthen the spleen and promote digestion. For severe distension and fullness, add areca nut; for nausea, add pinellia; for severe cold, add evodia; for severe heat, add bamboo shavings.

〔Interpretation〕 Food accumulation is inherently an excess condition; treatment strategies are dispersion and purgation. When the spleen is weak, both dispersion and tonification are applied. Additionally, there is another principle, namely "emesis to disperse accumulation," which is not included here. When food pathogens are in the upper epigastrium, for a short time, with a sense of nausea, restlessness, and disharmony between cold and heat, emesis can be used to disperse them. However, this method is difficult to master; improper use will only damage stomach qi without eliminating pathogens, so it is not routine. When applied appropriately, it is a shortcut to expel food pathogens, which must be known.

Section 12 Pestilence

Suwen • *Cifa Lun* states: "When the five pestilences arrive, they are all contagious, regardless of age, with similar disease manifestations," referring to highly contagious diseases. There are names such as cold pestilence, warm pestilence, pestilential rash, pestilential toxin, and pestilential dysentery. Investigating their etiology, they are all transmitted by pestilential qi, arising from damp turbidity in the intestines and stomach steaming and stagnating. In latent pestilence, there is slight aversion to cold in the back, dizziness and distension in the head and forehead, chest fullness and stuffiness, and soreness and numbness in the fingertips. In external outbreak of pestilence, there is high fever with clouded consciousness, convulsions and rash, swollen and ulcerated throat, and rapid gingival erosion. In inward collapse of pestilence, there is restlessness, excessive diarrhea, bleeding, and reversal cold.

Treatment principles for pestilence are categorized into cold and warm types.

1. Disperse Filth and Transform Turbidity Principle

〔Indications〕 Applicable to contraction of cold pestilence or mountain miasma toxin. This syndrome is mostly inhaled through the mouth and nose, directly attacking the middle jiao, with symptoms such as chest and diaphragm fullness, dizziness and muzziness, restlessness, and a white greasy tongue coating.

〔Medications〕 Sichuan notopterygium, fragrant angelica dahurica, broad agastache, roasted amomum tsao-ko, Sichuan magnolia bark, green tangerine peel, tangerine peel, areca nut

〔Explanation〕 These medicines are warm and aromatic, penetrating and releasing from the middle jiao, resolving both exterior and interior, focusing on the spleen and stomach. Warmth allows cold-damp turbidity pathogens to reach the exterior. Notopterygium is pungent and warm, dispelling wind-cold-damp pathogens to exit through the exterior. Angelica dahurica, agastache, amomum tsao-ko, and magnolia bark are aromatic, transforming dampness and awakening the spleen, resolving from the interior. Green tangerine peel and tangerine peel regulate qi, promoting spleen and stomach function. Areca nut regulates qi, moves water, and penetrates the triple jiao.

2. Clear Pestilence and Eliminate Turbidity Principle

〔Indications〕 Applicable to all pestilences. Symptoms include heat in both exterior and interior, foul breath, sore throat, or even mania, rash, with a white greasy or yellow dirty tongue coating.

〔Medications〕 Isatis root, raw gypsum, fresh bamboo leaf, light scutellaria, Sichuan coptis, rhinoceros horn, small raw rehmannia

〔Explanation〕 Isatis root clears pestilence and toxins, and clears the throat. Gypsum directly enters the lung and stomach to reduce excessive heat. Bamboo leaf clears heat and promotes diuresis. Scutellaria and coptis drain heart and lung fire in the upper jiao.

For mania and rash, rhinoceros horn, salty and cold, enters the nutrient and blood aspects, excelling at clearing fire and heat in the heart, liver, and stomach channels, with a clear and penetrating nature, cold without stagnation, penetrating pathogenic heat in the pericardium and toxic heat in the nutrient aspect. Raw rehmannia specializes in cooling blood and clearing heat without retaining pathogens.

〔Interpretation〕 Pestilence has various names, but treatment is roughly divided into two categories: cold pestilence, a severe form of damp-warmth, treated with aromatic transformation and filth dispersion; pox pestilence, a severe form of warm-heat, treated with clearing and penetration, resuscitation, rash transformation, and blood cooling.

Section 13 Worms

Worm syndromes are all caused by improper hunger and satiety, sluggish spleen transportation, and accumulation of damp-heat. Manifestations include: epigastric discomfort, abdominal pain, vomiting of saliva, sallow complexion, emaciation, abdominal distension, sparse hair, dark color under the eyes, or craving for rice, paper, mud, charcoal, or silence as if half-asleep, or unbearable anal itching, or excretion of worms of various sizes.

The two principles for treating worms are as follows.

1. Disperse Accumulation and Kill Worms Principle

〔Indications〕 Applicable to worm accumulation obstructing the middle jiao. Symptoms include abdominal pain and distension, emaciation, teeth grinding in sleep, red and white spots inside the lips, sallow complexion, reduced appetite; or craving for foreign objects, or anal itching, or worms in the stool.

〔Medications〕 Jiang aurantium, stir-fried atractylodes, hawthorn flesh, grain worms, quisqualis, white omphalia, old carpesium

〔Explanation〕 Worms arise from accumulation; the medicinal approach is twofold: disperse accumulation and kill worms. Aurantium descends qi and transforms stagnation, resolving stuffiness and fullness; atractylodes strengthens the spleen and dispels dampness to aid transportation; hawthorn disperses all food accumulations, especially good at dispersing meat and greasy accumulations. Quisqualis, omphalia, and carpesium expel worms and dispel malnutrition. Grain worms, being agile insect-like substances, disperse various accumulations.

2. Acrid-Sour-Bitter Descending Principle

〔Indications〕 Indicated for every form of parasitic accumulation and roundworm reversal. Manifestations include vexation and agitation, vomiting, epigastric and abdominal pain, a sensation of qi rushing upward to the heart, attacks that come and go, frequent spontaneous vomiting of roundworms, and cold reversal of the extremities.

〔Medications〕 Mume fruit, stir-fried Sichuan pepper, northern asarum, light dried ginger, cinnamon heart, stir-fried Sichuan coptis, medicated leaven

〔Explanation〕 Worms move when encountering sweetness, lie dormant when encountering sourness, stop when encountering acridness, and calm down when encountering bitterness. Mume is sour, calming worms and relieving pain. Sichuan pepper, asarum, dried ginger, cinnamon is acrid and warm, expelling worms and warming the viscera. Coptis is bitter and cold; bitterness can descend worms, and cold clears stomach heat. Medicated leaven assists by promoting digestion and strengthening the spleen. The medicines are a combination of cold and heat, with immediate effect in clinical practice.

〔Interpretation〕 Dispelling accumulation and killing worms acts on the intestines and stomach, mainly using worm-killing medicines assisted by spleen-strengthening agents, which is the direct worm-expelling method in Chinese medicine. Acrid-sour-bitter descending acts on Jueyin, using acrid to subdue worms, sour to contract worms, bitter to descend worms, which is the indirect worm-expelling method by regulating bodily functions. Understanding this subtlety allows mastery in treating worm syndromes.

Made in the USA
Monee, IL
05 November 2026

67914384R00380